P9-CCX-929

NURSE'S POCKET DRUG GUIDE 2012

EDITOR
Judith A. Barberio, PhD, APN, C, ANP, FNP, GNP

CONSULTING EDITOR
Leonard G. Gomella, MD, FACS

ASSOCIATE EDITORS
Steven A. Haist, MD, MS, FACP
Aimee Gelhot Adams, PharmD

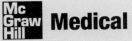

New York Chicago San Francisco Lisbon
London Madrid Mexico City Milan New Delhi
San Juan Seoul Singapore Sydney Toronto

The McGraw·Hill Companies

Nurse's Pocket Drug Guide 2012

Copyright © 2012 by Judith A. Barberio. Based on *Clinician's Pocket Drug Reference 2012* Copyright © 2012 by Leonard G. Gomella. Published by the McGraw-Hill Companies, Inc. All rights reserved. Printed in Canada. Except as permitted under the United States Copyright Act of 1976, no part of this publication may be reproduced or distributed in any form or by any means, or stored in a data base or retrieval system, without the prior written permission of the publisher.

1 2 3 4 5 6 7 8 9 0   QLM/QLM   15 14 13 12 11

ISBN 978-0-07-176930-3
MHID 0-07-176930-7
ISSN 1550-2554

Notice

Medicine is an ever-changing science. As new research and clinical experience broaden our knowledge, changes in treatment and drug therapy are required. The authors and the publisher of this work have checked with sources believed to be reliable in their efforts to provide information that is complete and generally in accord with the standards accepted at the time of publication. However, in view of the possibility of human error or changes in medical sciences, neither the authors nor the publisher nor any other party who has been involved in the preparation or publication of this work warrants that the information contained herein is in every respect accurate or complete, and they disclaim all responsibility for any errors or omissions or for the results obtained from use of the information contained in this work. Readers are encouraged to confirm the information contained herein with other sources. For example and in particular, readers are advised to check the product information sheet included in the package of each drug they plan to administer to be certain that the information contained in this work is accurate and that changes have not been made in the recommended dose or in the contraindications for administration. This recommendation is of particular importance in connection with new or infrequently used drugs.

The book was set in Times by Cenveo Publisher Services.
The editors were Joseph Morita and Christie Naglieri.
The production supervisor was Sherri Souffrance.
The text designer was Marsha Cohen/Parallelogram Graphics.
Project management was provided by Harleen Chopra, Cenveo Publisher Services.
The indexer was Cenveo Publisher Services.
Quad/Graphics Leominster was printer and binder.
This book is printed on acid-free paper.

McGraw-Hill books are available at special quantity discounts to use as premiums and sales promotions, or for use in corporate training programs. To contact a representative please e-mail us at bulksales@mcgraw.com.

CONTENTS

EDITOR

Judith A. Barberio, PhD, APN, C, ANP, FNP, GNP
Assistant Professor
Speciality Director: Adult/Geriatric Nurse Practitioner Track
Rutgers, The State University of New Jersey
College of Nursing
Newark, New Jersey

CONSULTING EDITOR

Leonard G. Gomella, MD, FACS
The Bernard W. Godwin, Jr., Professor
Chairman, Department of Urology
Jefferson Medical College
Associate Director of Clinical Affairs
Kimmel Cancer Center
Thomas Jefferson University
Philadelphia, Pennsylvania

ASSOCIATE EDITORS

Steven A. Haist, MD, MS, FACP
Clinical Professor
Department of Medicine
Drexel University College of Medicine
Philadelphia, Pennsylvania

Aimee Gelhot Adams, PharmD
Clinical Pharmacist Specialist, Ambulatory Care
Adjunct Assistant Professor
College of Pharmacy and Department of Internal Medicine
University of Kentucky Health Care
Lexington, Kentucky

PREFACE

I am pleased to present the eighth edition of the *Nurse's Pocket Drug Guide*. The goal is to identify the most frequently used and clinically important medications, including branded, generic, and OTC products. The book includes over 1200 generic medications and is designed to represent a cross-section of commonly used products in healthcare practices across the country.

The style of drug presentation includes key "must know" facts of commonly used medications and herbs, essential information for the student, practicing nurse, and healthcare provider. The inclusion of common uses of medications rather than just the official FDA-labeled indications are based on the uses of the medication and herbs supported by publications and community standards of care. All uses have been reviewed by our editorial board.

It is essential that students, registered nurses, and advanced-practice nurses learn more than the name and dose of the medications they administer and prescribe. Certain common side effects and significant warnings and contraindications are associated with prescription medications and herbs. Although nurses and other healthcare providers should ideally be completely familiar with the entire package insert of any medication prescribed, such a requirement is unreasonable. References such as the *Physicians' Desk Reference* and the drug manufacturers' Web sites make package inserts readily available for many medications, but may not highlight clinically significant facts or key data for generic drugs and those available over the counter.

The limitations of difficult-to-read package inserts were acknowledged by the Food and Drug Administration in early 2001, when it noted that healthcare providers do not have time to read the many pages of small print in the typical package insert. Newer drugs are producing more user-friendly package insert summaries that highlight important drug information for easier nursing reference. Although useful, these summaries do not commingle with similarly approved generic or "competing" similar products.

The editorial board has analyzed the information on both brand and generic medications and has made this key prescribing information available in this pocket-sized book. Information in this book is meant for use by healthcare professionals who are familiar with these commonly prescribed medications and herbs.

This 2012 edition has been completely reviewed and updated by our editorial board. Over 110 new drugs and herbs have been added, and dozens of changes in other medications based on FDA actions have been incorporated, including deletions of discontinued brand names and compounds.

Where appropriate, emergency cardiac care (ECC) guidelines are provided based on the latest recommendations for the American Heart Association (*Circulation*, Volume 112, Issue 24 Supplement; December 13, 2005 and Volume 122, Issue 25; December 2010) with the ECC emergency medication summary at the back of the book for rapid reference. Editions of this book are also available in a variety of electronic or eBook formats. Visit www.eDrugbook.com for a link to the electronic versions currently available. Additionally, this Web site has enhanced content features such as a comprehensive listing of "look alike–sound alike" medications that can contribute to prescribing errors.

I want to express a special thanks to my husband Marc Schweitzer and my family for their long-term support for this book. The contributions of the members of the editorial board, Joe Morita, and the entire team at McGraw-Hill are deeply appreciated. Your comments and suggestions are always welcome and encouraged because improvements to this book would be impossible without the interest and feedback of our readers. I hope this book will help you learn some of the key elements in prescribing medications and allow you to care for your patients in the best way possible.

Judith A. Barberio, PhD, APN, C, ANP, FNP, GNP
Newark, New Jersey
jabphd83@aol.com

MEDICATION KEY

Medications are listed by prescribing class, and the individual medications are then listed in alphabetical order by generic name. Some of the more commonly recognized trade names are listed for each medication (in parentheses after the generic name) or if available without prescription, noted as OTC (over the counter).

Generic Drug Name (Selected Common Brand Names [Controlled Substance]) **WARNING:** Summarized versions of the "Black Box" precautions deemed necessary by the FDA. These are significant precautions and contraindications concerning the individual medication. **Therapeutic and/or Pharmacologic Class:** Class is presented in brackets immediately following the brand name drug. The therapeutic drug class appears first and describes the disease state that the drug treats. The pharmacologic drug class follows and is based on the drug's mechanism of action. **Uses:** This includes both FDA-labeled indications bracketed by * and other "off-label" uses of the medication. Because many medications are used to treat various conditions based on the medical literature and not listed in their package insert, we list common uses of the medication in addition to the official "labeled indications" (FDA approved) based on input from our editorial board. **Action:** How the drug works. This information is helpful in comparing classes of drugs and understanding side effects and contraindications. *Spectrum:* Specifies activity against selected microbes for antimicrobials. **Dose:** *Adults.* Where no specific pediatric dose is given, the implication is that this drug is not commonly used or indicated in that age group. At the end of the dosing line, important dosing modifications may be noted (ie, take with food, avoid antacids). *Peds.* If appropriate dosing for children and infants is included with age ranges as needed. **Caution:** [Pregnancy/fetal risk categories, breast-feeding (as noted above)] cautions concerning the use of the drug in specific settings. **CI:** Contraindications. **Disp:** Common dosing forms. **SE:** Common or significant side effects. **Notes:** Other key information about the drug. **Interactions:** Common drug–drug, drug–herb, and drug–food interactions that may change the drug response. **Labs:** Common laboratory test results that are changed by the drug or significant laboratory monitoring requirements. **NIPE:** (Nursing Indications and/or Patient Education) Significant information that the nurse must be aware of with administration of the drug or information that should be given to any patient taking the drug.

CONTROLLED SUBSTANCE CLASSIFICATION

Medications under the control of the US Drug Enforcement Agency (DEA) (Schedule I–V controlled substances) are indicated by the symbol [C]. Most medications are "uncontrolled" and do not require a DEA prescriber number on the prescription. The following is a general description for the schedules of DEA-controlled substances:

Schedule (C–I) I: All nonresearch use forbidden (eg, heroin, LSD, mescaline).

Schedule (C–II) II: High addictive potential; medical use accepted. No telephone call-in prescriptions; no refills. Some states require special prescription form (eg, cocaine, morphine, methadone).

Schedule (C–III) III: Low to moderate risk of physical dependence, high risk of psychologic dependence; prescription must be rewritten after 6 months or five refills (eg, acetaminophen plus codeine).

Schedule (C–IV) IV: Limited potential for dependence; prescription rules same as for schedule III (eg, benzodiazepines).

Schedule (C–V) V: Very limited abuse potential; prescribing regulations often same as for uncontrolled medications; some states have additional restrictions.

FDA FETAL RISK CATEGORIES

Category A: Adequate studies in pregnant women have not demonstrated a risk to the fetus in the first trimester of pregnancy; there is no evidence of risk in the last two trimesters.

Category B: Animal studies have not demonstrated a risk to the fetus, but no adequate studies have been done in pregnant women.

or

Animal studies have shown an adverse effect, but adequate studies in pregnant women have not demonstrated a risk to the fetus during the first trimester of pregnancy and there is no evidence of risk in the last two trimesters.

Category C: Animal studies have shown an adverse effect on the fetus, but no adequate studies have been done in humans. The benefits from the use of the drug in pregnant women may be acceptable despite its potential risks.

or

No animal reproduction studies and no adequate studies in humans have been done.

Category D: There is evidence of human fetal risk, but the potential benefits from the use of the drug in pregnant women may be acceptable despite its potential risks.

Category X: Studies in animals or humans or adverse reaction reports, or both, have demonstrated fetal abnormalities. The risk of use in pregnant women clearly outweighs any possible benefit.

Category ?: No data available (not a formal FDA classification; included to provide complete data set).

BREAST-FEEDING

No formally recognized classification exists for drugs and breast-feeding. This shorthand was developed for the *Nurse's Pocket Drug Guide*.

+	Compatible with breast-feeding
M	Monitor patient or use with caution
±	Excreted, or likely excreted, with unknown effects or at unknown concentrations
?/−	Unknown excretion, but effects likely to be of concern
−	Contraindicated in breast-feeding
?	No data available

ABBREVIATIONS

▲: change
✓: check, follow, or monitor
↓: decrease/decreased
↑: increase/increased
>: greater than; older than
<: less than; younger than
⊘: not recommended; do not take; avoid
÷/%: divided dose
≠: not equal to; not equivalent to
AA: African American
Ab: antibody
Abd: abdominal
ABGs: arterial blood gases
ABMT: autologous bone marrow transplantation
ac: before meals (*ante cibum*)
ACE: angiotensin-converting enzyme
ACEI: angiotensin-converting enzyme inhibitor
ACH: acetylcholine
ACLS: advanced cardiac life support
ACS: acute coronary syndrome; American Cancer Society; American College of Surgeons
ACT: activated coagulation time
ADH: antidiuretic hormone
ADHD: attention-deficit hyperactivity disorder
ADR: adverse drug reaction
AF: atrial fibrillation
AF/A flutter: atrial fibrillation/atrial flutter
AHA: American Heart Association
Al: aluminum
alk phos: alkaline phosphate

ALL: acute lymphocytic leukemia
ALT: alanine aminotransferase
AMI: acute myocardial infarction
AML: acute myelogenous leukemia
amp: ampule
ANA: antinuclear antibody
ANC: absolute neutrophil count
antiplt: antiplatelet
antiSz: antiseizure
APACHE: acute physiology and chronic health evaluation
APAP: acetaminophen (*N*-acetyl-*p*-aminophenol)
APN: Advanced Practice Nurse
aPTT: activated partial thromboplastin time
ARB: angiotensin II receptor blocker
ARDS: adult respiratory distress syndrome
ARF: acute renal failure
AS: aortic stenosis
ASA: aspirin (acetylsalicylic acid)
ASAP: as soon as possible
AST: aspartate aminotransferase
ATP: adenosine triphosphate
AUB: abnormal uterine/vaginal bleeding
AUC: area under the curve
AV: atrioventricular
AVM: arteriovenous malformation
BBB: bundle branch block
BBs: beta blockers
BCL: B-cell lymphoma
bid: twice daily
BM: bone marrow; bowel movement

↓ BM: bone marrow suppression, myelosuppression
BMI: body mass index
BMD: bone mineral density
BMT: bone marrow transplantation
BOO: bladder outlet obstruction
BP: blood pressure
↓ BP: hypotension
BPH: benign prostatic hyperplasia
BPM: beats per minute
BS: blood sugar
BSA: body surface area
BUN: blood urea nitrogen
Ca: calcium
CA: cancer
CABG: coronary artery bypass graft
CaCl: calcium chloride
CAD: coronary artery disease
CAP: community-acquired pneumonia
caps: capsule(s)
cardiotox: cardiotoxicity
CBC: complete blood count
CCB: calcium channel blocker
CDC: Centers for Disease Control and Prevention
CF: cystic fibrosis
CHD: coronary heart disease
CHF: congestive heart failure
CI: contraindicated
CIDP: chronic inflammatory demyelinating polyneuropathy
CK: creatine kinase
CLA: *Cis*-linoleic acid
CLL: chronic lymphocytic leukemia
CML: chronic myelogenous leukemia
CMV: cytomegalovirus
CNS: central nervous system
c/o: complains of
combo: combination
comp: complicated

COMT: catechol-*O*-methyltransferase
conc: concentration(s)
cont: continuous
Contra: contraindicated
COPD: chronic obstructive pulmonary disease
COX: cyclooxygenase
CP: chest pain
CPK: creatine phosphokinase
CPP: central precocious puberty
CPR: cardiopulmonary resuscitation
CR: controlled release
CrCl: creatinine clearance
CRF: chronic renal failure
CSF: cerebrospinal fluid
CV: cardiovascular
CVA: cerebrovascular accident; costovertebral angle
CVD: cardiovascular disease
CVH: common variable hypergammaglobulinemia
CYP: cytochrome P-450 enzyme(s)
cytotox: cytotoxicity
CXR: chest X-ray
D: diarrhea
d: day
/d: per day
DA: dopamine
D_5LR: 5% dextrose in lactated Ringer's solution
D_5NS: 5% dextrose in normal saline
D_5W: 5% dextrose in water
DBP: diastolic blood pressure
D/C: discontinue; stop
derm: dermatologic
DI: diabetes insipidus
Disp: dispensed as; how the drug is supplied
DKA: diabetic ketoacidosis
dL: deciliter
DM: diabetes mellitus

DMARD: Disease-modifying antirheumatic drug; drugs defined in randomized trials to decrease erosions and joint space narrowing in rheumatoid arthritis (eg, D-penicillamine, methotrexate, azathioprine)

DN: diabetic nephropathy

DOC: drug of choice

DOT: directly observed therapy

dppr: dropper

DR: delayed release

d/t: due to

DVT: deep venous thrombosis

dx: diagnosis

Dz: disease

EC: enteric coated

ECC: emergency cardiac care

ECG: electrocardiogram

ED: erectile dysfunction

EGFR: epidermal growth factor receptor

EIB: exercise-induced bronchoconstriction

ELISA: enzyme-linked immunosorbent assay

EMG: electromyelogram

EMIT: enzyme-multiplied immunoassay test

epi: epinephrine

EPS: extrapyramidal symptoms (tardive dyskinesia, tremors and rigidity, restlessness [akathisia], muscle contractions [dystonia], changes in breathing and heart rate)

ER: extended release

ESA: erythropoiesis-stimulating agents

esp: especially

ESR: erythrocyte sedimentation rate

ESRD: end-stage renal disease

ET: endotracheal

EtOH: ethanol

eval: evaluation

exam (s):examination/s

externa: external

extrav: extravasation

FAP: familial adenomatous polyposis

FBS: fasting blood sugar

Fe: iron

fib: fibrillation

FiO_2: fraction of inspired oxygen

FSH: follicle-stimulating hormone

5-FU: fluorouracil

FVC: forced vital capacity

fx: fracture(s)

Fxn: function

g: gram

GABA: gamma-aminobutyric acid

GAD: generalized anxiety disorder

GBM: glioblastoma multiforme

GC: gonorrhea

G-CSF: granulocyte colony-stimulating factor

gen: generation

GERD: gastroesophageal reflux disease

GF: growth factor

GFR: glomerular filtration rate

GGT: gamma-glutamyl transferase

GH: growth hormone

GI: gastrointestinal

GIST: gastrointestinal stromal tumor

GLA: gamma-linoleic acid

GM-CSF: granulocyte-macrophage colony-stimulating factor

GnRH: gonadotropin-releasing hormone

G6PD: glucose-6-phosphate dehydrogenase

gt, gtt: drop, drops (*gutta*)

GTT: glucose tolerance test

GU: genitourinary

GVHD: graft-versus-host disease

h: hour(s)

HA: headache

HBsAg: hepatitis B surface antigen

HBV: hepatitis B virus
HCG: human chorionic gonadotropin
HCL: hairy cell leukemia
Hct: hematocrit
HCTZ: hydrochlorothiazide
HD: hemodialysis
HDAC: histone deacetylase
HDL-C: high-density lipoprotein
    cholesterol
hematotox: hematotoxicity
heme: hemoglobin
hep: hepatitis
hepatotox: hepatotoxicity
HF: heart failure
Hgb: hemoglobin
5-HIAA: 5-hydroxyindoleacetic acid
HIT: heparin-induced
    thrombocytopenia
HITTS: heparin-induced thrombosis-
    thrombocytopenia syndrome
HIV: human immunodeficiency virus
HMG-CoA: hydroxymethylglutaryl
    coenzyme A
H1N1: swine flu strain
h/o: history of
H_2O: water
HPV: human papillomavirus
HR: heart rate
↑ HR: increased heart rate (tachycardia)
hs: at bedtime (*hora somni*)
HSV: herpes simplex virus
5-HT: 5-hydroxytryptamine
HTN: hypertension
Hx: history
IBD: irritable bowel disease
IBS: irritable bowel syndrome
IBW: ideal body weight
ICP: intracranial pressure
I&D: incision & drainage
IFIS: intraoperative floppy iris syndrome
Ig: immunoglobulin
IGF: insulin-like growth factor

IGIV: Immune Globulin, IV
IHSS: idiopathic hypertrophic
    subaortic stenosis
IL: interleukin
IM: intramuscular
impair: impairment
Inf: infusion
info: information
Infxn/Infxns: infection/infections
Inh: inhalation
INH: isoniazid
Inhib/Inhibs: inhibitor(s)
Inj: injection
INR: international normalized ratio
Insuff: insufficiency
intra-Abd: intra-abdominal
intravag: intravaginal
IO: intraosseous
I&O: intake & output
IOP: intraocular pressure
IR: immediate release
ISA: intrinsic sympathomimetic activity
IT: intrathecal
ITP: idiopathic/immune
    thrombocytopenic purpura
IU: international units
IUD: intrauterine device
IV: intravenous
JIA: juvenile idiopathic arthritis
JME: juvenile myoclonic epilepsy
JRA: juvenile rheumatoid arthritis
Jt: joint
K: Klebsiella
K^+: potassium
KCl: potassium chloride
KI: potassium iodide
KOH: potassium hydroxide
L&D: labor and delivery
LA: long acting
L/d: liters per day
LDL: low-density lipoprotein
LDL-C:

LFT: liver function test
LH: luteinizing hormone
LHRH: luteinizing hormone–releasing
  hormone
Li: lithium
Liq: liquid
LMW: low molecular weight
LP: lumbar puncture
LUQ: left upper quadrant
LVD: left ventricular dysfunction
LVEF: left ventricular ejection fraction
LVSD: left ventricular systolic
  dysfunction
lyte(s): electrolyte(s)
MAC: *Mycobacterium avium* complex
maint: maintenance dose/drug
MAO/MAOI: monoamine oxidase/
  inhibitor
max: maximum
mcg: micrograms
mcL: microliter
mcm: micrometer
mcmol: micromole
MDD: major depressive disorder
MDI: multidose inhaler
MDS: myelodysplasia syndrome
meds: medicines
mEq: milliequivalent
met: metastatic
mg: milligram(s)
Mg^{2+}: magnesium
$MgOH_2$: magnesium hydroxide
MI: myocardial infarction; mitral
  insufficiency
mill: million
min: minute(s)
mL: milliliter
mo: month(s)
MoAb: monoclonal antibody(s)
mod: moderate
MRSA: methicillin-resistant
  Staphylococcus aureus

MS: multiple sclerosis; musculoskeletal
ms: millisecond(s)
MSSA: methicillin-sensitive
  Staphylococcus aureus
MTT: monotetrazolium
MTX: methotrexate
MU: million units
MyG: myasthenia gravis
N: nausea
N/A: not applicable
N/D: nausea/diarrhea
Na: sodium
NA: narrow angle
NAG: narrow angle glaucoma
$NaHCO_3$: sodium bicarbonate
NaI: sodium iodide
NEC: necrotizing enterocolitis
nephrotox: nephrotoxicity
neurotox: neurotoxicity
ng: nanogram
NG: nasogastric
NHL: non–Hodgkin lymphoma
NIAON: nonischemic arterial optic
  neuritis
NIDDM: non–insulin-dependent
  diabetes mellitus
nl: normal
NMDA: *N*-methyl-D-aspartate
NNRTI: nonnucleoside reverse
  transcriptase inhibitor
NO: nitric oxide
NPO: nothing by mouth (*nil per os*)
NRTI: nucleoside reverse transcriptase
  inhibitor
NS: normal saline
NSAID: nonsteroidal anti-
  inflammatory drug
NSCLC: non–small-cell lung cancer
NSTEMI: Non–ST elevation
  myocardial infarction
N/V: nausea and vomiting
N/V/D: nausea, vomiting, diarrhea

NYHA: New York Heart Association
OA: osteoarthritis
OAB: overactive bladder
obst: obstruction
OCD: obsessive compulsive disorder
OCP: oral contraceptive pill
OD: overdose
ODT: orally disintegrating tablets
OJ: orange juiceoint: ointment
OK: recommended
once/wk
ophthal: ophthalmic
OSAHS: obstructive sleep apnea/
  hypopnea syndrome
OTC: over the counter
ototox: ototoxicity
oz: ounces
P: phosphorus
PABA: para-amino benzoic acid
PAH: pulmonary arterial hypertension
PAT: paroxysmal atrial tachycardia
pc: after eating (*post cibum*)
PCa: cancer of the prostate
PCI: percutaneous coronary intervention
PCN: penicillin
PCP: *Pneumocystis jiroveci* (formerly
  carinii) pneumonia
PCWP: pulmonary capillary wedge
  pressure
PDE5: phosphodiesterase type 5
PDGF: platelet-derived growth factor
PE: pulmonary embolus; physical
  examination; pleural effusion
PEA: pulseless electrical activity
Ped: pediatrics
PFT: pulmonary function test
pg: picogram(s)
Ph: Philadelphia chromosome
Pheo: pheochromocytoma
PHN: post-herpetic neuralgia
photosens: Photosensitivity
phototox: phototoxicity

PID: pelvic inflammatory disease
PKU: phenylketonuria
plt(s): platelet(s)
↓ plt: decreased platelets
  (thrombocytopenia)
PMDD: premenstrual dysphoric disorder
PML: progressive multifocal
  leukoencephalopathy
PMS: premenstrual syndrome
PNA: penicillin
PO: by mouth (*per os*)
PPD: purified protein derivative
PPI: proton pump inhibitor(s)
PR: by rectum
Prep: preparation(s)
PRG: pregnancy
PRN: as often as needed (*pro re nata*)
PSA: prostate-specific antigen
PSVT: paroxysmal supraventricular
  tachycardia
pt(s): patient(s)
PT: prothrombin time
PTCA: percutaneous transluminal
  coronary angioplasty
PTH: parathyroid hormone
PTT: partial thromboplastin time
PUD: peptic ulcer disease
pulm: pulmonary
PVC: premature ventricular contraction
PVD: peripheral vascular disease
PWP: pulmonary wedge pressure
Px: prophylaxis
pyelo: pyelonephritis
q: every (*quaque*)
qd: every day
qh: every hour
q_h: every_hours
qhs: every hour of sleep (before bedtime)
qid: four times a day (*quater in die*)
qmo: every month
q_mo: every_month
qod: every other day

qowk: every other week
qwk: every week
RA: rheumatoid arthritis
RAS: renin–angiotensin system
RBC: red blood cell(s) (count)
RCC: renal cell carcinoma
RDA: recommended dietary allowance
RDS: respiratory distress syndrome
rec: recommends
recons: reconstitution
reeval: reevaluation
REMS: Risk Evaluation and
   Mitigation Strategy
resp: respiratory
RHuAb: recombinant human
   antibody
RIA: radioimmune assay
RLS: restless leg syndrome
RR: respiratory rate
RSI: rapid-sequence intubation
RSV: respiratory syncytial virus
RT: reverse transcriptase
RTA: renal tubular acidosis
Rx: prescription
Rxn(s): reaction(s)
s: second(s)
s/p: status/post
SAD: social anxiety disorder or
   seasonal affective disorder
SAE: serious adverse event
SBE: subacute bacterial endocarditis
SBP: systolic blood pressure
SCLC: small-cell lung cancer
SCr: serum creatinine
SD: single dose
SDV: single-dose vial
SE: side effect(s)
see package insert: see the
   manufacturer's insert
SIADH: syndrome of inappropriate
   antidiuretic hormone
sig: significant

SJIA: systemic juvenile idiopathic
   arthritis
SJS: Stevens–Johnson syndrome
SL: sublingual
SLE: systemic lupus erythematosus
SNRIs: serotonin–norepinephrine
   reuptake inhibitors
SOB: shortness of breath
Sol/soln: solution
sp: species
SPAG: small particle aerosol generator
SQ: subcutaneous
SR: sustained release
SSRI: selective serotonin reuptake
   inhibitor
SSS: sick sinus syndrome
S/Sxs: signs & symptoms
stat: immediately (*statim*)
STD: sexually transmitted disease
STEMI: ST elevation myocardial
   infarction
subsp: subspecies
supl(s): supplement(s)
supp: suppository
susp: suspension
SVR: systemic vascular resistance
SVT: supraventricular tachycardia
SWFI: sterile water for injection
SWSD: shift work sleep disorder
synd: syndrome
synth: synthesis
Sx: symptom(s)
Sz: seizure
tab/tabs: tablet/tablets
TB: tuberculosis
tbsp: tablespoon
TCA: tricyclic antidepressant
TFT: thyroid function test
TIA: transient ischemic attack
tid: three times a day (*ter in die*)
tinc: tincture
TKI: tyrosine kinase inhibitors

TMP: trimethoprim
TMP–SMX: trimethoprim–
    sulfamethoxazole
TNF: tumor necrosis factor
TOUCH: Tysabri Outreach Unified
    Commitment to Health
tox: toxicity
TPA: tissue plasminogen activator
tri: trimester
TSH: thyroid-stimulating hormone
tsp: teaspoon
TRALI: transfusion-related acute
    lung injury
TTP: thrombotic thrombocytopenic
    purpura
TTS: transdermal therapeutic system
Tx: treatment
UC: ulcerative colitis
UGT: uridine 5'
    diphosphoglucuronosyl transferase
ULN: upper limits of normal
uncomp: uncomplicated
UPA: pyrrolizidine alkaloids
URI: upper respiratory infection
UTI: urinary tract infection
UV: ultraviolet
V: vomiting
VAERS: Vaccine Adverse Events
    Reporting System

Vag: vaginal
VEGF: vascular endothelial growth factor
VF: ventricular fibrillation
vit: vitamin
VLDL: very low-density lipoprotein
vol: volume
VPA: valproic acid
VRE: vancomycin-resistant
    Enterococcus
VT: ventricular tachycardia
VTE: venous thromboembolism
w/: with
W/: with
w/hold: withhold
W/P: Warnings and Precautions
WBC: white blood cell(s) (count)
wgt: weight
WHI: Women's Health Initiative
w/in: within
wk: week
/wk: per week
WNL: within normal limits
w/o: without
WPW: Wolff–Parkinson–White
    syndrome
XL: extended release
XR: extended release
ZE: Zollinger–Ellison (syndrome)
Zn^{2+}: zinc

CLASSIFICATION (Generic and common brand names)

ALLERGY

Antihistamines

Azelastine (Astelin, Optivar)
Cetirizine (Zyrtec, Zyrtec D)
Chlorpheniramine (Chlor-Trimeton)
Clemastine Fumarate (Tavist)
Cyproheptadine (Periactin)
Desloratadine (Clarinex)
Diphenhydramine (Benadryl)
Fexofenadine (Allegra)
Hydroxyzine (Atarax, Vistaril)
Levocetirizine (Xyzal)
Loratadine (Alavert, Claritin)

Miscellaneous Antiallergy Agents

Budesonide (Rhinocort, Pulmicort)
Cromolyn Sodium (Intal, NasalCrom, Opticrom)
Montelukast (Singulair)
Phenylephrine, Oral (Sudafed PE, SudoGest PE, Nasop, Lusonal, AH-Chew D, Sudafed PE Quick Dissolve)

ANTIDOTES

Acetylcysteine (Acetadote, Mucomyst)
Amifostine (Ethyol)
Atropine/Pralidoxime (DuoDote)
Atropine, Systemic (AtroPen) Auto-Injector)
Charcoal (SuperChar, Actidose, Liqui-Char Activated)
Deferasirox (Exjade)
Dexrazoxane (Totect, Zinecard)
Digoxin Immune Fab (Digibind, DigiFab)
Flumazenil (Romazicon)
Hydroxocobalamin (Cyanokit)
Iodine (Potassium Iodide) [Lugol Soln] (SSKI, Thyro-Block, ThyroSafe, ThyroShield)
Ipecac Syrup (OTC Syrup)
Mesna (Mesnex)
Naloxone (Generic)
Physostigmine (Antilirium)
Succimer (Chemet)

ANTIMICROBIAL AGENTS

Antibiotics

AMINOGLYCOSIDES

Amikacin (Amikin)
Gentamicin (Garamycin, G-Myticin)

Neomycin Sulfate (Neofradin, Generic)

Streptomycin
Tobramycin (Nebcin)

CARBAPENEMS

Doripenem (Doribax)
Ertapenem (Invanz)

Imipenem-Cilastatin (Primaxin)

Meropenem (Merrem)

CEPHALOSPORINS, FIRST GENERATION

Cefadroxil (Duricef, Ultracef)

Cefazolin (Ancef, Kefzol)

Cephalexin (Keflex, Panixine DisperDose)
Cephradine (Velosef)

CEPHALOSPORINS, SECOND GENERATION

Cefaclor (Ceclor, Raniclor)
Cefotetan (Cefotan)

Cefoxitin (Mefoxin)
Cefprozil (Cefzil)

Cefuroxime (Ceftin [Oral], Zinacef [Parenteral])

CEPHALOSPORINS, THIRD GENERATION

Cefdinir (Omnicef)
Cefditoren (Spectracef)
Cefixime (Suprax)
Cefoperazone (Cefobid)
Cefotaxime (Claforan)

Cefpodoxime (Vantin)
Ceftazidime (Fortaz, Ceptaz, Tazidime, Tazicef)
Ceftibuten (Cedax)

Ceftizoxime (Cefizox)
Ceftriaxone (Rocephin)

CEPHALOSPORINS, FOURTH GENERATION

Cefepime (Maxipime)

CEPHALOSPORINS, UNCLASSIFIED, ("FIFTH GENERATION")

Ceftaroline (Teflaro)

FLUOROQUINOLONES

Ciprofloxacin (Cipro, Cipro XR, Proquin XR)
Gemifloxacin (Factive)

Levofloxacin (Levaquin)
Moxifloxacin (Avelox)

Norfloxacin (Noroxin, Chibroxin Ophthalmic)
Ofloxacin (Floxin)

KETOLIDE

Telithromycin (Ketek)

MACROLIDES

Azithromycin (Zithromax)
Clarithromycin (Biaxin, Biaxin XL)
Erythromycin (E-Mycin, E.E.S., Ery-Tab, EryPed, Ilotycin)
Erythromycin & Sulfisoxazole (Eryzole, Pediazole)

PENICILLINS

Amoxicillin (Amoxil, Polymox)
Amoxicillin & Clavulanic Acid (Augmentin, Augmentin 600 ES, Augmentin XR)
Ampicillin (Amcill, Omnipen)
Ampicillin-Sulbactam (Unasyn)
Dicloxacillin (Dynapen, Dycill)
Nafcillin (Nallpen, Unipen)
Oxacillin (Bactocill, Prostaphlin)
Penicillin G Aqueous (Potassium or Sodium) (Pfizerpen, Pentids)
Penicillin G Benzathine (Bicillin)
Penicillin G Procaine (Wycillin, Others)
Penicillin V (Pen-Vee K, Veetids, Others)
Piperacillin (Pipracil)
Piperacillin-Tazobactam (Zosyn)
Ticarcillin/Potassium Clavulanate (Timentin)

TETRACYCLINES

Doxycycline (Adoxa, Periostat, Oracea, Vibramycin, Vibra-Tabs)
Minocycline (Dynacin, Minocin, Solodyn)
Tetracycline (Achromycin V, Sumycin)
Tigecycline (Tygacil)

Miscellaneous Antibiotic Agents

Aztreonam (Azactam)
Clindamycin (Cleocin, Cleocin-T, Others)
Fosfomycin (Monurol)
Linezolid (Zyvox)
Metronidazole (Flagyl, MetroGel)
Mupirocin (Bactroban, Bactroban Nasal)
Neomycin Topical (see Bacitracin, Neomycin, & Polymyxin B, Topical [Neosporin Ointment], Bacitracin,
Neomycin, Polymyxin B, & Hydrocortisone, Topical [Cortisporin], Bacitracin, Neomycin, Polymyxin B, & Lidocaine, Topical [Clomycin])
Nitrofurantoin (Furadantin, Macrodantin, Macrobid)
Quinupristin-Dalfopristin (Synercid)
Retapamulin (Altabax)
Rifaximin (Xifaxan)
Telavancin (Vibativ)
Trimethoprim (Primsol, Proloprim)
Trimethoprim (TMP)–Sulfamethoxazole (SMX) [Co-Trimoxazole] (Bactrim, Septra)
Vancomycin (Vancocin, Vancoled)

ANTIFUNGALS

Amphotericin B (Amphocin, Fungizone)
Amphotericin B Cholesteryl (Amphotec)
Amphotericin B Lipid Complex (Abelcet)
Amphotericin B Liposomal (AmBisome)
Anidulafungin (Eraxis)
Caspofungin (Cancidas)
Clotrimazole (Lotrimin, Mycelex, Others OTC)
Clotrimazole & Betamethasone (Lotrisone)
Econazole (Spectazole)
Fluconazole (Diflucan)
Itraconazole (Sporanox)
Ketoconazole, Oral (Nizoral)
Ketoconazole, Topical (Extina, Kuric, Xolegel, Nizoral AD Shampoo) [Shampoo OTC]
Miconazole (Monistat 1 Combo, Monistat 3, Monistat 7) [OTC] (Monistat-Derm)
Miconazole, Buccal (Oravig)
Nystatin (Mycostatin)
Oxiconazole (Oxistat)
Posaconazole (Noxafil)
Sertaconazole (Ertaczo)
Terbinafine (Lamisil, Lamisil AT)
Triamcinolone & Nystatin (Mycolog-II)
Voriconazole (VFEND)

Antimycobacterials

Dapsone, Oral
Ethambutol (Myambutol)
Isoniazid (INH)
Pyrazinamide (Generic)
Rifabutin (Mycobutin)
Rifampin (Rifadin)
Rifapentine (Priftin)
Streptomycin

Antiparasitics

Benzyl Alcohol (Ulesfia)
Lindane (Kwell, Others)
Spinosad (Natroba)

Antiprotozoals

Artemether & Lumefantrine (Coartem)
Atovaquone (Mepron)
Atovaquone/Proguanil (Malarone)
Nitazoxanide (Alinia)
Tinidazole (Tindamax)

ANTIRETROVIRALS

Abacavir (Ziagen)
Daptomycin (Cubicin)
Darunavir (Prezista)
Delavirdine (Rescriptor)
Didanosine [ddI] (Videx)
Efavirenz (Sustiva)
Efavirenz/Emtricitabine/ Tenofovir (Atripla)
Etravirine (Intelence)
Fosamprenavir (Lexiva)
Indinavir (Crixivan)
Lamivudine (Epivir, Epivir-HBV, 3TC [Many Combo Regimens])
Lopinavir/Ritonavir (Kaletra)
Maraviroc (Selzentry)
Nelfinavir (Viracept)
Nevirapine (Viramune)
Raltegravir (Isentress)
Ritonavir (Norvir)

Saquinavir (Fortovase, Invirase)
Stavudine (Zerit)

Tenofovir (Viread)
Tenofovir/Emtricitabine (Truvada)

Zidovudine (Retrovir)
Zidovudine & Lamivudine (Combivir)

Antivirals

Acyclovir (Zovirax)
Adefovir (Hepsera)
Amantadine (Symmetrel)
Atazanavir (Reyataz)
Boceprevir (Victrelis)
Cidofovir (Vistide)
Emtricitabine (Emtriva)
Enfuvirtide (Fuzeon)
Famciclovir (Famvir)
Foscarnet (Foscavir)

Ganciclovir (Cytovene, Vitrasert)
Interferon Alfa-2b & Ribavirin Combo (Rebetron)
Oseltamivir (Tamiflu)
Palivizumab (Synagis)
Peginterferon Alfa-2b (Peg Intron)
Penciclovir (Denavir)

Ribavirin (Virazole, Copegus)
Rimantadine (Flumadine)
Telbivudine (Tyzeka)
Valacyclovir (Valtrex)
Valganciclovir (Valcyte)
Zanamivir (Relenza)

Miscellaneous Antiviral Agents

Daptomycin (Cubicin)
Pentamidine (Pentam 300, NebuPent)

Trimetrexate (NeuTrexin)

ANTINEOPLASTIC AGENTS

Alkylating Agents

Altretamine (Hexalen)
Bendamustine (Treanda)
Busulfan (Myleran, Busulfex)
Carboplatin (Paraplatin)

Cisplatin (Platinol, Platinol AQ)
Oxaliplatin (Eloxatin)
Procarbazine (Matulane)
Tapentadol (Nucynta)

Triethylene-Thiophosphoramide (Thiotepa, Thioplex, Tespa, TSPA)

NITROGEN MUSTARDS

Chlorambucil (Leukeran)
Cyclophosphamide (Cytoxan, Neosar)

Ifosfamide (Ifex, Holoxan)
Mechlorethamine (Mustargen)

Melphalan [L-PAM] (Alkeran)

NITROSOUREAS

Carmustine [BCNU] (BiCNU, Gliadel)

Streptozocin (Zanosar)

Antibiotics

Bleomycin Sulfate
  (Blenoxane)
Dactinomycin
  (Cosmegen)

Daunorubicin
  (Daunomycin,
  Cerubidine)
Doxorubicin
  (Adriamycin, Rubex)

Epirubicin (Ellence)
Idarubicin (Idamycin)
Mitomycin (Mutamycin)

Antimetabolites

Clofarabine (Clolar)
Cytarabine [ARA-C]
  (Cytosar-U)
Cytarabine Liposome
  (DepoCyt)
Floxuridine (FUDR)
Fludarabine
  Phosphate (Flamp,
  Fludara)

Fluorouracil [5-FU]
  (Adrucil)
Fluorouracil, Topical
  [5-FU] (Efudex)
Gemcitabine
  (Gemzar)
Mercaptopurine [6-MP]
  (Purinethol)

Methotrexate
  (Rheumatrex Dose
  Pack, Trexall)
Nelarabine (Arranon)
Pemetrexed (Alimta)
Pralatrexate (Folotyn)
Romidepsin (Istodax)
6-Thioguanine [6-TG]
  (Tabloid)

Hormones

Anastrozole (Arimidex)
Bicalutamide (Casodex)
Degarelix (Firmagon)
Estramustine Phosphate
  (Emcyt)
Exemestane (Aromasin)
Flutamide (Eulexin)
Fulvestrant (Faslodex)

Goserelin (Zoladex)
Leuprolide (Lupron,
  Lupron DEPOT,
  Lupron DEPOT-Ped,
  Viadur, Eligard)
Levamisole (Ergamisol)
Megestrol Acetate
  (Megace, Megace-ES)

Nilutamide (Nilandron)
Tamoxifen
Triptorelin (Trelstar 3.75,
  Trelstar 11.25, Trelstar
  22.5)

Mitotic Inhibitors (Vinca Alkaloids)

Etoposide [VP-16]
  (VePesid, Toposar)
Vinblastine (Velban,
  Velbe)

Vincristine (Oncovin,
  Vincasar PFS)
Vinorelbine (Navelbine)

Monoclonal Antibodies

Alemtuzumab (Campath)
Bevacizumab (Avastin)
Cetuximab (Erbitux)
Erlotinib (Tarceva)

Gemtuzumab Ozogamicin
  (Mylotarg)
Ipilimumab (Yervoy)
Lapatinib (Tykerb)

Ofatumumab (Arzerra)
Panitumumab (Vectibix)
Trastuzumab (Herceptin)

Proteasome Inhibitor

Bortezomib (Velcade)

Taxanes

Cabazitaxel (Jevtana)
Docetaxel (Taxotere)

Paclitaxel (Taxol, Abraxane)

Tyrosine Kinase Inhibitors (TKIs)

Dasatinib (Sprycel)
Everolimus (Afinitor)
Gefitinib (Iressa)
Imatinib (Gleevec)

Nilotinib (Tasigna)
Pazopanib Hydrochloride (Votrient)
Sorafenib (Nexavar)

Sunitinib (Sutent)
Temsirolimus (Torisel)

Miscellaneous Antineoplastic Agents

Abiraterone (Zytiga)
Aldesleukin [Interleukin-2, IL-2] (Proleukin)
Aminoglutethimide (Cytadren)
L-Asparaginase (Elspar, Oncaspar)
BCG [Bacillus Calmette-Guérin] (TheraCys, Tice BCG)
Cladribine (Leustatin)

Dacarbazine (DTIC)
Eribulin (Halaven)
Hydroxyurea (Hydrea, Droxia)
Irinotecan (Camptosar)
Ixabepilone Kit (Ixempra)
Letrozole (Femara)
Leucovorin (Wellcovorin)
Mitoxantrone (Novantrone)

Panitumumab (Vectibix)
Pemetrexed (Alimta)
Rasburicase (Elitek)
Sipuleucel-T (Provenge)
Thalidomide (Thalomid)
Topotecan (Hycamtin)
Tretinoin, Topical [Retinoic Acid] (Retin-A, Avita, Renova, Retin-A Micro)

CARDIOVASCULAR (CV) AGENTS

Aldosterone Antagonist

Eplerenone (Inspra)
Spironolactone (Aldactone)

Alpha-1-Adrenergic Blockers

Doxazosin (Cardura, Cardura XL)

Prazosin (Minipress)
Terazosin (Hytrin)

Angiotensin-Converting Enzyme (ACE) Inhibitors

Benazepril (Lotensin)
Captopril (Capoten, Others)
Enalapril (Vasotec)
Fosinopril (Monopril)
Lisinopril (Prinivil, Zestril)
Moexipril (Univasc)
Perindopril Erbumine (Aceon)
Quinapril (Accupril)
Ramipril (Altace)
Trandolapril (Mavik)

Angiotensin II Receptor Antagonists/Blockers

Amlodipine/Olmesartan (Azor)
Amlodipine/Valsartan (Exforge)
Candesartan (Atacand)
Eprosartan (Teveten)
Irbesartan (Avapro)
Losartan (Cozaar)
Telmisartan (Micardis)
Valsartan (Diovan)

Antiarrhythmic Agents

Adenosine (Adenocard)
Amiodarone (Cordarone, Nexterone, Pacerone)
Atropine, Systemic (AtroPen Auto-Injector)
Digoxin (Digitek, Lanoxin, Lanoxicaps)
Disopyramide (Norpace, Norpace CR)
Dofetilide (Tikosyn)
Dronedarone (Multaq)
Esmolol (Brevibloc)
Flecainide (Tambocor)
Ibutilide (Corvert)
Lidocaine, Systemic (Xylocaine, Others)
Mexiletine (Mexitil)
Procainamide (Pronestyl, Pronestyl SR, Procanbid)
Propafenone (Rythmol)
Quinidine (Quinidex, Quinaglute)
Sotalol (Betapace, Betapace AF)

Beta-Adrenergic Blockers

Acebutolol (Sectral)
Atenolol (Tenormin)
Atenolol & Chlorthalidone (Tenoretic)
Betaxolol (Kerlone)
Bisoprolol (Zebeta)
Carvedilol (Coreg, Coreg CR)
Labetalol (Trandate, Normodyne)
Metoprolol Succinate (Toprol XL)
Metoprolol Tartrate (Lopressor)
Nadolol (Corgard)
Nebivolol (Bystolic)
Penbutolol (Levatol)
Pindolol (Visken)
Propranolol (Inderal)
Timolol (Blocadren)

Calcium Channel Antagonists/Blockers (CCBs)

Amlodipine (Norvasc)
Amlodipine/Olmesartan (Azor)
Amlodipine/Valsartan (Exforge)
Clevidipine (Cleviprex)
Diltiazem (Cardizem, Cardizem CD, Cardizem LA, Cardizem SR, Cartia
XT, Dilacor XR, Diltia XT, Taztia XT, Tiamate, Tiazac)
Felodipine (Plendil)
Isradipine (DynaCirc)

Nicardipine (Cardene)
Nifedipine (Procardia, Procardia XL, Adalat CC)

Nimodipine (Nimotop)
Nisoldipine (Sular)

Verapamil (Calan, Caover HS, Isoptin, Verelan)

Centrally Acting Antihypertensive Agents

Clonidine, Oral (Catapres)
Clonidine, Oral, Extended Release (Kapvay)

Clonidine, Transdermal (Catapres TTS)
Guanfacine (Tenex)
Methyldopa (Aldomet)

Combination Antihypertensive Agents

Aliskiren & Amlodipine (Tekamlo)
Aliskiren, amlodipine, & Hydrochlorothiazide (Amturnide)
Aliskirin & Valsartan (Valturna)
Amlodipine, Valsartan, & Hydrochlorothiazide (Exforge HCT)

Isosorbide Dinitrate Hydralazine HCl (BiDil)
Lisinopril & Hydrochlorothiazide (Prinzide, Zestoretic, Generic)
Olmesartan, Amlodipine, & Hydrochlorothiazide (Tribenzor)

Olmesartan, Olmesartan, & Hydrochlorothiazide (Benicar, Benicar HCT)
Telmisartan & Amlodipine (Twynsta)

Diuretics

Acetazolamide (Diamox)
Amiloride (Midamor)
Bumetanide (Bumex)
Chlorothiazide (Diuril)
Chlorthalidone (Hygroton, Others)
Furosemide (Lasix)
Hydrochlorothiazide (HydroDIURIL, Esidrix, Others)

Hydrochlorothiazide & Amiloride (Moduretic)
Hydrochlorothiazide & Spironolactone (Aldactazide)
Hydrochlorothiazide & Triamterene (Dyazide, Maxzide)
Indapamide (Lozol)
Mannitol (Various)

Metolazone (Zaroxolyn)
Spironolactone (Aldactone)
Torsemide (Demadex)
Triamterene (Dyrenium)

Inotropic/Pressor Agents

Digoxin (Digitek, Lanoxin, Lanoxicaps)
Dobutamine (Dobutrex)
Dopamine (Intropin)
Epinephrine (Adrenalin, Sus-Phrine, EpiPen, EpiPen Jr, Others)

Inamrinone (Amrinone, Inocor)
Isoproterenol (Isuprel)
Milrinone (Primacor)
Nesiritide (Natrecor)

Norepinephrine (Levophed)
Phenylephrine, Systemic (Neo-Synephrine)

Lipid-Lowering Agents

Cholestyramine (Questran, Questran Light, Prevalite)
Colesevelam (WelChol)
Colestipol (Colestid)
Ezetimibe (Zetia)
Fenofibrate (TriCor, Antara, Lofibra, Lipofen, Triglide)

Fenofibric Acid (Trilipix)
Gemfibrozil (Lopid)
Niacin (Nicotinic Acid) (Niaspan, Slo-Niacin, Niacor, Nicolar) (OTC Forms)
Niacin & Lovastatin (Advicor)

Niacin & Simvastatin (Simcor)
Omega-3 Fatty Acid [Fish Oil] (Lovaza)

Lipid-Lowering/Antihypertensive Combos

Amlodipine/Atorvastatin (Caduet)

Statins

Atorvastatin (Lipitor)
Fluvastatin (Lescol)

Lovastatin (Mevacor, Altoprev)
Pitavastatin (Livalo)

Pravastatin (Pravachol)
Rosuvastatin (Crestor)
Simvastatin (Zocor)

Vasodilators

Alprostadil [Prostaglandin E_1] (Prostin VR)
Epoprostenol (Flolan)
Fenoldopam (Corlopam)
Hydralazine (Apresoline, Others)
Iloprost (Ventavis)
Isosorbide Dinitrate (Isordil, Sorbitrate, Dilatrate-SR)

Isosorbide Mononitrate (Ismo, Imdur)
Minoxidil, Oral
Nitroglycerin (Nitrostat, Nitrolingual, Nitro-Bid Ointment, Nitro-Bid IV, Nitrodisc, Transderm-Nitro, NitroMist, Others)

Nitroprusside (Nipride, Nitropress)
Tolazoline (Priscoline)
Treprostinil Sodium (Remodulin) Tyvaso

Miscellaneous Cardiovascular Agents

Aliskiren (Tekturna)
Aliskiren/
  Hydrochlorothiazide
  (Tekturna HCT)
Ambrisentan (Letairis)
Conivaptan (Vaprisol)

Dabigatran (Pradaxa)
Prasugrel hydrochloride
  (Effient)

Ranolazine (Ranexa)
Sildenafil (Viagra,
  Revatio)

CENTRAL NERVOUS SYSTEM AGENTS

Alzheimer Agents

Donepezil (Aricept)
Galantamine
  (Razadyne,
  RazadyneER)

Memantine (Namenda,
  Namenda XR)
Rivastigmine
  (Exelon)

Rivastigmine
  Transdermal
  (Exelon Patch)
Tacrine (Cognex)

Antianxiety Agents

Alprazolam (Xanax,
  Niravam)
Buspirone (BuSpar)
Chlordiazepoxide
  (Librium, Mitran,
  Libritabs)

Clorazepate (Tranxene)
Diazepam (Diastat,
  Valium)
Doxepin (Sinequan,
  Adapin)

Hydroxyzine (Atarax,
  Vistaril)
Lorazepam (Ativan,
  Others)
Meprobamate (Various)
Oxazepam

Anticonvulsants

Carbamazepine (Tegretol
  XR, Carbatrol, Epitol,
  Equetro)
Clonazepam (Klonopin)
Diazepam (Diastat,
  Valium)
Ethosuximide (Zarontin)
Fosphenytoin (Cerebyx)
Gabapentin (Neurontin)
Lacosamide (Vimpat)
Lamotrigine (Lamictal)

Lamotrigine Extended
  Release (Lamictal
  XR)
Levetiracetam (Keppra)
Lorazepam (Ativan,
  Others)
Magnesium Sulfate
  (Various)
Oxcarbazepine
  (Trileptal)

Pentobarbital (Nembutal,
  Others)
Phenobarbital
Phenytoin (Dilantin)
Rufinamide (Banzel)
Tiagabine (Gabitril)
Topiramate (Topamax)
Valproic Acid
  (Depakene, Depakote)
Vigabatrin (Sabril)
Zonisamide (Zonegran)

Antidepressants

Amitriptyline (Elavil)
Bupropion Hydrobromide (Aplenzin)
Bupropion Hydrochloride (Wellbutrin, Wellbutrin SR, Wellbutrin XL, Zyban)
Citalopram (Celexa)
Desipramine (Norpramin)
Desvenlafaxine (Pristiq)
Doxepin (Adapin)
Duloxetine (Cymbalta)
Escitalopram (Lexapro)
Fluoxetine (Prozac, Sarafem)
Fluvoxamine (Luvox)
Imipramine (Tofranil)
Milnacipran (Savella)
Mirtazapine (Remeron, Remeron SolTab)
Nefazodone (Serzone)
Nortriptyline (Pamelor)
Paroxetine (Paxil, Paxil CR, Pexeva)
Phenelzine (Nardil)
Selegiline Transdermal (Emsam)
Sertraline (Zoloft)
Tranylcypromine (Parnate)
Trazodone (Desyrel, Oleptro)
Venlafaxine (Effexor, Effexor XR)
Viibryd (Vilazodone)

Antiparkinson Agents

Amantadine (Symmetrel)
Apomorphine (Apokyn)
Benztropine (Cogentin)
Bromocriptine (Parlodel)
Carbidopa/Levodopa (Sinemet, Parcopa)
Entacapone (Comtan)
Pramipexole (Mirapex, Mirapex ER)
Rasagiline Mesylate (Azilect)
Rivastigmine Transdermal (Exelon Patch)
Ropinirole (Requip)
Selegiline (Eldepryl, Zelapar)
Tolcapone (Tasmar)
Trihexyphenidyl (Artane)

Antipsychotics

Aripiprazole (Abilify, Abilify DISCMELT)
Asenapine Maleate (Saphris)
Chlorpromazine (Thorazine)
Clozapine (Clozaril, FazaClo)
Fluphenazine (Prolixin, Permitil)
Haloperidol (Haldol)
Iloperidone (Fanapt)
Lithium Carbonate (Eskalith, Lithobid, Others)
Lurasidone (Latuda)
Molindone (Moban)
Olanzapine (Zyprexa, Zyprexa Zydis)
Olanzapine, LA Parenteral (Zyprexa Relprevv)
Paliperidone (Invega, Invega Sustenna)
Perphenazine (Trilafon)
Pimozide (Orap)
Prochlorperazine (Compazine)
Quetiapine (Seroquel, Seroquel XR)
Risperidone, Oral (Risperdal, Risperdal Consta, Risperdal M-Tab)
Risperidone, Parenteral (Risperdal Consta)
Thioridazine (Mellaril)
Thiothixene (Navane)
Trifluoperazine (Stelazine)
Ziprasidone (Geodon)

Sedative Hypnotics

Chloral Hydrate (Aquachloral, Supprettes)
Dexmedetomidine (Precedex)
Diphenhydramine (Benadryl [OTC])
Doxepin (Silenor)
Etomidate (Amidate)
Estazolam (ProSom)
Eszopiclone (Lunesta)
Flurazepam (Dalmane)
Hydroxyzine (Atarax, Vistaril)
Midazolam (various) [C-IV]
Pentobarbital (Nembutal, Others)
Phenobarbital
Propofol (Diprivan)
Ramelteon (Rozerem)
Secobarbital (Seconal)
Temazepam (Restoril)
Thiopental Sodium (Pentothal)
Triazolam (Halcion)
Zaleplon (Sonata)
Zolpidem (Ambien, Ambien CR, Edluar, ZolpiMist)

Stimulants

Armodafinil (Nuvigil)
Atomoxetine (Strattera)
Dexmethylphenidate (Focalin, Focalin XR)
Dextroamphetamine (Dexedrine)
Guanfacine (Intuniv)
Lisdexamfetamine (Vyvanse)
Methylphenidate, Oral (Concerta, Metadate CD, Methylin Ritalin, Ritalin LA, Ritalin SR, Others) [CII]
Methylphenidate, Transdermal (Daytrana)
Modafinil (Provigil)
Rivastigmine (Exelon)
Sibutramine (Meridia)

Miscellaneous CNS Agents

Clomipramine (Anafranil)
Clonidine, Oral, Extended Release (Kapvay)
Dalfampridine (Ampyra)
Fingolimod (Gilenya)
Interferon Beta-1a (Rebif)
Meclizine (Antivert) (Bonine, Dramamine OTC)
Natalizumab (Tysabri)
Nimodipine (Nimotop)
Rizatriptan (Maxalt, Maxalt MLT)
Sodium Oxybate (Xyrem)
Tetrabenazine (Xenazine)

DERMATOLOGIC AGENTS

Acitretin (Soriatane)
Acyclovir (Zovirax)
Adapalene (Differin)
Adapalene & Benzoyl Peroxide (Epiduo Gel)
Alefacept (Amevive)
Anthralin (Anthra-Derm)
Amphotericin B (Amphocin, Fungizone)
Bacitracin, Topical (Baciguent)
Bacitracin & Polymyxin B, Topical (Polysporin)

Bacitracin, Neomycin, & Polymyxin B, Topical (Neosporin Ointment)

Bacitracin, Neomycin, Polymyxin B, & Hydrocortisone, Topical (Cortisporin)

Bacitracin, Neomycin, Polymyxin B, & Lidocaine, Topical (Clomycin)

Botulinum Toxin Type A [Abobotulinumtoxin A] (Dysport)

Botulinum Toxin Type A [Incobotulinumtoxin A] (Xeomin)

Botulinum Toxin Type A [Onabotulinumtoxin A] (Botox, Botox Cosmetic)

Botulinum Toxin Type B [Rimabotulinumtoxin B] (Myobloc)

Calcipotriene (Dovonex)

Calcitriol Ointment (Vectical)

Capsaicin (Capsin, Zostrix, Others)

Ciclopirox (Loprox, Penlac)

Ciprofloxacin (Cipro, Cipro XR, Proquin XR)

Clindamycin (Cleocin, Cleocin T, Others)

Clindamycin & Tretinoin (Veltin Gel)

Clotrimazole & Betamethasone (Lotrisone)

Dapsone Topical (Aczone)

Dibucaine (Nupercainal)

Diclofenac, Topical (Solaraze)

Doxepin, Topical (Zonalon, Prudoxin)

Econazole (Spectazole)

Erythromycin, Topical (A/T/S, Eryderm, Erycette, T-Stat)

Erythromycin & Benzoyl Peroxide (Benzamycin)

Finasteride (Propecia)

Fluorouracil, Topical [5-FU] (Efudex)

Gentamicin, Topical (Garamycin, G-Myticin)

Imiquimod Cream, 5% (Aldara)

Isotretinoin [13-*cis* Retinoic Acid] (Accutane, Amnesteem, Claravis, Sotret)

Ketoconazole (Nizoral)

Kunecatechins [Sinecatechins] (Veregen)

Lactic Acid & Ammonium Hydroxide [Ammonium Lactate] (Lac-Hydrin)

Lindane (Kwell, Others)

Lisdexamfetamine (Vyvanse)

Metronidazole (Flagyl, MetroGel)

Miconazole (Monistat 1 Combo, Monistat 3, Monistat 7) [OTC] (Monistat-Derm)

Miconazole/Zinc Oxide/Petrolatum (Vusion)

Minocycline (Dynacin, Minocin, Solodyn)

Minoxidil, Topical (Theroxidil, Rogaine) [OTC]

Mupirocin (Bactroban, Bactroban Nasal)

Naftifine (Naftin)

Nystatin (Mycostatin)

Oxiconazole (Oxistat)

Penciclovir (Denavir)

Permethrin (Nix, Elimite)

Pimecrolimus (Elidel)

Podophyllin (Podocon-25, Condylox Gel 0.5%, Condylox)

Pramoxine (Anusol Ointment, ProctoFoam-NS)

Pramoxine & Hydrocortisone (Enzone, ProctoFoam-HC)

Selenium Sulfide (Exsel Shampoo, Selsun Blue Shampoo, Selsun Shampoo)

Silver Sulfadiazine (Silvadene, Others)

Steroids, Topical (Table 3)

Tacrolimus [FK506] (Prograf, Protopic)

Tazarotene (Tazorac, Avage)
Terbinafine (Lamisil, Lamisil AT [OTC])
Tolnaftate (Tinactin, Others [OTC])

Tretinoin, Topical [Retinoic Acid] (Avita, Retin-A, Retin-A Micro, Renova)

Ustekinumab (Stelara)
Vorinostat (Zolinza)

DIETARY SUPPLEMENTS

Calcium Acetate (Calphron, Phos-Ex, PhosLo)
Calcium Glubionate (Neo-Calglucon)
Calcium Salts (Chloride, Gluconate, Gluceptate)
Cholecalciferol [Vitamin D_3] (Delta D)
Cyanocobalamin [Vitamin B_{12}] (Nascobal)
Ferric Gluconate Complex (Ferrlecit)

Ferrous Gluconate (Fergon [OTC], Others)
Ferrous Sulfate
Ferumoxytol (Feraheme)
Fish Oil (Lovaza, Others [OTC])
Folic Acid
Iron Dextran (Dexferrum, INFeD)
Iron Sucrose (Venofer)
Magnesium Oxide (Mag-Ox 400, Others [OTC])

Magnesium Sulfate (Various)
Multivitamins, Oral [OTC] (Table 12)
Phytonadione [Vitamin K] (Aqua-MEPHYTON, Others)
Potassium Supplements (Kaon, Kaochlor, K-Lor, Slow-K, Micro-K, Klorvess)
Pyridoxine [Vitamin B_6]
Sodium Bicarbonate [$NaHCO_3$]
Thiamine [Vitamin B_1]

EAR (OTIC) AGENTS

Acetic Acid & Aluminum Acetate (Otic Domeboro)
Benzocaine & Antipyrine (Auralgan)
Ciprofloxacin, Otic (Cetraxal)
Ciprofloxacin & Dexamethasone, Otic (Ciprodex Otic)
Ciprofloxacin & Hydrocortisone, Otic (Cipro HC Otic)

Neomycin, Colistin, & Hydrocortisone (Cortisporin-TC Otic Drops)
Neomycin, Colistin, Hydrocortisone, & Thonzonium (Cortisporin-TC Otic Suspension)
Ofloxacin Otic (Floxin Otic, Floxin Otic Singles)

Polymyxin B & Hydrocortisone (Otobiotic Otic)
Sulfacetamide & Prednisolone (Blephamide, Others)
Triethanolamine (Cerumenex [OTC])

ENDOCRINE SYSTEM AGENTS

Antidiabetic Agents

Acarbose (Precose)
Bromocriptine
  Mesylate
  (Cycloset)
Chlorpropamide
  (Diabinese)
Exenatide (Byetta)
Glimepiride (Amaryl)
Glimepiride/Pioglitazone
  (Duetact)
Glipizide (Glucotrol,
  Glucotrol XL)
Glyburide (DiaBeta,
  Micronase, Glynase)

Glyburide/Metformin
  (Glucovance)
Insulins, Injectable
  (Table 4)
Liraglutide Recombinant
  (Victoza)
Metformin
  (Glucophage,
  Glucophage XR)
Miglitol (Glyset)
Nateglinide (Starlix)
Pioglitazone (Actos)
Pioglitazone/Metformin
  (ACTOplus Met)

Repaglinide (Prandin)
Repaglinide &
  Metformin
  (PrandiMet)
Rosiglitazone (Avandia)
Rosiglitazone/Metformin
  (Avandamet)
Sitagliptin (Januvia)
Sitagliptin & Metformin
  (Janumet)
Tolazamide (Tolinase)
Tolbutamide (Orinase)

DPP-4 Inhibitors

Linagliptin
  (Tradjenta)
Saxagliptin (Onglyza)

Saxagliptin & Metformin
  (Kombiglyze XR)
Sitagliptin (Januvia)

Sitagliptin/Metformin
  (Janumet)

Hormone & Synthetic Substitutes

Calcitonin (Fortical,
  Miacalcin)
Calcitriol (Rocaltrol,
  Calcijex)
Cortisone Systemic &
  Topical
Desmopressin (DDAVP,
  Stimate)
Dexamethasone,
  Systemic & Topical
  (Decadron)

Fludrocortisone Acetate
  (Florinef)
Fluoxymesterone
  (Halotestin, Androxy)
Glucagon
Hydrocortisone Topical
  & Systemic (Cortef,
  Solu-Cortef)
Methylprednisolone
  (Solu-Medrol)
Prednisolone

Prednisone
Testosterone (AndroGel
  1%, AndroGel 1.62%,
  Androderm, Axiron,
  Fortesta, Striant,
  Testim)
Vasopressin (Antidiuretic
  Hormone [ADH])
  (Pitressin)

Hypercalcemia/Osteoporosis Agents

Alendronate (Fosamax, Fosamax Plus D)
Denosumab (Prolia, Xgeva)
Etidronate Disodium (Didronel)

Gallium Nitrate (Ganite)
Ibandronate (Boniva)
Pamidronate (Aredia)
Raloxifene (Evista)
Risedronate (Actonel, Actonel w/ Calcium)

Risedronate, Delayed Release (Atelvia)
Teriparatide (Forteo)
Zoledronic Acid (Zometa, Reclast)

Obesity Management

Orlistat (Xenical, Alli [OTC])

Thyroid/Antithyroid Agents

Levothyroxine (Synthroid, Levoxyl, Others)
Liothyronine (Cytomel, Triostat, T_3)

Methimazole (Tapazole)
Potassium Iodide [Lugol Soln] (Iosat, SSKI, Thyro-Block,

ThyroSafe, ThyroShield) [OTC]
Propylthiouracil [PTU]

Miscellaneous Endocrine Agents

Cinacalcet (Sensipar)
Demeclocycline (Declomycin)

Diazoxide (Proglycem)
Somatropin (Serostim)

Tesamorelin (Egrifta)

EYE (OPHTHALMIC) AGENTS

Glaucoma Agents

Acetazolamide (Diamox)
Apraclonidine (Iopidine)
Betaxolol, Ophthalmic (Betoptic)
Brimonidine (Alphagan P)
Brimonidine/Timolol (Combigan)
Brinzolamide (Azopt)

Carteolol (Ocupress, Carteolol Ophthalmic)
Dipivefrin (Propine)
Dorzolamide (Trusopt)
Dorzolamide & Timolol (Cosopt)
Echothiophate Iodine (Phospholine Ophthalmic)
Latanoprost (Xalatan)

Levobunolol (AK-Beta, Betagan)
Lodoxamide (Alomide)
Rimexolone (Vexol Ophthalmic)
Timolol, Ophthalmic (Timoptic)
Trifluridine, Ophthalmic (Viroptic)

Ophthalmic Antibiotics

Azithromycin Ophthalmic 1% (AzaSite)

Bacitracin, Ophthalmic (AK-Tracin Ophthalmic)

Bacitracin & Polymyxin B, Ophthalmic (AK-Poly-Bac Ophthalmic, Polysporin Ophthalmic)

Bacitracin, Neomycin, & Polymyxin B (AK-Spore Ophthalmic, Neosporin Ophthalmic)

Bacitracin, Neomycin, Polymyxin B, & Hydrocortisone, Ophthalmic (AK-Spore HC Ophthalmic, Cortisporin Ophthalmic)

Besifloxacin (Besivance)

Ciprofloxacin, Ophthalmic (Ciloxan)

Erythromycin, Ophthalmic (Ilotycin Ophthalmic)

Gentamicin, Ophthalmic (Garamycin, Genoptic, Gentacidin, Gentak, Others)

Gentamicin & Prednisolone, Ophthalmic (Pred-G Ophthalmic)

Levofloxacin Ophthalmic (Quixin, Iquix)

Moxifloxacin Ophthalmic (Vigamox Ophthalmic)

Neomycin & Dexamethasone (AK-Neo-Dex Ophthalmic, NeoDecadron Ophthalmic)

Neomycin, Polymyxin, & Hydrocortisone (Cortisporin Ophthalmic & Otic)

Neomycin, Polymyxin B, & Dexamethasone (Maxitrol)

Neomycin, Polymyxin B, & Prednisolone (Poly-Pred Ophthalmic)

Norfloxacin Ophthalmic (Chibroxin Ophthalmic)

Ofloxacin Ophthalmic (Ocuflox Ophthalmic)

Silver Nitrate (Dey-Drop, Others)

Sulfacetamide (Bleph-10, Cetamide, Sodium Sulamyd)

Sulfacetamide & Prednisolone (Blephamide, Others)

Tobramycin Ophthalmic (AKTob, Tobrex)

Tobramycin & Dexamethasone Ophthalmic (TobraDex)

Trifluridine Ophthalmic (Viroptic)

Miscellaneous Ophthalmic Agents

Alcaftadine (Lastacaft)

Artificial Tears (Tears Naturale [OTC])

Atropine, Ophthalmic (Isopto Atropine, Generic)

Bepotastine Besilate (Bepreve)

Cromolyn Sodium (Opticrom)

Cyclopentolate Ophthalmic (Cyclogyl, Cyclate)

Cyclopentolate w/ Phenylephrine (Cyclomydril)

Cyclosporine Ophthalmic (Restasis)

Dexamethasone, Ophthalmic (AK-Dex Ophthalmic, Decadron Ophthalmic)

Diclofenac Ophthalmic (Voltaren Ophthalmic)

Emedastine (Emadine)
Epinastine (Elestat)
Ganciclovir, Ophthalmic Gel (Zirgan)
Ketorolac Ophthalmic (Acular, Acular LS, Acular PF)
Ketotifen Ophthalmic (Alaway, Zaditor) [OTC]
Levocabastine (Livostin)

Lodoxamide (Alomide)
Naphazoline (Albalon, Naphcon, Others)
Naphazoline & Pheniramine Acetate (Naphcon A, Visine A)
Nepafenac (Nevanac)
Olopatadine Ophthalmic (Patanol, Pataday)
Pemirolast (Alamast)

Phenylephrine, Ophthalmic (Neo-Synephrine Ophthalmic, AK-Dilate, Zincfrin [OTC])
Ranibizumab (Lucentis)
Rimexolone (Vexol Ophthalmic)
Scopolamine Ophthalmic

GASTROINTESTINAL AGENTS

Antacids

Alginic Acid + Aluminum Hydroxide & Magnesium Trisilicate (Gaviscon) [OTC]
Aluminum Hydroxide (Amphojel, AlternaGEL, Dermagran) [OTC]
Aluminum Hydroxide w/ Magnesium Carbonate (Gaviscon Extra Strength, Liquid) [OTC]

Aluminum Hydroxide w/ Magnesium Hydroxide (Maalox)
Aluminum Hydroxide w/ Magnesium Hydroxide & Simethicone (Mylanta, Mylanta II, Maalox Plus) [OTC]
Aluminum Hydroxide w/ Magnesium Trisilicate (Gaviscon, Regular Strength) [OTC]

Calcium Carbonate (Tums, Alka-Mints) [OTC]
Magaldrate (Riopan-Plus) [OTC]
Simethicone (Mylicon, Others) [OTC]

Antidiarrheals

Bismuth Subsalicylate (Pepto-Bismol)
Diphenoxylate w/ Atropine (Lomotil, Lonox)
Kaolin-Pectin (Kaodene, Kao-Spen, Kapectolin)

Lactobacillus (Lactinex Granules)
Loperamide (Diamode, Imodium) [OTC]
Octreotide (Sandostatin, Sandostatin LAR)

Paregoric (Camphorated Tincture of Opium)
Rifaximin (Xifaxan, Xifaxan550)

Antiemetics

Aprepitant (Emend)
Chlorpromazine (Thorazine)
Dimenhydrinate (Dramamine, Others) [OTC]
Dolasetron (Anzemet)
Dronabinol (Marinol)
Droperidol (Inapsine)
Fosaprepitant (Emend, Injection)
Granisetron (Kytril)

Meclizine (Antivert, Bonine, Dramamine [OTC])
Metoclopramide (Reglan, Clopra, Octamide)
Nabilone (Cesamet)
Ondansetron (Zofran, Zofran ODT)
Ondansetron, Oral Soluble Film (Zuplenz)

Palonosetron (Aloxi)
Prochlorperazine (Compazine)
Promethazine (Phenergan)
Scopolamine (Scopace, Transderm-Scop)
Thiethylperazine (Torecan)
Trimethobenzamide (Tigan)

Antisecretory/GI Protectant Agents

Bismuth Subcitrate/ Metronidazole/ Tetracycline (Pylera)
Cimetidine (Tagamet, Tagamet HB [OTC], Tagamet DS [OTC])
Dexlansoprazole (Dexilant)
Esomeprazole (Nexium)
Famotidine (Pepcid, Pepcid AC [OTC])

Lansoprazole (Prevacid, Prevacid IV)
Nizatidine (Axid, Axid AR [OTC])
Omeprazole (Prilosec, Prilosec OTC)
Omeprazole & Sodium Bicarbonate (Zegerid, Zegerid OTC)
Omeprazole, Sodium Bicarbonate, &

Magnesium Hydroxide (Zegerid with Magnesium Hydroxide)
Pantoprazole (Protonix)
Rabeprazole (AcipHex)
Ranitidine Hydrochloride (Zantac, Zantac OTC)
Sucralfate (Carafate)

Cathartics/Laxatives

Bisacodyl (Dulcolax [OTC])
Docusate Calcium (Surfak)
Docusate Potassium (Dialose)
Docusate Sodium (DOSS, Colace)
Glycerin Suppository
Lactulose (Constulose, Generlac, Chronulac, Cephulac, Enulose, Others)

Magnesium Citrate (Citroma, Others) [OTC]
Magnesium Hydroxide (Milk of Magnesia) [OTC]
Mineral Oil [OTC]
Mineral Oil Enema (Fleet Mineral Oil) [OTC]
Mineral Oil-Pramoxine HCl-Zinc Oxide [OTC]

Polyethylene Glycol (PEG)-Electrolyte Solution (GoLYTELY, CoLyte)
Polyethylene Glycol (PEG) 3350 (MiraLAX)
Psyllium (Metamucil, Serutan, Effer-Syllium)
Sodium Phosphate (Visicol)
Sorbitol (Generic)

Enzymes

Pancrelipase (Pancrease, Cotazym, Creon, Ultrase)

Miscellaneous GI Agents

Alosetron (Lotronex)
Alvimopan (Entereg)
Apriso (Salix)
Balsalazide (Colazal)
Budesonide (Entocort EC)
Certolizumab Pegol (Cimzia)
Dexpanthenol (Ilopan-Choline Oral, Ilopan)
Dibucaine (Nupercainal)
Dicyclomine (Bentyl)
Fidaxomicin (Dificid)
Hydrocortisone, Rectal (Anusol-HC Suppository, Cortifoam Rectal, Proctocort, Others)
Hyoscyamine (Anaspaz, Cystospaz, Levsin, Others)
Hyoscyamine, Atropine, Scopolamine, &

Phenobarbital (Donnatal, Others)
Infliximab (Remicade)
Lubiprostone (Amitiza)
Mesalamine (Asacol, Canasa, Lialda, Pentasa, Rowasa)
Methylnaltrexone Bromide (Relistor)
Metoclopramide (Reglan, Clopra, Octamide)
Mineral Oil-Pramoxine HCl-Zinc Oxide (Tucks Ointment) [OTC]
Misoprostol (Cytotec)
Neomycin Sulfate (Neo-Fradin, Generic)
Olsalazine (Dipentum)
Oxandrolone (Oxandrin)

Pramoxine (Anusol Ointment, ProctoFoam-NS, Others)
Pramoxine w/ Hydrocortisone (Enzone, ProctoFoam-HC)
Propantheline (Pro-Banthine)
Starch, Topical, Rectal (Tucks Suppositories) [OTC]
Sulfasalazine (Azulfidine, Azulfidine EN)
Vasopressin (Antidiuretic Hormone [ADH]) (Pitressin)
Witch Hazel (Tucks Pads, Others [OTC])

HEMATOLOGIC AGENTS

Anticoagulants

Antithrombin, Recombinant (Atryn)
Argatroban (Acova)
Bivalirudin (Angiomax)
Dalteparin (Fragmin)

Desirudin (Iprivask)
Enoxaparin (Lovenox)
Fondaparinux (Arixtra)
Heparin
Lepirudin (Refludan)

Protamine (Generic)
Tinzaparin (Innohep)
Warfarin (Coumadin)

Antiplatelet Agents

Abciximab (ReoPro)
Aspirin (Bayer, Ecotrin, St. Joseph's [OTC])
Clopidogrel (Plavix)
Dipyridamole (Persantine)

Dipyridamole & Aspirin (Aggrenox)
Eptifibatide (Integrilin)
Prasugrel Hydrochloride (Effient)

Ticlopidine (Ticlid)
Tirofiban (Aggrastat)

Antithrombotic Agents

Alteplase, Recombinant [tPA] (Activase)
Aminocaproic Acid (Amicar)
Anistreplase (Eminase)

Dextran 40 (Gentran 40, Rheomacrodex)
Reteplase (Retavase)
Streptokinase (Streptase, Kabikinase)

Tenecteplase (TNKase)
Urokinase (Abbokinase)

Hematopoietic Stimulants

Darbepoetin Alfa (Aranesp)
Eltrombopag (Promacta)
Epoetin Alfa [Erythropoietin, EPO] (Epogen, Procrit)

Filgrastim [G-CSF] (Neupogen)
Iron Dextran (Dexferrum, INFeD)
Iron Sucrose (Venofer)
Oprelvekin (Neumega)

Pegfilgrastim (Neulasta)
Plerixafor (Mozobil)
Romiplostim (Nplate)
Sargramostim [GM-CSF] (Leukine)

Volume Expanders

Albumin (Albuminar, Albutein, Buminate)
Dextran 40 (Gentran 40, Rheomacrodex)

Hetastarch (Hespan)
Plasma Protein Fraction (Plasmanate, Others)

Miscellaneous Hematologic Agents

Antihemophilic Factor VIII (Monoclate)
Antihemophilic Factor (Recombinant) (Xyntha)

Decitabine (Dacogen)
Desmopressin (DDAVP, Stimate)
Fibrinogen Concentrate, Human (Riastap)

Lenalidomide (Revlimid)
Pentoxifylline (Trental)

IMMUNE SYSTEM AGENTS

Immunomodulators

Interferon Alfa
  (Roferon-A, Intron A)
Interferon Alfacon-1
  (Infergen)
Interferon Beta-1a
  (Rebif)

Interferon Beta-1b
  (Betaseron, Extavia)
Interferon Gamma-1b
  (Actimmune)
Natalizumab
  (Tysabri)

Peginterferon Alfa-2a
  [Pegylated Interferon]
  (Pegasys)
Peginterferon Alfa-2b
  [Pegylated Interferon]
  (PEG-Intron)

Immunomodulators: Disease-Modifying Antirheumatic Drugs (DMARDs)

Abatacept (Orencia)
Adalimumab (Humira)
Anakinra (Kineret)

Certolizumab Pegol
  (Cimzia)
Etanercept (Enbrel)

Golimumab (Simponi)
Infliximab (Remicade)
Tocilizumab (Actemra)

Immunosuppressive Agents

Azathioprine (Imuran)
Basiliximab (Simulect)
Cyclosporine
  (Sandimmune,
  Gengraf, Neoral)
Daclizumab (Zenapax)
Everolimus (Zortress)
Lymphocyte Immune
  Globulin

Antithymocyte
  Globulin, ATG
  (Atgam)
Muromonab-CD3
  (Orthoclone OKT3)
Mycophenolate Mofetil
  (CellCept)

Mycophenolic Acid
  (Myfortic)
Sirolimus (Rapamune)
Steroids, Systemic
  (Table 2)
Tacrolimus [FK506]
  (Prograf, Protopic)

Vaccines/Serums/Toxoids

Cytomegalovirus
  Immune Globulin
  [CMV-IG IV]
  (CytoGam)
Diphtheria & Tetanus
  Toxoids (Td)
  (Decavac
  for > 7 y)
Diphtheria & Tetanus
  Toxoids (DT)
  (Generic Only
  for < 7 y)

Diphtheria, Tetanus
  Toxoids, & Acellular
  Pertussis Adsorbed
  (DTaP) (Ages < 7 y)
  (Daptacel, Infanrix,
  Tripedia)
Diphtheria, Tetanus
  Toxoids, & Acellular
  Pertussis Adsorbed
  (Tdap) (Ages > 10–11 y)
  (Boosters: Adacel,
  Boostrix)

Diphtheria, Tetanus
  Toxoids, Acellular
  Pertussis Adsorbed,
  Hep B (Recombinant),
  & Inactivated
  Poliovirus Vaccine
  (IPV) Combined
  (Pediarix)
Haemophilus B
  Conjugate Vaccine
  (ActHIB, HibTITER,
  PedvaxHIB, Prohibit,
  TriHIBit, Others)

Hepatitis A (Inactivated) & Hepatitis B Recombinant Vaccine (Twinrix)

Hepatitis A Vaccine (Havrix, Vaqta)

Hepatitis B Immune Globulin (HyperHep, HepaGam B, Nabi-HB, H-BIG)

Hepatitis B Vaccine (Engerix-B, Recombivax HB)

Human Papillomavirus (Types 6, 11, 16, 18) Recombinant Vaccine (Gardasil)

Immune Globulin, IV (Gamimune N, Sandoglobulin, Gammar IV)

Immune Globulin, Subcutaneous (Vivaglobin)

Influenza Monovalent Vaccine (H1N1), Inactivated (CSL, Novartis, Sanofi, Pasteur)

Influenza Vaccine, Inactivated (Afluria, Fluarix, FluLaval, Fluvirin, Fluzone)

Influenza Virus Vaccine Live, Intranasal (FluMist)

Measles, Mumps, & Rubella Vaccine Live [MMR] (M-M-R II)

Measles, Mumps, Rubella, & Varicella Virus Vaccine Live [MMRV] (ProQuad)

Meningococcal Conjugate Vaccine [Quadrivalent, MCV4] (Menactra)

Meningococcal Polysaccharide Vaccine [MPSV4] (Menomune A/C/Y/W-135)

Pneumococcal 7-Valent Conjugate Vaccine (Prevnar)

Pneumococcal Vaccine, Polyvalent (Pneumovax-23)

Rotavirus Vaccine, Live, Oral, Monovalent (Rotarix)

Rotavirus Vaccine, Live, Oral, Pentavalent (RotaTeq)

Smallpox Vaccine

Tetanus Immune Globulin

Tetanus Toxoid (TT)

Varicella Immune Globulin (VarZIG)

Varicella Virus Vaccine (Varivax)

Zoster Vaccine, Live (Zostavax)

MUSCULOSKELETAL AGENTS

Antigout Agents

Allopurinol (Zyloprim, Lopurin, Aloprim)

Colchicine

Febuxostat (Uloric)

Pegloticase (Krystexxa)

Probenecid (Benemid, Others)

Sulfinpyrazone

Muscle Relaxants

Baclofen (Lioresal Intrathecal, Generic)
Carisoprodol (Soma)
Chlorzoxazone (Paraflex, Parafon Forte DSC, Others)
Cyclobenzaprine (Flexeril)
Cyclobenzaprine, Extended Release (Amrix)
Dantrolene (Dantrium)
Diazepam (Diastat, Valium)
Metaxalone (Skelaxin)
Methocarbamol (Robaxin)
Orphenadrine (Norflex)
Tizanidine Hydrochloride (Zanaflex)

Neuromuscular Blockers

Atracurium (Tracrium)
Botulinum Toxin Type A [Incobotulinumtoxin A] (Xeomin)
Botulinum Toxin Type A [Onabotulinumtoxin A] (Botox, Botox Cosmetic)
Botulinum Toxin Type B [Rimabotulinumtoxin B] (Myobloc)
Pancuronium (Pavulon)
Rocuronium (Zemuron)
Succinylcholine (Anectine, Quelicin, Sucostrin, Others)
Vecuronium (Norcuron)

Miscellaneous Musculoskeletal Agents

Edrophonium (Tensilon, Reversol)
Leflunomide (Arava)
Methotrexate (Rheumatrex Dose Pack, Trexall)
Sulfasalazine (Azulfidine, Azulfidine EN)
Tizanidine (Zanaflex)

OB/GYN AGENTS

Contraceptives

Copper IUD Contraceptive (ParaGard T 380A)
Estradiol Cypionate & Medroxyprogesterone Acetate (Lunelle)
Ethinyl Estradiol & Norelgestromin (Ortho Evra)
Etonogestrel/Ethinyl Estradiol Vaginal Insert (NuvaRing)
Etonogestrel Implant (Implanon)
Levonorgestrel Intrauterine Device (IUD) (Mirena)

Medroxyprogesterone (Provera, Depo Provera, Depo-Sub Q Provera)

Oral Contraceptives, Extended Cycle Combination (Table 5)

Oral Contraceptives, Monophasic (Table 5)

Oral Contraceptives, Multiphasic (Table 5)

Oral Contraceptives, Progestin-Only (Table 5)

Emergency Contraceptives

Levonorgestrel (Plan B, One Step, Next Choice)

Ulipristal Acetate (Ella)

Estrogen Supplementation

ESTROGEN ONLY

Esterified Estrogens (Estratab, Menest)

Estradiol (Estrace, Femtrace, Delestrogen)

Estradiol Gel (Divigel)

Estradiol Gel (Elestrin)

Estradiol, Oral (Delestrogen, Estrace, Femtrace, Others)

Estradiol, Spray (Evamist)

Estradiol, Transdermal (Estraderm, Climara, Vivelle Dot)

Estradiol, Vaginal (Estring, Femring, Vagifem)

Estrogen, Conjugated (Premarin)

Estrogen, Conjugated-Synthetic (Cenestin, Enjuvia)

Ethinyl Estradiol (Estinyl, Feminone)

COMBINATION ESTROGEN/PROGESTIN

Ethinyl Estradiol & Drospirenone (YAZ)

Ethinyl Estradiol/ Levonorgestrel (Seasonale)

Ethinyl Estradiol & Norelgestromin (Ortho Evra)

Esterified Estrogens w/ Methyltestosterone (Estratest, Estratest HS, Syntest DS, HS)

Estrogen, Conjugated w/ Medroxyprogesterone (Prempro, Premphase)

Estrogen, Conjugated w/ Methylprogesterone (Premarin w/ Methyl progesterone)

Estrogen, Conjugated w/ Methyltestosterone (Premarin w/ Methyltestosterone)

Estradiol/Levonorgestrel, Transdermal (Climara Pro)

Estradiol/ Medroxyprogesterone (Lunelle)

Estradiol/Norethindrone Acetate (Femhrt, Activella)

Norethindrone Acetate/ Ethinyl Estradiol (Femhrt, Activella)

Vaginal Preparations

Amino-Cerv pH 5.5 Cream
Miconazole (Monistat 1 Combo, Monistat 3,

Monistat 7) [OTC] (Monistat-Derm)
Nystatin (Mycostatin)

Terconazole (Terazol 7)
Tioconazole (Vagistat)

Miscellaneous Ob/Gyn Agents

Clomiphene (Clomid)
Dinoprostone (Cervidil Vaginal Insert, Prepidil Vaginal Gel, Prostin E2)
Gonadorelin (Factrel)
Leuprolide (Lupron)
Lutropin Alfa (Luveris)

Lysteda (Tranexamic Acid)
Magnesium Sulfate (Various)
Medroxyprogesterone (Provera, Depo Provera, Depo-Sub Q Provera)

Methylergonovine (Methergine)
Mifepristone [RU 486] (Mifeprex)
Oxytocin (Pitocin)
Terbutaline (Brethine, Bricanyl) Tranexamic Acid (Lysteda)

PAIN MEDICATIONS

Local Anesthetics (Table 1)

Benzocaine (Americaine, Lanacaine, Hurricane, Various [OTC])
Benzocaine & Antipyrine (Auralgan)
Bupivacaine (Marcaine)
Capsaicin (Capsin, Zostrix, Others [OTC])
Cocaine

Dibucaine (Nupercainal)
Lidocaine; Lidocaine w/ Epinephrine (Anestacon Topical, Xylocaine, Xylocaine Viscous, Xylocaine MPF Others)
Lidocaine, Powder Intradermal Injection System (Zingo)

Lidocaine & Prilocaine (EMLA, LMX)
Mepivacaine (Carbocaine)
Procaine (Novocaine)
Pramoxine (Anusol Ointment, ProctoFoam-NS, Others)

Migraine Headache Medications

Acetaminophen w/ Butalbital w/ & w/o Caffeine (Fioricet, Medigesic, Repan, Sedapap-10, Two-Dyne, Triapine, Axocet, Phrenilin Forte)
Almotriptan (Axert)
Aspirin & Butalbital Compound (Fiorinal)

Aspirin w/ Butalbital, Caffeine, & Codeine (Fiorinal w/ Codeine)
Eletriptan (Relpax)
Frovatriptan (Frova)
Naratriptan (Amerge)
Sumatriptan (Alsuma, Imitrex Injection, Imitrex Nasal Spray, Imitrex Oral)

Sumatriptan & Naproxen Sodium (Treximet)
Sumatriptan Needleless System (Sumavel DosePro)
Zolmitriptan (Zomig)

Narcotic Analgesics

Acetaminophen w/
  Codeine (Tylenol
  No. 2, 3, 4)
Alfentanil (Alfenta)
Aspirin w/ Codeine
  (Empirin No. 2, 3, 4)
Buprenorphine (Buprenex)
Buprenorphine,
  Transdermal
  (Butrans)
Buprenorphine &
  Naloxone (Suboxone)
Butorphanol (Stadol)
Codeine
Fentanyl (Sublimaze)
Fentanyl Iontophoretic
  Transdermal System
  (Ionsys)
Fentanyl, Transdermal
  (Duragesic)
Fentanyl, Transmucosal
  (Abstral, Actiq,
  Fentora, Onsolis)
Hydrocodone &
  Acetaminophen
  (Lorcet, Vicodin,
  Hycet, Others)

Hydrocodone & Aspirin
  (Lortab ASA, Others)
Hydrocodone &
  Ibuprofen
  (Vicoprofen)
Hydromorphone
  (Dilaudid,
  Dilaudid HP)
Hydromorphone,
  Extended Release
  (Exalgo)
Levorphanol (Levo-
  Dromoran)
Meperidine (Demerol,
  Meperitab) [C–II]
Methadone (Dolophine,
  Methadose) [C–II]
Morphine (Avinza XR,
  Astramorph/PF,
  Duramorph,
  Infumorph, MS
  Contin, Kadian SR,
  Oramorph SR,
  Roxanol) [C–II]
Morphine, Liposomal
  (DepoDur)

Morphine & Naltrexone
  (Embeda)
Nalbuphine (Nubain)
Oxycodone [Dihydro
  Hydroxycodeinone]
  (OxyContin,
  Roxicodone)
Oxycodone &
  Acetaminophen
  (Percocet, Tylox)
Oxycodone & Aspirin
  (Percodan)
Oxycodone/Ibuprofen
  (Combunox)
Oxymorphone (Opana,
  Opana ER)
Pentazocine (Talwin,
  Talwin Compound,
  Talwin NX)

Nonnarcotic Analgesics

Acetaminophen [APAP,
  N-acetyl-p-
  aminophenol]
  (Acephen, Tylenol,
  Other Generic)
Acetaminophen +
  Butalbital ± Caffeine
  (Fioricet, Medigesic,
  Repan, Sedapap-10,
  Two-Dyne, Triapin,
  Axocet, Phrenilin
  Forte)

Aspirin (Bayer, Ecotrin,
  St. Joseph's [OTC])
Tramadol (Ultram,
  Ultram ER)
Tramadol/
  Acetaminophen
  (Ultracet)

Nonsteroidal Anti-Inflammatory Agents (NSAIDs)

Celecoxib (Celebrex)
Diclofenac, Oral (Cataflam, Voltaren, Voltaren XR)
Diclofenac, Topical (Flector Patch, Pennsaid, Voltaren gel)
Diclofenac & Misoprostol (Arthrotec)
Diflunisal (Dolobid)
Etodolac

Fenoprofen (Nalfon)
Flurbiprofen (Ansaid, Ocufen)
Ibuprofen (Motrin, Rufen, Advil)
Ibuprofen, Parenteral (Caldolor)
Indomethacin (Indocin)
Ketoprofen (Orudis, Oruvail)
Ketorolac (Toradol)
Ketorolac Nasal (Sprix)
Meloxicam (Mobic)

Nabumetone (Relafen)
Naproxen (Aleve [OTC], Anaprox, Naprosyn)
Naproxen & Esomeprazole (Vimovo)
Oxaprozin (Daypro, Daypro ALTA)
Piroxicam (Feldene)
Sulindac (Clinoril)
Tolmetin (Tolectin)

Miscellaneous Pain Medications

Amitriptyline (Elavil)
Imipramine (Tofranil)
Pregabalin (Lyrica)

Tapentadol (Nucynta)
Tramadol (Ultram, Ultram ER)

Ziconotide (Prialt)

RESPIRATORY AGENTS

Antitussives, Decongestants, & Expectorants

Acetylcysteine (Acetadote, Mucomyst)
Benzonatate (Tessalon Perles)
Codeine
Dextromethorphan (Benylin DM, Delsym, Mediquell, PediaCare 1, Others [OTC])
Guaifenesin (Robitussin, Others)
Guaifenesin & Codeine (Robitussin AC, Brontex, Others)

Guaifenesin & Dextromethorphan (Many OTC Brands)
Hydrocodone & Guaifenesin (Hycotuss Expectorant)
Hydrocodone & Homatropine (Hycodan, Hydromet, Others)
Hydrocodone & Pseudoephedrine (Detussin, Histussin-D, Others)

Hydrocodone, Chlorpheniramine, Phenylephrine, Acetaminophen, & Caffeine (Hycomine Compound)
Potassium Iodide [Lugol Soln] (SSKI), Pseudoephedrine (Sudafed, Novafed, Afrinol, Others [OTC])

Bronchodilators

Albuterol (Proventil, Ventolin, Volmax)

Albuterol & Ipratropium (Combivent, DuoNeb)

Aminophylline

Arformoterol (Brovana)

Ephedrine

Epinephrine (Adrenalin, Sus-Phrine, EpiPen, EpiPen Jr, Others)

Formoterol Fumarate (Foradil, Perforomist)

Isoproterenol (Isuprel)

Levalbuterol (Xopenex, Xopenex HFA)

Metaproterenol (Alupent, Metaprel)

Pirbuterol (Maxair)

Salmeterol (Serevent, Serevent Diskus)

Terbutaline (Brethine, Bricanyl)

Theophylline (Theo24, Theochron)

Respiratory Inhalants

Acetylcysteine (Acetadote, Mucomyst)

Beclomethasone (QVAR)

Beclomethasone Nasal (Beconase AQ)

Beractant (Survanta)

Budesonide (Rhinocort Aqua, Pulmicort)

Budesonide/Formoterol (Symbicort)

Calfactant (Infasurf)

Ciclesonide, Inhalation (Alvesco)

Ciclesonide, Nasal (Omnaris)

Cromolyn Sodium (Intal, NasalCrom, Opticrom, Others)

Dexamethasone, Nasal (Dexacort Phosphate Turbinaire)

Flunisolide (AeroBid, Aerospan, Nasarel)

Fluticasone Furoate Nasal (Veramyst)

Fluticasone Propionate, Inhalation (Flovent HFA, Flovent Diskus)

Fluticasone Propionate, Nasal (Flonase)

Fluticasone Propionate & Salmeterol Xinafoate (Advair Diskus, Advair HFA)

Formoterol Fumarate (Foradil Aerolizer, Perforomist)

Ipratropium (Atrovent HFA, Atrovent Nasal)

Mometasone & Formoterol (DULERA)

Mometasone, Inhaled (Asmanex Twisthaler)

Mometasone, Nasal (Nasonex)

Olopatadine Nasal (Patanase)

Phenylepherine, Nasal (Neo-Syeenphrine Nasal OTC)

Tiotropium (Spiriva)

Triamcinolone (Azmacort)

Miscellaneous Respiratory Agents

Alpha-1-Protease Inhibitor (Prolastin)

Aztreonam, Inhaled

Dornase Alfa (Pulmozyme, DNase)

Montelukast (Singulair)

Omalizumab (Xolair)

Tadalafil (Adcirca)

Zafirlukast (Accolate)

Zileuton (Zyflo, Zyflo CR)

URINARY/GENITOURINARY AGENTS

Benign Prostatic Hyperplasia

Alfuzosin (Uroxatral)
Doxazosin (Cardura, Cardura XL)
Dutasteride (Avodart)

Finasteride (Propecia, Proscar)
Silodosin (Rapaflo)

Tamsulosin (Flomax)
Terazosin (Hytrin)

Bladder Agents (Overactive Bladder, Other Anticholinergics)

Belladonna & Opium Suppositories (B & O Supprettes)
Bethanechol (Duvoid, Urecholine, Others)
Butabarbital-Hyoscyamine Hydrobromide-Phenazopyridine (Pyridium Plus)
Darifenacin (Enablex)
Fesoterodine Fumarate (Toviaz)
Flavoxate (Urispas)

Hyoscyamine (Anaspaz, Cystospaz, Levsin)
Hyoscyamine, Atropine, Scopolamine, & Phenobarbital (Donnatal, Others)
Methenamine Hippurate (Hiprex)
Methenamine Mandelate (UROQUID-Acid No. 2)
Oxybutynin (Ditropan, Ditropan XL)

Oxybutynin Transdermal System (Oxytrol)
Oxybutynin, Topical (Gelnique)
Phenazopyridine (Pyridium, Azo-Standard, Urogesic, Many Others)
Solifenacin (Vesicare)
Tolterodine (Detrol, Detrol LA)
Trospium Chloride (Sanctura, Sanctura XR)

Erectile Dysfunction

Alprostadil, Intracavernosal (Caverject, Edex)
Alprostadil, Urethral Suppository (Muse)

Sildenafil (Viagra, Revatio)
Tadalafil (Cialis)

Vardenafil (Levitra, Stayxn)
Yohimbine (Yocon, Yohimex)

Urolithiasis

Potassium Citrate (Urocit-K)
Potassium Citrate & Citric Acid (Polycitra-K)

Sodium Citrate/Citric Acid (Bicitra, Oracit)

Trimethoprim (Trimpex, Proloprim)

Miscellaneous Urology Agents

Ammonium Aluminum Sulfate [Alum] [OTC]

Atropine, Benzoic Acid, Hyoscyamine Sulfate, Methenamine, Methylene Blue, Phenyl Salicylate (Urised)

Dimethyl Sulfoxide [DMSO] (Rimso-50)

Neomycin-Polymyxin Bladder Irrigant [Neosporin GU Irrigant]

Nitrofurantoin (Macrodantin, Furadantin, Macrobid)

Pentosan Polysulfate Sodium (Elmiron)

WOUND CARE

Becaplermin (Regranex Gel)

Silver Nitrate (Dey-Drop, Others)

MISCELLANEOUS THERAPEUTIC AGENTS

Acamprosate (Campral)

Alglucosidase Alfa (Myozyme)

C1 Esterase Inhibitor, Human (Berinert, Cinryze)

Cilostazol (Pletal)

Dextrose 50%/25%

Drotrecogin Alfa (Xigris)

Ecallantide (Kalbitor)

Eculizumab (Soliris)

Lanthanum Carbonate (Fosrenol)

Mecasermin (Increlex, Iplex)

Megestrol Acetate (Megace, Megace-ES)

Naltrexone (Depade, ReVia, Vivitrol)

Nicotine Gum (Nicorette, Others)

Nicotine Nasal Spray (Nicotrol NS)

Nicotine Transdermal (Habitrol, Nicoderm CQ [OTC], Others)

Palifermin (Kepivance)

Potassium Iodide [Lugol Solution] (SSKI, Thyro-Block, ThyroSafe, Thyroshield)

Sevelamer Carbonate (Renvela)

Sevelamer HCl (Renagel)

Sodium Polystyrene Sulfonate (Kayexalate)

Talc (Sterile Talc Powder)

Varenicline (Chantix)

NATURAL AND HERBAL AGENTS

Aloe Vera (*Aloe barbadensis*)

Arnica (*Arnica montana*)

Bilberry (*Vaccinium myrtillus*)

Black Cohosh (*Cimicifuga racemosa*)

Bogbean (*Menyanthes trifoliate*)

Borage (*Borago officinalis*)

Bugleweed (*Lycopus virginicus*)

Butcher's Broom (*Ruscus aculeatus*)

Capsicum (*Capsicum frutescens*)

Cascara Sagrada (*Rhamnus purshiana*)

Chamomile (*Matricaria recutita*)

Chondroitin Sulfate

Comfrey (*Symphytum officinale*)

Coriander (*Coriandrum sativum*)

Cranberry (*Vaccinium macrocarpon*)

Dong Quai (*Angelica polymorpha, sinensis*)

Echinacea (*Echinacea purpurea*)

Ephedra/Ma Huang

Evening Primrose Oil (*Oenothera biennis*)

Feverfew (*Tanacetum parthenium*)

Fish Oil Supplements (Omega-3 Polyunsaturated Fatty Acid)

Garlic (*Allium sativum*)

Gentian (*Gentiana lutea*)

Ginger (*Zingiber officinale*)

Ginkgo (*Ginkgo biloba*)

Ginseng (*Panax quinquefolius*)

Glucosamine Sulfate (Chitosamine)

Green Tea (*Camellia sinensis*)

Guarana (*Paullinia cupana*)

Hawthorn (*Crataegus laevigata*)

Horsetail (*Equisetum arvense*)

Kava Kava (*Piper methysticum*)

Licorice (*Glycyrrhiza glabra*)

Melatonin (MEL)

Milk Thistle (*Silybum marianum*)

Nettle (*Urtica dioica*)

Red Yeast Rice

Resveratrol

Rue (*Ruta graveolens*)

Saw Palmetto (*Serenoa repens*)

Spirulina (*Spirulina* spp)

Stevia (*Stevia rebaudiana*)

St. John's wort (*Hypericum perforatum*)

Tea Tree (*Melaleuca alternifolia*)

Valerian (*Valeriana officinalis*)

Yohimbine (*Pausinystalia yohimbe*) Yocon, Yohimex

GENERIC AND SELECTED BRAND DRUG DATA

Abacavir (Ziagen) [Antiretroviral/NRTI] **WARNING:** Allergy (fever, rash, fatigue, GI, resp) reported; D/C drug stat & do not rechallenge; lactic acidosis & hepatomegaly/steatosis reported **Uses:** *HIV Infxn* **Action:** NRTI **Dose:** *Adults.* 300 mg PO bid or 600 mg PO daily *Peds.* 8 mg/kg bid/300 mg bid max **Caution:** [C, –] CDC rec HIV-infected mothers not breast-feed (transmission risk) **Disp:** Tabs 300 mg; soln 20 mg/mL **SE:** See Warning **Interactions:** EtOH ↓ drug elimination & ↑ drug exposure; many drug interactions **Labs:** ↑ LFTs, fat redistribution; monitor LFTs, FBS, CBC, & differential, BUN & Cr, triglycerides **NIPE:** ⊘ EtOH; monitor & teach pt about hypersensitivity Rxns; HLA-B*5701 at ↑ risk for fatal hypersensitivity Rxn, genetic screen before use; allergic Rxn usually appears w/in first 6 wk of Tx if pt is allergic; D/C drug stat if hypersensitivity Rxn occurs and ⊘ rechallenge; take w/ or w/o food

Abatacept (Orencia) [Immunomodulator] **Uses:** *Mod/severe RA w/ inadequate response to one or more DMARDs, JIA* **Action:** Selective costimulation modulator, ↓ T-cell activation **Dose:** *Adults.* Initial 500 mg (< 60 kg), 750 mg (60–100 kg); 1 g (> 100 kg) IV over 30 min; repeat at 2 & 4 wk, then q4wk *Peds. 6–17 y.* 10 mg/kg (< 75 kg), 750 mg (75–100 kg), IV × 1 wk 0, 2, 4, then q4wk (> 100 kg, adult dose) **Caution:** [C, ?/–] w/ TNF blockers; COPD; h/o recurrent/ localized/chronic/predisposition to Infxn; w/ immunosuppressants **Disp:** IV powder: 250 mg/10 mL **SE:** HA, URI, N, nasopharyngitis, Infxn, malignancy, Inf Rxns/hypersensitivity (dizziness, HA, HTN), COPD exacerbations, cough, dyspnea **Interactions:** Do not give W/ live vaccines or w/ or w/in 3 mo D/C abatacept **NIPE:** Screen for TB prior to use; D/C if serious Infxn occurs; may worsen COPD Sxs

Abciximab (ReoPro) [Platelet-Aggregation Inhibitor/Antiplatelet] **Uses:** *Prevent acute ischemic comps in PTCA*, MI* **Action:** ↓ plt aggregation (glycoprotein IIb/IIIa Inhib) **Dose:** *ECC 2010: ACS w/ immediate PCI:* 0.25 mg/ kg IV bolus 10–60 min before PCI, then 0.125 mcg/kg/min IV for 12 h w/ heparin *ACS w/ planned PCI w/in 24 h:* 0.25 mcg/kg IV bolus, then 10 mcg/min IV over 18–24 h concluding 1 h post PCI **Caution:** [C, ?/–] **CI:** Active/recent (w/in 6 wk) internal hemorrhage, CVA w/in 2 y or CVA w/ sig neuro deficit, bleeding diathesis, or PO anticoagulants w/in 7 d (unless PT < 1.2 ×control), ↓ plt (< 100,000/mm³), recent trauma or major surgery (w/in 6 wk), CNS tumor, AVM, aneurysm, severe uncontrolled HTN, vasculitis, use of dextran use w/ PTCA, allergy to murine proteins, w/ other glycoprotein IIb/IIIa Inhibs **Disp:** Inj 2 mg/mL **SE:** ↓ BP, CP, allergic Rxns, bleeding **Notes:** Use w/ heparin/ASA **Interactions:** May ↑ bleeding **W/** anticoagulants, antiplts, NSAIDs, thrombolytics **Labs:** ↓ plt; monitor CBC, PT, PTT, INR, guaiac stools, urine for blood **NIPE:** Monitor for ↑ bleeding & bruising; ⊘ shake vial or mix w/ another drug; ⊘ contact sports

Abiraterone (Zytiga) [CYP17 Inhibitor] Uses: *Castrate-resistant metastatic PCa s/p docetaxel* **Action:** CYP17 Inhib; ↓ testosterone **Dose:** 1000 mg PO qd w/ 5 mg prednisone bid; w/o food 2 h ac and 1 h pc; ↓ w/ hepatic impair **Caution:** [X, N/A] w/ Severe CHF, monitor for adrenocortical insuff/excess, w/ CYP2D6 inhib/CYP3A4 inhib or inducers **CI:** PRG **Disp:** Tabs 250 mg **SE:** ↑ LFTs, Jt swell, ↓ K⁺, edema, muscle pain, hot flush, D, UTI, cough, ↑ BP, ↑ URI, urinary frequency, dyspepsia **Labs:** ✓ LFTs **NIPE:** CYP17 inhib may ↑ mineralocorticoid SEs; prednisone; ↓ ACTH-limiting SEs

Acamprosate (Campral) [Hypoglycemic/Alpha-Glucosidase Inhibitor] Uses: *Maint abstinence from EtOH* **Action:** ↓ Glutamatergic transmission; modulates neuronal hyperexcitability; related to GABA **Dose:** 666 mg PO tid; CrCl 30–50 mL/min: 333 mg PO tid **Caution:** [C, ?/–] **CI:** CrCl < 30 mL/min **Disp:** Tabs 333 mg EC **SE:** N/D, depression, anxiety, insomnia **Interactions:** None **Labs:** ↑ BS, LFTs, uric acid; ↑ Hgb, Hct, plts **NIPE:** Does not eliminate EtOH withdrawal Sx; continue even if relapse occurs; caution w/ elderly & pts w/ h/o suicide ideations or depression; take w/o regard to food & swallow whole; N make up missed dose or take > 3 doses in 24 h

Acarbose (Precose) [Hypoglycemic/Alpha-Glucosidase Inhibitor] Uses: *Type 2 DM* **Action:** a-Glucosidase Inhib; delays carbohydrates digestion to ↓ glucose **Dose:** 25–100 mg PO tid w/ 1st bite each meal; 50 mg tid (< 60 kg); 100 mg tid (> 60 kg); usual maint 50–100 mg PO tid **Caution:** [B, ?] w/ CrCl < 25 mL/min; can affect digoxin levels **CI:** IBD, colonic ulceration, partial intestinal obst; cirrhosis **Disp:** Tabs 25, 50, 100 mg **SE:** Abd pain, D, flatulence, hypersensitivity Rxn **Interactions:** OK **W/** sulfonylureas; ↑ hypoglycemic effect **W/** juniper berries, ginseng, garlic, coriander, celery; ↓ effects **W/** intestinal absorbents, digestive enzyme preps, diuretics, corticosteroids, phenothiazines, estrogens, phenytoin, INH, sympathomimetics, CCBs, thyroid hormones; ↓ conc **OF** digoxin **Labs:** ↑ LFTs, ✓ LFTs q3mo for 1st y, FBS, HbA1c, Hgb & Hct, monitor digoxin levels **NIPE:** Take drug w/ 1st bite of food, ↓ GI SE by ↓ dietary starch, treat hypoglycemia w/ dextrose instead of sucrose, continue diet, & exercise program

Acebutolol (Sectral) [Antihypertensive, Antiarrhythmic, Beta-Blocker] Uses: *HTN, arrhythmias* chronic stable angina **Action:** Blocks β-adrenergic receptors, β₁, & ISA **Dose:** *HTN:* 400–800 mg/d 2 ÷ doses *Arrhythmia:* 400–1200 mg/d 2 ÷ doses; ↓ w/ CrCl < 50 mL/min or elderly; ideally initial 200–400 mg/d; max 800 mg/d **Caution:** [B, D in 2nd & 3rd tri, +] Can exacerbate ischemic heart Dz, do not D/C abruptly **CI:** 2nd-, 3rd-degree heart block **Disp:** Caps 200, 400 mg **SE:** Fatigue, HA, dizziness, bradycardia **Interactions:** ↓ Antihypertensive effect

W/ NSAIDs, salicylates, thyroid preps, anesthetics, antacids, α-adrenergic stimulants, ma huang, ephedra, licorice; ↓ hypoglycemic effect *OF* glyburide; ↑ hypotensive response *W/* other antihypertensives, nitrates, EtOH, diuretics, black cohosh, hawthorn, goldenseal, parsley; ↑ bradycardia *W/* digoxin, amiodarone; ↓ hypoglycemic effect *OF* insulin **Labs:** Monitor lipids, uric acid, K⁺, FBS, LFTs, thyroxin, ECG **NIPE:** Teach pt to monitor BP, pulse, S/Sxs CHF; ⊘ D/C abruptly—can ↑ angina or cause MI

Acetaminophen [APAP, N-Acetyl-p-Aminophenol] (Acephen, Tylenol, Other Generic) [OTC] [Analgesic, Antipyretic] Uses: *Mild–mod pain, HA, fever* **Action:** Nonnarcotic analgesic; ↓ CNS synth of prostaglandins & hypothalamic heat-regulating center **Dose: Adults.** 650 mg PO or PR q4–6h or 1000 mg PO q6h; max 4 g/24 h **Peds < 12 y.** 10–15 mg/kg/dose PO or PR q4–6h; max 2.6 g/24 h. Administer q6h if CrCl 10–50 mL/min & q8h if CrCl < 10 mL/min **Caution:** [B, +] Hepatotoxic in elderly & w/ EtOH use w/ > 4 g/d; EtOH liver Dz, G6PD deficiency, liver damage in children w/ 5 suppositories in 24 h **CI:** Hypersensitivity **Disp:** Tabs melt away/dissolving 160 mg *Tabs:* 325, 500, 650 mg *Chewtabs:* 80, 160 mg *Liq:* 100 mg/mL, 120 mg/2.5 mL, 120 mg/5 mL, 160 mg/ 5 mL, 167 mg/5 mL, 325 mg/5 mL, 500 mg/15 mL, 80 mg/0.8 mL *Supp:* 80, 120, 125, 325, 650 mg **SE:** OD hepatotoxic at 10 g; 15 g can be lethal; Rx w/ *N*-acetyl-cysteine **Interactions:** ↑ Hepatotox *W/* EtOH, barbiturates, carbamazepine, INH, rifampin, phenytoin; ↑ risk of bleeding *W/* NSAIDs, salicylates, warfarin, feverfew, ginkgo, red clover; ↓ absorption *W/* antacids, cholestyramine, colestipol **Labs:** Monitor LFTs, CBC, BUN, Cr, PT, INR; false ↑ urine 5-HIAA, urine glucose, serum uric acid; false ↓ serum glucose, amylase **NIPE:** No anti-inflammatory or plt-inhibiting action; ⊘ EtOH; teach S/Sxs hepatotox; consult healthcare provider if temp ↑ 103°F/> 3 d; delayed absorption if given w/ food

Acetaminophen + Butalbital ± Caffeine (Fioricet, Medigesic, Repan, Sedapap-10, Two-Dyne, Triaprin, Axocet, Phrenilin Forte) [C-III] [Analgesic, Antipyretic/Barbiturate] Uses: *Tension HA*, mild pain **Action:** Nonnarcotic analgesic w/ barbiturate **Dose:** 1–2 tabs or caps PO q4–6h PRN; ↓ in renal/hepatic impair; 4 g/24 h APAP max **Caution:** [C, D, +] Alcoholic liver Dz, G6PD deficiency **CI:** Hypersensitivity **Disp:** Caps: *DolgicPlus:* butalbital 50 mg, caffeine 40 mg, APAP 750 mg Caps: *Medigesic, Repan, Two-Dyne:* butalbital 50 mg, caffeine 40 mg, + APAP 325 mg Caps: *Axocet, Phrenilin Forte:* butalbital 50 mg + APAP 650 mg Caps: *Esgic-Plus, Zebutal:* butalbital 50 mg, caffeine 40 mg, APAP 500 mg Liq: *DolgicLQ:* butalbital 50 mg, caffeine 40 mg, APAP 325 mg/15 mL Tabs: *Medigesic, Fioricet, Repan:* butalbital 50 mg, caffeine 40 mg, APAP 325 mg Tabs: *Phrenilin:* butalbital 50 mg + APAP 325 mg Tabs: *Sedapap-10:* butalbital 50 mg + APAP 650 mg **SE:** Drowsiness, dizziness, "hangover" effect, N/V **Interactions:** ↑ Effects *OF* benzodiazepines, opiate analgesics, sedatives/hypnotics, EtOH, methylphenidate hydrochloride; ↓ effects *OF* MAOIs, TCAs, corticosteroids, theophylline, OCPs,

BBs, doxycycline **NIPE:** ⊘ EtOH & CNS depressants, may impair coordination, monitor for depression, use barrier protection contraception; butalbital is habit forming

Acetaminophen + Codeine (Tylenol No. 2, 3, No. 4) [C-III, C-V] [Analgesic, Antipyretic/Opiate] Uses: *Mild–mod pain (No. 2–3); mod–severe pain (No. 4)* **Action:** Combined APAP & narcotic analgesic **Dose:** *Adults.* 1–2 tabs q3–4h PRN or 30–60 mg/codeine q4–6h based on codeine content (max dose APAP = 4 g/d) *Peds.* APAP 10–15 mg/kg/dose; codeine 0.5–1 mg/kg dose q4–6h (*guide:* 3–6 y, 5 mL/dose; 7–12 y, 10 mL/dose) max 2.6 g/d if < 12 y; ↓ in renal/hepatic impair **Caution:** [C, +] Alcoholic liver Dz; G6PD deficiency **CI:** Hypersensitivity **Disp:** Tabs 300 mg APAP + codeine (No. 2 = 15 mg, No. 3 = 30 mg, No. 4 = 60 mg); caps 325 mg APAP + codeine; susp (C-V) APAP 120 mg + codeine 12 mg/5 mL **SE:** Drowsiness, dizziness, N/V **Interactions:** ↑ Effects *OF* benzodiazepines, opiate analgesics, sedatives/hypnotics, EtOH, methylphenidate hydrochloride; ↓ effects *OF* MAOIs, TCAs, corticosteroids, theophylline, OCPs, BBs, doxycycline **NIPE:** ⊘ EtOH & CNS depressants, may impair coordination, monitor for depression, use barrier protection contraception; codeine may be habit forming

Acetazolamide (Diamox) [Anticonvulsant, Diuretic/Carbonic Anhydrase Inhibitor] Uses: *Diuresis, drug and CHF edema, glaucoma, prevent high-altitude sickness, refractory epilepsy* metabolic alkalosis **Action:** Carbonic anhydrase Inhib; ↓ renal excretion of hydrogen & ↑ renal excretion of Na^+, K^+, HCO_3^-, & H_2O **Dose:** *Adults.* 250–375 mg IV or PO q24h *Glaucoma:* 250–1000 mg PO q24h in ÷ doses *Epilepsy:* 8–30 mg/kg/d PO in ÷ doses *Altitude sickness:* 250 mg PO q8–12h or SR 500 mg PO q12–24h start 24–48 h before & 48 h after highest ascent *Metabolic alkalosis:* 250 mg IV q6h × 4 or 500 mg IV × 1 *Peds.* *Epilepsy:* 8–30 mg/kg/24 h PO in ÷ doses; max 1 g/d *Diuretic:* 5 mg/kg/24 h PO or IV *Alkalinization of urine:* 5 mg/kg/dose PO bid–tid *Glaucoma:* 8–30 mg/kg/24 h PO in 3 ÷ doses; max 1 g/d; ↓ dose w/ CrCl 10–50 mL/min; avoid if CrCl < 10 mL/min **Caution:** [C, +] Renal/hepatic/adrenal failure, sulfa allergy, hyperchloremic acidosis **Disp:** Tabs 125, 250 mg; ER caps 500 mg; Inj 500 mg/vial, powder for recons **SE:** Malaise, metallic taste, drowsiness, photosensitivity, hyperglycemia **Interactions:** Causes ↑ effects *OF* amphetamines, quinidine, procainamide, TCAs, ephedrine; ↓ effects *OF* Li, phenobarbital, salicylates, barbiturates; ↑ K^+ loss w/ corticosteroids and amphotericin B **Labs:** Monitor serum lytes esp Na^+ & K^+, CBC, Cr, plt, & IOP; false(+) for urinary protein, urinary urobilinogen; ↓ I uptake; ↑ serum & urine glucose, uric acid, Ca^{2+}, serum ammonia **NIPE:** ↓ GI distress w/ food, monitor for S/Sxs metabolic acidosis, ↑ fluid to ↓ risk of kidney stones; SR forms not for epilepsy

Acetic Acid & Aluminum Acetate (Otic Domeboro) [Astringent/Anti-Infective] Uses: *Otitis externa* **Action:** Anti-infective **Dose:** 4–6 gtt in ear(s) q2–3h **Caution:** [C, ?] **CI:** Perforated tympanic membranes **Disp:** 2% otic soln **SE:** Local irritation **NIPE:** Burning w/ instillation or irrigation

Acetylcysteine (Acetadote, Mucomyst) [Mucolytic/Amino Acid Derivative] **Uses:** *Mucolytic, antidote to APAP hepatotox/OD* adjuvant Rx chronic bronchopulmonary Dzs & CF* prevent contrast-induced renal dysfunction **Action:** Splits mucoprotein disulfide linkages; restores glutathione in APAP OD to protect liver **Dose:** ***Adults & Peds.*** *Nebulizer:* 3–5 mL of 20% soln diluted w/ equal vol of H_2O or NS tid–qid *Antidote:* PO or NG: 140 mg/kg load, then 70 mg/kg q4h ×17 doses (dilute 1:3 in carbonated beverage or OJ), repeat if emesis w/in 1 h of dosing *Acetadote:* 150 mg/kg IV over 60 min, then 50 mg/kg over 4 h, then 100 mg/kg over 16 h; prevent renal dysfunction: 600–1200 mg PO bid ×2 d **Caution:** [B, ?] **Disp:** Soln, inhaled and oral 10%, 20%; Acetadote IV soln 20% **SE:** Bronchospasm (inhaled), N/V, drowsiness, anaphylactoid Rxns w/ IV **Notes:** Activated charcoal absorbs PO acetylcysteine for APAP ingestion; start Rx for APAP OD w/in 6–8 h **Interactions:** Discolors rubber, Fe, Cu, Ag; incompatible *W/* multiple antibiotics—administer drugs separately **Labs:** Monitor ABGs & pulse oximetry w/ bronchospasm **NIPE:** Inform pt of ↑ productive cough; clear airway before aerosol administration; ↑ fluids to liquefy secretions; unpleasant odor will disappear & may cause N/V

Acitretin (Soriatane) [Retinoid] **WARNING:** Not to be used by women who are PRG or who intend to become PRG during/for 3 y following drug D/C; no EtOH during/2 mo following D/C; no blood donation for 3 y following D/C; hepatotoxic **Uses:** *Severe psoriasis*; other keratinization Dz (lichen planus, etc) **Action:** Retinoid-like activity **Dose:** 25–50 mg/d PO, w/ main meal; ↑ if no response by 4 wk to 75 mg/d **Caution:** [X, –] Renal/hepatic impair; in women of reproductive potential **CI:** See Warning; ↑ serum lipids; w/ MTX or tetracyclines **Disp:** Caps 10, 25 mg **SE:** Hyperesthesia,cheilitis, skin peeling, alopecia, pruritus, rash, arthralgia, GI upset,photosens, thrombocytosis **Interactions:** ↑ risk of hep *W/* methotrexate; ↑ risk of ICP *W/* tetracycline; EtOH prolongs teratogenic potential for 2 mo > therapy; ↑ effects *OF* phenytoin, sulfonylureas; ↓ effects *OF* progestin OC and possibly all OC **Labs:** ↑ triglycerides, ↑ Na, K, PO_4; ✓ LFTs/lytes/lipids; **NIPE:** response takes up to 2–3 mo; informed consent & FDA guide w/ each Rx required

Acyclovir (Zovirax) [Antiviral/Synthetic Purine Nucleoside] **Uses:** *Herpes simplex (HSV) (genital/mucocutaneous, encephalitis, keratitis), varicella zoster, herpes zoster (shingles) Infxns* **Action:** Interferes w/ viral DNA synth **Dose:** ***Adults.*** Dose on IBW if obese > 125% IBW PO: *Initial genital HSV:* 200 mg PO q4h while awake (5 caps/d) × 10 d or 400 mg PO tid × 7–10 d *Chronic HSV suppression:* 400 mg PO bid *Intermittent HSV Rx:* As initial Rx, except Rx for 5 d, or 800 mg PO bid, at prodrome *Topical:Initial herpes genitalis:* Apply q3h (6×/d) for 7 d *HSV encephalitis:* 10 mg/kg IV q8h × 10 d *Herpes zoster:* 800 mg PO 5×/d for 7–10 d *IV:* 5–10 mg/kg/dose IV q8h *Peds. Genital HSV: 3 mo–2 y:* 15 mg/kg/ IV ÷ q8h × 5–7 d, 60 mg/kg/d max *2–12y:* 1200 mg/d PO ÷ q8h × 7–10 d > *12 y:* 1000–1200 mg PO ÷ q8h × 7–10 d *HSV encephalitis: 3 mo–12 y:* 60 mg/kg/d IV ÷ q8h × 10 d > *12 y:* 30 mg/kg/d IV ÷ q8h × 10d *Chickenpox: = 2y:* 20 mg/kg/ dose PO qid × 5 d *Shingles: < 12 y:* 30 mg/kg/d PO or 1500 mg/m²/d IV ÷ q8h × 7–10 d; ↓ w/ CrCl < 50 mL/min **Caution:** [B, +] **CI:** Hypersensitivity to compound **Disp:** Caps 200 mg; tabs 400, 800 mg; susp 200 mg/5 mL; Inj 500 & 1000 mg/vial; Inj soln 25 mg/mL, 50 mg/mL oint 5%, and cream 5% **SE:** Dizziness, lethargy, malaise, confusion, rash, IV site inflammation **Interactions:** ↑ CNS SE **W/** MTX w/ zidovudine, ↑ blood levels **W/** probenecid **Labs:** Monitor BUN, SCr, LFTs, CBC; transient ↑ Cr/BUN **NIPE:** Start stat w/ Sxs; ↑ hydration w/ IV dose; ↑ risk cervical CA w/ genital herpes; ↑ length of Rx in immunocompromised pts; PO better than topical for herpes genitalis

Adalimumab (Humira) [Antirheumatic/TNF Alpha-Blocker]

WARNING: Cases of TB have been observed; ✓ TB skin test prior to use; hep B reactivation possible, invasive fungal and other opportunistic Infxns reported; lymphoma/other CAs possible in children and adolescents **Uses:** *Mod–severe RA w/ an inadequate response to one or more DMARDs, psoriatic arthritis (PA), JIA, plaque psoriasis, ankylosing spondylitis (AS), Crohn Dz* **Action:** TNF-α Inhib **Dose:** *RA,PA,AS:* 40 mg SQ q owk; may ↑ 40 mg qwk if not on MTX. JIA 15–30 kg 20 mg qowk *Crohn Dz:* 160 mg d 1, 80 mg 2 wk later, then 2 wk later maint 40 mg qowk **Caution:** [B, ?/–] See Warning, do not use w/ live vaccines **CI:** None **Disp:** Prefilled 0.4 mL (20 mg) & 0.8 mL (40 mg) syringe **SE:** Inj site Rxns, anaphylaxis, cytopenias demyelinating Dz, new onset psoriasis **Interactions:** ↑ Effects **W/** MTX **Labs:** May ↑ lipids, alk phos **NIPE:** ⊘ Exposure to Infxn; ⊘ admin live virus vaccines; refrigerate prefilled syringe, rotate Inj sites, OK w/ other DMARDs

Adapalene (Differin) [Retinoid]

Uses: *Acne vulgaris* **Action:** Retinoid-like, modulates cell differentiation/keratinization/inflammation **Dose:** *Adults & Peds > 12 y:* Apply 1 × daily to clean/dry skin **Caution:** [C, ?/–] Products w/ sulfur/resorcinol/salicylic acid ↑ irritation **Disp:** Top lotion, gel, cream 0.1%; gel 0.3% **SE:** Skin redness, dryness, burning, stinging, scaling, itching, sunburn **NIPE:** Avoid exposure to sunlight/sunlamps; wear sunscreen; avoid waxing-treated areas

Adapalene & Benzoyl Peroxide (Epiduo Gel) [Retinoid + Antibacterial/Keratolytic]

Uses: *Acne vulgaris* **Action:** Retinoid-like, modulates cell differentiation, keratinization, and inflammation w/ antibacterial. **Dose:** *Adults & Peds > 12 y.* Apply 1 × daily to clean/dry skin **Caution:** [C, ?] Bleaching effects, photosensitivity **Contra:** Component sensitivity **Disp:** Topical gel adapalene 0.1% and benzoyl peroxide 2.5% (45g) **SE:** Local irritation, dryness, erythema, burning, stinging **Interactions:** ⊘ Concomitantly **W/** topical irritants and waxed areas; ↑ risk of irritation w/ sulfur, resorcinol, salicylic acid, and other topical acne meds **NIPE:** Vit A may ↑ SE; ⊘ use on open skin/wounds or sunburned areas. Avoid eyes, lips, mucous membranes

Adefovir (Hepsera) [Antiviral/Acyclic Nucleotide Analogue]
WARNING: Acute exacerbations of hep seen after D/C therapy (monitor LFTs); nephrotoxic w/ underlying renal impair w/ chronic use (monitor renal Fxn); HIV resistance/untreated may emerge; lactic acidosis & severe hepatomegaly w/ steatosis reported **Uses:** *Chronic active hep B* **Action:** Nucleotide analog **Dose:** *CrCl > 50 mL/min:* 10 mg PO daily *CrCl 20–49 mL/min:* 10 mg PO q48h;*CrCl 10–19 mL/min:* 10 mg PO q72h; *HD:* 10 mg PO q7d postdialysis; adjust w/ CrCl < 50 mL/min **Caution:** [C, –] **Disp:** Tabs 10 mg **SE:** Asthenia, HA, Abd pain; see Warning **Interactions:** See Warning **Labs:** LFTs, BUN, Cr, CK, amylase **NIPE:** Effects on fetus & baby not known; N breast-feed; use barrier contraception; ✓ HIV status before using

Adenosine (Adenocard) [Antiarrhythmic/Nucleoside]
Uses: *PSVT*; including w/ WPW **Action:** Class IV antiarrhythmic; slows AV node conduction **Dose:** *Adults. ECC 2010:* 6-mg rapid IV push, then 20-mL NS bolus. Elevate extremity; repeat 12 mg in 1–2 min PRN. *Peds. ECC 2010:* Symptomatic SVT: 0.1 mg/kg rapid IV/IO push (max dose 6 mg); can follow w/ 0.2 mg/kg rapid IV/IO push (max dose 12 mg); follow each dose w/ 10 mL NS flush **Caution:** [C, ?] h/o Bronchospasm **CI:** 2nd-/3rd-degree AV block or SSS (w/o pacemaker); arterial flutter, AF, V, tachycardia, recent MI or CNS bleed **Disp:** Inj 3 mg/mL **SE:** Facial flushing, HA, dyspnea, chest pressure, ↓ BP; **Interactions:** ↓ Effects W/, guarana; ↑ effects W/ dipyridamole, theophylline, caffeine; ↑ risk of hypotension & CP W/ nicotine; ↑ risk of bradycardia W/ BBs; ↑ risk of heart block W/ carbamazepine; ↑ risk of VF W/ digitalis glycosides **Labs:** Monitor ECG during administration **NIPE:** Monitor BP & pulse during therapy; monitor resp status ↑ risk of bronchospasm in asthmatics; discard unused or unclear soln; doses > 12 mg not OK; can cause momentary asystole when administered; caffeine, theophylline antagonize effects

Albumin (Albuminar, Buminate, Albutein) [Plasma Volume Expander]
Uses: *Plasma vol expansion for shock* (eg, burns, hemorrhage) **Action:** Maintain plasma colloid oncotic pressure **Dose:** *Adults.* Initial 25 g IV; then based on response; 250 g/48 h max *Peds.* 0.5–1 g/kg/dose; Inf at 0.05–0.1 g/min; max 6 g/kg/d **Caution:** [C, ?] Severe anemia; cardiac, renal, or hepatic Insuff d/t protein load & hypervolemia **CI:** CHF, severe anemia **Disp:** Soln 5%, 25% **SE:** Chills, fever, CHF, tachycardia, ↓ BP, hypervolemia **Interactions:** Atypical Rxns W/ ACEI withhold 24 h prior to plasma administration **Labs:** ↑ Alk phosp, monitor HMG, Hct, lytes, serum protein **NIPE:** Monitor BP & D/C if hypervolemia; monitor I&O; admin to all blood types; contains 130–160 mEq Na⁺/L; may cause pulm edema-monitor resp status & lung sounds

Albuterol (Proventil, Ventolin, Volmax) [Bronchodilator/Adrenergic]
Uses: *Asthma, COPD, prevent exercise-induced bronchospasm*

Action: β-Adrenergic sympathomimetic bronchodilator; relaxes bronchial smooth muscle **Dose:** *Adults. Inhaler:* 2 Inh q4–6h PRN; 1 Rotacaps inhaled q4–6h *PO:* 2–4 mg PO tid–qid *Nebulizer:* 1.25–5 mg (0.25–1 mL of 0.5% soln in 2–3 mL of NS) tid–qid *Prevent exercise-induced asthma:* 2 puffs 5–30 min prior to activity *Peds. Inhaler:* 2 Inh q4–6h. *PO:* 0.1–0.2 mg/kg/dose PO; max 2–4 mg PO tid *Nebulizer:* 0.05 mg/kg (max 2.5 mg) in 2–3 mL of NS tid–qid; 2–6 y 12 mg/d max, 6–12 y 24 mg/d max **Caution:** [C, +] **Disp:** Tabs: 2, 4 mg; XR tabs: 4, 8 mg; syrup: 2 mg/5 mL; 90 mcg/dose metered-dose inhaler; soln for nebulizer 0.083, 0.5% **SE:** Palpitations, tachycardia, nervousness, GI upset **Interactions:** ↑ Effects *W/* other sympathomimetics; ↑ CV effects *W/* MAOI, TCA, inhaled anesthetics; ↓ effects *W/* BBs; ↓ effectiveness *OF* insulin, oral hypoglycemics, digoxin **Labs:** Transient ↑ in serum glucose after Inh; transient ↓ K^+ after Inh **NIPE:** Monitor HR, BP, ABGs, S/Sxs bronchospasm & CNS stimulation; instruct on use of inhaler; must use as 1st inhaler & rinse mouth after use

Albuterol & Ipratropium (Combivent, DuoNeb) [Bronchodilator/ Adrenergic, Anticholinergic] **Uses:** *COPD* **Action:** Combo of β-adrenergic bronchodilator & quaternary anticholinergic **Dose:** 2 Inh qid; nebulizer 3 mL q6h; max 12/Inh/24 h or 3 mL q4h **Caution:** [C, +] **CI:** Peanut/soybean allergy **Disp:** Metered-dose inhaler, 18 mcg ipratropium & 103 mcg albuterol/puff; nebulization soln (DuoNeb) ipratropium 0.5 mg & albuterol 2.5 mg/3 mL 0.042%, 0.21% **SE:** Palpitations, tachycardia, nervousness, GI upset, dizziness, blurred vision **Interactions:** ↑ Effects *W/* anticholinergics, including ophthal meds; ↓ effects *W/* herb jaborandi tree, pill-bearing spurge **NIPE:** See Albuterol; may cause transient blurred vision/irritation or urinary changes

Alcaftadine (Lastacaft) [Antihistamine/mast cell stabilizer] **Uses:** *Allergic conjunctivitis* **Action:** Histamine H_1-receptor antag **Dose:** 1 gtt in eye(s) daily **Caution:** [B, ?] **Disp:** Ophth Sol 0.25% **SE:** Eye irritation **NIPE:** Remove contacts before use

Aldesleukin [IL-2] (Proleukin) [Immunomodulator/Antineo-Plastic] WARNING: High dose associated w/ capillary leak synd w/ hypotension and ↓ organ perfusion; ↑ Infxn d/t poor neutrophil activity; D/C w/ mod–severe lethargy, may progress to coma **Uses:** *Met RCC & melanoma* **Action:** Acts via IL-2 receptor; many immunomodulatory effects **Dose:** 600,000 IU/kg q8h × 14 doses d 1–5 and d 15–19 of 28-d cycle (FDA-approved dose/schedule for RCC); other schedules (eg, "high dose" $24 × 10^6$ IU/m² IV q8h on days 1–5 & 12–16) **Caution:** [C, ?/–] **CI:** Organ allografts **Disp:** Powder for recons $22 × 10^6$ IU, when reconstituted 18 mill IU/mL = 1.1 mg/mL **SE:** Flu-like Sxs (malaise, fever, chills), N/V/D, ↑ bilirubin; capillary leak synd; ↓ BP, tachycardia, pulm & peripheral edema, fluid retention, & wgt gain; renal & mild hematologic tox (↓ HgB, plt, WBC), eosinophilia; cardiac tox (ischemia, atrial arrhythmias); neurotox (CNS depression, somnolence, delirium, rare coma); pruritic rashes, urticaria, & erythroderma common **Interactions:** May ↑ tox *OF* cardiotox, hepatotox, myelotoxic, & nephrotoxic drugs; ↑ hypotension

W/ antihypertensive drugs; ↓ effects W/ corticosteroids; acute Rxn W/ iodinated contrast media up to several mo after Inf; CNS effects W/ psychotropics **Labs:** May cause ↑ alk phos, bilirubin, BUN, SCr, LFTs **NIPE:** Thoroughly explain serious SE of drug (hypotension, pulm edema, arrhythmias, and neurotox) & that some SE are expected; N EtOH, NSAIDs, ASA

Alefacept (Amevive) [Antipsoriatic/Immunosuppressive] WARNING: Monitor CD4 before each dose; w/hold if < 250; D/C if < 250 × 1 mo **Uses:** *Mod/severe chronic plaque psoriasis* **Action:** Fusion protein Inhib **Dose:** 7.5 mg IV or 15 mg IM once/wk × 12 wk **Caution:** [B, ?/–] PRG registry; associated w/ serious Infxn **CI:** Lymphopenia, HIV **Disp:** 15-mg powder for recons **SE:** Pharyngitis, myalgia, Inj site Rxn, malignancy **Interactions:** No studies performed **Labs:** Monitor WBCs, CD4 + T lymphocyte counts **NIPE:** ↑ Risk of Infxn; N exposure to Infxns; Inj site inflammation; rotate sites; IV and IM different formulations; may repeat course 12 wk later if CD4 OK

Alemtuzumab (Campath) [Monoclonal Antibody, CD52 (Recombinant, Humanized)] WARNING: Serious, including fatal, cytopenias, Inf Rxns, and Infxns can occur; limit dose to 30 mg (single) & 90 mg (weekly), higher doses ↑ risk of pancytopenia; ↑ dose gradually & monitor during Inf, D/C for Grade 3 or 4 Inf Rxns; give prophylaxis for PCP & herpes virus Infxn **Uses:** *B-cell CLL* **Action:** CD52-directed cytolitic Ab **Dose:** *Adults.* ↑ dose to 30 mg/d IV 3 ×/wk for 12 wks (see label for escalation strategy); infuse over 2 h; premedicate w/ oral antihistamine & APAP **Caution:** [C, –] Do not give live vaccines; D/C for autoimmune/severe hematologic Rxns **Disp:** Inj **SE:** Cytopenias, Infxns, Inf Rxns, N/V/D, insomnia, anxiety **Interactions:** Avoid live virus vaccines > recent therapy **Labs:** ✓ CBC & plt weekly & CD4 counts after Rx until ≥ 200 cells/mL

Alendronate (Fosamax, Fosamax Plus D) [Antiosteoporotic] **Uses:** *Rx & prevent osteoporosis male & postmenopausal female, Rx steroid-induced osteoporosis, Paget Dz* **Action:** ↓ nl & abnormal bone resorption, ↓ osteoclast action **Dose:** *Osteoporosis:* Rx: 10 mg/d PO or 70 mg qwk; Fosamax plus D 1 tab qwk *Steroid-induced osteoporosis:* Rx: 5 mg/d PO, 10 mg/d postmenopausal not on estrogen *Prevention:* 5 mg/d PO or 35 mg qwk *Paget Dz:* 40 mg/d PO **Caution:** [C, ?] Not OK if CrCl < 35 mL/min, w/ NSAID use **CI:** Esophageal anomalies, inability to sit/stand upright for 30 min, ↓ Ca²⁺ **Disp:** Tabs 5, 10, 35, 40, 70 mg, soln 70 mg/75 mL *Fosamax Plus D:* Alendronate 70 mg w/ cholecalciferol (vit D₃) 2800 or 5600 IU **SE:** Abd pain, acid regurgitation, constipation, D/N, dyspepsia, musculoskeletal pain, jaw osteonecrosis (w/ dental procedures, chemo) **Notes:** Take 1st thing in AM w/ H₂O (8 oz) > 30 min before 1st food/beverage of the day; do not lie down for 30 min after **Interactions:** ↓ Absorption W/ antacids, Ca supls, Fe, food; ↑ risk of upper GI bleed W/ ASA & NSAIDs **Labs:** May cause transient ↑ serum Ca & phosphate **NIPE:** May cause cardiac conduction changes d/t ↑ Ca²⁺—use Ca²⁺ & vit D supl w/ regular tab; ↑ wgt-bearing activity; ↓ smoking & EtOH use; ↑ risk of jaw fx—esp w/ dental procedures; may ↑ atypical subtrochanteric femur fxs

Alfentanil (Alfenta) [C-II] [Narcotic Analgesic] Uses: *Adjunct in maint of anesthesia; analgesia* **Action:** Short-acting narcotic analgesic **Dose: Adults & Peds > 12 y.** 3–75 mcg/kg (IBW) IV Inf; total depends on duration of procedure **Caution:** [C, +/–] ↑ ICP, resp depression **Disp:** Inj 500 mcg/mL **SE:** Bradycardia, ↓ BP arrhythmias, peripheral vasodilation, ↑ ICP, drowsiness, resp depression, N/V/constipation **Interactions:** ↓ Effect W/ phenothiazines; ↑ effects W/ BBs, CNS depressants, erythromycin **NIPE:** Monitor HR, BP, resp rate

Alfuzosin (Uroxatral) [Selective Alpha-Adrenergic Antagonist] **WARNING:** May prolong QTc interval **Uses:** *Symptomatic BPH* **Action:** α-Blocker **Dose:** 10 mg PO daily stat after the same meal **Caution:** [B, –] **CI:** w/ CYP3A4 Inhibs; mod–severe hepatic impair **Disp:** Tabs 10 mg ER **SE:** Postural ↓ BP, dizziness, HA, fatigue; **Interactions:** ↑ Effects W/ atenolol, azole antifungals, cimetidine, ritonavir; ↑ effects OF antihypertensives **NIPE:** Not indicated for use in women or children; take w/ food; ↑ risk of postural hypotension; ⊘ take other meds that prolong QT interval. Do not cut or crush; ⊘ ejaculatory disorders compared w/ similar drugs

Alginic Acid + Aluminum Hydroxide & Magnesium Trisilicate (Gaviscon) [OTC] [Antacid] Uses: *Heartburn*; hiatal hernia pain **Action:** Protective layer blocks gastric acid **Dose:** Chew 2–4 tabs or 15–30 mL PO qid followed by H₂O **Caution:** [B, –] Avoid w/ renal impair or Na⁺-restricted diet **Disp:** Chew tabs, susp **SE:** D, constipation; **Interactions:** ↓ Absorption OF tetracyclines

Alginic Acid + Aluminum Hydroxide & Magnesium Trisilicate (Soriatane) [Retinoid] **WARNING:** Must not be used by females who are pregnant or who intend to become pregnant during or for 3 y following D/C of therapy; EtOH must not be ingested during or for 2 mo following cessation; do not donate blood for 3 y following cessation; hepatotoxic **Uses:** *Severe psoriasis*; other keratinization disorders (lichen planus, etc) **Action:** Retinoid-like activity **Dose:** 25–50 mg/d PO, w/ main meal; ↑ if no response by 4 wk to 75 mg/d **Caution:** [X, –] Renal/hepatic impair; in women of reproductive potential **CI:** See Warning; ↑ serum lipids; w/ MTX or tetracyclines **Disp:** Caps 10, 25 mg **SE:** Hyperesthesia, cheilitis, skin peeling, alopecia, pruritus, rash, arthralgia, GI upset, photosensitivity, thrombocytosis, ↑ triglycerides, ↑ Na, K, PO₄⁻ **Interactions:** ↑ 1/2-life W/ EtOH use, ↑ hepatotox W/ MTX, ↓ effects OF progestin-only contraceptives **Labs:** Monitor LFTs, lipids, lytes, FBS, HbA1c; response takes up to 2–3 mo **NIPE:** Use effective contraception; N donate blood for 3 y after Rx; teach pt S/Sxs pancreatitis; pt agreement/ informed consent prior to use; FDA guide w/ each Rx

Alglucosidase Alfa (Myozyme) [Recombinant Acid Alpha-Glucosidase] **WARNING:** Life-threatening anaphylactic Rxns seen w/ Inf; medical support measures should be stat available **Uses:** *Rx Pompe DZ* **Action:** Recombinant acid α-glucosidase; degrades glycogen in lysosomes **Dose: Peds 1 mo–3.5 y.** 20 mg/kg IV q2wk over 4 h (see package insert) **Caution:**

[B, ?/−] Illness at time of Inf may ↑ Inf Rxns **CI:** None **Disp:** Powder 50 mg/vial **SE:** Hypersensitivity, fever, rash, D, V, gastroenteritis, pneumonia, URI, cough, resp distress/failure, Infxns, cardiac arrhythmia w/ general anesthesia, tachy/brady-cardia, flushing, anemia **NIPE:** Anaphylactic Rxns commonly reported

Aliskiren (Tekturna) [Direct Renin Inhibitor] **WARNING:** May cause injury and death to a developing fetus; D/C stat when PRG detected **Uses:** *HTN* **Action:** First direct renin Inhib **Dose:** 150–300 mg/d PO **Caution:** [C (1st tri), D (2nd & 3rd tri), ?]; avoid w/ CrCl < 30 mL/min **CI:** Anuria, sulfur sensitivity **Disp:** Tabs 150, 300 mg **SE:** D, Abd pain, dyspepsia, GERD, cough, angioedema, ↓ BP, dizziness **Interactions:** ↑ Effects & levels W/ atorvastatin, ketoconazole, & other CYP3A4 Inhibs; ↓ effects W/ irbesartan; ↑ effects OF furosemide plasma levels; caution w/ max doses of ACE Inhibs **Labs:** ↑ K⁺, uric acid **NIPE:** D/C once pregnant—may cause fetal death; not recommended for < 18 y or during breast-feeding

Aliskiren & Amlodipine (Tekamlo) [Renin Inhibitor + Dihydropyridine (DHP) Calcium Channel Blocker (CCB)] **WARNING:** May cause fetal injury & death; D/C stat when PRG detected **Uses:** *HTN* **Action:** Renin Inhib w/ dihydropyridine CCB **Dose:** *Adult.* 150/5 mg PO 1 × daily; max 300/10 mg/d); max effect in 2 wk **Caution:** [D, −] Do not use w/ cyclosporine/itraconazole **Disp:** Tabs (aliskiren mg/amlodipine mg) 150/5, 150/10, 300/5, 300/10 **SE:** ↓ BP, angioedema, peripheral edema, D, dizziness, angina, MI **Interactions:** ↑ effects W/ atorvastatin, ketoconazole; ↓ effects W/ irbesartan; ↓ effects OF furosemide; Caution W/ ACEI, K⁺ supls, K⁺-sparing diuretics, K⁺-containing salt substitutes **Labs:** ↑ K⁺, monitor lytes **NIPE:** Give consistently w/ regard to meals; absorption reduced w/ high-fat meal

Aliskiren, Amlodipine, Hydrochlorothiazide (Amturnide) [Renin Inhibitor + Dihydropyridine Calcium Channel Blocker (CCB) + Thiazide Diuretic] **WARNING:** May cause fetal injury & death; D/C stat when PRG detected **Uses:** *HTN* **Action:** Renin Inhib, dihydropyridine CCB, & thiazide diuretic **Dose:** *Adult.* Titrate q2wk PRN to 300/10/25 mg PO max/d **Caution:** [D, −] Avoid w/ CrCl ≤ 30 mL/min; do not use w/ cyclosporine/itraconazole; ↓ BP in salt/vol depleted pts; HCTZ may exacerbate/activate SLE; D/C if myopia or NAG **CI:** Anuria, sulfonamide allergy **Disp:** Tabs (aliskiren mg/amlodipine mg/ HCTZ mg) 150/5/12.5, 300/5/12.5, 300/5/25, 300/10/12.5, 300/10/25 **SE:** ↓ BP, hyperuricemia, angioedema, peripheral edema, D, HA, dizziness, angina, MI, nasopharyngitis **Interactions:** ↑ effects W/ atorvastatin, ketoconazole, EtOH; ↓ effects W/ NSAIDs, irbesartan; ↓ effects OF furosemide; Caution W/ ACEI, K⁺ supls, K⁺-sparing diuretics, K⁺-containing salt substitutes **Labs:** ↑ K⁺, monitor lytes **NIPE:** Titrate at 2 wk intervals; may need to adjust hypoglycemic agents

Aliskiren/Hydrochlorothiazide (Tekturna Hct) [Direct Renin Inhibitor with Thiazide Diuretic] **WARNING:** May cause injury and death to a developing fetus; D/C stat when PRG detected **Uses:** *HTN, not primary Rx* **Action:** Renin Inhib w/ diuretic **Dose:** *Monotherapy failure:* 150 mg/ 12.5 mg PO qd; may ↑ to 150 mg/25 mg, 300 mg/12.5 mg qd after 24 wk *Max:* 300 mg/25 mg **Caution:** [D, ?]; Avoid w/ CrCl ΙЗ0 mL/min **Disp:**Tab:Aliskirenmg/HCTZ mg:· 150/12.5, 150/25, 300/12.5, 300/25 **SE:** Dizziness, influenza, D, cough, vertigo, asthenia, arthralgia, angioedema **Interactions:** ↑ effects *OF* antihypertensives and possibly nondepolarizing muscle relaxants; ↑ effects *W/* ketoconazole, atorvastatin, & other CYP3A4 Inhibs as it may ↑ aliskirin levels; ↓ effects *W/* irbesartan, NSAIDs; ↓ effects *OF* furosemide; ACTH & corticosteroids ↑ the risk of hypokalemia; adjust antidiabetic drugs. Orthostatic hypotension potentiated by alcohol, CNS depressants. ↑ Risk of Li tox (avoid) **Labs:** ↑ ALT, BUN/creatinine, uric acid **NIPE:** ↓ Drug absorption w/ high-fat meal; not recommended for < 18 y or during breast-feeding; not for initial therapy

Aliskiren & Valsartan (Valturna) [Direct Renin Inhibitor + Angiotensin II Receptor Blocker]   WARNING: May cause fetal injury & death; D/C stat w/ PRG **Uses:** *HTN* **Action:** Renin Inhib w/ ARB **Dose:** *Adult.* 150/160 mg PO once daily; max 300/320 mg/d; max effect in 2 wk **Caution:** [D, –] do not use w/ cyclosporine or itraconazole; ↓ BP in salt/vol depleted pts **Disp:** Tabs (aliskiren mg/valsartan mg) 150/160, 300/320 **SE:** ↓ BP, angioedema, D, HA, dizziness, nasopharyngitis, fatigue **Interactions:** ↑ effects *W/* atorvastatin, ketoconazole, EtOH; ↓ effects *W/* irbesartan; ↓ effects *OF* furosemide; Caution *W/* ACEI, K⁺ supls, K⁺-sparing diuretics, K⁺-containing salt substitutes **Labs:** ↑ K⁺, ↑ SCr; **NIPE:** Take consistently w/ regard to meals; absorption reduced w/ high-fat meal

Allopurinol (Zyloprim, Lopurin, Aloprim) [Xanthine Oxidase Inhibitor]   **Uses:** *Gout, hyperuricemia of malignancy, uric acid urolithiasis* **Action:** Xanthine oxidase Inhib; ↓ uric acid production **Dose:** *Adults.* PO: Initial 100 mg/d; usual 300 mg/d; max 800 mg/d; ÷ dose if > 300 mg/d IV: 200–400 mg/m²/d (max 600 mg/24 h); (after meal w/ plenty of fluid) *Peds. Only for hyperuricemia of malignancy if < 10 y:* 10 mg/kg/24 h PO or 200 mg/m²/d IV ÷ q6–8h; max 600 mg/ 24 h; ↓ in renal impair **Caution:** [C, M] **Disp:** Tabs 100, 300 mg; Inj 500 mg/30 mL (Aloprim) **SE:** Rash, N/V, renal impair, angioedema **Notes:** Aggravates acute gout; begin after acute attack resolves; IV dose of 6 mg/mL final conc as single daily Inf or ÷ 6-, 8-, or 12-h intervals **Interactions:** ↑ Effect *OF* theophylline, oral anticoagulants; ↑ hypersensitivity Rxns *W/* ACEIs, thiazide diuretics; ↑ risk of rash *W/* ampicillin/ amoxicillin; ↑ BM depression *W/* cyclophosphamide, azathioprine, mercaptopurine; ↓ effects *W/* EtOH **Labs:** ↑ Alk phos, bilirubin, LFTs **NIPE:** ↑ Fluids to 2–3 L/d; take pc; may ↑ drowsiness; ↑ risk of acute gout attack in 1st 6 wk of Tx

Almotriptan (Axert) [Serotonin 5-HT₁ Receptor Agonist]   **Uses:** *Rx acute migraine* **Action:** Vascular serotonin receptor agonist **Dose:** *Adults.* PO: 6.25–12 mg PO, repeat in 2 h PRN; 2 dose/24 h max PO dose; max 12 or 24 mg/d; w/ hepatic/renal impair 6.25 mg single dose (max 12.5 mg/d) **Caution:**

[C, ?/–] **CI:** Angina, ischemic heart Dz, coronary artery vasospasm, hemiplegic, or basilar migraine, uncontrolled HTN, ergot use, MAOI use w/in 14 d **Disp:** Tabs 6.25, 12.5 mg **SE:** somnolence, paresthesias, HA, dry mouth, weakness, numbness, coronary vasospasm, HTN **Interactions:** ↑ Serotonin effects *OF* SSRIs, ↑ vasoactive action *OF* ergot derivatives & 5-HT agonists, ↑ effects *W/* erythromycin, ketoconazole, itraconazole, MAOIs, ritonavir, verapamil **NIPE:** N Ergot compounds or 5-HT agonist w/in 24 h of almotriptan; N use if pregnant or breast-feeding; concurrent use w/ SSRIs may cause serotonin synd (shivering, sweating, tremors/twitching, agitation, ↑ HA); use only during migraine HA attack; avoid driving if drug causes drowsiness

Alosetron (Lotronex) [Selective 5-HT₃ Receptor Antagonist]
WARNING: Serious GI SEs, some fatal, including ischemic colitis reported. Prescribed only through participation in the prescribing program **Uses:** *Severe D—predominant IBS in women who fail conventional therapy* **Action:** Selective 5-HT₃ receptor antagonist **Dose:** *Adults.* 0.5 mg PO bid; ↑ to 1 mg bid max after 4 wk; D/C after 8 wk not controlled **Caution:** [B, ?/–] **CI:** h/o chronic/severe constipation, GI obst, strictures, toxic megacolon, GI perforation, adhesions, ischemic colitis/UC, Crohn Dz, diverticulitis, thrombophlebitis, hypercoagulability **Disp:** Tabs 0.5, 1 mg **SE:** Constipation, Abd pain, N **Notes:** D/C stat if constipation or Sxs of ischemic colitis develop; pt must sign informed consent prior to use **Interactions:** ↑ Risk constipation *W/* other drugs that ↓ GI motility, inhibits *N*-acetyltransferase, & may influence metabolism of INH, procainamide, hydralazine **Labs:** Monitor for ↑ ALT, AST, alk phos, bilirubin **NIPE:** Administer w/o regard to food, eval effectiveness > 4 wk

Alpha-1-Protease Inhibitor (Prolastin) [Respiratory Agent/Alpha Protease Inhibitor Replacement] **Uses:** *α₁-Antitrypsin deficiency*; panacinar emphysema **Action:** Replace human α₁-protease Inhib **Dose:** 60 mg/kg IV once/wk **Caution:** [C, ?] **CI:** Selective IgA deficiencies w/ known IgA antibodies **Disp:** Inj 500 mg/20 mL, 1000 mg/40 mL powder for Inj **SE:** HA, MS discomfort, fever, dizziness, flu-like Sxs, allergic Rxns **Labs:** Monitor for ↑ ALT, AST **NIPE:** Inf over 30 min, N mix w/ other drugs, use w/in 3 h of reconstitution

Alprazolam (Xanax, Niravam) [C-IV] [Anxiolytic/Benzodiazepine] **Uses:** *Anxiety & panic disorders*; anxiety w/ depression **Action:** Benzodiazepine; antianxiety agent **Dose:** *Anxiety:* Initial, 0.25–0.5 mg tid; ↑ to 4 mg/d max ÷ doses *Panic:* Initial, 0.5 mg tid; may gradually ↑ to response; ↓ in elderly, debilitated, & hepatic impair **Caution:** [D, –] **CI:** NAG, concomitant itra/ketoconazole **Disp:** Tabs 0.25, 0.5, 1, 2 mg *Xanax XR:* 0.5, 1, 2, 3 mg *Niravam* (ODT): 0.25, 0.5, 1, 2 mg; soln 1 mg/mL **SE:** Drowsiness, fatigue, irritability, memory impair, sexual dysfunction, paradoxical Rxns **Interactions:** ↑ CNS depression *W/* EtOH, other CNS depressants, narcotics, MAOIs, anesthetics, antihistamines, theophylline; herbs: kava kava, valerian; ↑ effect *W/* OCPs, cimetidine, INH, disulfiram, omeprazole, valproic acid, ciprofloxacin, erythromycin, clarithromycin, phenytoin, verapamil, grapefruit juice; ↑ risk *OF* ketoconazole, itraconazole, digitalis tox, ↓ effectiveness *OF* levodopa; ↓ effect *W/* carbamazepine, rifampin, rifabutin, barbiturates, cigarette smoking **Labs:** ↑ Alk phos, may cause ↓ Hct & neutropenia **NIPE:** Monitor for resp depression; avoid abrupt D/C after prolonged use

Alprostadil [Prostaglandin E₁] (Prostin VR) [Vasodilator/Prostaglandin] **WARNING:** Apnea in up to 12% of neonates esp < 2 kg at birth **Uses:** *Conditions ductus arteriosus blood flow must be maint* sustain pulm/systemic circulation until OR (eg, pulm atresia/stenosis, transposition) **Action:** Vasodilator (ductus arteriosus very sensitive), plt Inhib **Dose:** 0.05 mcg/kg/min IV; ↓ to lowest that maint response **Caution:** [X, –] **CI:** Neonatal resp distress synd **Disp:** Inj 500 mcg/mL **SE:** Cutaneous vasodilation, Sz-like activity, jitteriness, ↑ temp, thrombocytopenia, ↓ BP; may cause apnea **Interactions:** ↑ Effects *OF* anticoagulants & antihypertensives, ↓ effects *OF* cyclosporine **Labs:** ↓ Ca²⁺, fibrinogen **NIPE:** Dilute drug before administration, refrigerate & discard > 24 h, central line preferred, flushing indicates catheter malposition, apnea & bradycardia indicates drug OD, keep intubation kit at bedside; administered to hospitalized newborns

Alprostadil, Intracavernosal (Caverject, Edex) [GU Agent/Prostaglandin] **Uses:** *ED* **Action:** Relaxes smooth muscles, dilates cavernosal arteries, ↑ lacunar spaces w/ blood entrapment **Dose:** 2.5–60 mcg intracavernosal; titrate in office **Caution:** [X, –] **CI:** ↑ Risk of priapism (eg, sickle cell); penile deformities/implants; men in whom sexual activity inadvisable **Disp:** *Caverject:* 5, 10, 20, 40 mcg powder for Inj vials ± diluent syringes 10, 20, 40 mcg amp *Caverject Impul* **SE:** Self-contained syringe (29 gauge) 10, 20 mcg *Edex:* 10, 20, 40 mcg cartridges **SE:** Local pain w/ Inj **Interactions:** ↑ Effects *OF* anticoagulants & antihypertensives, ↓ effects *OF* cyclosporine **Labs:** ↓ Fibrinogen **NIPE:** Vag itching and burning in female partners, ⊘ Inj > 3 ×/wk or closer than 24 h/dose; counsel about priapism, penile fibrosis, hematoma risks, titrate dose in office

Alprostadil, Urethral Suppository (Muse) [GU Agent/Prostaglandin] **Uses:** *ED* **Action:** Urethral absorption; vasodilator, relaxes smooth muscle of corpus cavernosa **Dose:** 125–1000 mcg system 5–10 min prior to sex; repeat × 1/24 h; titrate in office **Caution:** [X, –] **CI:** ↑ Priapism risk (esp sickle cell, myeloma, leukemia) penile deformities/implants; men in whom sex is inadvisable **Disp:** 125, 250, 500, 1000 mcg w/ transurethral system **SE:** ↓ BP, dizziness, syncope, penile/testicular pain, urethral burning/bleeding, priapism **Interactions:** ↑ Effects *OF* anticoagulants & antihypertensives, ↓ effects *OF* cyclosporine **Labs:** ↓ Fibrinogen **NIPE:** No more than 2 supp/24 h, counsel about priapism, urinate prior to use; titrate dose in office, dizziness 30–60 min

Alteplase, Recombinant [tPA] (Activase) [Plasminogen Activator/Thrombolytic Enzyme] **Uses:** *AMI, PE, acute ischemic stroke, & CV cath occlusion* **Action:** Thrombolytic; binds fibrin in thrombus, initiates fibrinolysis **Dose:** *ECC 2101:* STEMI 15-mg bolus; then 0.75 mg/kg over 30 min (50 mg max); then 0.50 mg/kg over next 60 min (35 mg max; max total dose 100 mg) *Acute* *ischemic stroke:* 0.9 mg/kg IV (max 90 mg) over 60 min give 10% of total dose over 1 min; remaining 90% over 1 h (or 3-h Inf). *Cath occlusion:* 10–29 kg 1 mg/mL: = 30 kg 2 mg/mL **Caution:** [C, ?] **CI:** Active internal bleeding; uncontrolled HTN (SBP = > 185 mm Hg/DBP = > 110 mm Hg); recent (w/in 3 mo) CVA, GI bleed, trauma; intracranial or intraspinal surgery or Dzs (AVM/aneurysm/subarachnoid hemorrhage/neoplasm), prolonged cardiac massage; intracranial neoplasm, suspected aortic dissection, w/ anticoagulants or INR > 1.7, heparin w/in 48 h, plts < 100,000, Sz at the time of stroke **Disp:** Powder for Inj 2, 50, 100 mg **SE:** Bleeding, bruising (eg, venipuncture sites), ↓ BP **Interactions:** ↑ Risk of bleeding **W/** heparin, ASA, NSAIDs, abciximab, dipyridamole, eptifibatide, tirofiban; ↓ effects **W/** nitroglycerine **Labs:** ↓ Fibrinogen, monitor PT/PTT **NIPE:** Compress venipuncture site at least 30 min, bed rest during Inf; give heparin to prevent reocclusion; in AMI, doses of > 150 mg associated w/ intracranial bleeding

Altretamine   (Hexalen)   [Antineoplastic/Alkylating   Agent]
WARNING:↓ BM, neurotox common **Uses:** *Epithelial ovarian CA* **Action:** Unknown; cytotoxic/alkylating agent, ↓ nucleotide incorporation into DNA/RNA **Dose:** 260 mg/m²/d in 4 ÷ doses for 14–21 d of a 28-d Rx cycle; dose ↑ to 150 mg/m²/d for 14 d in multiagent regimens (per protocols); after meals & hs **Caution:** [D, ?/–] **CI:** Preexisting BM depression or neurotox **Disp:** Gel caps 50 mg **SE:** N/V/D, cramps; neurotox (neuropathy, CNS depression); minimal myelosuppression **Interactions:** ↓ Effect **W/** phenobarbital, ↓ Ab response **W/** live virus vaccines, ↑ risk of tox **W/** cimetidine & hypotension **W/** MAOIs, ↑ BM depression **W/** radiation **Labs:** Monitor CBC, ↑ alk phos, BUN, SCr **NIPE:** Use barrier contraception, take w/ food, routine neuro exams—neurotox common

Aluminum Hydroxide (Amphojel, ALternaGEL, Dermagran) [OTC]
Uses: *Relief of heartburn, upset or sour stomach, or acid indigestion*; supl to Rx of hyperphosphatemia; *minor cuts, burns (Dermagran)* **Action:** Neutralizes gastric acid; binds PO₄²⁻ **Dose: Adults.** 10–30 mL or 300–1200 mg PO q4–6h **Peds.** 5–15 mL PO q4–6h or 50–150 mg/kg/24 h PO ÷ q4–6h (hyperphosphatemia) **Caution:** [C, ?] **Disp:** Tabs 300, 600 mg; susp 320, 600 mg/5 mL; oint 0.275% (*Dermagran*) **SE:** Constipation **Interactions:** ↓ Absorption & effects *OF* allopurinol, benzodiazepines, corticosteroids, chloroquine, cimetidine, digoxin, INH, phenytoin, quinolones, ranitidine, tetracycline **Labs:** ↑ Serum gastrin, ↓ serum phosphate **NIPE:** Separate other drug administration by 2 h, ↓ effectiveness of Liq form; OK in renal failure

Aluminum Hydroxide + Magnesium Carbonate (Gaviscon Extra Strength, Liquid) [Antacid/Aluminum & Magnesium Salts] [OTC]
Uses: *Relief of heartburn, acid indigestion* **Action:** Neutralizes gastric acid **Dose: Adults.** 15–30 mL PO pc & hs; 2–4 chew tabs up to qid **Peds.** 5–15 mL PO qid or PRN; avoid in renal impair **Caution:** [C, ?] ↑ Mg²⁺, avoid w/ renal impair **Disp:** Liq w/ AlOH 95 mg/Mg carbonate 358 mg/15 mL; extra strength Liq AlOH 254 mg/Mg carbonate 237 mg/15 mL; chew tabs AlOH 160 mg/Mg carbonate 105 mg

SE: Constipation, D **Interactions:** In addition to AlOH ↓ effects *OF* histamine blockers, hydantoins, nitrofurantoin, phenothiazine, ticlopidine, ↑ effects *OF* quinidine, sulfonylureas **NIPE:** ↓ Fiber; qid doses best given pc & hs; may ↓ absorption of some drugs, take 2–3 h apart to ↓ effect

Aluminum Hydroxide + Magnesium Hydroxide (Maalox) [Antacid/ Aluminum & Magnesium Salts] [OTC] Uses: *Hyperacidity* (peptic ulcer, hiatal hernia, etc) **Action:** Neutralizes gastric acid **Dose:** *Adults.* 10–20 mL or 2–4 tabs PO qid or PRN *Peds.* 5–15 mL PO qid or PRN **Caution:** [C, ?] **Disp:** Chew tabs, susp **SE:** May ↑ Mg^{2+} w/ renal Insuff, constipation, D **Interactions:** In addition to AlOH, ↓ effects *OF* digoxin, quinolones, phenytoin, Fe supl, & keto-conazole **NIPE:** ⊘ Concurrent drug use—separate by 2 h; doses qid best given pc & hs

Aluminum Hydroxide + Magnesium Hydroxide & Simethicone (Mylanta, Mylanta II, Maalox Plus) [Antacid/Aluminum & Magnesium Salts] [OTC] Uses: *Hyperacidity w/ bloating* **Action:** Neutralizes gastric acid & defoaming **Dose:** *Adults.* 10–20 mL or 2–4 tabs PO qid or PRN *Peds.* 5–15 mL PO qid or PRN; avoid in renal impair **Caution:** [C, ?] **Disp:** Tabs, susp, Liq **SE:** ↑ Mg^{2+} in renal Insuff, D, constipation **Interactions:** In addition to AlOH, ↓ effects *OF* digoxin, quinolones, phenytoin, Fe supl, & ketoconazole **NIPE:** ⊘ Concurrent drug use—separate by 2 h; may affect absorption of some drugs; Mylanta II contains 2× Al & Mg of Mylanta

Aluminum Hydroxide + Magnesium Trisilicate (Gaviscon, Regular Strength) [Antacid/Aluminum & Magnesium Salts] [OTC] Uses: *Relief of heartburn, upset or sour stomach, or acid indigestion* **Action:** Neutralizes gastric acid **Dose:** Chew 2–4 tabs qid; avoid in renal impair **Caution:** [C, ?] **CI:** Mg^{2+}, sensitivity **Disp:** AlOH 80 mg/Mg trisilicate 20 mg/tab **SE:** ↑ Mg^{2+} in renal Insuff, constipation, D **Interactions:** In addition to Al, ↓ effects *OF* digoxin, quinolones, phenytoin, Fe supl, & ketoconazole **NIPE:** ⊘ Concurrent drug use—separate by 2 h; may affect absorption of some drugs

Alvimopan (Entereg) [Opioid Antagonist] **WARNING:** For short-term hospital use only (max 15 doses) Uses: *↓↓ Time to GI recovery w/ bowel resection and primary anastomosis* **Action:** Opioid (mu) receptor antagonist; selectively binds GI receptors, antagonizes effects of opioids on GI motility/secretion **Dose:** 12 mg 30 min–5 h pre op PO, then 12 mg bid up to 7 d; max 15 doses **Caution:** [B, ±] Not recommended in complete bowel obst surgery, hepatic/renal impair **Contra:** Therapeutic opioids > 7 consecutive days prior **Disp:** Caps 12 mg **SE:** dyspepsia, constipation, flatulence, urinary retention, anemia, back pain **Labs:** ↓ K^+, monitor LFTs & BUN/Cr for hepatic/renal impair; ⊘ **NIPE:** Hospitals must be registered in Entereg Access & Support Program to use; D/C if adverse Rxns

Amantadine (Symmetrel) [Antiviral, Antiparkinsonian/AntiCholinergic-Like Medium] Uses: *Rx/prophylaxis influenza A, Parkinsonism, & drug-induced EPS* (Note: Not for influenza, not for use in US d/t resistance including H1N1) **Action:** Prevents infectious viral nucleic acid release into host cell; releases DA & blocks reuptake of DA in presynaptic nerves **Dose:** *Adults. Influenza A:* 200 mg/d PO or 100 mg PO bid w/in 48 h of Sx *Parkinsonism:* 100 mg PO daily–bid *Peds 1–9 y.* 4.4–8.8 mg/kg/24 h to 150 mg/24 h max ÷ doses daily–bid *10–12 y:* 100–200 mg/d in 1–2 ÷ doses; ↓ in renal impair **Caution:** [C, M] **Disp:** Caps 100 mg; tabs 100 mg; soln 50 mg/5 mL **SE:** Orthostatic ↓ BP, edema, insomnia, depression, irritability, hallucinations, dream abnormalities, N/D, dry mouth **Interactions:** ↑ Effects *W/* HCTZ, triamterene, amiloride, pheasant's eye herb, Scopolia root, benztropine **Labs:** ↑ BUN, SCr, CPK, alk phos, bilirubin, LDH, AST, ALT **NIPE:** ⊘ D/C abruptly, take at least 4 h before sleep if insomnia occurs, eval for mental status changes, take w/ meals, ⊘ EtOH

Ambrisentan (Letairis) [Endothelin Receptor Antagonist] **WARNING:** May cause ↑ AST/ALT to > 3× ULN, LFTs monthly. CI in PRG; ✓ monthly PRG tests **Uses:** *Pulm arterial HTN* **Action:** Endothelin receptor antagonist **Dose:** *Adults.* 5 mg PO/d, max 10 mg/d; not recommended w/ hepatic impair **Caution:** [X, –] **CI:** PRG **Disp:** Tabs 5, 10 mg **SE:** Edema, nasal congestion, sinusitis, dyspnea, flushing, constipation, HA, palpitations, hepatotoxic **Interactions:** Caution *W/* cyclosporine, strong CYP3A or 2C19 Inhib, inducers of P-glycoprotein, CYPs, & UGTs **Labs:** D/C AST/ALT > 5 × ULN or bilirubin > 2× ULN or S/Sx of liver dysfunction **NIPE:** Available only through the Letairis Education and Access Program (LEAP); childbearing females must use 2 methods of contraception

Amifostine (Ethyol) [Antineoplastic/Thiophosphate Cytoprotective] **Uses:** *Xerostomia prophylaxis during RT (head, neck, etc) where parotid is in radiation field; ↓ renal tox w/ repeated cisplatin* **Action:** Prodrug, dephosphorylated by alk phos to active thiol metabolite; binds cisplatin metabolites **Dose:** 910 mg/m²/d 15-min IV Inf 30 min prechemotherapy **Caution:** [C, +/–] CV Dz **Disp:** 500-mg vials powder, reconstitute in NS **SE:** Transient ↓ BP (> 60%), N/V, flushing w/ hot or cold chills, dizziness, somnolence, sneezing **Interactions:** ↑ Effects *W/* antihypertensives **Labs:** ↓ Ca levels **NIPE:** Monitor BP for hypotension; ensure adequate hydration; infuse over 15 min w/ pt supine; does not ↓ effectiveness of cyclophosphamide + cisplatin chemotherapy

Amikacin (Amikin) [Antibiotic/Aminoglycoside] **Uses:** *Serious gram(–) bacterial Infxns* & mycobacteria **Action:** Aminoglycoside; ↓ protein synth **Spectrum:** Good gram(–) bacterial coverage: *Pseudomonas* & *Mycobacterium* sp **Dose:** *Adults & Peds. Conventional:* 5–7.5 mg/kg/dose q8h; *once daily:* 15–20 mg/kg q24h; ↑ interval w/ renal impair *Neonates < 1200 g.0–4 wk:* 7.5 mg/kg/dose q18h–24h *Age < 7 d,1200–2000 g:* 7.5 mg/kg/dose q12h > *2000 g:* 10 mg/kg/dose q12h *Age > 7d, 1200–2000g:* 7 mg/kg/dose q8h > *2000g:* 7.5–10 mg/kg/dose q8h **Caution:** [C, +/–] Avoid w/ diuretics **Disp:** 50 & 250 mg/mL Inj **SE:** Nephro-/oto-/neurotox, neuromuscular blockage, renal damage, resp paralysis **Notes:** May be effective in gram(–) resistance to gentamicin & tobramycin; follow Cr; *Levels: Peak* 30 min after Inf *Trough* < 0.5 h before next dose *Therapeutic: Peak* 20–30 mcg/mL *Trough*

< 8 mcg/mL *Toxic:* Peak > 35 mcg/mL *1/2-life:* 2 h **Interactions:** ↑ Risk of ototox and nephrotox **W/** acyclovir, amphotericin B, cephalosporins, cisplatin, loop diuretics, methoxyflurane, polymyxin B, vancomycin; ↑ neuromuscular blocking effect **W/** muscle relaxants & anesthetics **Labs:** ↑ BUN, SCr, AST, ALT, serum alk phos, bilirubin, LDH **NIPE:** ↑ Fluid consumption; may cause resp depression

Amiloride (Midamor) [Potassium-Sparing Diuretic] Uses: *HTN, CHF, & thiazide-induced ↓ K$^+$* **Action:** K$^+$-sparing diuretic; interferes w/ K$^+$/Na$^+$ exchange in distal tubule **Dose:** *Adults.* 5–10 mg PO daily **Peds.** 0.625 mg/kg/d; ↓ w/ renal impair **Caution:** [B, ?] **CI:** ↑ K$^+$, SCr > 1.5 mg/dL, BUN > 30 mg/100 mL, diabetic neuropathy, w/ other K$^+$-sparing diuretics **Disp:** Tabs 5 mg **SE:** ↑ K$^+$; HA, dizziness, dehydration, impotence **Interactions:** ↑ Risk of hyperkalemia **W/** ACE-I, K-sparing diuretics, NSAIDs, & K-salt substitutes; ↑ effects **OF** Li, digoxin, antihypertensives, amantadine; ↑ risk of *F* hypokalemia **W/** licorice **Labs:** Monitor K$^+$-monitor ECG for hyperkalemia (peaked T waves) **NIPE:** Take w/ food, I&O, daily wgt, ⊘ salt substitutes, bananas, oranges

Aminocaproic Acid (Amicar) [Antithrombotic Agent/Carboxylic Acid Derivative] Uses: *Excessive bleeding from systemic hyperfibrinolysis & urinary fibrinolysis* **Action:** ↓ Fibrinolysis; inhibits TPA, inhibits conversion of plasminogen to plasmin **Dose:** *Adults.* 5 g IV or PO (1st h) followed by 1–1.25 g/h IV or PO × 8 h or until bleeding controlled; 30 g/d max **Peds.** 100 mg/kg IV (1st h) then 1 g/m^2/h; max 18 g/m^2/d; ↓ w/ renal Insuff **Caution:** [C, ?] Not for upper urinary tract bleeding **CI:** DIC **Disp:** Tabs 500, syrup 250 mg/mL; Inj 250 mg/mL **SE:** ↓ BP, bradycardia, dizziness, HA, fatigue, rash, GI disturbance, ↓ plt Fxn **Notes:** Administer × 8 h or until bleeding controlled; not for upper urinary tract bleeding **Interactions:** ↑ Coagulation **W/** estrogens & OCP **Labs:** ↑ K$^+$ levels, false ↑ urine amino acids **NIPE:** CK monitoring w/ long-term use, eval for thrombophlebitis & difficulty urinating

Amino-Cerv pH 5.5 Cream [Cervical Hydrating Agent] Uses: *Mild cervicitis*, postpartum cervicitis/cervical tears, postcauterization, post-cryosurgery, & postconization **Action:** Hydrating agent; removes excess keratin in hyperkeratotic conditions **Dose:** 1 Applicator-full intravag hs × 2–4 wk **Caution:** [C, ?] w/ Viral skin Infxn **Disp:** Vag cream **SE:** Stinging, local irritation **NIPE:** AKA carbamide or urea; contains 8.34% urea, 0.5% sodium propionate, 0.83% methionine, 0.35% cystine, 0.83% inositol, & benzalkonium chloride

Aminoglutethimide (Cytadren) [Adrenal Steroid Inhibitor] Uses: *Cushing synd* Adrenocortical carcinoma, breast CA & PCa **Action:** ↓ Adrenal steroidogenesis & conversion of androgens to estrogens; 1st gen aromatase Inhib **Dose:** Initial 250 mg PO 4 × d, titrate q1–2wk max 2 g/d; w/ hydrocortisone 20–40 mg/d; ↓ w/ renal Insuff **Caution:** [D, ?] **Disp:** Tabs 250 mg **SE:** Adrenal Insuff ("medical adrenalectomy"), hypothyroidism, masculinization, ↓ BP, N/V, rare hepatotox, rash, myalgia, fever, drowsiness, lethargy, anorexia **Interactions:** ↑ Effects **W/** dexamethasone & hydrocortisone, ↓ effects **OF** warfarin, theophylline, medroxyprogesterone **NIPE:** Masculinization reversible after D/C drug, ⊘ PRG; give q6h to ↓ N

Aminophylline (Generic) [Bronchodilator/Xanthine Derivative]

Uses: *Asthma, COPD*, & bronchospasm **Action:** Relaxes smooth muscle (bronchi, pulm vessels); stimulates diaphragm **Dose:** *Adults. Acute asthma:* Load 6 mg/kg IV, then 0.4–0.9 mg/kg/h IV cont Inf, not > than 25 mg/min *Chronic asthma:* 24 mg/kg/24 h PO ÷ q6h *Peds.* Load 6 mg/kg IV, then 6 wk–6 mo 0.5 mg/kg/h, 6 mo–1 y 0.6–0.7 mg/kg/h, 1–9 y 1 mg/kg/h IV Inf; ↓ w/ hepatic Insuff & w/ some drugs (macrolide & quinolone antibiotics, cimetidine, propranolol) **Caution:** [C, +] Uncontrolled arrhythmias, HTN, Sz disorder, hyperthyroidism, peptic ulcers **Disp:** Tabs 100, 200 mg; PR tabs 100 mg, 200 mg, soln 105 mg/5 mL, Inj 25 mg/mL **SE:** N/V, irritability, tachycardia, ventricular arrhythmias, Szs **Notes:** Individualize dosage *Level:* 10–20 mcg/mL, toxic > 20 mcg/mL; aminophylline 85% theophylline; erratic rectal absorption **Interactions:** ↓ Effects *OF* Li, phenytoin, adenosine; ↓ effects *W/* phenobarbital, aminoglutethimide, barbiturates, rifampin, ritonavir, thyroid meds, tobacco; ↑ effects *W/* cimetidine, ciprofloxacin, erythromycin, INH, OCP, verapamil, charcoal-broiled foods, St. John's wort **Labs:** ↑ Uric acid levels, falsely ↑ levels w/ furosemide, probenecid, APAP, coffee, tea, cola, chocolate **NIPE:** ⊘ Chew or crush time-released caps & take on empty stomach, IR can be taken w/ food, ↑ fluids 2 L/d, tobacco ↑ drug elimination; narrow therapeutic range

Amiodarone (Cordarone, Pacerone, Nexterone) [Ventricular Antiarrhythmic/Adrenergic Blocker] WARNING: Liver tox, exacerbation of arrhythmias and lung damage reported

Uses: *Recurrent VF or hemodynamically unstable VT*, supraventricular arrhythmias, AF **Action:** Class III antiarrhythmic (Table 9) **Dose:** *Adults. Ventricular arrhythmias: IV:* 15 mg/min for 10 min, then 1 mg/min × 6 h, maint 0.5 mg/min cont Inf or *PO:* Load: 800–1600 mg/d PO × 1–3 wk *Maint:* 600–800 mg/d PO for 1 mo, then 200–400 mg/d *Supraventricular arrhythmias: IV:* 300 mg IV over 1 h, then 20 mg/kg for 24 h, then 600 mg PO daily for 1 wk, maint 100–400 mg daily or *PO:* Load 600–800 mg/d PO for 1–4 wk *Maint:* Slow ↓ to 100–400 mg daily *ECC 2010:* **VF/VT Cardiac arrest refractory to CPR, Shock and Pressor:** 300 mg IV/IO push; can give additional 150 mg IV/IO once; life-threatening arrhythmias: Max dose 2.2 g IV/24 h Rapid Inf: 150 mg IV over first 10 min (15 mg/min); can repeat 150 mg IV q10 min PRN. Slow Inf: 360 mg IV over 60 min (1 mg/min) Maint: 540 mg IV over 18 h (0.5 mg/min) *Peds.* 10–15 mg/kg/24 h ÷ q12h PO for 7–10 d, then 5 mg/kg/24 h ÷ q12h or daily (infants require ↑ loading); *ECC 2010:* **Pulseless VT/refractory VF:** 5 mg/kg IV/IO bolus, repeat PRN to 15 mg/kg (2.2 g in adolescents)/24 h; max single dose 300 mg; perfusing SVT/ventricular arrhythmias: 5 mg/kg IV/IO load over 20–60min; repeat PRN to 15 mg/kg (2.2 g in adolescents)/24 h **Caution:** [D, −] May require ↓ digoxin/warfarin dose, ↓ w/ liver Insuff, many drug interactions **CI:** Sinus node dysfunction, 2nd-/3rd-degree AV block, sinus brady (w/o pacemaker), iodine sensitivity **Disp:** Tabs 100, 200, 400 mg; Inj 50 mg/mL **SE:** Pulm fibrosis, exacerbation of arrhythmias, ↑ QT interval; CHF, hypo-/hyperthyroidism, ↑ LFTs, liver failure, corneal microdeposits, optic neuropathy/neuritis, peripheral neuropathy, photosensitivity **Notes:** IV conc > 2.0 mg/mL only via central line *Levels: Trough:* Just before next dose *Therapeutic:* 1–2.5 mcg/mL *Toxic:* > 2.5 mcg/mL *1/2-life:* 30–100 h **Interactions:** ↑ Serum levels *OF* digoxin, quinidine, procainamide, flecainide, phenytoin, warfarin, theophylline, cyclosporine; ↑ levels *W/* cimetidine, indinavir, ritonavir; ↑ levels *W/* cholestyramine, rifampin, St. John's wort; ↑ cardiac effects *W/* BBs, CCB **Labs:** ↑ LFTs, ↑ T₄ & RT₃, ANA titer, ↓ T₃ **NIPE:** Monitor cardiac rhythm, BP, LFTs, thyroid Fxn, ophthalmologic exam; may cause bradycardia; ↑ photosensitivity—use sunscreen; take w/ food

Amitriptyline (Elavil) [Antidepressant/TCA]   WARNING: Antidepressants may ↑ suicide risk; consider risks/benefits of use. Monitor pts closely **Uses:** *Depression (not bipolar depression)* peripheral neuropathy, chronic pain, tension HAs **Action:** TCA; ↓ reuptake of serotonin & norepinephrine by presynaptic neurons **Dose:** *Adults. Initial:* 30–50 mg PO hs; may ↑ to 300 mg hs *Peds.* Not OK < 12 y unless for chronic pain *Initial:* 0.1 mg/kg PO hs, ↑ over 2–3 wk to 0.5–2 mg/kg PO hs; taper to D/C **Caution:** CV Dz, Szs [D,+/−] NAG, hepatic impair **CI:** w/ MAOIs or w/in 14 d of use, during AMI recovery **Disp:** Tabs 10, 25, 50, 75, 100, 150 mg; Inj 10 mg/mL **SE:** Strong anticholinergic SEs; OD may be fatal; urine retention, sedation, ECG changes, photosensitivity **Notes:** *Levels: Therapeutic:* 120–150 ng/mL *Toxic:* > 500 ng/mL; levels may not correlate w/ effect **Interactions:** ↓ Effects *W/* carbamazepine, phenobarbital, rifampin, cholestyramine, colestipol, tobacco; ↑ effects *W/* cimetidine, quinidine, indinavir, ritonavir, CNS depressants, SSRIs, haloperidol, OCPs, BBs, phenothiazines, EtOH, evening primrose oil; ↑ effects *OF* amphetamines, anti-cholinergics, epinephrine, hypoglycemics, phenylephrine **Labs:** ↑ Glucose, false ↑ carbamazepine levels **NIPE:** ↑ Photosensitivity—use sunscreen; ↑ appetite & craving for sweets; ⊘ D/C abruptly; may turn urine blue-green

Amlodipine (Norvasc) [Antihypertensive, Antianginal/CCB]   Uses: *HTN, stable or unstable angina* **Action:** CCB; relaxes coronary vascular smooth muscle **Dose:** 2.5–10 mg/d PO; ↓ w/ hepatic impair **Caution:** [C, ?] **Disp:** Tabs 2.5, 5, 10 mg **SE:** edema, HA, palpitations, flushing, dizziness **Interactions:** ↑ Effect of hypotension *W/* antihypertensives, fentanyl, nitrates quinidine, EtOH, grapefruit juice; ↑ risk of neurotox *W/* Li; ↓ effects *W/* NSAIDs **Labs:** Monitor BUN, Cr, LFTs **NIPE:** Take w/o regard to meals; monitor for peripheral edema

Amlodipine/Atorvastatin (Caduet) [Antianginal, Antihypertensive, Antilipemic/Calcium Channel Blocker, HMG-CoA Reductase Inhibitor]   Uses: *HTN, chronic stable/vasospastic angina, control cholesterol & triglycerides* **Action:** CCB & HMG-CoA reductase Inhib **Dose:** Amlodipine 2.5–10 mg w/ atorvastatin 10–80 mg PO daily **Caution:** [X, −] **CI:** Active liver Dz, ↑ LFTs **Disp:** Tabs amlodipine mg/atorvastatin mg: 2.5/10, 2.5/20, 2.5/40,

5/10, 5/20, 5/40, 5/80, 10/10, 10/20, 10/40, 10/80 **SE:** Edema, HA, palpitations, flushing, myopathy, arthralgia, myalgia, GI upset, liver failure **Interactions:** ↑ Hypotension W/ fentanyl, nitrates, EtOH, quinidine, other antihypertensives, grapefruit juice; ↑ effects W/ diltiazem, erythromycin, H₂-blockers, PPI, quinidine; ↓ effects W/ NSAIDs, barbiturates, rifampin **Labs:** Monitor LFTs & CPK **NIPE:** ⊘ D/C abruptly, ↑ photosensitivity—use sunscreen; rare risk of rhabdomyolysis; instruct pt to report muscle pain/weakness

Amlodipine/Olmesartan (Azor) [Calcium Channel Blocker + Angiotensin II Receptor Blocker] **WARNING:** Use of renin-angiotensin agents in PRG can cause injury and death to fetus, D/C stat when PRG detected **Uses:** *HTN* **Action:** CCB w/ ARB **Dose:** *Adults.* Initial 2 mg/ 20 mg, max 10 mg/40 mg qd **Caution:** [C (1st tri), D (2nd, 3rd tri), −] w/ K⁺ supl or K⁺-sparing diuretics, renal impair, RAS, severe CAD, AS **CI:** PRG **Disp:** Tab amlodipine mg/olmesartan mg: 5/20, 10/20, 5/40, 10/40 **SE:** Edema, vertigo, dizziness, ↓ BP **Labs:** ↓ Hmg & Hct; monitor LFTs & BUN/Cr **NIPE:** May need ↓ dose in elderly; not recommended in children

Amlodipine/Valsartan (Exforge) [Calcium Channel Blocker (Dihydropyridine) + Angiotensin II Receptor Blocker] **WARNING:** Use of renin-angiotensin agents in PRG can cause fetal injury and death, D/C stat when PRG detected **Uses:** *HTN* **Action:** CCB w/ ARB **Dose:** *Adults.* Initial 5 mg/160 mg, may ↑ after 1–2 wk, max 10 mg/320 mg qd, start elderly at 1/2 initial dose **Caution:** [C (1st tri), D (2nd, 3rd tri), −] w/ K⁺ supl or K⁺-sparing diuretics, renal impair, RAS, severe CAD **CI:** PRG **Disp:** Tabs amlodipine mg/valsartan mg: 5/160, 10/160, 5/320,10/320 **SE:** Edema, vertigo, nasopharyngitis, URI, dizziness, ↓ BP **Interactions:** ↑ Risk of hyperkalemia W/ concomitant K⁺ supls, K⁺-sparing diuretics, K⁺-containing salt substitutes; ↑ SCr in HF **NIPE:** ⊘ PRG or breastfeeding; max effects w/in 2 wk after dose change

Amlodipine/Valsartan/HCTZ (Exforge Hct) [Calcium Channel Blocker + Angiotensin Receptor Blocker + Diuretic] **WARNING:** Use of renin-angiotensin agents in PRG can cause fetal injury and death, D/C stat when PRG detected **Uses:** *HTN* **Action:** CCB, ARB, & thiazide diuretic **Dose:** 1 tab 1 × d, may ↑ dose after 2 wk; max dose 10/320/25 mg **Caution:** [D, −] w/ Severe hepatic or renal impair **CI:** Anuria, sulfonamide allergy **Disp:** Tabs amlodipine mg/valsartan mg/HCTZ mg: 5/160/12.5, 10/160/12.5, 5/160/25, 10/160/25, 10/320/25 **SE:** Edema, dizziness, HA, fatigue, nasopharyngitis, dyspepsia, N, back pain, muscle spasm, ↓ BP **Interactions:** ↑ Risk of hypotension W/ diuretics, antihypertensives **NIPE:** Monitor BP for hypotension; ⊘ PRG or breast-feeding; ↑ risk of hyperkalemia w/ concomitant K⁺ supls, K⁺-sparing diuretics, K⁺-containing salt substitutes; ↑ SCr in HF

Ammonium Aluminum Sulfate [Alum] [GU Astringent] [OTC] **Uses:** *Hemorrhagic cystitis when saline bladder irrigation fails* **Action:** Astringent **Dose:** 1–2% soln w/ constant NS bladder irrigation **Caution:** [+/−] **Disp:**

Powder for recons **SE:** Encephalopathy possible; can precipitate & occlude catheters **Labs:** Monitor Al levels, esp in renal Insuff **NIPE:** Safe to use w/o anesthesia & w/ vesicoureteral reflux

Amoxicillin (Amoxil, Polymox) [Antibiotic/Aminopenicillin] Uses: *Ear, nose, & throat, lower resp, skin, UTI from susceptible gram(+) bacteria* endocarditis prophylaxis, H pylori eradication w/ other agents (gastric ulcers) **Action:** β-Lactam antibiotic; ↓ cell wall synth *Spectrum:* Gram(+) (*Streptococcus* sp, *Enterococcus* sp); some gram(−) (*H influenzae, E coli, N gonorrhoeae, H pylori,* & *P mirabilis*) **Dose:** *Adults.* 250–500 mg PO tid or 500–875 mg bid *Peds.* 25–100 mg/kg/24 h PO ÷ q8h, 200–400 mg PO bid (equivalent to 125–250 mg tid); ↓ in renal impair **Caution:** [B, +] **Disp:** Caps 250, 500 mg; chew tabs 125, 200, 250, 400 mg; susp 50, 125, 200, 250 mg/mL, & 400 mg/5 mL; tabs 500, 875 mg **SE:** D; skin rash **Interactions:** ↑ Effects *OF* warfarin, ↑ effects *W/* probenecid, disulfiram, ↑ risk of rash *W/* allopurinol, ↓ effects *OF* OCP, ↓ effects *W/* tetracyclines, chloramphenicol **Labs:** ↑ Serum alk phos, LDH, LFTs, false(+) direct Coombs test **NIPE:** Space med over 24 h; eval for super Infxn; use barrier contraception; cross hypersensitivity w/ PCN; many E coli strains resistant; chew tabs contain phenylalanine

Amoxicillin & Clavulanic Acid (Augmentin, Augmentin 600 ES, Augmentin XR) [Antibiotic/Aminopenicillin, Beta-Lactamase Inhibitor] Uses: *Ear, lower resp, sinus, urinary tract, skin Infxns caused by β-lactamase-producing H influenzae, S aureus, & E coli* **Action:** β-lactam antibiotic w/ β-lactamase Inhib *Spectrum:* Gram(+) same as amoxicillin alone, MSSA; gram(−) as w/ amoxicillin alone, β-lactamase-producing H influenzae, Klebsiella sp, M catarrhalis **Dose:** *Adults.* 250–500 mg PO q8h or 875 mg q12h; XR 2000 mg PO q12h *Peds.* 20–40 mg/kg/d as amoxicillin PO ÷ q8h or 45 mg/kg/d ÷ q12h; ↓ in renal impair; take w/ food **Caution:** [B, enters breast milk] **Disp:** Supplied as (amoxicillin/clavulanic): Tabs (mg/mg) 250/125, 500/125, 875/125; chew tabs (mg/mg) 125/31.25, 200/28.5, 250/62.5, 400/57; susp 125/31.25, 250/62.5, 200/28.5, 400/57 mg/5 mL; susp: ES 600 mg/42.9 mg/5 mL; XR tab 1000 mg/62.5 mg **SE:** Abd discomfort, N/V/D, allergic Rxn, vaginitis **Interactions:** ↑ Effects *OF* warfarin, ↑ effects *W/* probenecid, disulfiram, ↑ risk of rash *W/* allopurinol, ↓ effects *OF* OCP, ↓ effects *W/* tetracyclines, chloramphenicol **Labs:** ↑ Serum alk phos, LDH, LFTs, false(+) direct Coombs test **NIPE:** Space med over 24 h, eval for super Infxn, use barrier contraception; do not substitute two 250-mg tabs for one 500-mg tab (OD of clavulanic acid); max clavulanic acid 125 mg/dose

Amphotericin B (Amphocin, Fungizone) [Antifungal/Polyene Macrolide] Uses: *Severe, systemic fungal Infxns; oral & cutaneous candidiasis* **Action:** Binds ergosterol in the fungal membrane to alter permeability **Dose:** *Adults & Peds. Test Dose:* 1 mg IV adults or 0.1 mg/kg to 1 mg IV in children; then 0.25–1.5 mg/kg/24 h IV over 2–6 h (25–50 mg/d or qod). Total varies w/ indication *PO:* 1 mL qid **Caution:** [B, ?] **Disp:** Powder (Inj) 50 mg/vial **SE:** ↓ K⁺/Mg²⁺

from renal wasting; anaphylaxis, HA, fever, chills, nephrotox, ↓ BP, anemia, rigors SE Interactions: ↑ Nephrotoxic effects W/ antineoplastics, cyclosporine, furosemide, vancomycin, aminoglycosides, ↑ hypokalemia W/ corticosteroids, skeletal muscle relaxants Labs: Monitor Cr/LFTs/K/Mg; ↑ serum bilirubin, serum cholesterol NIPE: Monitor CNS effects & ⊘ take hs; ↓ in renal impair; pretreatment w/ APAP & antihistamines (Benadryl) ⊘ SE

Amphotericin B Cholesteryl (Amphotec) [Antifungal/Polyene Macrolide] Uses: *Aspergillosis if intolerant/refractory to conventional amphotericin B*, systemic candidiasis Action: Binds ergosterol in fungal membrane, alters permeability Dose: *Adults & Peds. Test Dose*: 1.6–8.3 mg, over 15–20 min, then 3–4 mg/kg/d; 1 mg/kg/h Inf, 7.5 mg/kg/d max; ↓ w/ renal Insuff Caution: [B, ?] Disp: Powder for Inj 50 mg, 100 mg/vial SE: Anaphylaxis; fever, chills, HA, nephrotox, ↓ BP, anemia Interactions: See Amphotericin B Labs: Monitor LFTs, lytes; ↓ K+, ↓ Mg2+ NIPE: Do not use inline filter

Amphotericin B Lipid Complex (Abelcet) [Antifungal/Polyene Macrolide] Uses: *Refractory invasive fungal Infxn in pts intolerant to conventional amphotericin B* Action: Binds ergosterol in fungal membrane, alters permeability Dose: *Adults & Peds*. 5 mg/kg/d IV single daily dose Caution: [B, ?] Disp: Inj 5 mg/mL SE: Anaphylaxis; fever, chills, HA, nephrotox, ↓ BP, anemia Interactions: See Amphotericin B Labs: ↓ K+, ↓ Mg2+ NIPE: Filter w/ 5-mcm needle; do not mix in lyte-containing solns; if Inf > 2 h, manually mix bag

Amphotericin B Liposomal (AmBisome) [Antifungal/Polyene Macrolide] Uses: *Refractory invasive fungal Infxn w/ intolerance to conventional amphotericin B; cryptococcal meningitis in HIV; empiric for febrile neutropenia; visceral leishmaniasis* Action: Binds ergosterol in fungal membrane, alters membrane permeability Dose: *Adults & Peds*. 3–6 mg/kg/d, Inf 60–120 min; dose varies by indication; ? ↓ in renal Insuff Caution: [B, ?] Disp: Powder Inj 50 mg SE: Anaphylaxis, fever, chills, HA, nephrotox, ↓ BP, anemia Interactions: See amphotericin B Labs: ↓ K+, ↓ Mg2+; NIPE: Do not use < 1-mcg filter

Ampicillin (Amcill, Omnipen) [Antibiotic/Aminopenicillin] Uses: *Resp, GU, or GI tract Infxns, meningitis d/t gram(−) & (+) bacteria; SBE prophylaxis* Action: β-Lactam antibiotic; ↓ cell wall synth Spectrum: Gram(+) (*Streptococcus* sp, *Staphylococcus* sp, *Listeria*); gram(−) (*Klebsiella* sp, *E coli, H influenzae, P mirabilis, Shigella* sp, *Salmonella* sp) Dose: *Adults*. 500 mg–2 g IM or IV q6h or 250–500 mg PO q6h; varies by indication *Peds Neonates*.< 7 d: 50–100 mg/kg/24 h IV ÷ q8h *Term infants*: 75–150 mg/kg/24 h ÷ q6–8h IV or PO *Children* ≥ 1 mo: 100–200 mg/kg/24 h ÷ q4–6h IM or IV; 50–100 mg/kg/24 h ÷ q6h PO up to 250 mg/dose *Meningitis*: 200–400 mg/kg/24 h ÷ q4–6h IV; ↓ w/ renal impair; take on empty stomach Caution: [B, M] Cross-hypersensitivity w/ PCN Disp: Caps 250, 500 mg; susp 100 mg/mL (reconstituted gtt); 125/5, 250/5 mg/mL powder (Inj) 125, 250, 500 mg, 1, 2, 10 g/vial SE: D, rash, allergic Rxn Notes: Many *E coli* resistant Interactions: ↓ Effects *OF* OCP & atenolol, ↓ effects *W/* chloramphenicol, erythromycin, tetracycline, & food; ↑ effects *OF* anticoagulants & MTX; ↑ risk of rash *W/* allopurinol; ↑ effects *W/* probenecid & disulfiram **Labs:** ↑ LFTs, serum protein, serum theophylline, serum uric acid; ↓ serum estrogen, serum cholesterol, serum folate; false(+) direct Coombs test, urine glucose, & urine amino acids **NIPE:** Take on empty stomach & around the clock; may cause candial vaginitis; use barrier contraception

Ampicillin-Sulbactam (Unasyn) [Antibiotic/Aminopenicillin & Beta-Lactamase Inhibitor] Uses: *Gynecologic, intra-Abd, skin Infxns d/t β-lactamase-producing *S aureus*, *Enterococcus*, *H influenzae*, *P mirabilis*, & *Bacteroides* sp* **Action:** β-Lactam antibiotic & β-lactamase Inhib *Spectrum:* Gram(+) & (−) as for amp alone; includes *Enterobacter*, *Acinetobacter*, *Bacteroides* **Dose:** *Adults.* 1.5–3 g IM or IV q6h *Peds.* 100–400 mg ampicillin/kg/d (150–300 mg Unasyn) q6h; ↓ w/ renal Insuff **Caution:** [B, M] **Disp:** Powder for Inj 1.5, 3 g/vial, 15 g bulk package **SE:** Allergic Rxns, rash, D, Inj site pain **Notes:** A 2:1 ratio ampicillin:sulbactam **Interactions:** ↓ Effects *OF* OCP & atenolol, ↓ effects *W/* chloramphenicol, erythromycin, tetracycline, & food; ↑ effects *OF* anticoagulants & MTX; ↑ risk of rash *W/* allopurinol; ↑ effects *W/* probenecid & disulfiram **Labs:** ↑ LFTs, serum protein, serum theophylline, serum uric acid; ↓ serum estrogen, serum cholesterol, serum folate; false(+) direct Coombs test, urine glucose, & urine amino acids **NIPE:** Take around the clock; may cause candial vaginitis; use barrier contraception

Anakinra (Kineret) [Antirheumatic/Immunomodulator] WARNING: Associated w/ ↑ incidence of serious Infxn; D/C w/ serious Infxn Uses: *Reduce S/Sxs of mod/severe active RA, failed 1 or more DMARD* **Action:** Human IL-1 receptor antagonist **Dose:** 100 mg SQ daily; w/ CrCl < 30 mL/min, qod **Caution:** [B, ?] **CI:** *E coli*–derived proteins allergy, active Infxn; < 18 y **Disp:** 100-mg prefilled syringes; 100 mg (0.67 mL/vial) **SE:** ↓ WBC esp w/ TNF-blockers, Inj site Rxn (may last up to 28 d), Infxn, N/D, Abd pain, flu-like Sxs, HA **Interactions:** ↓ Effects *OF* immunizations; ↑ risk of Infxns if combined *W/* TNF-blocking drugs **Labs:** ↓ WBCs, plts, ANC **NIPE:** Store drug in refrigerator; ⊘ light exposure, & discard unused portion; ⊘ use soln if discolored or has particulate matter

Anastrozole (Arimidex) [Antineoplastic/Nonsteroidal Aromatase Inhibitor] Uses: *Breast CA: postmenopausal w/ met breast CA, adjuvant Rx postmenopausal early hormone-receptor(+) breast CA* **Action:** Selective nonsteroidal aromatase Inhib, ↓ circulatory estradiol **Dose:** 1 mg/d **Caution:** [D, ?] **CI:** PRG **Disp:** Tabs 1 mg **SE:** May ↑ cholesterol; N/V/D, HTN, flushing, ↑ bone/tumor pain, HA, somnolence, mood disturbance, depression, rash **Interactions:** None noted **Labs:** ↑ GTT, LFTs, alk phos, total & LDL cholesterol; no effect on adrenal steroids or aldosterone **NIPE:** May ↓ fertility & cause fetal damage; eval for pain & administer adequate analgesia; may cause Vag bleeding 1st few wk

Anidulafungin (Eraxis) [Antifungal/Echinocandin] Uses: *Candidemia, esophageal candidiasis, other *Candida* Infxn (peritonitis, intra-Abd abscess)* **Action:** Echinocandin; ↓ cell wall synth *Spectrum: C albicans, C glabrata, C parapsilosis, C tropicalis* **Dose:** *Candidemia, others:* 200 mg IV × 1, then 100 mg IV daily (Tx = 14 d after last + culture); *esophageal candidiasis:* 100 mg IV × 1, then 50 mg IV daily (Tx > 14 d and 7 d after resolution of Sx); 1.1 mg/min max Inf rate **Caution:** [C, ?/–] **CI:** Echinocandin hypersensitivity **Disp:** Powder 50, 100 mg/vial **SE:** Histamine-mediated Inf Rxns (urticaria, flushing, ↓ BP, dyspnea, etc), fever, N/V/D, ↓ K+, hep, ↑ LFTs, hep, worsening hepatic failure **Labs:** ↑ LFTs, ↓ K+ **NIPE:** ↓ Inf rate to < 1.1 mg/min w/ Inf Rxns; monitor ECG for hypokalemia (flattened T waves)

Anistreplase (Eminase) [Antithrombotic Agent/Plasminogen Activator] Uses: *AMI* Action: Thrombolytic; activates conversion of plasminogen to plasmin, ↑ thrombolysis Dose: *ECC 2010:* ACS: 30 units IV over 2–5 min Caution: [C, ?] CI: Active internal bleeding, h/o CVA, recent (< 2 mo) intracranial or intraspinal surgery/trauma/neoplasm, AVM, aneurysm, bleeding diathesis, severe HTN Disp: 30 units/vial SE: Bleeding, ↓ BP, hematoma Notes: Ineffective if readministered > 5 d after the previous dose of anistreplase or streptokinase, or streptococcal Infxn (production of antistreptokinase Ab) Interactions: ↑ Risk of hemorrhage W/ warfarin, oral anticoagulants, ASA, NSAIDs, dipyridamole; ↓ effectiveness W/ aminocaproic acid Labs: ↓ Plasminogen & fibrinogen, ↓ transaminase level, thrombin time, aPTT & PT NIPE: Store powder in refrigerator & use w/in 30 min of reconstitution; initiate therapy ASAP after MI; monitor S/Sxs internal bleeding

Anthralin (Anthra-Derm) [Keratolytic Dermatologic Agent] Uses: *Psoriasis* Action: Keratolytic Dose: Apply daily Caution: [C, ?] CI: Acutely inflamed psoriatic eruptions, erythroderma Disp: Cream, oint 0.1%, 0.25%, 0.4%, 0.5%, 1% SE: Irritation; hair/fingernails/skin discoloration Interactions: ↑ Tox if used stat after long-term topical corticosteroid therapy NIPE: May stain fabric; external use only; ⊘ sunlight-medicated areas

Antihemophilic Factor [AHF, Factor VIII] (Monoclate) [Antihemophilic] Uses: *Classic hemophilia A, von Willebrand Dz* Action: Provides factor VIII needed to convert prothrombin to thrombin Dose: *Adults & Peds.* 1 AHF unit/kg ↑ factor VIII level by 2 IU/dL; units required = (wgt in kg) (desired factor VIII ↑ as % nl) × (0.5); prevent spontaneous hemorrhage = 5% nl; hemostasis after trauma/surgery = 30% nl; head injuries, major surgery, or bleeding = 80–100% nl Caution: [C, ?] Disp: ✓ Each vial for units contained, powder for recons SE: Rash, fever, HA, chills, N/V Notes: Determine % nl factor VIII before dosing Interactions: None Labs: Monitor CBC & direct Coombs test NIPE: ⊘ ASA; immunize against hep B; D/C if tachycardic

Antihemophilic Factor (Recombinant) (Xyntha) [Clotting Factor] Uses: *Control/prevent bleeding & surgical prophylaxis in hemophilia A* Action: ↑ Levels of factor VIII Dose: *Adults.* Required units = body wgt (kg) × desired factor VIII rise (IU/dL or % of nl) × 0.5 (IU/kg per IU/dL); frequency/duration determined by type of bleed (see package insert) Caution: [C, ?/–] Severe hypersensitivity Rxn possible CI: None Disp: Inj powder: 250, 500, 1000, 2000 IU SE:

HA, fever, N/V/D, weakness, allergic Rxn **NIPE:** Monitor for the development of factor VIII neutralizing antibodies

Antithrombin, Recombinant (Atryn) [Antithrombin] Uses: * Prevent peri-op/peri-partum thromboembolic events w/ hereditary antithrombin (AT) deficiency* **Action:** Inhibits thrombin and factor Xa **Dose: Adults.** Based on pre-Rx AT level, BW (kg) and drug monitoring; see package insert. Goal AT levels 0.8–1.2 IU/mL **Caution:** [C, –/] Hypersensitivity Rxns; **CI:** Hypersensitivity to goat/goat milk proteins **Disp:** Powder 1750 IU/vial **SE:** Bleeding, Inf site Rxn **Interactions:** ↑effects *OF* heparin, LMW heparins **Labs:** ✓ aPTT and antifactor Xa **NIPE:** Monitor for bleeding or thrombosis

Antithymocyte Globulin (See Lymphocyte Immune Globulin) [Immunosuppressive Agent]

Apomorphine (Apokyn) [Antiparkinsonian/Dopamine Agonist] **WARNING:** Do not administer IV **Uses:** *Acute, intermittent hypomobility ("off") episodes of Parkinson Dz* **Action:** DA agonist **Dose: Adults.** 0.2 mL SQ supervised test dose; if BP OK, initial 0.2 mL (2 mg) SQ during "off" periods; only 1 dose per "off" period; titrate dose; 0.6 mL (6 mg) max single doses; use w/ antiemetic; ↓ in renal impair **Caution:** [C, +/–] Avoid EtOH; antihypertensives, vasodilators, cardio- or cerebrovascular Dz, hepatic impair **CI:** 5-HT$_3$ antagonists, sulfite allergy **Disp:** Inj 10 mg/mL, 3-mL pen cartridges; 2-mL amp **SE:** Emesis, syncope, ↑ QT, orthostatic ↓ BP, somnolence, ischemia, Inj site Rxn, abuse potential, dyskinesia, fibrotic conditions, priapism, CP/angina, yawning, rhinorrhea **Interactions:** ↑ Risk of hypotension *W/* alosetron, dolasetron, granisetron, ondansetron, Palonosetron **Labs:** ECG—monitor for prolongation of QT interval **NIPE:** Daytime somnolence may limit activities; trimethobenzamide 300 mg tid PO or other non–5-HT$_3$ antagonist antiemetic given 3 d prior to & up to 2 mo following initiation

Apraclonidine (Iopidine) [Glaucoma Agent/Alpha-Adrenergic Agonist] Uses: *Glaucoma, intraocular HTN* **Action:** α$_2$-Adrenergic agonist **Dose:** 1–2 gtt of 0.5% tid; 1 gtt of 1% before and after surgical procedure **Caution:** [C, ?] **CI:** w/in 14 d of or w/ MAOI **Disp:** 0.5%, 1% soln **SE:** Ocular irritation, lethargy, xerostomia **Interactions:** ↓ IOP *W/* pilocarpine or topical BBs **NIPE:** Monitor CV status of pts w/ CAD; potential for dizziness

Aprepitant (Emend, Oral) [Centrally Acting Antiemetic] Uses: *Prevents N/V associated w/ emetogenic CA chemotherapy (eg, cisplatin) (use in combo w/ other antiemetics)*, post-op N/V **Action:** Substance P/neurokinin 1 (NK$_1$) receptor antagonist **Dose:** 125 mg PO day 1, 1 h before chemotherapy, then 80 mg PO qAM days 2 & 3; post-op N/V: 40 mg w/in 3 h of induction **Caution:** [B, ?/–] Substrate & mod CYP3A4 Inhib; CYP2C9 inducer (Table 10) **CI:** Use w/ pimozide **Disp:** Caps 40, 80, 125 mg **SE:** Fatigue, asthenia, hiccups **Interactions:** ↑ Effects *W/* clarithromycin, diltiazem, itraconazole, ketoconazole, nefazodone, nelfinavir, ritonavir, troleandomycin; ↑ effects *OF* alprazolam, astemizole, cisapride, dexamethasone, methylprednisolone, midazolam, pimozide, terfenadine, triazolam,

& chemotherapeutic agents, eg, docetaxel, etoposide, ifosfamide, imatinib, irinotecan, paclitaxel, vinblastine, vincristine, vinorelbine; ↓ effects W/ paroxetine, rifampin; ↓ effects OF OCPs, paroxetine, phenytoin, tolbutamide, warfarin Labs: ↑ ALT, AST, BUN, alk phos, leukocytes NIPE: Use barrier contraception; take w/o regard to food; see also Fosaprepitant (Emend, Inj)

Apriso (Salix) [Aminosalicylate] Uses: *Maintenance of UC remission* Action: Locally acting aminosalicylate Dose: 1.5 g (0.375 g caps × 4) PO daily in AM; not w/ antacids Caution: [B, ±] May cause renal impair, exacerbation of colitis CI: Hypersensitivity to salicylates/aminosalicylates Disp: Caps ER 0.375 g SE: HA, N/D, Abd pain, nasopharyngitis, influenza, sinusitis, acute intolerance synd (cramping, Abd pain, bloody D, fever, HA, rash) Labs: Monitor CBC, SCr NIPE: For pts w/ PKU product contains aspartame; in elderly—monitor CBC. Assess renal function before Tx & periodically during Tx; ⊘ take w/ antacids.

Arformoterol (Brovana) [Long-Acting Beta-2 Agonist] WARNING: LA β_2-adrenergic agonists may ↑ the risk of asthma-related death. Use only for pts not adequately controlled on other asthma-controller meds Uses: *Maint in COPD* Action: Selective LA β_2-adrenergic agonist Dose: *Adults.* 15 mcg bid nebulization Caution: [C, ?] CI: Hypersensitivity Disp: Soln: 15 mcg/2 mL SE: Pain, back pain, CP, D, sinusitis, nervousness, palpitations, allergic Rxn Interactions: ↑ Risk of prolonged QT interval W/ MAOIs, TCAs; ↑ risk of hypokalemia W/ steroids; ↓ effects W/ aminophylline, BBs, K⁺-depleting diuretics, theophylline Labs: Monitor K⁺ NIPE: Not for acute bronchospasm; refrigerate, use stat after opening

Argatroban (Acova) [Anticoagulant/Thrombin Inhibitor] Uses: *Prevent/Tx thrombosis in HIT, PCI in pts w/ HIT risk* Action: Anticoagulant, direct thrombin Inhib Dose: 2 mcg/kg/min IV; adjust until a PTT 1.5–3 × baseline not to exceed 100 s; 10 mcg/kg/min max; ↓ w/ hepatic impair Caution: [B, ?] Avoid PO anticoagulants, ↑ bleeding risk; avoid use w/ thrombolytics CI: Overt major bleed Disp: Inj 100 mg/mL SE: AF, cardiac arrest, cerebrovascular disorder, ↓ BP, VT, N/V/D, sepsis, cough, renal tox Interactions: ↑ Risk of bleeding W/ anticoagulants, feverfew, garlic, ginger, ginkgo, ↑ risk of intracranial bleed W/ thrombolytics Labs: ↑ aPTT, PT, INR, ACT, thrombin time; ✓ aPTT w/ Inf start and after each dose change ↓ Hgb NIPE: Report ↑ bruising & bleeding; ⊘ breastfeed; steady state in 1–3 h

Aripiprazole (Abilify, Abilify Discmelt) [Antipsychotic/Psychotropic] WARNING: ↑ Mortality in elderly w/ dementia-related psychosis; ↑ suicidal thinking in children, adolescents, & young adults w/ MDD Uses: *Schizophrenia adults & peds 13–17 y, mania or mixed episodes associated w/ bipolar disorder, MDD in adults, agitation w/ schizophrenia* Action: DA & serotonin antagonist Dose: *Adults. Schizophrenia:* 10–15 mg PO/d *Acute agitation:* 9.75 mg/ 1.3 mL IM *Bipolar:* 15 mg MDD adjunct w/ other anti-depressants initial 2 mg/d, 10 mg/d OK *Peds. Schizophrenia: 13–17 y:* Start 2 mg/d, usual 10 mg/d; max 30 mg/d for all adult and peds uses; ↓ dose w/ CYP3A4/CYP2D6 Inhibs (Table 10); ↑ dose w/ CYP3A4 inducer **Caution:** [C, –] w/ low WBC **Disp:** Tabs 2, 5, 10, 15, 20, 30 mg; Discmelt (disintegrating tabs 10, 15, 20, 30 mg) soln 1 mg/mL; Inj 7.5 mg/mL **SE:** Neuroleptic malignant synd, tardive dyskinesia, orthostatic ↓ BP, cognitive & motor impair **Interactions:** ↑ Effects **W/** ketoconazole, quinidine, fluoxetine, paroxetine, ↓ effects **W/** carbamazepine **Labs:** ↑ Glucose, monitor CBC, monitor for leukopenia, neutropenia, & agranulocytosis **NIPE:** ⊘ Breast-feed, consume EtOH, or use during PRG; use barrier contraception; ↑ fluid intake; Discmelt contains phenylalanine

Armodafinil (Nuvigil) [Binds Dopamine Receptor] Uses: *Narcolepsy, SWSD, and OSAHS* **Action:** ?; binds DA receptor, ↓ DA reuptake **Dose:** *Adults. OSAHS/narcolepsy:* 150 or 250 mg PO daily in AM *SWSD:* 150 mg PO qd 1 h prior to start of shift; ↓ w/ hepatic impair **Caution:** [C, ?] w/ renal impair **CI:** Hypersensitivity to modafinil/armodafinil **Disp:** Tabs 50, 150, 200 mg **SE:** HA, N, dizziness, insomnia, xerostomia, rash including SJS, angioedema, anaphylactoid Rxns, multiorgan hypersensitivity Rxns **Interactions:** *Avoid:* May significantly ↑ effects **W/** fosamprenavir, itraconazole, ketoconazole, lopinavir, nelfinavir, ritonavir, telithromycin, tipranavir; ↑ effects **W/** chloramphenicol, clarithromycin, conivaptan, erythromycin, fluvoxamine, imatinib, nefazodone, posaconazole, voriconazole; ↑ effects **OF** carisoprodol, clomipramine, desipramine, diazepam, doxepin, ifosfamide, imipramine, propranolol, phenytoins, pentamidine, tiagabine, warfarin, caffeine; ↑ effects of CV &/or CNS stimulation **W/** caffeine, ergotamine, stimulants/ anorexiants; ↑ effects of HTN crisis **W/** linezolid, MAOIs; ↓ effects **W/** barbiturates, carbamazepine, nevirapine, phenytoins, rifampin, rifapentine, warfarin, St. John's wort *Avoid:* May significantly ↓ effects **OF** atazanavir, clopidogrel, OC, darunavir, dasatinib, delavirdine, dronedarone, erlotinib, everolimus, indinavir, irinotecan, itraconazole, ixabepilone, ketoconazole, lapatinib, lopinavir, nelfinavir, nilotinib, pazopanib, ritonavir, saquinavir, sunitinib, telithromycin, temsirolimus, tipranavir, tolvaptan; ↓ effects **OF** alfentanil, amiodarone, aprepitant, aripiprazole, bexarotene, bortezomib, bosentan, buprenorphine, buspirone, carbamazepine, CCBs, cinacalcet, cisapride, clozapine, colchicine, conivaptan, corticosteroids, cyclosporine, dapsone, darifenacin, disopyramide, docetaxel, doxorubicins, efavirenz, eplerenone, ethosuximide, fentanyl, gefitinib, maraviroc, meperidine, methadone, nevirapine, quinidine, paclitaxel, pimozide, proguanil, propoxyphene, repaglinide, risperidone, sildenafil, sirolimus, statins, sufentanil, tacrolimus, tandalafil, theophylline, tramadol, trazadone, zaleplon, ziprasidone, zonisamide **NIPE:** Monitor BP, ↑ risk for psychosis, suicidal ideation, mania; may cause dependency; lower doses in elderly

Artemether & Lumefantrine (Coartem) [Antiprotozoal/ Antimalarial] Uses: *Acute, uncomplicated malaria (Plasmodium falciparum)* **Action:** Antiprotozoal/antimalarial **Dose:** *Adults> 16 y:25–< 35 kg:* 3 tabs h 0 & h 8 day 1, then 3 tabs bid day 2 & 3 (18 tabs/course) = *35 kg:* 4 tabs h 0 & h 8 day 1, then 4 tabs bid day 2 & 3 (24 tabs/course) *Peds .2 mo–< 16 y. 5–< 15 kg:* 1 tab at h 0 & h 8 day 1, then 1 tab bid day 2 & 3 (6 tabs/course) *15–< 25 kg:* 2 tabs h 0 & h 8 day 1, then 2 tabs bid day 2 & 3 (12 tabs/course); 25–< 35 kg: 3 tabs at h 0 & h 8 day 1, then 3 tabs bid on day 2 & 3 (18 tabs/course) = 35 kg: See Adult dose **Caution:** [C, ?] ↑ QT, hepatic/renal impair, CYP3A4 Inhibs **Contra:** Component hypersensitivity **Disp:** Tabs artemether 20 mg/lumefantrine 120 mg **SE:** Palp, HA, dizziness, chills, sleep disturb, fatigue, anorexia, N/V/D, Abd pain, weakness, arthralgia, myalgia, cough, splenomegaly, hepatomegaly **Labs:** ↑ AST, ↑ QT **NIPE:** Not recommended w/ other agents that ↑ QT—monitor ECG

Artificial Tears (Tears Naturale) [Ocular Lubricant] [OTC] Uses: *Dry eyes* **Action:** Ocular lubricant **Dose:** 1–2 gtt tid–qid **Disp:** OTC soln **SE:** Mild stinging, temperature blurred vision

Asenapine Maleate (Saphris) [Atypical Antipsychotic (Dibenzo-Oxepino Pyrrole)] **WARNING:** ↑ Mortality in elderly w/ dementia-related psychosis **Uses:** *Schizophrenia; manic/mixed bipolar disorder* **Action:** DA/serotonin antagonist **Dose:** *Adults. Schizophrenia:* 5 mg tid *Bipolar disorder:* 10 mg tid **Caution:** [C, ?/–] **Disp:** SL Tabs 5, 10 mg **SE:** Dizziness, somnolence, akathisia, oral hypoesthesia, EPS, ↑wgt, ↓ BP, ↑ QT interval, hyperprolactinemia, neuroleptic malignant synd **Interactions:** Avoid drugs that ↑ QT interval (eg, Class Ia or Class III antiarrhythmics, ziprasidone, chlorpromazine, thioridazine, moxifloxacin, alcohol), ↑ effects *OF* antihypertensives; ↓ effects *W/* fluvoxamine **Labs:** ↑ glucose, ↓ WBC **NIPE:** Do not swallow/crush/chew tab; avoid eating/drinking 10 min after dose

L-Asparaginase (Elspar, Oncaspar) [Antineoplastic/Protein Synthesis Inhibitor] Uses: *ALL* (in combo w/ other agents) **Action:** Protein synth Inhib **Dose:** 500–20,000 IU/m²/d for 1–14 d (per protocols) **Caution:** [C, ?] CI: Active/Hx pancreatitis; h/o allergic Rxn, thrombosis or hemorrhagic event w/ prior Rx w/ asparaginase **Disp:** Powder (Inj) 10,000 units/vial **SE:** Allergy 20–35% (urticaria to anaphylaxis); fever, chills, N/V, anorexia, Abd cramps, depression, agitation, Sz, pancreatitis, coagulopathy **Interactions:** ↑ Effects *W/* prednisone, vincristine; ↓ effects *OF* MTX, sulfonylureas, insulin **Labs:** ✓ Glucose, coagulation studies, LFTs; ↓ ↑ T₄- & T₄-binding globulin, serum albumin, total cholesterol, plasma fibrinogen; ↑ BUN, glucose, uric acid, LFTs, alk phos **NIPE:** ↑ Fluid intake; monitor for bleeding; monitor I&O & wgt; ⊘ EtOH or ASA; test dose OK

Aspirin (Bayer, Ecotrin, St. Joseph's) [Antipyretic, Analgesic/Salicylate] [OTC] Uses: *Angina, CABG, PTCA, carotid endarterectomy, ischemic stroke, TIA, ACS/MI, arthritis, pain*, HA, *fever*, inflammation, Kawasaki Dz **Action:** Prostaglandin Inhib **Dose:** *Adults. Pain, fever:* 325–650 mg q4–6h PO or PR (4 g/d max) *RA:* 3–6 g/d PO in ÷ doses *Plt Inhib:* 81–325 mg PO daily *Prevent MI:* 81 (preferred)–325 mg PO daily *ECC 2010:* ACS: 160–325 mg non-enteric coated PO ASAP (chewing preferred at ACS onset) *Peds. Antipyretic:* 10–15 mg/kg/dose PO or PR q4–6h up to 80 mg/kg/24 h *RA:* 60–100 mg/kg/24 h PO ÷ q4–6h (keep levels 15–30 mg/dL) *Kawasaki Dz:* 80–100 mg/kg/d ÷ q6h, 3–5 mg/kg/d after fever resolves; for all uses 4 g/d max; avoid w/ CrCl < 10 mL/min, severe liver Dz

Caution: [C, M] Linked to Reye synd; avoid w/ viral illness in peds < 16 y **CI:** Allergy to ASA, chickenpox/flu Sxs, synd of nasal polyps, angioedema, & bronchospasm to NSAIDs **Disp:** Tabs 325, 500 mg; chew tabs 81 mg; EC tabs 81, 162, 325, 500, 650, 975 mg; SR tabs 650, 800 mg; effervescent tabs 325, 500 mg; supp 125, 200, 300, 600 mg **SE:** GI upset, erosion, & bleeding **Notes:** Salicylate levels: *Therapeutic:* 100–250 mcg/mL *Toxic:*> 300 mcg/mL **Interactions:** ↑ Effects W/ anticoagulants, ammonium chloride, antibiotics, ascorbic acid, furosemide, methionine, nizatidine, NSAIDs, verapamil, EtOH, feverfew, garlic, ginkgo, horse chestnut, kelpware (black-tang), prickly ash, red clover; ↓ effects W/ antacids, activated charcoal, corticosteroids, griseofulvin, NaHCO₃, ginseng, food; ↑ effects OF ACEI, hypoglycemics, insulin, Li, MTX, phenytoin, sulfonamides, valproic acid; ↓ effects OF BBs, probenecid, spironolactone, sulfinpyrazone **Labs:** False(−) of urinary glucose & urinary ketone tests, serum albumin, total serum phenytoin, T_3, & T_4 **NIPE:** D/C 1 wk prior to surgery; avoid/limit EtOH; Chronic ASA use may result in ↓ folic acid, Fe-deficiency anemia, & hypernatremia; ⊘ foods ↑ salicylate (eg, curry powder, paprika, licorice, prunes, raisins, tea; take ASA w/ food or milk); report S/Sxs bleeding/GI pain/ringing in ears

Aspirin & Butalbital Compound (Fiorinal) [C-III] [Analgesic & Barbiturate] **Uses:** *Tension HA*, pain **Action:** Barbiturate w/ analgesic **Dose:** 1–2 PO q4h PRN, max 6 tabs/d; avoid w/ CrCl < 10 mL/min or severe liver Dz **Caution:** [C (D w/ prolonged use or high doses at term), ?] **CI:** ASA allergy, GI ulceration, bleeding disorder, porphyria, synd of nasal polyps, angioedema, & bronchospasm to NSAIDs **Disp:** Caps (*Fiorgen PF, Lanorinal*), tabs (*Lanorinal*) ASA 325 mg/butalbital 50 mg/caffeine 40 mg **SE:** Drowsiness, dizziness, GI upset, ulceration, bleeding; see Aspirin **Interactions:** ↑ Effect OF benzodiazepines, CNS depressants, chloramphenicol, methylphenidate, propoxyphene, valproic acid; ↓ effects OF BBs, corticosteroids, chloramphenicol, cyclosporines, doxycycline, griseofulvin, haloperidol, OCPs, phenothiazines, quinidine, TCAs, theophylline, warfarin **NIPE:** Butalbital habit-forming; D/C 1 wk prior to surgery; use barrier contraception, avoid or limit EtOH

Aspirin + Butalbital, Caffeine, & Codeine (Fiorinal + Codeine) [C-III] [Analgesic & Barbiturate & Narcotic] **Uses:** Mild *pain*, HA, esp tension HA w/ stress **Action:** Sedative & narcotic analgesic **Dose:** 1–2 tabs/ caps PO q4–6h PRN max 6/d **Caution:** [C, ?] **CI:** Allergy to ASA & codeine; synd of nasal polyps, angioedema, & bronchospasm to NSAIDs, bleeding diathesis, peptic ulcer or sig GI lesions, porphyria **Disp:** Caps/tabs contain 325 mg ASA, 40 mg caffeine, 50 mg butalbital, 30 mg codeine **SE:** Drowsiness, dizziness, GI upset, ulceration, bleeding; see Aspirin + Butalbital **Interactions:** ↑ Effects W/ narcotic analgesics, MAOIs, neuromuscular blockers; ↓ effects W/ tobacco smoking; ↑ effects OF digitoxin, phenytoin, rifampin; ↓ resp & CNS depression W/ cimetidine **Labs:** ↑ Plasma amylase & lipase **NIPE:** D/C 1 wk prior to surgery, avoid/limit EtOH; may cause constipation, ↑ fluids & fiber; take w/ milk to ↓ GI distress

Aspirin + Codeine (Empirin No. 3, 4) [C-III] [Narcotic Analgesic]
Uses: Mild–*mod pain*, symptomatic nonproductive cough **Action:** Combined effects of ASA & codeine **Dose:** *Adults.* 1–2 tabs PO q4–6h PRN *Peds.* ASA 10 mg/kg/dose; codeine 0.5–1 mg/kg/dose q4h **Caution:** [D, M] **CI:** Allergy to ASA/ codeine, PUD, bleeding, anticoagulant Rx, children w/ chickenpox or flu Sxs, synd of nasal polyps, angioedema, & bronchospasm to NSAIDs **Disp:** Tabs 325 mg of ASA & codeine (codeine in No. 3 = 30 mg, No. 4 = 60 mg) **SE:** Drowsiness, dizziness, GI upset, ulceration, bleeding; see Aspirin **Interactions** ↑ Effects *W/* narcotic analgesics, MAOIs, neuromuscular blockers, ↓ effects *W/* tobacco smoking; ↓ effects *OF* digitoxin, phenytoin, rifampin; ↑ resp & CNS depression *W/* cimetidine **Labs:** ↑ Plasma amylase & lipase **NIPE:** D/C 1 wk prior to surgery; avoid/limit EtOH; May cause constipation, ↑ fluids & fiber; take w/ milk ↓ GI distress

Atazanavir (Reyataz) [Antiretroviral/HIV-1 Protease Inhibitor]
WARNING: Hyperbilirubinemia may require drug D/C **Uses:** *HIV-1 Infxn* **Action:** Protease Inhib **Dose:** Antiretroviral naïve 400 mg PO daily w/ food; experienced pts 300 mg w/ ritonavir 100 mg; when given w/ efavirenz 600 mg, administer atazanavir 300 mg + ritonavir 100 mg once/d; separate doses from buffered didanosine administration; ↓ w/ hepatic impair **Caution:** CDC rec HIV-infected mothers not breast-feed [B, –]; ↑ levels of statins (avoid use) sildenafil, antiarrhythmics, warfarin, cyclosporine, TCAs; ↓ w/ St. John's wort, H$_2$-receptor antagonists **CI:** w/ midazolam, triazolam, ergots, pimozide **Disp:** Caps 100, 150, 200, 300 mg **SE:** HA, N/V/D, rash, Abd pain, DM, photosensitivity, ↑ PR interval **Interactions:** May have less adverse effect on cholesterol; if given w/ H$_2$-blocker, give together or at least 10 h after H$_2$; if given w/ PPI, separate by 12 h; concurrent use not recommended in experienced pts; ↑ effects *W/* amprenavir, clarithromycin, indinavir, lamivudine, lopinavir, ritonavir, saquinavir, stavudine, tenofovir, zalcitabine, zidovudine; ↑ effects *OF* amiodarone, atorvastatin, CCBs, clarithromycin, cyclosporine, diltiazem, irinotecan, lidocaine, lovastatin, OCPs, rifabutin, quinidine, saquinavir, sildenafil, simvastatin, sirolimus, tacrolimus, warfarin; ↓ effects *W/* antacids, antimycobacterials, efavirenz, esomeprazole, H$_2$-receptor antagonists, lansoprazole, omeprazole, rifampin, St. John's wort **Labs:** ↑ ALT, AST, total bilirubin, amylase, lipase, serum glucose; ↑ Hgb, neutrophils **NIPE:** CDC rec HIV-infected mothers not to breast-feed; take w/ food; will not cure HIV or ↓ risk of transmission; use barrier contraception; ↑ risk of skin and/or scleral yellowing

Atenolol (Tenormin) [Antihypertensive, Antianginal/Beta-Blocker]
Uses: *HTN, angina, MI* **Action:** Selective β-adrenergic receptor blocker **Dose:** 25–50 qd up to 100 mg/d; *HTN & angina:* 50–100 mg/d PO *ECC 2010: AMI:* 5 mg IV over 5 min; in 10 min, 5 mg slow IV; if tolerated in 10 min, start 50 mg PO, titrate; ↓ in renal impair **Caution:** [D, M] DM, bronchospasm; abrupt D/C can exacerbate angina & ↑ MI risk **CI:** Bradycardia, cardiogenic shock, cardiac failure, 2nd-/3rd-degree AV block, sinus node dysfunction, pulm edema **Disp:** Tabs 25, 50, 100 mg; Inj 5 mg/10 mL **SE:** Bradycardia, ↓ BP, 2nd-/3rd-degree AV block, dizziness, fatigue

Interactions: ↑ Effects *W/* other antihypertensives esp diltiazem & verapamil, nitrates, EtOH; ↑ bradycardia *W/* adenosine, digitalis glycosides, dipyridamole, physostigmine, tacrine; ↓ effects *W/* ampicillin, antacids, NSAIDs, salicylates; ↑ effects *OF* lidocaine; ↓ effects *OF* DA, glucagons, insulin, sulfonylureas **Labs:** ↑ ANA titers, BUN, glucose, serum lipoprotein, K⁺, triglyceride, uric acid levels; ↓ HDL **NIPE:** May mask S/sxs hypoglycemia; may ↑ sensitivity to cold; may ↑ depression, wheezing, orthostatic hypotension

Atenolol & Chlorthalidone (Tenoretic) [Antihypertensive, Antianginal/Beta-Blocker & Diuretic] Uses: *HTN* Action: β-Adrenergic blockade w/ diuretic **Dose:** 50–100 mg/d PO based on atenolol; ↓ dose w/ CrCl < 35 mL/min **Caution:** [D, M] DM, bronchospasm **CI:** See Atenolol; anuria, sulfonamide cross-sensitivity **Disp:** *Tenoretic 50:* Atenolol 50 mg/chlorthalidone 25 mg; *Tenoretic 100:* Atenolol 100 mg/chlorthalidone 25 mg **SE:** Bradycardia, ↓ BP, 2nd-/3rd-degree AV block, dizziness, fatigue; see Atenolol **Interactions:** ↑ Effects *W/* other antihypertensives; ↓ effects *W/* cholestyramine, NSAIDs; ↑ effects *OF* Li, digoxin, ↓ effects of sulfonylureas **Labs:** ↑ CPK, serum ammonia, amylase, Ca²⁺, cholesterol, glucose; ↓ serum Cl⁻, Mg²⁺, K⁺, Na⁻ **NIPE:** Take in AM to prevent nocturia, use sunblock > SPF 15, photosensitivity, monitor S/Sxs gout

Atomoxetine (Strattera) [ADHD/Selective Norepinephrine Reuptake Inhibitor] WARNING: Severe liver injury may rarely occur; D/C w/ jaundice or ↑ LFTs, ↑ frequency of suicidal thinking; monitor closely Uses: *ADHD* Action: Selective norepinephrine reuptake Inhib **Dose:** *Adults & children > 70 kg.* 40 mg PO/d, after 3 d minimum, ↑ to 80–100 mg ÷ daily–bid *Peds < 70 kg.* 0.5 mg/kg × 3 d, then ↑ 1.2 mg/kg daily or bid (max 1.4 mg/kg or 100 mg); ↓ dose w/ hepatic Insuff or in combo w/ CYP2D6 Inhibs (Table 10) **Caution:** w/ Known structural cardiac anomalies, cardiac Hx [C, ?/–] **CI:** NAG, w/ or w/in 2 wk of D/C w/ MAOI **Disp:** Caps 5, 10, 18, 25, 40, 60, 80, 100 mg **SE:** HA, insomnia, dry mouth, Abd pain, N/V, anorexia ↑ BP, tachycardia, wgt loss, sexual dysfunction, jaundice **Labs:** ↑ LFTs **NIPE:** AHA rec all children receiving stimulants for ADHD receive CV assessment before therapy initiated; D/C stat w/ jaundice

Atorvastatin (Lipitor) [Antilipemic/HMG-CoA Reductase Inhibitor] Uses: *↑ Cholesterol & triglycerides* Action: HMG-CoA reductase Inhib **Dose:** Initial 10 mg/d, may ↑ to 80 mg/d **Caution:** [X, –] **CI:** Active liver Dz, unexplained ↑ LFTs **Disp:** Tabs 10, 20, 40, 80 mg **SE:** Myopathy, HA, arthralgia, myalgia, GI upset, CP, edema, insomnia dizziness, liver failure **Interactions:** ↑ Effects *W/* azole antifungals, erythromycin, nefazodone, protease Inhibs, grapefruit juice; ↓ effects *W/* antacids, bile acid sequestrants; ↑ effects *OF* digoxin, levothyroxine, OCPs **Labs:** Monitor LFTs; ↑ LFTs, CPK; ↑ lipid levels **NIPE:** Instruct pt to report unusual muscle pain or weakness; ⊘ EtOH, breast-feeding, or while PRG

Atovaquone (Mepron) [Antiprotozoal] Uses: *Rx & prevention PCP & Toxoplasmagondii encephalitis* Action: ↓ Nucleic acid & ATP synth **Dose:** *Rx:* 750 mg PO bid for 21 d *Prevention:* 1500 mg PO once/d (w/ meals) **Caution:** [C, ?]

Disp: Susp 750 mg/5 mL **SE:** Fever, HA, anxiety, insomnia, rash, N/V, cough **Interactions:** ↓ Effects *W/* metoclopramide, rifabutin, rifampin, tetracycline **Labs:** Monitor LFTs w/ long-term use **NIPE:** ↑ Absorption w/ meal esp high-fat meal

Atovaquone/Proguanil (Malarone) [Antimalarial] Uses: *Prevention or Rx *Plasmodium falciparum* malaria* **Action:** Antimalarial **Dose:** *Adults: Prevention:* 1 tab PO 2 d before, during, & 7 d after leaving endemic region; *Rx:* 4 tabs PO single dose daily ×3 d **Peds.** See package insert **Caution:** [C, ?] **CI:** Prophylactic use when CrCl < 30 mL/min **Dose:** Tabs atovaquone 250 mg/proguanil 100 mg; peds atovaquone 62.5 mg/ proguanil 25 mg **SE:** HA, fever, myalgia, N/V **Interactions:** ↓ Effects *W/* metoclopramide, rifabutin, rifampin, tetracycline **Labs:** ↑ LFTs, monitor LFTs w/ long-term use **NIPE:** ↑ Absorption w/ meal esp high-fat meal

Atracurium (Tracrium) [Skeletal Muscle Relaxant/Neuromuscular Blocker] Uses: *Anesthesia adjunct to facilitate ET intubation* **Action:** Non-depolarizing neuromuscular blocker **Dose:** *Adults & Peds > 2 y.* 0.4–0.5 mg/kg IV bolus, then 0.08–0.1 mg/kg q20–45min PRN **Caution:** [C, ?] **Disp:** Inj 10 mg/mL **SE:** Flushing **Interactions:** ↑ Effects *W/* general anesthetics, aminoglycosides, bacitracin, BBs, β-agonists, clindamycin, CCBs, diuretics, lidocaine, Li, MgSO₄, narcotic analgesics, procainamide, quinidine, succinylcholine, trimethaphan, verapamil; ↓ effects *W/* Ca, carbamazepine, phenytoin, theophylline, caffeine **Labs:** Monitor BUN, Cr, LFTs **NIPE:** Drug does not affect consciousness or pain; inability to speak until drug wears off; pt must be intubated & on controlled ventilation; use adequate amounts of sedation & analgesia

Atropine, Benzoic Acid, Hyoscyamine Sulfate, Methenamine, Methylene Blue, Phenyl Salicylate (Urised) [Urinary Tract Analgesic/Antispasmodic/Antiseptic] Uses: *Lower urinary tract discomfort* **Action:** Methenamine in acid urine releases formaldehyde (antiseptic), methylene blue/benzoic acid mild antiseptic, phenyl salicylate mild analgesic, hyoscyamine, & atropine parasympatholytic ↓ muscle spasm **Dose:** *Adults.* 2 tabs PO qid *Peds > 6 y.* Individualize **Caution:** [C, ?/–] **CI:** NAG, pyloric/duodenal obst, BOO, coronary artery spasm **Disp:** Tabs: Atropine 0.03 mg/benzoic acid 4.5 mg/hyoscyamine 0.03 mg/methenamine 40.8 mg/methylene blue 5.4 mg/phenyl salicylate 18.1 mg **SE:** Rash, dry mouth, flushing, ↑ pulse, dizziness, blurred vision, voiding difficulty **Interactions:** Avoid *W/* sulfonamides **Labs:** Interferes w/ colorimetric urine tests **NIPE:** Take w/ plenty of fluid, can cause crystalluria; inform pt about urine/feces discoloration

Atropine, Ophthalmic (Isopto Atropine, Generic) [Antiarrhythmic/Anticholinergic] Uses: *Cycloplegic refraction, uveitis, amblyopia* **Action:** Antimuscarinic; cycloplegic, dilates pupils **Dose:** *Adults. Refraction:* 1–2 gtt 1 h before *Uveitis:* 1–2 gtt daily–qid *Peds.* 1 gtt in nonamblyopic eye daily **Caution:** [C, +] **CI:** NAG, adhesions between iris & lens **Disp:** 2.5- & 15-mL bottle 1% ophthal soln, 1% oint **SE:** Local irritation, burning, blurred vision, light sensitivity **Interactions:** ↑ Effects *W/* amantadine, antihistamines, disopyramide, procainamide, quinidine, TCA, thiazides, betel palm, squaw vine; ↓ effects *W/* antacids, levodopa; ↓ effects *OF* phenothiazines **NIPE:** Compress lacrimal sac 2–3 min after instillation; effects can last 1–2 wk; ↑ risk of photophobia

Atropine, Systemic (AtroPen Auto-Injector) [Antiarrhythmic/ Anticholinergic] WARNING: Primary protection against exposure to chemical nerve agent & insecticide poisoning is the wearing of specially designed protective garments **Uses:** *Preanesthetic; symptomatic bradycardia & asystole, AV block, organophosphate (insecticide) & acetylcholinesterase (nerve gas) Inhib antidote; cycloplegic* **Action:** Antimuscarinic; blocks ACH at parasympathetic sites, cycloplegic **Dose: Adults. ECC 2010: Asystole or PEA:** Routine use for asystole or PEA no longer recommended. *Bradycardia:* 0.5 mg IV q3–5min PRN; max 3 mg or 0.04 mg/kg; ET 2–3 mg in 10 mL NS *Preanesthetic:* 0.3–0.6 mg IM *Poisoning:* 1–2 mg IV bolus, repeat q3–5min PRN to reverse effects **Peds. ECC 2010: Symptomatic bradycardia:** 0.2 mg/kg IV/IO (minium dose 0.1 mg, max single dose 0.5 mg); repeat PRN × 1; max total dose 1 mg child, 3 mg adolescent *Toxins/ OD (Organophosphates):* < 12 y 0.02–0.05 mg/kg IV/IO repeat PRN q20–30 min; > 12 y 2 mg IV/IO then 1–2 mg IV/IO PRN *RSI:* 0.01–0.02 mg/kg IV/IO or 0.02 mg/kg IM (minimum dose 0.1 mg, max 0.5 mg) **Caution:** [C, +] **CI:** NAG, adhesions between iris & lens, tachycardia, GI obst, ileus, severe UC, obstructive uropathy, Mobitz II block **Disp:** Inj 0.05, 0.1, 0.3, 0.4, 0.5, 0.8, 1 mg/mL; AtroPen Auto-Injector: 0.25, 0.5, 1, 2 mg/dose; tabs 0.4 mg, MDI 0.36 mg/Inh **SE:** Flushing, mydriasis, tachycardia, dry mouth & nose, blurred vision, urinary retention, constipation psychosis **Notes:** SLUDGE (Salivation, Lacrimation, Urination, Diaphoresis, Gastrointestinal motility, Emesis) are Sx of organophosphate poisoning; Auto-Injector limited distribution; see also Atropine Opthalmic **Interactions:** ↑ Effects *W/* amantadine, antihistamines, disopyramide, procainamide, quinidine, TCA, thiazides, betel palm, squaw vine; ↓ effects *W/* antacids, levodopa; ↓ effects *OF* phenothiazines **Labs:** ↓ Gastric motility & emptying may affect results of upper GI series **NIPE:** Monitor I&O, ↑ fluids & oral hygiene, wear dark glasses to ↓ photophobia

Atropine/Pralidoxime (DuoDote) [Antiarrhythmic/Anticholinergic/ Antidote] WARNING: For use by personnel w/ appropriate training; wear protective garments; do not rely solely on medication, evacuation, & decontamination ASAP **Uses:** *Nerve agent (tabun, sarin, & others) & insecticide poisoning* **Action:** Atropine blocks effects of excess ACH; pralidoxime reactivates acetylcholinesterase inactivated by poisoning **Dose:** 1 Inj in midlateral thigh; wait 10–15 min for effect; w/ severe Sx give 2 additional Inj; if alert & oriented no additional doses **Caution:** [C, ?] **CI: Disp:** Auto-injector 2.1 mg atropine/600 mg pralidoxime **SE:** Dry mouth, blurred vision, dry eyes, photophobia, confusion, HA, tachycardia, ↑ BP, flushing, urinary retention, constipation, Abd pain N, V, emesis **Interactions:** ↑ Effects *W/* amantadine, antihistamines, disopyramide, procainamide, quinidine, TCA, thiazides, betel palm, squaw vine; ↑ effects *OF* barbiturates; ↓ effects *W/* antacids, levodopa; ↓ effects *OF* phenothiazines **Labs:** ↑ ALT,

AST, Cr **NIPE:** Severe Sx of poisoning: confusion, dyspnea w/ copious secretions, weakness, twitching, involuntary urination & defecation, convulsions, unconsciousness; limited distribution

Azathioprine (Imuran) [Immunosuppressant/Purine Antagonist] WARNING: May ↑ neoplasia w/ chronic use; mutagenic & hematologic tox possible **Uses:** *Adjunct to prevent renal transplant rejection, RA*, SLE, Crohn Dz, UC **Action:** Immunosuppressive; antagonizes purine metabolism **Dose:** *Adults: Crohn & UC:* Start 50 mg/d, ↑ 25 mg/d q1–2wk, target dose 2–3 mg/kg/d *Adults & Peds. Renal transplant:* 3–5 mg/kg/d IV/PO single daily dose, taper by 0.5 mg/kg q4wk to lowest effective dose; RA 1 mg/kg/d once daily k ÷ bid × 6–8 wk, ↑ 0.5 mg/kg/d q4wk to 2.5 mg/kg/d; ↓ w/ renal Insuff **Caution:** [D, ?] **CI:** PRG **Disp:** Tabs, 50, 75, 100 mg; powder for Inj 100 mg **SE:** GI intolerance, fever, chills, leukopenia, thrombocytopenia **Interactions:** ↑ Effects W/ allopurinol; ↓ effects OF antineoplastic drugs, cyclosporine, myelosuppressive drugs, MTX; ↑ risk of severe leucopenia W/ ACEI; ↓ effects OF nondepolarizing neuromuscular blocking drugs, warfarin **Labs:** Monitor BUN, Cr, CBC, LFTs during therapy **NIPE:** Handle Inj w/ cytotoxic precautions; do not administer live vaccines on drug; dose per local transplant protocol, usually start 1–3 d pretransplant; ⊘ PRG, breast-feeding

Azelastine (Astelin, Astepro, Optivar) [Antihistamine/H₁-Receptor Antagonist] Uses: *Allergic rhinitis (rhinorrhea, sneezing, nasal pruritus); vasomotor rhinitis; allergic conjunctivitis* **Action:** Histamine H₁-receptor antagonist **Dose:** *Adults & Peds > 12 y. Nasal:* 1–2 sprays/nostril bid *Ophthal:* 1 gtt in each affected eye bid *Peds 5–11 y.* 1 spray/nostril 1× d **Caution:** [C, ?/–] **CI:** Component sensitivity **Disp:** Nasal 137 mcg/spray; ophthal soln 0.05% **SE:** Somnolence, bitter taste, HA, cold Sx (rhinitis, cough) **Interactions:** ↑ Effects W/ cimetidine; ↑ effects OF EtOH, CNS depressants **Labs:** ↑ AST, ↓ skin Rxns to antigen skin tests **NIPE:** Systemically absorbed; clear nares before administration; prime pump before use

Azilsartan medoxomil (Edarbi) [Angiotensin II receptor blocker] Uses: antihypertensive; **Action:** ARB ; **Dose:** 80 mg qd, 40 mg qd for pts treated with high doses of diuretics; **Caution:** [C (1st tri), D (2nd & 3rd tri), –] w/ severe CHF; w/ renal artery stenosis; **Disp:** Tabs 40 mg, 80 mg.; **SE:** D, N, dizziness, fatigue, muscle spasm, cough **Interactions:** ↑ risk of renal toxicity W/ NSAIDS, COX-2 inhibitors **Labs:** Monitor Serum Cr esp in elderly and volume depleted pts **NIPE:** If pt salt/volume depleted, correct before starting drug; may be used alone or in combination with other antihypertensives

Azithromycin (Zithromax) [Antibiotic/Macrolide] Uses: *Community-acquired pneumonia, pharyngitis, otitis media, skin Infxns, nongonococcal (chlamydial) urethritis, chancroid & PID; Rx & prevention of MAC in HIV** **Action:** Macrolide antibiotic; bacteriostatic; ↓ protein synth *Spectrum: Chlamydia, H ducreyi, H influenzae, Legionella, Mcatarrhalis, M pneumoniae, M hominis, N gonorrhoeae, S aureus, S agalactiae, S pneumoniae, S pyogenes* **Dose:** *Adults. Resp tract Infxns:*

PO: Caps 500 mg/d 1, then 250 mg/d PO × 4 d; *sinusitis* 500 mg/d PO × 3 d; *IV:* 500 mg × 2 d, then 500 mg PO × 7–10 d or 500 mg IV daily × 2 d, then 500 mg/d PO × 7–10 d *Nongonococcal urethritis:* 1 g PO × 1 *GC, uncomp:* 2 g PO × 1 *Prevent MAC:* 1200 mg PO once/wk *Peds. Otitis media:* 10 mg/kg PO day 1, then 5 mg/kg/d days 2–5 *Pharyngitis:* 12 mg/kg/d PO × 5 d; take susp on empty stomach; tabs OK w/ or w/o food; ↓ w/ CrCl < 10 mL/min **Caution:** [B, +] **Disp:** Tabs 250, 500, 600 mg; Z-Pack (5 d, 250 mg); Tri-Pak (500-mg tabs × 3); susp 1 g; single-dose packet (ZMAX) ER susp. (2 g); susp 100, 200 mg/5 mL; Inj powder 500 mg; 2.5 mL ophthal soln 1% **SE:** GI upset, metallic taste **Interactions:** ↓ Effects *W/* Al- & Mg-containing antacids, atovaquone, food (suspension); ↑ effects *OF* alfentanil, barbiturates, bromocriptine, carbamazepine, cyclosporine, digoxin, dysopyramide, ergot alkaloids, phenytoin, pimozide, terfenadine, theophylline, triazolam, warfarin; ↓ effects *OF* penicillins **Labs:** May ↑ serum bilirubin, alk phos, BUN, Cr, CPK, glucose, K+, LFTs, LDH, PT; may ↓ WBC, plt count, serum folate **NIPE:** Monitor S/Sxs super Infxns; use sunscreen & protective clothing

Azithromycin Ophthalmic 1% (AzaSite) [Antibiotic/Macrolide]
Uses: *Bacterial conjunctivitis* **Adults.** 1 gtt bid, q8–12 h × 2 d, then 1 gtt qd × 5 d. *Peds = 1 y.* 1 gtt bid, q8–12h × 2 d , then 1 gtt qd × 5 d. **Caution:** [B, +/–] **CI:** None **Disp:** 1% in 2.5 mL bottle **SE:** Irritation, burning, stinging, contact dermatitis, corneal erosion, dry eye, dysgeusia, nasal congestion, sinusitis, ocular discharge, keratitis **NIPE:** Avoid contact w/ use

Aztreonam (Azactam) [Antibiotic/Monobactam]
Uses: *Aerobic gram(−)* UTIs, lower resp, intra-Abd, skin, gynecologic Infxns & septicemia* **Action:** Monobactam; ↓ cell wall synth. *Spectrum:* Gram(−) (*Pseudomonas, E coli, Klebsiella, H influenzae, Serratia, Proteus, Enterobacter, Citrobacter*) **Dose:** **Adults.** 1–2 g IV/IM q6–8h *UTI:* 500 mg–1 g IV q8–12h *Meningitis:* 2 g IV q6–8h **Peds.** *Premature:* 30 mg/kg/dose IV q12h *Term & children:* 30 mg/kg/dose q6–8h; ↓ in renal impair **Caution:** [B, +] **Disp:** Inj (soln), 1, 2 g/50 mL Inj powder for recons 500 mg, 1, 2 g **SE:** N/V/D, rash, pain at Inj site **Interactions:** ↑ Effects *W/* probenecid, aminoglycosides, β-lactam antibiotics; ↓ effects *W/* cefoxitin, chloramphenicol, imipenem **Labs:** ↑ LFTs, alk phos, SCr, PT, PTT, & (+)direct Coombs test **NIPE:** No gram(+) or anaerobic activity; OK in PCN-allergic pts; monitor S/Sxs super Infxn; taste changes w/ IV administration

Aztreonam, Inhaled (Cayston) [Monobactam]
Uses: *Improve resp Sx in CF pts w/ P aeruginosa* **Action:** Monobactam; ↓ Cell wall synth **Dose:** **Adults & Peds ≥ 7 y.** 1 dose 3 × d 28 d (space doses q4h) **Caution:** [B, +] w/ β-lactam allergy **CI:** Allergy to aztreonam **Disp:** Lyophilized aztreonam w/NaCl **SE:** Allergic Rxn, bronchospasm, cough, nasal congestion, wheezing, pharyngolaryngeal pain, V, Abd pain, chest discomfort, pyrexia, rash **NIPE:** Use stat after reconstitution, use only w/ Altera nebulizer system; bronchodilator prior to use

Bacitracin, Ophthalmic (AK-Tracin Ophthalmic); Bacitracin & Polymyxin B, Ophthalmic (AK Poly Bac Ophthalmic, Polysporin

Ophthalmic); Bacitracin, Neomycin, & Polymyxin B, Ophthalmic (AK Spore Ophthalmic, Neosporin Ophthalmic); Bacitracin, Neomycin, Polymyxin B, & Hydrocortisone, Ophthalmic (AK Spore HC Ophthalmic, Cortisporin Ophthalmic) [Antibiotic/Anti-Inflammatory] Uses: *Steroid-responsive inflammatory ocular conditions* **Action:** Topical antibiotic w/ anti-inflammatory **Dose:** Apply q3–4h into conjunctival sac **Caution:** [C, ?] **CI:** Viral, mycobacterial, fungal eye Infxn **Disp:** See Bacitracin, Topical equivalents, next **Interactions:** ↑ Effects **W/** neuromuscular blocking agents, anesthetics, nephrotoxic drugs **NIPE:** May cause blurred vision

Bacitracin, Topical (Baciguent); Bacitracin & Polymyxin B, Topical (Polysporin); Bacitracin, Neomycin, & Polymyxin B, Topical (Neosporin); Bacitracin, Neomycin, Polymyxin B, & Hydrocortisone, Topical (Cortisporin); Bacitracin, Neomycin, Polymyxin B, & Lidocaine, Topical (Clomycin) [Antibiotic/Anti-Inflammatory/Analgesic] Uses: Prevent/Rx of *minor skin Infxns* **Action:** Topical antibiotic w/ added components (anti-inflammatory & analgesic) **Dose:** Apply sparingly bid–qid **Caution:** [C, ?] Not for deep wounds, puncture, or animal bites **Disp:** Bacitracin 500 units/g oint; bacitracin 500 units/polymyxin B sulfate 10,000 units/g oint & powder; bacitracin 400 units/neomycin 3.5 mg/polymyxin B 5000 units/g oint; bacitracin 400 units/neomycin 3.5 mg/polymyxin B 5000 units/hydrocortisone 10 mg/g oint; bacitracin 500 units/neomycin 3.5 mg/polymyxin B 5000 units/lidocaine 40 mg/g oint **NIPE:** Ophthal, systemic, & irrigation forms available, not generally used d/t potential tox

Baclofen (Lioresal Intrathecal, Generic) [Antispasmodic/Skeletal Muscle Relaxant] **WARNING:** If abrupt discontinuation can lead to organ failure, rhabdomyolysis, & death **Uses:** *Spasticity d/t severe chronic disorders (eg, MS, amyotrophic lateral sclerosis, or spinal cord lesions)*, trigeminal neuralgia, intractable hiccups **Action:** Centrally acting skeletal muscle relaxant; ↓ transmission of monosynaptic & polysynaptic cord reflexes **Dose:** Adults. Initial, 5 mg PO tid; ↑ q3d to effect; max 80 mg/d. IT: Via implantable pump (see package insert) **Peds 2–7 y.** 10–15 mg/d ÷ q8h; titrate, max 40 mg/d > 8 y. max 60 mg/d IT: Via implantable pump (see package insert); ↓ in renal impair; take w/ food or milk **Caution:** [C, +] Epilepsy, neuropsychological disturbances **Disp:** Tabs 10, 20 mg; IT Inj 50 mcg/mL, 10 mg/5 mL, 10 mg/20 mL **SE:** Dizziness, drowsiness, insomnia, ataxia, weakness, ↓ BP **Interactions:** ↑ CNS depression **W/** CNS depressants, MAOIs, EtOH, antihistamines, opioid analgesics, sedatives, hypnotics; ↑ effects **OF** antihypertensives, clindamycin, guanabenz; ↑ risk of resp paralysis & renal failure **W/** aminoglycosides **Labs:** ↑ Serum glucose, AST, ammonia, alk phos; ↓ bilirubin **NIPE:** Take oral meds w/ food; ⊘ EtOH

Balsalazide (Colazal) [Anti-Inflammatory/GI Drug] Uses: *UC* **Action:** 5-ASA derivative, anti-inflammatory, ↓ leukotriene synth **Dose:** 2.25 g (3 caps) tid × 8–12 wk **Caution:** [B, ?] Severe renal failure **CI:** Mesalamine or salicylate hypersensitivity **Disp:** Caps 750 mg **SE:** Dizziness, HA, N, Abd pain, agranulocytosis, renal impair, allergic Rxns **Notes:** Daily dose of 6.75 g = 2.4 g mesalamine **Interactions:** Oral antibiotics may interfere W/ mesalamine release in the colon **Labs:** ↑ Bilirubin, CPK, LFTs, LDH **NIPE:** ✓ If ASA allergy; take w/ food & swallow caps whole

Basiliximab (Simulect) [Immunosuppressant/Monoclonal Antibody]
WARNING: Administer only under the supervision of a physician experienced in immunosuppression therapy in an appropriate facility **Uses:** *Prevent acute transplant rejection* **Action:** IL-2 receptor antagonists **Dose:** *Adults & Peds > 35 kg.* 20 mg IV 2 h before transplant, then 20 mg IV 4 d posttransplant. *Peds < 35 kg.* 10 mg 2 h prior to transplant; same dose IV 4 d posttransplant **Caution:** [B, ?/–] **CI:** Hypersensitivity to murine proteins **Disp:** Inj powder 10, 20 mg **SE:** Edema, HTN, HA, dizziness, fever, pain, Infxn, GI effects, lytes disturbances **Notes:** A murine/ human MoAb **Interactions:** May ↑ immunosuppression W/ other immunosuppressive drugs **Labs:** ↑ Cholesterol, BUN, Cr, lipids, uric acid; ↓ serum Mg phosphate, plts, Hgb, Hct, Ca²⁺, ↑ or ↓ glucose, K⁺ **NIPE:** Monitor for Infxns—hypersensitivity Rxns—can occur up to 24 h following administration, IV dose over 20–30 min

BCG [Bacillus Calmette-Guérin] (TheraCys, Tice BCG) [Antineoplastic, Antituberculotic] **WARNING:** Contains live, attenuated mycobacteria; risk for transmission; handle as a biohazard; nosocomial Infxns reported in immunosuppressed; fatal Rxns reported **Uses:** *Bladder CA (superficial)*, TB prophylaxis **Action:** Attenuated live BCG culture, immunomodulator **Dose:** *Bladder CA:* 1 vial prepared & instilled in bladder for 2 h; repeat once/wk × 6 wk; then 1 Tx at 3, 6, 12, 18, & 24 mo after **Caution:** [C, ?] Asthma **CI:** Immunocompromised, steroid use, febrile illness, UTI, gross hematuria, w/ traumatic catheterization or UTI **Disp:** Powder for recons 81 mg (10.5 ± 8.7 × 108 CFU vial) (TheraCys), 50 mg (1–8 × 10⁸ CFU/vial) (Tice BCG) **SE:** *Intravesical:* Hematuria, urinary frequency, dysuria, bacterial UTI, rare BCG sepsis **Interactions:** ↓ Effects W/ antimicrobials, immunosuppressives, radiation **Labs:** Prior BCG may cause false(+) PPD **NIPE:** PPD is not contra in BCG vaccinated persons; monitor for S/Sxs systemic Infxn, report persistent pain on urination or blood in urine; routine US adult BCG immunization not recommended. Use for children who are PPD(–) & continually exposed to untreated/ineffectively treated adults or whose TB strain is INH/ rifampin resistant. Used for healthcare workers in high-risk environments; intravesical use, dispose/void in toilet w/ chlorine bleach

Becaplermin (Regranex Gel) [Growth Factor] **WARNING:** ↑ Mortality d/t malignancy reported; use w/ caution in known malignancy **Uses:** Local wound care adjunct w/ *diabetic foot ulcers* **Action:** Recombinant PDGF, enhances granulation tissue **Dose:** *Adults.* Based on lesion: calculate the length of gel, measure the greatest length of ulcer by the greatest width; tube size & measured result determine the formula used in the calculation. Recalculate q1–2wk based on change in lesion size *15-g tube:* (length × width) × 0.6 = length of gel (in inches) or for *2-g tube:* (length × width) × 1.3 = length of gel (in inches); rinse after 12 h; do not reapply w/in 24 h; repeat in 12 h *Peds.* See package insert **Caution:** [C, ?] **CI:** Neoplasmatic site **Disp:** 0.01% gel in 2-, 15-g tubes **SE:** Rash **Interactions:** None known **NIPE:** Dosage recalculated q1–2wk; Use w/ good wound care; wound must be vascularized; reassess after 10 wk if ulcer not ↓ by 30% or not healed by 20 wk

Beclomethasone (QVAR) [Antiasthmatic/Synthetic Corticosteroid]
Uses: Chronic *asthma* **Action:** Inhaled corticosteroid **Dose:** *Adults & Peds 5–11 y.* 40–160 mcg 1–4 Inh bid; initial 40–80 mcg Inh bid if on bronchodilators alone; 40–160 mcg w/ other inhaled steroids; 320 mcg bid max; taper to lowest effective dose bid; rinse mouth/throat after **Caution:** [C, ?] **CI:** Acute asthma **Disp:** PO metered-dose inhaler; 40, 80 mcg/Inh **SE:** HA, cough, hoarseness, oral candidiasis **Interactions:** None noted **NIPE:** Use inhaled bronchodilator prior to inhaled steroid, rinse mouth after inhaled steroid; not effective for acute asthma; effect in 1–2 d or as long as 2 wk

Beclomethasone Nasal (Beconase AQ) [Anti-Inflammatory/ Corticosteroid] **Uses:** *Allergic rhinitis* refractory to antihistamines & decongestants; *nasal polyps* **Action:** Inhaled steroid **Dose:** *Adults & Peds. Aqueous inhaler:* 1–2 sprays/nostril bid **Caution:** [C, ?] **Disp:** Nasal metered-dose inhaler 42 mcg/spray **SE:** Local irritation, burning, epistaxis **Interactions:** None noted **NIPE:** Prior use of decongestant nasal gtt if edema or secretions, may take several days for full steroid effect

Belladonna & Opium Suppositories (B&O Suppretes) [C-II] [Antispasmodic, Analgesic] **Uses:** *Bladder spasms; mod/severe pain* **Action:** Antispasmodic, analgesic **Dose:** 1 supp PR q6h PRN **Caution:** [C, ?] **CI:** Glaucoma, resp depression **Disp:** 15A = 30 mg opium/16.2 mg belladonna extract; 16A = 60 mg opium/16.2 mg belladonna extract **SE:** Anticholinergic (eg, sedation, urinary retention, constipation) **Interactions:** ↑ Effects *W/* CNS depressants, TCAs; ↓ effects *W/* phenothiazine **Labs:** ↑ LFTs **NIPE:** ⊘ Refrigerate; moisten finger & supp before insertion; may cause blurred vision

Benazepril (Lotensin) [Antihypertensive/ACEI] **Uses:** *HTN*, DN, CHF **Action:** ACE Inhib **Dose:** 10–80 mg/d PO **Caution:** [C (1st tri), D (2nd & 3rd tri), +] **CI:** Angioedema, h/o edema, bilateral RAS **Disp:** Tabs 5, 10, 20, 40 mg **SE:** Symptomatic ↓ BP w/ diuretics; dizziness, HA, ↑ K+, nonproductive cough **Interactions:** ↑ Effects *W/* α-blockers, diuretics, capsaicin; ↓ effects *W/* NSAIDs, ASA; ↑ effects *OF* insulin, Li; ↑ risk of hyperkalemia *W/* TMP & K+-sparing diuretics **Labs:** ↑ BUN, SCr, K+; ↓ Hgb; monitor ECG for signs of hyperkalemia (peaked T waves) **NIPE:** Persistent cough and/or taste changes may develop; ⊘ PRG, D/C if angioedema

Bendamustine (Treanda) [Alkylating Agent] **Uses:** *CLL* **Action:** Mechlorethamine derivative; alkylating agent **Dose:** *Adults.* 100 mg/m² IV over 30 min days 1 & 2 of 28-d cycle, up to 6 cycles (w/ tox see package insert for dose changes; do not use w/ CrCl < 40 mL/min, severe hepatic impair) **Caution:** [D, ?/−] **CI:** Hypersensitivity to bendamustine or mannitol **Disp:** Inj powder 100 mg **SE:** Pyrexia, N/V, dry mouth, fatigue, cough, stomatitis, rash, myelosuppression, Infxns, Inf Rxns & anaphylaxis, tumor lysis synd, skin Rxns **Interactions:** ↑ Effects *W/* CYP1A2 Inhibs; ↓ effects *W/* CYP1A2 inducers **Labs:** ↑ LFTs **NIPE:** Consider use of allopurinol to prevent tumor lysis synd; ⊘ PRG or breast-feeding

Benzocaine (Americaine, Hurricane Lanacaine, Aarious) [OTC Topical Anesthetic] **Uses:** *Topical anesthetic, lubricant on ET tubes, catheters, etc; pain relief in external otitis, cerumen removal, skin conditions, sunburn, insect bites, mouth & gum irritation, hemorrhoids* **Action:** Topical local anesthetic **Dose:** *Adults & Peds > 1 y.* Anesthetic lubricant: Apply evenly to tube/instrument *Cerumen removal:* Instill 3× d for 2–3 d *Otic drops:* 4–5 gtt in external canal, insert cotton plug, repeat q1–2h PRN; other uses per manufacturer instructions **Caution:** [C, −] Do not use on broken skin; see provider if condition does not respond; avoid in infants & those w/ pulm Dzs **Disp:** Many site-specific OTC forms creams, gels, Liq, sprays, 2–20% **SE:** Itching, irritation, burning, edema, erythema, pruritus, rash, stinging, tenderness, urticaria; methemoglobinemia (infants or in COPD) **NIPE:** Use minimum amount to obtain effect; methemoglobinemia S/Sxs: HA, lightheadedness, SOB, anxiety, fatigue, pale, gray or blue-colored skin, & tachycardia; treat w/ IV methylene blue

Benzocaine & Antipyrine (Auralgan) [Otic Anesthetic] **Uses:** *Analgesia in severe otitis media* **Action:** Anesthetic w/ local decongestant **Dose:** Fill ear & insert a moist cotton plug; repeat 1–2 h PRN **Caution:** [C, ?] **CI:** w/ perforated eardrum **Disp:** Soln 5.4% antipyrine, 1.4% benzocaine **SE:** Local irritation **Interactions:** May ↓ Effects *OF* sulfonamides

Benzonatate (Tessalon Perles) [Antitussive] **Uses:** Symptomatic relief of *cough* **Action:** Anesthetizes the stretch receptors in the resp passages **Dose:** *Adults & Peds > 10 y.* 100 mg PO tid (max 600 mg/d) **Caution:** [C, ?] **Disp:** Caps 100, 200 mg **SE:** Sedation, dizziness, GI upset **Interactions:** ↑ CNS depression *W/* antihistamines, EtOH, hypnotics, opioids, sedatives **NIPE:** ↑ Fluid intake to liquefy secretions; do not chew or puncture the caps

Benztropine (Cogentin) [Antiparkinsonian/Anticholinergic] **Uses:** *Parkinsonism & drug-induced extrapyramidal disorders* **Action:** Partially blocks striatal cholinergic receptors **Dose:** *Adults. Parkinsonism:* Initial 0.5–1 mg PO/IM/IV qhs, ↑ q5–6d PRN by 0.5 mg, usual dose 1–2 mg, 6 mg/d max *Extrapyramidal:* 1–4 mg PO/IV/IM qd–bid *Acute dystonia:* 1–2 mg IM/IV, then 1–2 mg PO bid *Peds > 3 y.* 0.02–0.05 mg/kg/dose 1–2/d **Caution:** [C, ?] w/ urinary Sxs, NAG, hot environments, CNS or mental disorders, other phenothiazines or TCA **CI:** < 3 y **Disp:** Tabs 0.5, 1, 2 mg; Inj 1 mg/mL **SE:** Anticholinergic (tachycardia, ileus, N/V, etc), anhidrosis, heat stroke **Notes:** Physostigmine 1–2 mg SQ/IV to reverse severe Sxs **Interactions:** ↑ Sedation & depressant effects *W/* EtOH & CNS depressants; ↑ anticholinergic effects *W/* antihistamine, phenothiazine, quinidine, disopyramide,

TCAs, MAOIs; ↑ effect *OF* digoxin; ↓ effect *OF* levodopa; ↓ effects *W/* antacids & antidiarrheal drugs **NIPE:** May ↑ susceptibility to heat stroke, take w/ meals to avoid GI upset

Benzyl Alcohol (Ulesfia) [Pediculicide] Uses: *Head lice* **Action:** pediculicide **Dose:** < 6 mo. Not recommended > 6 mo. Apply w/ for hair length to dry hair; saturate the scalp; leave on 10 min; rinse w/ H_2O; repeat in 7 d *Hair length 0–2 in:* 4–6 oz *2–4 in:* 6–8 oz *4–8 in:* 8–12 oz *8–16 in:* 12–24 oz *16–22 in:* 24–32 oz *> 22 in:* 32–48 oz **Caution:** [B, ?] Avoid eyes **Contra:** None **Disp:** 5% lotion 4, 8 oz bottles **SE:** Pruritus, erythema, irritation (local, eyes) **NIPE:** Use fine-tooth/ nit comb to remove nits & dead lice; avoid contact w/ eyes; wash hands after application; does not have ovicidal activity

Bepotastine Besilate (Bepreve) [Antihistamine/Mast Cell Stabilizer] Uses: *Allergic conjunctivitis* **Action:** H_1-receptor antagonist **Dose:** *Adults.* 1 gtt into affected eye(s) bid **Caution:** [C, ?/?] **Disp:** Soln 1.5% **SE:** Mild taste, eye irritation, HA, nasopharyngitis **NIPE:** Do not use while wearing contacts, reinsert 10 min > dosing if eye not red

Beractant (Survanta) [Lung Surfactant] Uses: *Prevention & Rx of RDS in premature infants* **Action:** Replaces pulm surfactant **Dose:** 100 mg/kg via ET tube; repeat 3 × q6h PRN; max 4 doses/48 h **Disp:** Susp 25 mg of phospholipid/mL **SE:** Transient bradycardia, desaturation, apnea **Notes:** Administer via 4-quadrant method **Interactions:** None noted **NIPE:** ↑ Risk of nosocomial sepsis after Rx w/ this drug

Besifloxacin (Besivance) [Antibiotic/Quinolone] Uses: *Bacterial conjunctivitis* **Action:** Inhibits DNA gyrase & topoisomerase IV **Dose:** *Adults & Peds > 1 y.* 1 gtt into eye(s) tid 4–12 h apart × 7 d **Caution:** [C, ?] Remove contacts during Tx **Contra:** None **Disp:** 0.6% susp **SE:** HA, redness, blurred vision, irritation, HA, super Infxn **NIPE:** ⊘ Wear contact lenses during therapy or if symptomatic

Betaxolol (Kerlone) [Antihypertensive/Beta-Blocker] Uses: *HTN* **Action:** Competitively blocks β-adrenergic receptors, $β_1$ **Caution:** [C (1st tri), D (2nd/3rd tri), +/–] **CI:** Sinus bradycardia, AV conduction abnormalities, uncompensated cardiac failure **Dose:** 5–20 mg/d **Disp:** Tabs 10, 20 mg **SE:** Dizziness, HA, bradycardia, edema, CHF **Interactions:** ↑ Effects *W/* anticholinergics, verapamil, general anesthetics; ↓ effects *W/* thyroid drugs, amphetamine, cocaine, ephedrine, epinephrine, norepinephrine, phenylephrine, pseudoephedrine, NSAIDs; ↑ effects *OF* insulin, digitalis glycosides; ↓ effects *OF* theophylline, DA, glucagon **Labs:** ↑ BUN, serum lipoprotein, glucose, K^+, triglyceride, uric acid, ANA titers **NIPE:** May ↑ sensitivity to cold, ⊘ D/C abruptly

Betaxolol, Ophthalmic (Betoptic) [Beta-Blocker] Uses: Open-angle glaucoma **Action:** Competitively blocks β-adrenergic receptors **Dose:** 1–2 gtt bid **Caution:** [C (1st tri), D (2nd/3rd tri), ?/–] **Disp:** Soln 0.5%; susp 0.25% **SE:** Local irritation, photophobia; see Betaxolol **Additional NIPE:** Use sunglasses to ↓ exposure; may cause photophobia, review installation procedures

Bethanechol (Duvoid, Urecholine, Others) [Urinary Tract Stimulant/ Cholinergic Agonist] Uses: *Acute post-op/postpartum nonobstructive urinary retention; neurogenic bladder w/ retention* **Action:** Stimulates cholinergic smooth muscle in bladder & GI tract **Dose:** *Adults.* Initial 5–10 mg then repeat qh until response or 50 mg, typical 10–50 mg tid–qid, 200 mg/d max tid–qid; 2.5–5 mg SQ tid–qid & PRN *Peds.* 0.3–0.6 mg/kg/24 h PO ÷ tid–qid or 0.15–2 mg/kg/d SQ ÷ 3–4 doses; take on empty stomach **Caution:** [C, –] **CI:** BOO, PUD, epilepsy, hyperthyroidism, bradycardia, COPD, AV conduction defects, Parkinsonism, ↓ BP, vasomotor instability **Disp:** Tabs 5, 10, 25, 50 mg; Inj 5 mg/mL **SE:** Abd cramps, D, salivation, ↓ BP **Interactions:** ↑ Effects *W/* BBs, tacrine, cholinesterase Inhibs; ↓ effects *W/* atropine, anticholinergic drugs, procainamide, quinidine, epinephrine **Labs:** ↑ In serum AST, ALT, amylase, lipase, bilirubin **NIPE:** Do not use IM/IV; may cause blurred vision; monitor I&O; take on an empty stomach

Bevacizumab (Avastin) [Antineoplastic/Monoclonal Antibody] WARNING: Associated w/ GI perforation, wound dehiscence, & fatal hemoptysis **Uses:** *Met colorectal CA w/ 5-FU, NSCLC w/ paclitaxel & carboplatin; met RCC w/ IFN-α* **Action:** VE GF Inhib **Dose:** *Adults. Colon:* 5 mg/kg or 10 mg/kg IV q14d *NSCLC:* 15 mg/kg q21d; 1st dose over 90 min; 2nd over 60 min, 3rd over 30 min if tolerated *RCC:* 10 mg/kg IV q2wk w/ IFN-α **Caution:** [C, –] Do not use w/in 28 d of surgery if time for separation of drug & anticipated surgical procedures is unknown; D/C w/ serious adverse effects **CI:** Serious hemorrhage or hemoptysis **Disp:** 100 mg/4 mL, 400 mg/16 mL vials **SE:** Wound dehiscence, GI perforation, tracheoesophageal fistula, arterial thrombosis, hemoptysis, hemorrhage, HTN, proteinuria, CHF, Inf Rxns, D, leucopenia **Labs:** Monitor for ↑ proteinuria **NIPE:** Monitor for ↑ BP

Bicalutamide (Casodex) [Antineoplastic/Nonsteroidal Antiandrogen] Uses: *Advanced PCa w/ GnRH agonists (eg, leuprolide, goserelin)* **Action:** Nonsteroidal antiandrogen **Dose:** 50 mg/d **Caution:** [X, ?] **CI:** Women **Disp:** Caps 50 mg **SE:** Hot flashes, loss of libido, impotence, D/N/V, gynecomastia **Interactions:** ↑ Effects *OF* anticoagulants, TCAs, phenothiazides; ↓ effects *OF* antipsychotic drugs **Labs:** ↑ LFTs, alk phos, bilirubin, BUN, Cr; ↓ Hgb, WBCs **NIPE:** Monitor PSA, may experience hair loss

Bicarbonate (See Sodium Bicarbonate)

Bisacodyl (Dulcolax) [OTC] [Stimulant Laxative] Uses: *Constipation; pre-op bowel prep* **Action:** Stimulates peristalsis **Dose:** *Adults.* 5–15 mg PO or 10 mg PR PRN *Peds < 2 y.* 5 mg PO or 10 mg PR PRN *> 2 y.* 5 mg PO or 10 mg PR PRN (do not chew tabs or give w/in 1 h of antacids or milk) **Caution:** [C, ?] **CI:** Acute Abd or bowel obst, appendicitis, gastroenteritis **Disp:** EC tabs 5 mg; tabs 5 mg; supp 10 mg, enema soln 10 mg/30 mL **SE:** Abd cramps, proctitis, & inflammation w/ suppositories **Interactions:** Antacids & milk ↑ dissolution of EC causing Abd irritation **Labs:** ↑ Phosphate, Na; ↓ Ca, Mg, K⁺ **NIPE:** ↑ Fluid intake & high-fiber foods, ⊘ take w/ milk or antacids

Bismuth Subcitrate/Metronidazole/Tetracycline (Pylera) [Antibacterial/Antiprotozoal] WARNING: Metronidazole possibly carcinogenic based on animal studies Uses: *H pylori Infxn w/ omeprazole* Action: Eradicates H pylori Dose: 3 caps qid w/ omeprazole 20 mg bid for 10 d Caution: [D, –] CI: PRG, peds < 8 y (tetracycline-induced teeth discoloration), w/ renal/hepatic impair, component hypersensitivity Disp: Caps w/ 140 mg bismuth subcitrate potassium, 125 mg metronidazole, & 125 mg tetracycline hydrochloride SE: Stool abnormality, D, dyspepsia, Abd pain, HA, flu-like synd, taste perversion, vaginitis, dizziness Interactions: See multiple drug interactions for each component Labs: ↓ Neutrophils, WBC NIPE: EtOH use may cause disulfiram-like Rxn; possible occurrence of metallic taste & reddish-brown urine; take w/ food; see SE for each component

Bismuth Subsalicylate (Pepto-Bismol) [Antidiarrheal/Adsorbent] [OTC] Uses: Indigestion, N, & *D*; combo for Rx of *H pylori Infxn* Action: Antisecretory & anti-inflammatory Dose: **Adults.** 2 tabs or 30 mL PO PRN (max 8 doses/24 h) **Peds** (all max 8 doses/24 h) *3–6 y.* 1/3 tabs or 5 mL PO PRN *6–9 y.* 2/3 tabs or 10 mL PO PRN *9–12 y.* 1 tab or 15 mL PO PRN Caution: [C, D (3rd tri), –] Avoid w/ renal failure; h/o severe GI bleed CI: Influenza or chickenpox (↑ risk of Reye synd), ASA allergy (see Aspirin) Disp: Chew tabs; caplets 262 mg; Liq 262, 525 mg/15 mL; susp 262 mg/15 mL SE: May turn tongue & stools black Interactions: ↑ Effects *OF* ASA, MTX, valproic acid; ↓ effects *OF* tetracyclines; ↓ effects *W/* corticosteroids, probenecid Labs: ↑ Lipid levels; may interfere w/ GI tract x-rays NIPE: Chew tabs, ⊘ swallow whole; may darken tongue & stool to black

Bisoprolol (Zebeta) [Antihypertensive/Beta-Blocker] Uses: *HTN* Action: Competitively blocks β_1-adrenergic receptors Dose: 2.5–10 mg/d (max dose 20 mg/d); ↓ w/ renal impair Caution: [C (1st tri), D (2nd & 3rd tri), +/–] CI: Sinus bradycardia, AV conduction abnormalities, uncompensated cardiac failure Disp: Tabs 5, 10 mg SE: Fatigue, lethargy, HA, bradycardia, edema, CHF Notes: Not dialyzed Interactions: ↑ Bradycardia *W/* adenosine, amiodarone, digoxin, dipyridamole, neostigmine, physostigmine, tacrine; ↑ effects *W/* cimetidine, fluoxetine, prazosin; ↓ effects *W/* NSAIDs, rifampin; ↓ effects *OF* theophylline, glucagon Labs: ↑ Alk phos, BUN, cholesterol, glucose, K+, triglycerides, uric acid NIPE: ⊘ D/C abruptly, may mask S/Sxs hypoglycemia, take w/o regard to food

Bivalirudin (Angiomax) [Anticoagulant/Direct Thrombin Inhibitor] 0020aa Uses: *Anticoagulant w/ ASA in unstable angina undergoing PTCA, PCI, or in pts undergoing PCI w/ or at risk of HIT/HITTS* Action: Anticoagulant, thrombin Inhib Dose: 0.75 mg/kg IV bolus, then 1.75 mg/kg/h for duration of procedure & up to 4 h postprocedure; ✓ ACT 5 min after bolus, may repeat 0.3 mg/kg bolus if necessary (give w/ ASA 300–325 mg/d; start pre-PTCA) Caution: [B, ?] CI: Major bleeding Disp: Powder 250 mg for Inj SE: Bleeding, back pain, N, HA Interactions: ↑ Risk of bleeding *W/* heparin, warfarin, oral anticoagulants Labs: ↑ PT, PTT NIPE: Monitor venipuncture site for bleeding; instruct pt to watch for bleeding, bruising, or tarry stool

Bleomycin Sulfate (Blenoxane) [Antineoplastic/Antibiotic] Uses: *Testis CA; Hodgkin Dz & NHLs; cutaneous lymphomas; & squamous cell CA (head & neck, larynx, cervix, skin, penis); malignant PE sclerosing agent* **Action:** Induces DNA breakage (scission) **Dose:** (Per protocols); ↓ w/ renal impair **Caution:** [D, ?] **CI:** Severe pulm Dz (pulm fibrosis) **Disp:** Powder (Inj) 15, 30 units **SE:** Hyperpigmentation & allergy (rash to anaphylaxis); fever in 50%; lung tox (idiosyncratic & dose related); pneumonitis w/ fibrosis; Raynaud phenomenon, N/V **Notes:** Test dose 1 units, esp in lymphoma pts; lung tox w/ total dose > 400 units or single dose > 30 units; avoid high FiO₂ in general anesthesia to ↓ tox **Interactions:** ↑ Effects *W/* cisplatin & other antineoplastic drugs; ↓ effects *OF* digoxin & phenytoin **Labs:** ↑ Uric acid, WBC; monitor BUN, Cr, pulm Fxn tests **NIPE:** Eval lungs for adventitious sounds; transient hair loss; ⊘ immunizations, breast-feeding; use contraception method

Boceprevir (Victrelis) [HCV NS3/4A Protease Inhibitor] Uses: *Chronic hep C genotype 1 combo w/ peginterferon alfa & ribavirin* **Action:** NS3/4A protease Inhib **Dose:** 800 mg PO tid w/ food w/ peginterferon alfa (*PEG-Intron*) & ribavirin (*Rebetol*) (See individual products) **Caution:** [B (but treat as X d/t ribavirin use), ?/–]w/ CYP3A4/5 metabolized drugs; **CI:** PRG, same as for peginterferon alfa & ribavirin **Disp:** caps 200 mg **SE:** Fatigue, anemia, N, HA, dysgeusia; **Interactions:** ↑ Effects *OF* CYP3A4/5 substrates (eg, amiodarone, bepridil, propafenone, quinidine, flecainide, trazodone, desipramine, azole antifungals, clarithromycin) ↓ effect *OF* ethinyl estradiol; ↓ effects *W/* CYP3A4/5 Inhibs **Labs:** ↓ Hct/WBC— monitor **NIPE:** Not a monotherapy; PRG test before; take w/ food

Bortezomib (Velcade) [Antineoplastic/Proteosome Inhibitor] WARNING: May worsen preexisting neuropathy Uses: *Rx multiple myeloma or mantel cell lymphoma w/ one failed previous Rx* **Action:** Proteasome Inhib **Dose:** 1.3 mg/m² bolus IV 2 ×/wk for 2 wk (days 1, 2, 8, 11), w/ 10-d rest period (= 1 cycle); ↓ dose w/ hematologic tox, neuropathy **Caution:** [D, ?/–] w/ drugs CYP450 metabolized (Table 10) **Disp:** 3.5-mg vial **SE:** Asthenia, GI upset, anorexia, dyspnea, HA, orthostatic ↓ BP, edema, insomnia, dizziness, rash, pyrexia, arthralgia, neuropathy **Interactions:** ↑ Risk of peripheral neuropathy *W/* amiodarone, antivirals, INH, nitrofurantoin, statins; ↑ risk hypotension *W/* antihypertensives; ↑ effects *W/* cimetidine, clarithromycin, diltiazem, disulfiram, erythromycin, fluoxetine, propoxyphene, verapamil, zafirlukast; ↓ effects *W/* amiodarone, carbamazepine, phenobarbital, phenytoin, rifampin **Labs:** ↓ HMG, Hct, neutrophils, plts **NIPE:** ⊘ PRG or breast-feeding; use contraception; caution w/ driving d/t fatigue/ dizziness; ↑ fluids if c/o N/V; may worsen neuropathy

Botulinum Toxin Type A [AbobotulinumtoxinA] (Dysport) [Neuromuscular Blocker/Neurotoxin] WARNING: Effects may spread beyond Tx area leading to swallowing & breathing difficulties (may be fatal); Sxs may occur h–wk after Inj Uses: *Cervical dystonia (adults), glabellar lines (cosmetic)* **Action:** Neurotoxin, ↓ ACH release from nerve endings, ↓ neuromuscular transmission **Dose:** *Cervical dystonia:* 500 units IM ÷ units into muscles; retreat no less than 12–16 wk PRN dose range 250–100 units based on response. *Glabellar lines:* 50 units ÷ in 10 units/Inj into muscles, repeat no less than q3mo **Caution:** [C, ?] Sedentary pt to resume activity slowly after Inj; aminoglycosides & nondepolarizing muscle blockers may {doubleup} effects; do not exceed dosing **CI:** Hypersensitivity to components (cow milk), Infxn at Inj site **Disp:** Inj **SE:** Anaphylaxis, erythema multiforme, dysphagia, dyspnea, syncope, HA, NAG, Inj site pain **Interactions:** ↑ effects **W/** aminoglycosides, other botulinum toxin products **NIPE:** Botulinum toxin products not interchangeable; Inj site pain

Botulinum Toxin Type A [IncobotulinumtoxinA] (Xeomin) [Neuromuscular Blocker/Neurotoxin]   WARNING: Effects may spread beyond Tx area leading to swallowing & breathing difficulties (may be fatal); Sxs may occur h–wk after Inj Uses: *Cervical dystonia (adults), blepharospasm* Action: Neurotoxin; ↓ ACH release from nerve endings, ↓ neuromuscular transmission Dose: *Cervical dystonia:* 120 units IM ÷ muscles *Blepharospasm:* 1.25–2.5 units IM/site; typical 5.6 units/Inj, 6 Inj/eye Caution: [C, ?] Sedentary pt to resume activity slowly after Inj; aminoglycosides & nondepolarizing muscle blockers may {doubleup} effects; do not exceed dosing CI: Hypersensitivity to components (cow milk), Infxn at Inj site Disp: Inj SE: *Cervical dystonia:* Dysphagia, neck/musculoskeletal pain, muscle weakness, Inj site pain *Blepharospasm:* Ptosis, dry eye/mouth, D,HA, visual impair, dyspnea, nasopharyngitis, URI Interactions: ↑ Effects W/ aminoglycosides, other botulinum toxin products NIPE: Effect 12–16 wk w/ 5000–10,000 units; botulinum toxin products not interchangeable; Inj site pain; for eye Inj, D/C if diplopia develops

Botulinum Toxin Type A [OnabotulinumtoxinA] (Botox, Botox Cosmetic) [Neuromuscular blocker/Neurotoxin]   WARNING : Effects may spread beyond Tx area leading to swallowing/breathing difficulties (may be fatal); Sxs may occur h–wk after Inj Uses: *Glabellar lines (cosmetic) < 65 y, blepharospasm, cervical dystonia, axillary hyperhidrosis, strabismus, chronic migraine, upper limb spasticity*, OAB Action: Neurotoxin; ↓ ACH release from nerve endings; denervates sweat glands/muscles Dose: *Adults. Glabellar lines (cosmetic):* 0.1 mL IM × 5 sites q3–4mo *Blepharospasm:* 1.25–2.5 units IM/site q3mo; max 200 units/30 d total *Cervical dystonia:* 198–300 units IM ÷ < 100 units into muscle *Hyperhidrosis:* 50 units intradermal/axilla *Strabismus:* 1.25–2.5 units IM/site q3mo; inject eye muscles w/ EMG guidance *Chronic migraine:* 155 units total, 0.1 mL (5 unit) Inj ÷ into 7 head/neck muscles *Upper limb spasticity:* Dose based on Hx; use EMG guidance *Peds. Blepharospasm:* > 12 y. Adult dose *Cervical dystonia:* > 16 y. 198–300 units IM ÷ among affected muscles; use < 100 units in sternocleidomastoid *Strabismus:* > 12 y. 1.25–2.5 units IM/site q3mo; 25 units/site max; inject eye muscles w/ EMG guidance Caution: [C, ?] w/ neurologic Dz; do not exceed dosing recommended; sedentary pt to resume activity slowly after Inj; aminoglycosides & nondepolarizing muscle blockers may {doubleup} effects;

do not exceed dosing **CI:** Hypersensitivity to components, Infxn at Inj site **Disp:** Inj powder, single use vial (dilute w/ NS); (*Botox cosmetic*) 50, 100 units; (*Botox*) 100, 200 unit vials **SE:** Anaphylaxis, erythema multiforme, dysphagia, dyspnea, syncope, HA, NAG **Interactions:** ↑ Effects *W/* aminoglycosides, other botulinum toxin products **NIPE:** Effect 12–16 wk w/ 5000–10,000 units; botulinum toxin products not interchangeable; Inj site pain; do not exceed total dose of 360 units q12–16wk

Botulinum Toxin Type B [RimabotulinumtoxinB] (Myobloc) [Neuromuscular blocker/Neurotoxin] WARNING: Effects may spread beyond Tx area leading to swallowing & breathing difficulties (may be fatal); Sxs may occur h–wk after Inj **Uses:** *Cervical dystonia adults* **Action:** Neurotoxin, ↓ ACH release from nerve endings, ↓ neuromuscular transmission **Dose:** *Cervical dystonia:* 2500–5000 units IM ÷ units into muscles; lower dose if näive **Caution:** [C, ?] Sedentary pt to resume activity slowly after Inj; aminoglycosides & nondepolarizing muscle blockers may {doubleup} effects; do not exceed dosing **CI:** Hypersensitivity to components, Infxn at Inj site **Disp: SE:** Anaphylaxis, erythema multiforme, dysphagia, dyspnea, syncope, HA, NAG, Inj site pain **Interactions:** ↑ Effects *W/* aminoglycosides, other botulinum toxin products **NIPE:** Effect 12–16 wk w/ 5000–10,000 units; botulinum toxin products not interchangeable; Inj site pain out

Brimonidine (Alphagan P) [Alpha Agonist/Glaucoma Agent] Uses: *Open-angle glaucoma, ocular HTN* **Action:** α_2-Adrenergic agonist **Dose:** 1 gtt in eye(s) tid (wait 15 min to insert contacts) **Caution:** [B, ?] **CI:** MAOI therapy **Disp:** 0.15%, 0.1% soln **SE:** Local irritation, HA, fatigue **Interactions:** ↑ Effects *OF* antihypertensives, BBs, cardiac glycosides, CNS depressants; ↓ effects *W/* TCAs **NIPE:** ⊘ EtOH, insert soft contact lenses 15+ min after drug use

Brimonidine/Timolol (Combigan) [Alpha-2 Agonist + Noncardioselective Beta-Blocker] Uses: *↓ IOP in glaucoma or ocular HTN* **Action:** Selective α_2-adrenergic agonist & nonselective β-adrenergic antagonist **Dose:** *Adults & Peds > 2 y.* 1 gtt bid ~q12h **Caution:** [C, –] **CI:** Asthma, severe COPD, sinus bradycardia, 2nd/3rd-degree AV block, CHF cardiac failure, cardiogenic shock, component hypersensitivity **Disp:** *Soln:* (2 mg/mL brimonidine, 5 mg/mL timolol) 5, 10, 15 mL **SE:** Allergic conjunctivitis, conjunctival folliculosis, conjunctival hyperemia, eye pruritus, ocular burning & stinging **Interactions:** ↑ Risk of conduction defects *W/* digoxin, CCBs; ↓ effects *OF* epinephrine; may ↑ or ↓ effects *W/* other CNS depressants, systemic BB, reserpine, quinidine, SSRIs, other CYP2D6 Inhibs **NIPE:** Instill other ophthal products 5 min apart

Brinzolamide (Azopt) [Carbonic Anhydrase Inhibitor/Glaucoma Agent] Uses: *Open-angle glaucoma, ocular HTN* **Action:** Carbonic anhydrase Inhib **Dose:** 1 gtt in eye(s) tid **Caution:** [C, ?] **CI:** Sulfonamide allergy **Disp:** 1% susp **SE:** Blurred vision, dry eye, blepharitis, taste disturbance **Interactions:** ↑ Effects *W/* oral carbonic anhydrase Inhibs **Labs:** Check LFTs, BUN, Cr **NIPE:** ⊘

Use drug if ↓ renal & hepatic studies or allergies to sulfonamides; shake well before use; insert soft contact lenses 15+ min after drug use; wait 10 min before use of other topical ophthal drugs; may caused blurred vision or taste changes

Bromocriptine (Parlodel) [Antiparkinson/Dopamine Receptor Agonist] Uses: *Parkinson Dz, hyperprolactinemia, acromegaly, pituitary tumors* **Action:** Agonist to striatal DA receptors; ↓ prolactin secretion **Dose:** Initial, 1.25 mg PO bid; titrate to effect, w/ food **Caution:** [B, ?] **CI:** Severe ischemic heart Dz or PVD **Disp:** Tabs 2.5 mg; caps 5 mg **SE:** ↓ BP, Raynaud phenomenon, dizziness, N, GI upset, hallucinations **Interactions:** ↑ Effects **W/** erythromycin, fluvoxamine, nefazodone, sympathomimetics; ↓ effects **W/** phenothiazines, antipsychotics **Labs:** ↑ BUN, AST, ALT, CPK, alk phos, uric acid **NIPE:** ⊘ Breastfeeding, PRG, OCPs; drug may cause intolerance to EtOH, return of menses & suppression of galactorrhea may take 6–8 wk; take drug w/ meals

Bromocriptine Mesylate (Cycloset) [Dopamine Receptor Agonist] Uses: *Improve glycemic control in adults w/ type 2 DM* **Action:** DA receptor agonist; ?? DM mechanism **Dose:** *Initial:* 0.8 mg PO daily, ↑ weekly by 1 tab; usual dose 1.6–4.8 mg 1 × d; w/in 2 h after waking w/ food **Caution:** [B, –] May cause orthostatic ↓ BP, psychotic disorders; not for type 1 DM or DKA; w/ strong inducers/Inhib of CYP3A4, avoid w/ DA antagonists/receptor agonists **CI:** Hypersensitivity to ergots drugs, w/ syncopal migraine, nursing mothers **Disp:** Tabs 0.8 mg **SE:** N/V, fatigue, HA, dizziness, somnolence **NIPE:** ↑ Risk of syncope; ↑ risk of hypotension; may restore fertility

Budesonide (Rhinocort Aqua, Pulmicort) [Anti-Inflammatory/ Glucocorticoid] Uses: *Allergic & nonallergic rhinitis, asthma* **Action:** Steroid **Dose:** *Adults. Rhinocort Aqua:* 1–4 sprays/nostril/d *Turbuhaler:* 1–4 Inh bid *Pulmicort Flexhaler:* 1–2 Inh bid **Peds.** *Rhinocort Aqua intranasal:* 1–2 sprays/ nostril/d *Pulmicort Turbuhaler:* 1–2 Inh bid **Respules:** 0.25–0.5 mg daily or bid (rinse mouth after PO use) **Caution:** [B, ?/–] **CI:** w/ Acute asthma **Disp:** Metered-dose *Turbuhaler,* 200 mcg/Inh; *Flexhaler,* 90, 180 mcg/Inh; *Respules,* 0.25, 0.5, 1 mg/2 mL; *Rhinocort Aqua,* 32 mcg/spray **SE:** HA, N, cough, hoarseness, *Candida* Infxn, epistaxis **Interactions:** ↑ Effects **W/** ketoconazole, itraconazole, ritonavir, indinavir, saquinavir, erythromycin, & grapefruit juice **NIPE:** Shake inhaler well before use, rinse mouth & wash inhaler after use, swallow caps whole, ⊘ exposure chickenpox or measles

Budesonide, Oral (Entocort EC) [Anti-Inflammatory, Corticosteroid] Uses: *Mild–mod Crohn Dz* **Action:** Steroid, anti-inflammatory **Dose:** *Adults.* Initial, 9 mg PO qAM to 8 wk max: maint 6 mg PO qAM taper by 3 mo; avoid grapefruit juice **CI:** Active TB & fungal Infxn **Caution:** [C, ?/–] DM, glaucoma, cataracts, HTN, CHF **Disp:** Caps 3 mg ER **SE:** HA, N, ↑ wgt, mood change, *Candida* Infxn, epistaxis **Interactions:** ↑ Effects **W/** erythromycin, indinavir, itraconazole, ketoconazole, ritonavir, saquinavir **Labs:** ↑ Alk phos, C-reactive protein, ESR, WBC; ↓ HMG, Hct **NIPE:** Do not cut/crush/chew caps; taper on D/C

Budesonide/Formoterol (Symbicort) [Anti-Inflammatory, Bronchodilator/Beta-2-Agonist] **WARNING:** LA β_2-adrenergic agonists may ↑ risk of asthma-related death. Use only for pts not adequately controlled on other meds **Uses:** *Maint Rx of asthma* **Action:** Steroid w/ LA selective β_2-adrenergic agonist **Dose:** *Adults & Peds = 12 y.* 2 Inh bid (use lowest effective dose), 640 mcg/18 mcg/d max **Caution:** [C, ?/–] **CI:** Status asthmaticus/acute episodes **Disp:** Inh (budesonide mcg/formoterol mcg) 80/4.5 mcg, 160/4.5 mcg **SE:** HA, GI discomfort, nasopharyngitis, palpitations, tremor, nervousness, URI, paradoxical bronchospasm, hypokalemia, cataracts, glaucoma **Interactions:** ↑ Effects *W/* adrenergics; ↑ hypokalemic effects *W/* cardiac glycosides, diuretics, steroids; ↑ risk of ventricular arrhythmias *W/* MAOIs, TCA, quinidine, phenothiazines; ↓ effects *W/* BBs **Labs:** ↑ Serum glucose; ↓ K⁺ **NIPE:** ⊘ EtOH; not for acute bronchospasm; not for transferring pt from chronic systemic steroids; rinse & spit w/ H_2O after each dose

Bumetanide (Bumex) [Diuretic/Loop] **Uses:** *Edema from CHF, hepatic cirrhosis, & renal Dz* **Action:** Loop diuretic; ↓ reabsorption of Na⁺ & Cl⁻, in ascending loop of Henle & the distal tubule **Dose:** *Adults.* 0.5–2 mg/d PO; 0.5–1 mg IV/IM q8–24h (max 10 mg/d) *Peds.* 0.015–0.1 mg/kg PO qd–24h (max 10 mg/d) **Caution:** [D,?] **CI:** Anuria, hepatic coma, severe lyte depletion **Disp:** Tabs 0.5, 1, 2 mg; Inj 0.25 mg/mL **SE:**, dizziness, ototox **Interactions:** ↑ Effects *W/* antihypertensives, thiazides, nitrates, EtOH, clofibrate; ↓ effects *OF* Li, warfarin, thrombolytic drugs, anticoagulants; ↑ K⁺ loss *W/* carbenoxolone, corticosteroids, terbutaline; ↑ ototox *W/* aminoglycosides, cisplatin; ↓ effects *W/* cholestyramine, colestipol, NSAIDs, probenecid, barbiturates, phenytoin **Labs:** ↑ Cr, uric acid; ↓ serum K⁺, Ca²⁺, Na⁺, Mg⁺ **NIPE:** Take drug w/ food, take early to prevent nocturia, daily wgt; monitor fluid & lytes; monitor ECG for hypokalemia (flattened T waves)

Bupivacaine (Marcaine) [Anesthetic] **WARNING:** Administration only by clinicians experienced in local anesthesia d/t potential tox; avoid 0.75% for OB anesthesia d/t reports of cardiac arrest & death **Uses:** *Local, regional, & spinal anesthesia, local & regional analgesia* **Action:** Local anesthetic **Dose:** *Adults & Peds.* Dose dependent on procedure (tissue vascularity, depth of anesthesia, etc) (Table 1) **Caution:** [C, ?] **CI:** Severe bleeding, ↓ BP, shock & arrhythmias, local Infxns at site, septicemia **Disp:** Inj 0.25%, 0.5%, 0.75% **SE:** ↓ BP, bradycardia, dizziness, anxiety **Interactions:** ↑ Effects *W/* BBs, hyaluronidase, ergot-type oxytocics, MAOI, TCAs, phenothiazines, vasopressors; ↓ effects *W/* chloroprocaine **NIPE:** Anesthetized area has temporary loss of sensation & Fxn

Buprenorphine (Buprenex) [C-III] [Analgesic/Opioid Agonist-Antagonist] **Uses:** *Mod/severe pain* **Action:** Opiate agonist–antagonist **Dose:** 0.3–0.6 mg IM or slow IV push q6h PRN **Caution:** [C, ?/–] **Disp:** 0.3 mg/mL **SE:** Sedation, ↓ BP, resp depression **Notes:** Withdrawal if opioid-dependent **Interactions:** ↑ Effects of resp & CNS depression *W/* EtOH, opiates, benzodiazepines, TCAs, MAOIs, other CNS depressants **Labs:** ↓ Alk phos, HMG, Hct, erythrocyte count **NIPE:** ⊘ EtOH & other CNS depressants

Buprenorphine, Transdermal (Butrans) [C-III] [Opioid Analgesic]
WARNING: Limit use to severe chronic pain; assess for opioid abuse/addiction before use; 20 mcg/h max d/t ↑ QTc; avoid heat on patch, may result in OD **Uses:** *Mod/severe chronic pain requiring around the clock opioid analgesic* **Action:** Opiate agonist–antagonist **Dose:** Wear patch × 7 d; if opioid naive start 5 mcg/h; see label for conversion from opioid; wait 72 h before Δ dose; wait 3 wk before using same application site **Caution:** [C, ?/–] **CI:** Resp depression, severe asthma, ileus, component hypersensitivity, short-term opioid need, post-op/mild/intermittent pain **Disp:** Transdermal patch 5,10,20 mcg/h **SE:** N/V, HA, site Rxns pruritus, dizziness, constipation, somnolence, dry mouth **Interactions:**↑ Effects W/ CNS & resp depressants (eg, benzodiazepines, muscle relaxants, tricyclics, phenothiazines), EtOH; do not give w/in 14 d of MAOIs; ↑ risk of cardiac effects W/ Class Ia (eg, quinidine, procainamide, disopyramide) or Class III antiarrhythmics (eg, sotalol, amiodarone, dofetilide) **NIPE:** Taper on D/C

Buprenorphine & Naloxone (Suboxone) [C-III] [Opioid (partial agonist–antagonist) + opioid antagonist] **Uses:** *Maint opioid withdrawal* **Action:** Opioid agonist–antagonist + opioid antagonist **Dose:** Opioid agonist–antagonist 2/0.5–24/6 mg SL daily; ↑/↓ by 2/0.5 mg or 4/1 mg to effect of S/Sxs **Caution:** [C, +/–] **CI:** Hypersensitivity **Disp:** SL film *Buprenorphine/naloxone:* 2/0.5, 8/2 mg **SE:** Oral hypoparesthesia, pain, constipation, diaphoresis **Interactions:** ↑ effects W/ CYP3A4 Inhibs (eg, azole antifungals, macrolides, HIV protease Inhibs) **NIPE:** Not for analgesia; dissolve under tongue, do not swallow tabs or film

Bupropion Hydrobromide (Aplenzin) [Aminoketone] **WARNING:** ↑ Suicide risk in pts < 24 y w/ major depressive/other psychiatric disorders; not for ped use **Uses:** *Depression* **Action:** Aminoketone, ? action **Dose:** *Adults.* 174 mg PO, qd qAM, ↑ PRN to 348 mg qd on day 4 if tolerated, max 522 mg/d; see package insert if switching from Wellbutrin; mild–mod hepatic/renal impair ↓ frequency/dose; severe hepatic impair 174 mg max qod **Caution:** [C, –] w/ drugs that ↓ Sz threshold, ↑ w/ CYP2D6-metabolized meds (Table 10) **CI:** Sz disorder, bulimia, anorexia nervosa, w/in 14 d of MAOIs, other forms of bupropion, abrupt D/C of EtOH, or sedatives **Disp:** ER tabs 174, 348, 522 mg **SE:** Dry mouth, N, Abd pain, insomnia, dizziness, pharyngitis, agitation, anxiety, tremor, palpitation, tremor, sweating, tinnitus, myalgia, anorexia, urinary frequency, rash **Interactions:** ↑ Effects W/ stimulants & meds metabolized by CYP2D6 **NIPE:** Do not cut/crush/chew, avoid EtOH, ⊘ D/C abruptly

Bupropion Hydrochloride (Wellbutrin, Wellbutrin SR, Wellbutrin XL, Zyban) [Aminoketone] **WARNING:** All pts being treated w/ bupropion for smoking cessation Tx should be observed for neuropsychiatric S/Sxs (hostility, agitation, depressed mood, & suicide-related events; most during/after; *Zyban*; Sxs may persist following D/C; closely monitor for worsening depression or emergence of suicidality, ↑ suicidal behavior in young adults **Uses:** *Depression, smoking cessation adjunct*, ADHD **Action:** Weak Inhib of neuronal uptake of serotonin & norepinephrine; ↓ neuronal DA reuptake **Dose:** *Depression:* 100–450 mg/d ÷ bid–tid; SR 150–200 mg bid; XL 150–450 mg daily *Smoking cessation (Zyban, Wellbutrin XR):* 150 mg/d × 3 d, then 150 mg bid × 8–12 wk, last dose before 6 PM; ↓ dose w/ renal/hepatic impair **Caution:** [C, ?/–] **CI:** Sz disorder, h/o anorexia nervosa or bulimia, MAOI, w/in 14 d, abrupt D/C of EtOH or sedatives **Disp:** Tabs 75, 100 mg; SR tabs 100, 150, 200 mg; XL tabs 150, 300 mg; Zyban 150 mg tabs **SE:** Szs, agitation, insomnia, HA, tachycardia, ↑ wgt **Interactions:** ↑ Effects *W/* cimetidine, levodopa, MAOIs; ↑ risk of Szs *W/* EtOH, phenothiazines, antidepressants, theophylline, TCAs, or abrupt withdrawal of corticosteroids, benzodiazepines **Labs:** ↓ Prolactin level **NIPE:** Drug may ↑ adverse events including Szs; take 3–4 wk for full effect; ⊘ EtOH or CNS depressants; ⊘ abrupt D/C; SR & XR do not cut/ chew/ crush

Buspirone (BuSpar) [Anxiolytic]   **WARNING:** Closely monitor for worsening depression or emergence of suicidality **Uses:** Short-term relief of *anxiety* **Action:** Antianxiety; antagonizes CNS serotonin & DA receptors **Dose:** *Initial:* 7.5 mg PO bid; ↑ by 5 mg q2–3d to effect; usual 20–30 mg/d; max 60 mg/d w/ MAOI **Caution:** [B, ?/–] Avoid w/ severe hepatic/renal Insuff **Disp:** Tabs ÷ dose 5, 10, 15, 30 mg **SE:** Drowsiness, dizziness, HA, N, EPS, serotonin synd, hostility, depression **Interactions:** ↑ Effects *W/* erythromycin, clarithromycin, itraconazole, ketoconazole, diltiazem, verapamil, grapefruit juice; ↓ effects *W/* carbamazepine, rifampin, phenytoin, dexamethasone, phenobarbital, fluoxetine **Labs:** ↑ Glucose; ↓ WBC, plts **NIPE:** ↑ Sedation w/ EtOH, therapeutic effects may take up to 4 wk; no abuse potential or physical/psychological dependence

Busulfan (Myleran, Busulfex) [Antineoplastic/Alkylating Drug] **WARNING:** Can cause severe BM **Uses:** *CML*, preparative regimens for allogeneic & ABMT in high doses **Action:** Alkylating agent **Dose:** (per protocol) **Caution:** [D, ?] **Disp:** Tabs 2 mg, Inj 60 mg/10 mL **SE:** BM suppression, ↓ BM, ↑ BP, pulm fibrosis, N (w/ high-dose), gynecomastia, adrenal Insuff, skin hyperpigmentation **Interactions:** ↑ Effects *W/* APAP; ↑ BM suppression *W/* anti-neoplastic drugs & radiation therapy; ↑ uric acid levels *W/* probenecid & sulfinpyrazone; ↓ effects *W/* itraconazole, phenytoin **Labs:** ↑ Glucose, ALT, bilirubin, BUN, Cr, uric acid; monitor CBC, LFTs **NIPE:** ⊘ Immunizations, PRG, breast-feeding; ↑ fluids; use barrier contraception; ↑ risk of hair loss, rash, darkened skin pigment; ↑ susceptibility to Infxn

Butabarbital, Hyoscyamine Hydrobromide, Phenazopyridine (Pyridium Plus) [Urinary Tract Analgesic & Sedative] Uses: *Relieve urinary tract pain w/ UTI, procedures, trauma* **Action:** Phenazopyridine (topical anesthetic), hyoscyamine (parasympatholytic, ↓ spasm) & butabarbital (sedative) **Dose:** 1 PO qid, pc, & hs; w/ antibiotic for UTI, 2 d max **Caution:** [C, ?] **Disp:** Tabs butabarbital 15 mg /hyoscyamine 0.3 mg /phenazopyridine 150 mg **SE:** HA, rash, itching, GI distress, methemoglobinemia, hemolytic anemia, anaphylactoid-like Rxns, dry mouth, dizziness, drowsiness, blurred vision **Labs:**

Effects urine test results **NIPE:** Colors urine orange, may tint skin, sclera; stains clothing/contacts

Butorphanol (Stadol) [C-IV] [Analgesic/Opiate Agonist–Antagonist]
Uses: *Anesthesia adjunct, pain* & migraine HA Action: Opiate agonist–antagonist w/ central analgesic actions Dose: 1–4 mg IM or IV q3–4h PRN *Migraine:* 1 spray in 1 nostril, repeat × 1, 60–90 min, then q3–4h ↓ in renal impair Caution: [C (D if high dose or prolonged use at term), +] Disp: Inj 1, 2 mg/mL; nasal 1 mg/spray (10 mg/mL) SE: Drowsiness, dizziness, nasal congestion Interactions: ↑ Effects W/ EtOH, antihistamines, cimetidine, CNS depressants, phenothiazines, barbiturates, skeletal-muscle relaxants, MAOIs; ↓ effects OF opiates Labs: ↑ Serum amylase & lipase NIPE: ⊘ EtOH or other CNS depressants; may induce withdrawal in opioid dependency

C1 Esterase Inhibitor, Human (Berinert, Cinryze) [C1 Inhibitor]
Uses: *Berinert: Rx acute Abd or facial attacks of hereditary angioedema (HAE)*, *Cinryze: Prophylaxis of HAE* Action: ↓ contact system by ↓ Factor XIIa & kallikrein activation Dose: Adults & Adolescents. *Berinert:* 20 units/kg IV × 1; *Cinryze:* 1000 units IV q3–4d Caution: [C, ?/–] Hypersensitivity Rxns, monitor for thrombotic events, may contain infectious agents CI: Hypersensitivity Rxns to C1 esterase Inhib Prep Disp: 500 units/vial SE: HA, Abd pain, N/V/D, muscle spasms, pain, subsequent HAE attack, anaphylaxis, thromboembolism NIPE: Contains human plasma, monitor for possible Infxn transmission

Cabazitaxel (Jevtana) [Taxane Antimicrotubule] WARNING: Neutropenic deaths reported; v CBCs, CI w/ ANC < 1500 cells/mm³; Severe hypersensitivity (rash/erythema, ↓ BP, bronchospasm) may occur, D/C drug & Tx; CI w/ Hx of hypersensitivity to cabazitaxel or others formulated w/ polysorbate 80 Uses: *Hormone refractory metastatic PCa* Action: Microtubule Inhib Dose: 25 mg/m² IV Inf (over 1 h) q3wk w/ prednisone 10 mg PO daily; Premedicate w/ antihistamine, corticosteroid, H₂ antagonist; do not use w/ bilirubin ≥ ULN, AST/ALT ≥ 1.5 × ULN Caution: [D, ?/–] w/ CYP3A Inhib/inducers CI: See box Disp: Inj SE: Sepsis, N/V/D, constipation, Abd/back/Jt pain, dysgeusia, fatigue, hematuria, neuropathy, anorexia, cough, dyspnea, alopecia, pyrexia, hypersensitivity Rxn, renal failure Interactions: ↑ Effects OF CYP3A4 Inhibs (eg, ketoconazole, clarithromycin, atazanavir, nefazodone, nelfinavir, ritonavir, saquinavir, voriconazole); ↓ effects OF CYP3A4 inducers (eg., phenytoin, carbamazepine, rifampin, phenobarbital) (may antagonize cabazitaxel). St. John's wort Labs: ↓ WBC, ↓ Hgb, ↓ plt NIPE: Monitor closely pts > 65 y

Calcipotriene (Dovonex) [Keratolytic] Uses: *Plaque psoriasis* Action: Keratolytic Dose: Apply bid Caution: [C, ?] CI: ↑ Ca²⁺; vit D tox; do not apply to face Disp: Cream; oint; soln 0.005% SE: Skin irritation, dermatitis Interactions: None noted Labs: Monitor serum Ca NIPE: Wash hands after application or wear gloves to apply, D/C drug if ↑ Ca

Calcitonin (Fortical, Miacalcin) [Hypocalcemic, Bone Resorption Inhibitor/Thyroid Hormone] Uses: *Miacalcin:* *Paget Dz, emergent Rx*

hypercalcemia, postmenopausal osteoporosis* *Fortical:* *Postmenopausal osteoporosis*; osteogenesis imperfecta **Action:** Polypeptide hormone (salmon source), inhibits osteoclasts **Dose:** *Paget Dz:* 100 units/d IM/SQ initial, 50 units/d or 50–100 units q1–3d maint *Hypercalcemia:* 4 units/kg IM/SQ q12h; ↑ to 8 units/kg q12h, max q6h *Osteoporosis:* 100 units/qod IM/SQ; intranasal 200 units = 1 nasal spray/d **Caution:** [C, ?] **Disp:** *Fortical, Miacalcin* nasal spray 200 IU/activation; Inj, *Miacalcin* 200 units/mL (2 mL) **SE:** Facial flushing, N, Inj site edema, nasal irritation, polyuria **Notes:** *Fortical* is rDNA derived from salmon **Interactions:** ↑ Effect Tx w/ alendronate, risedronate, etidronate or pamidronate may ↓ effects *OF* calcitonin **Labs:** May ↑ granular casts in urine; ↓ serum Li; monitor serum Ca & alk phos **NIPE:** Allergy skin test prior to use; take hs to < N/V; flushing > Inj is transient; N > Inj will < w/ continued Tx; for nasal spray alternate nostrils daily; ensure adequate Ca & vit D intake

Calcitriol (Rocaltrol, Calcijex) [Antihypocalcemic/Vitamin D Analog] Uses: *Predialysis reduction of ↑ PTH levels to treat bone Dz; ↑ Ca²⁺ on dialysis* **Action:** 1,25-Dihydroxycholecalciferol (vit D analog); ↑ Ca²⁺ & P absorption; ↑ bone mineralization **Dose:** *Adults. Renal failure:* 0.25 mcg/d PO, 0.25 mcg/d q4–6wk PRN; 0.5 mcg 3 ×/wk IV, ↑ PRN *Hypoparathyroidism:* 0.5–2 mcg/d *Peds. Renal failure:* 15 ng/kg/d, ↑ PRN; maint 30–60 ng/kg/d *Hypoparathyroidism:* < 5 y: 0.25–0.75 mcg/d > 6 y: 0.5–2 mcg/d **Caution:** [C, ?] ↑ Mg²⁺ possible w/ antacids **CI:** ↑ Ca²⁺; vit D tox **Disp:** Inj 1, mcg/mL (in 1 mL); caps 0.25, 0.5 mcg; soln 1 mcg/mL **SE:** ↑ Ca²⁺ possible **Interactions:** ↑ Effect *W/* thiazide diuretics; ↓ effect *W/* cholestyramine, colestipol, ketoconazole **Labs:** Monitor for ↑ Ca²⁺, cholesterol, BUN, AST, ALT; down} alk phos **NIPE:** ⊘ Mg-containing antacids or supls; use non-aluminum phosphate binders & low-phosphate diet to control serum phosphate

Calcitriol, Ointment (Vectical) [Vitamin D₃ Derivative] Uses: *Mild/mod plaque psoriasis* **Action:** Vit D₃ analog **Dose:** *Adults.* Apply to area bid; max 200 g/wk **Caution:** [C, ?/–] Avoid excess sunlight **CI:** None **Disp:** Oint 3 mcg/g (5-, 100-g tube) **SE:** Hypercalcemia, hypercalciuria, nephrolithiasis, worsening psoriasis, pruritus, skin discomfort **Interactions:** ↑ Risk of hypercalcemia *W/* thiazide diuretics, calcium supls or high doses of vit D **Labs:** Monitor for hypercalcemia **NIPE:** ↑ Absorption may occur w/ occlusive dressing; D/C Tx until normocalcemia returns; ⊘ apply to eyes, lips, facial skin; avoid excessive sunlight or artificial light

Calcium Acetate (PhosLo) [Calcium Supplement, Antiarrhythmic/ Mineral, Electrolyte] Uses: *ESRD-associated hyperphosphatemia* **Action:** Ca²⁺ supl w/o Al to ↓ PO₄²⁻ absorption **Dose:** 2–4 tabs PO w/ meals **Caution:** [C, ?] **CI:** ↑ Ca²⁺ **Disp:** Gelcap 667 mg **SE:** Can ↑ Ca²⁺, hypophosphatemia, constipation **Interactions:** ↑ Effects *OF* quinidine; ↓ effects *W/* large intake of dietary fiber, spinach, rhubarb; ↓ effects *OF* atenolol, CCB, etidronate, tetracyclines, fluoroquinolones, phenytoin, Fe salts, thyroid hormones **Labs:** Monitor for ↑ Ca²⁺; ↓ Mg²⁺ **NIPE:** ⊘ EtOH, caffeine, tobacco; separate Ca supls & other meds by 1–2 h

Calcium Carbonate (Tums, Alka-Mints) [Antacid, Calcium Supplement/Mineral, Electrolyte] [OTC] Uses: *Hyperacidity associated w/ PUD, hiatal hernia, etc* Action: Neutralizes gastric acid Dose: 500 mg–2 g PO PRN, 7 g/d max; ↓ w/ renal impair Caution: [C, ?] Disp: Chew tabs 350, 420, 500, 550, 750, 850 mg; susp SE: ↑ Ca^{2+}, ↓ PO_4^{2-}, constipation Interactions: ↓ Effect OF tetracyclines, fluoroquinolones, Fe salts, & ASA; ↓ Ca absorption W/ high intake of dietary fiber Labs: Monitor for↑↑ Ca^{2+}, ↓ Mg^{2+} NIPE: ↑ Fluids; may cause constipation; ⊘ EtOH, caffeine, tobacco; separate Ca supls & other meds by 1–2 h, chew tabs well

Calcium Glubionate (Neo-Calglucon) [Calcium Supplement, Antiarrhythmic/Mineral, Electrolyte] [OTC] Uses: *Rx & prevent calcium deficiency* Action: Ca^{2+} supls Dose: Adults. 6–18 g/d ÷ doses Peds. 600–2000 mg/kg/d ÷ qid (9 g/d max); ↓ in renal impair Caution: [C, ?] CI: ↑ Ca^{2+} Disp: OTC syrup 1.8 g/5 mL = elemental Ca 115 mg/5 mL SE: ↑ Ca^{2+}, ↓ PO_4^{2-}, constipation Interactions: ↑ Effects OF quinidine; ↓ effect OF tetracyclines; ↓ Ca absorption W/ high intake of dietary fiber Labs: ↑ Ca^{2+}, ↓ Mg^{2+} NIPE: ⊘ EtOH, caffeine, tobacco, separate Ca supls & other meds by 1–2 h

Calcium Salts (Chloride, Gluconate, Glucepate) [Calcium Supplement, Antiarrhythmic/Mineral, Electrolyte] Uses: *Ca^{2+} replacement*, VF, Ca^{2+} blocker tox, Mg^{2+} intoxication, tetany, *hyperphosphatemia in ESRD* Action: Ca^{2+} supls/replacement Dose: Adults. Replacement: 1–2 g/d PO Tetany: 1 g CaCl over 10–30 min; repeat in 6 h PRN ECC 2010: Hyperkalemia/hypermagnesemia/CCB OD: 500–1000 mg (5–10 mL of 10% soln) IV; repeat PRN; comparable dose of 10% Ca gluconate is 15–30 mL Peds. Replacement: 200–500 mg/kg/24 h PO or IV ÷ qid Tetany: 10 mg/kg CaCl over 5–10 min; repeat in 6 h or use Inf (200 mg/kg/d max) ECC 2010: Hypocalcemia/hyperkalemia/hypermagnesemia/CCB OD: CaCl or Ca gluconate 20 mg/kg (0.2 mL/kg) slow IV/IO, repeat PRN; central venous route preferred Adults & Peds. ↓ Ca^{2+} d/t citrated blood Inf: 0.45 mEq Ca/100 mL citrated blood Inf (↓ in renal impair) Caution: [C, ?] CI: ↑ Ca^{2+} Disp: CaCl Inj 10% = 100 mg/mL = Ca 27.2 mg/mL = 10-mL amp; Ca gluconate Inj 10% = 100 mg/mL = Ca 9 mg/mL; tabs 500 mg = 45 mg Ca, 650 mg = 58.5 mg Ca, 975 mg = 87.75 mg Ca, 1 g = 90 mg Ca; Ca gluceptate Inj 220 mg/mL = 18 mg/mL Ca SE: Bradycardia, cardiac arrhythmias, ↑ Ca^{2+}, constipation Notes: CaCl 270 mg (13.6 mEq) elemental Ca/g, & calcium gluconate 90 mg (4.5 mEq) Ca/g. RDA for Ca: Peds < 6 mo: 210 mg/d; 6 mo–1 y: 270 mg/d; 1–3 y: 500 mg/d; 4–9 y: 800 mg/d; 10–18 y: 1200 mg/d. Adults. 1000 mg/d; > 50 y: 1200 mg/d Interactions: ↑ Effects OF quinidine & digitalis; ↓ effects OF tetracyclines, quinolones, verapamil, CCBs, Fe salts, ASA, atenolol; ↓ Ca absorption W/ high intake of dietary fiber Labs: Monitor for ↑ Ca^{2+}, ↓ Mg^{2+} NIPE: ⊘ EtOH, caffeine, tobacco; separate Ca supls & other meds by 1–2 h

Calfactant (Infasurf) [RDS Agent/Surfactant] Uses: *Prevention & Rx of RSD in infants* Action: Exogenous pulm surfactant Dose: 3 mL/kg instilled into lungs. Can repeat 3 total doses given 12 h apart **Caution:** [?, ?] **Disp:** Intratracheal susp 35 mg/mL **SE:** Monitor for cyanosis, airway obst, ↓ HR during administration **Interactions:** None noted **NIPE:** Only for intratracheal use; ⊘ reconstitute, dilute, or shake vial; refrigerate & keep away from light; no need to warm soln prior to use

Candesartan (Atacand) [Antihypertensive/ARB] Uses: *HTN*, DN, CHF **Action:** Angiotensin II receptor antagonist **Dose:** 4–32 mg/d (usual 16 mg/d) **Caution:** [C (1st tri), D (2nd & 3rd tri), −] **CI:** Primary hyperaldosteronism; bilateral RAS **Disp:** Tabs 4, 8, 16, 32 mg **SE:** Dizziness, HA, flushing, angioedema **Interactions:** ↑ Effects *W/* cimetidine; ↑ risk of hyperkalemia *W/* amiloride, spironolactone, triamterene, K+ supls, TMP; ↑ effects *OF* Li; ↓ effects *W/* phenobarbital, rifampin **Labs:** ↑ BUN, Cr, K+, LFTs, uric acid; monitor for albuminuria, hyperglycemia, triglyceridemia, uricemia **NIPE:** ⊘ Breast-feeding or PRG, use barrier contraception, may take 4–6 wk for full effect, adequate fluid intake, take w/o regard to food

Capsaicin (Capsin, Zostrix, Others) [Topical Anesthetic/Analgesic] [OTC] Uses: Pain d/t *postherpetic neuralgia*, chronic neuralgia, *arthritis, diabetic neuropathy*, post-op pain, psoriasis, intractable pruritus **Action:** Topical analgesic **Dose:** Apply tid–qid **Caution:** [C, ?] **Disp:** OTC creams; gel; lotions; roll-ons **SE:** Local irritation, neurotox, cough **Interactions:** May ↑ cough *W/* ACEIs **NIPE:** External use only; wk to onset of action; ⊘ contact w/ eyes or broken/irritated skin; apply w/ gloves; transient stinging/burning

Capsaicin Patch (Qutenza) [Analgesic/TRPV1 Channel Agonist] Uses: Management of neuropathic pain associated w/ *postherpetic neuralgia* **Action:** Dermal patch w/ capsaicin causes a reduction in transient receptor potential vanilloid 1 (TRPV 1) expressing nociceptive nerve endings **Dose:** *Adults.* Application only by healthcare providers. Up to 4 patches can be applied to Tx area on clean, dry, intact skin for 60 min, then apply cleansing gel to area for 1 min, then wash & dry area of Tx. Repeat q3mo PRN, but not sooner than 3 mo intervals *Peds.* Not recommended < 18 y **Caution:** [B, − do not breast-feed on day of Tx]; **Disp:** Dermal patch 8% (179 mg) **SE:** Skin Rxns (burning, erythema, pain, pruritus, papules) & HTN during & a few h after Tx; **Interactions:** Drug can ↑ BP during Tx **NIPE:** Apply topical anesthetic to area for recommended time before application of patch; treated areas may be sensitive to heat (hot showers/baths, sun exposure, exercise) for few days > Tx; may need pain meds to minimize discomfort; apply patch w/in 2 h of opening package; rapid removal of patches may cause aerosolization of capsaicin—remove slowly, rolling inward; use nitrile gloves when handling patch & cleaning capsaicin residue from skin & stat dispose of patches

Captopril (Capoten, Others) [Antihypertensive/ACEI] Uses: *HTN, CHF, MI*, LVD, DN **Action:** ACE Inhib **Dose:** *Adults. HTN:* Initial, 25 mg PO bid–tid; ↑ to maint q1–2wk by 25-mg increments/dose (max 450 mg/d) to effect

CHF: Initial, 6.25–12.5 mg PO tid; titrate PRN *LVD:* 50 mg PO tid *DN:* 25 mg PO tid *Peds. Infants < 2 mo.* 0.05–0.5 mg/kg/dose PO q8–24h *Children.* Initial, 0.3–0.5 mg/kg/dose PO; ↑ to 6 mg/kg/d max in 2–4 ÷ doses; 1 h ac **Caution:** [C (1st tri), D (2nd & 3rd tri), +]; unknown effects in renal impair **CI:** h/o angioedema, bilateral RAS **Disp:** Tabs 12.5, 25, 50, 100 mg **SE:** Rash, proteinuria, cough, ↑ K+ **Interactions:** ↑ Effects *W/* antihypertensives, diuretics, nitrates, probenecid, black catechu; ↓ effects *W/* antacids, ASA, NSAIDs, food; ↑ effects *OF* digoxin, insulin, oral hypoglycemics, Li **Labs:** False(+) urine acetone; may ↑ urine protein, serum BUN, Cr, K+, prolactin, LFTs; may ↓ HMG, Hct, RBC, WBC, plt **NIPE:** ⊘ PRG, breast-feeding, K+-sparing diuretics; take w/o food, give 1 h < meals; may take 2 wk for full therapeutic effect

Carbamazepine (Tegretol XR, Carbatrol, Epitol, Equetro) [Anticonvulsant/Analgesic]
WARNING: Aplastic anemia & agranulocytosis have been reported w/ carbamazepine; pts w/ Asian ancestry should be tested to determine potential for skin Rxns **Uses:** *Epilepsy, trigeminal neuralgia, acute mania w/ bipolar disorder (Equetro)* EtOH withdrawal **Action:** Anticonvulsant **Dose:** *Adults. Initial:* 200 mg PO bid or 100 mg qid/d (as susp); ↑ by 200 mg/d; usual 800–1200 mg/d ÷ doses *Acute Mania (Equetro):* 400 mg/d, ↑ bid, adjust by 200 mg/d to response 1600 mg/d max *Peds < 6 y.* 5 mg/kg/d, ↑ to 10–20 mg/kg/d ÷ in 2–4 doses *6–12 y. Initial:* 100 mg PO bid or 10 mg/kg/24 h PO ÷ daily–bid; ↑ to maint 20–30 mg/kg/24 h ÷ tid–qid; ↓ in renal impair; take w/ food **Caution:** [D, +] **CI:** MAOI use, h/o BM suppression **Disp:** Tabs 100, 200, 300, 400 mg; chew tabs 100, 200 mg; XR tabs 100, 200, 400 mg; Equetro caps ER 100, 200, 300 mg; susp 100 mg/5 mL **SE:** Drowsiness, dizziness, blurred vision, N/V, rash, SJS/toxic epidermal necrolysis (TEN), ↓ Na+, leukopenia, agranulocytosis **Notes:** *Trough:* Just before next dose *Therapeutic peak:* 8–12 mcg/mL (monotherapy), 4–8 mcg/mL (polytherapy) *Toxic trough : >* 15 mcg/mL *1/2-life:* 15–20 h; generic products not interchangeable, many drug interactions, administer susp in 3–4 ÷ doses daily; skin tox (SJS/TEN) ↑ w/ HLA-B*1502 allele **Interactions:** ↑ Effects *W/* cimetidine, clarithromycin, danazol, diltiazem, felbamate, fluconazole, fluoxetine, fluvoxamine, INH, itraconazole, ketoconazole, macrolides, metronidazole, propoxyphene, protease Inhibs, valproic acid, verapamil, grapefruit juice; ↑ effects *OF* Li, MAOIs; ↓ effects *W/* phenobarbital, phenytoin, primidone, plantain; ↓ effects *OF* benzodiazepines, corticosteroids, cyclosporine, doxycycline, felbamate, haloperidol, OCPs, phenytoin, theophylline, thyroid hormones, TCAs, warfarin **Labs:** Monitor CBC & levels; ↑ eosinophil count; ↓ HMG, Hct, WBC, plts; ↓ LFTs, thyroid hormones; ↑ BUN **NIPE:** Take w/ food; may cause photosensitivity—use sunscreen; use barrier contraception; abrupt withdrawal may cause Sz; ⊘ breast-feeding or PRG

Carbidopa/Levodopa (Sinemet, Parcopa) [Antiparkinsonian/Dopamine Agonist]
Uses: *Parkinson Dz* **Action:** ↑ CNS DA levels **Dose:** 25/100 mg bid–qid; ↑ PRN (max 200/2000 mg/d) **Caution:** [C, ?] **CI:** NAG, suspicious skin lesion (may activate melanoma), melanoma, MAOI use **Disp:** Tabs

(carbidopa mg/levodopa mg) 10/100, 25/100, 25/250; tabs SR (carbidopa mg/levodopa mg) 25/100, 50/200; ODT (oral disintegrating tabs) (carbidopa mg/levodopa mg) 10/100, 25/100, 25/250 **SE:** Psychological disturbances, orthostatic ↓ BP, dyskinesias, cardiac arrhythmias **Interactions:** ↑ Risk of hypotension *W/* antihypertensives; ↑ risk of HTN *W/* MAOIs; ↓ effects *W/* antacids; ↓ effects *W/* anticholinergics, anticonvulsants, benzodiazepines, haloperidol, Fe, methionine, papaverine, phenothiazines, phenytoin, pyridoxine, reserpine, spiramycin, tacrine, thioxanthenes, high-protein food **Labs:** ↑ Alk phos, AST, bilirubin, BUN, uric acid ↓ HMG, plts, WBCs **NIPE:** Darkened urine & sweat may result; ⊘ crush or chew SR tabs; take w/o food; muscle or eyelid twitching may suggest tox

Carboplatin (Paraplatin) [Antineoplastic/Alkylating Agent]
WARNING: Administration only by physician experienced in CA chemotherapy; BM suppression possible; anaphylaxis may occur **Uses:** *Ovarian*, lung, head & neck, testicular, urothelial, & brain *CA, NHL* & allogeneic &ABMT in high doses **Action:** DNA cross-linker; forms DNA-platinum adducts **Dose:** 360 mg/m² (ovarian carcinoma); AUC dosing 4–8 mg/mL (Culvert formula: mg = AUC × [25 + calculated GFR]); adjust based on plt count, CrCl, & BSA (Egorin formula); up to 1500 mg/m² used in ABMT setting (per protocols) **Caution:** [D, ?] **CI:** Severe BM suppression, excessive bleeding **Disp:** Inj 50, 150, 450 mg vial (10 mg/mL) **SE:** Anaphylaxis, ↓ BM, N/V/D, nephrotox, hematuria, neurotox **Notes:** Physiologic dosing based on Culvert or Egorin formula allows ↑ doses w/ ↓ tox **Interactions:** ↑ Myelosuppression *W/* myelosuppressive drugs; ↑ hematologic effects *W/* BM suppressants; ↑ bleeding *W/* ASA; ↑ nephrotox *W/* nephrotoxic drugs; ↓ effects *OF* phenytoin **Labs:** Monitor for ↑ LFTs, BUN, Cr; ↓ Mg²⁺, lytes, CBC levels **NIPE:** ⊘ Use w/ Al needles or IV administration sets, PRG, breast-feeding; antiemetics prior to administration may prevent N/V, maint adequate food & fluid intake

Carisoprodol (Soma) [Skeletal Muscle Relaxant/Carbamate Derivative]
Uses: *Adjunct to sleep & physical Rx to relieve painful musculoskeletal conditions* **Action:** Centrally acting muscle relaxant **Dose:** 250–350 mg PO tid–qid **Caution:** [C, M] Tolerance may result; w/ renal/hepatic impair **CI:** Allergy to meprobamate; acute intermittent porphyria **Disp:** Tabs 250–350 mg **SE:** CNS depression, drowsiness, dizziness, HA, tachycardia **Interactions:** ↑ Effects *W/* CNS depressants, phenothiazines, EtOH **NIPE:** Avoid EtOH & other CNS depressants; available in combo w/ ASA or codeine; ⊘ breast-feeding; take w/ food if GI upset

Carmustine [BCNU] (BiCNU, Gliadel) [Antineoplastic, Alkylating Agent]
WARNING: BM suppression, dose-related pulm tox possible; administer under direct supervision of experienced physician **Uses:** *Primary or adjunct brain tumors, multiple myeloma, Hodgkin lymphoma & NHL * multiple myeloma, induction for allogeneic & ABMT high doses *surgery & RT adjunct high-grade glioma & recurrent glioblastoma (Gliadel implant)* **Action:** Alkylating agent; nitrosourea forms DNA cross-links to inhibit DNA **Dose:** 150–200 mg/m² q6–8wk single or ÷ dose daily Inj over 2 d; 20–65 mg/m² q4–6wk; 300–900 mg/m² in BMT

(per protocols); up to 8 implants in CNS op site; ↓ w/ hepatic & renal impair **Caution:** [D, ?] Renal/hepatic impair **CI:** ↓ BM, PRG **Disp:** Inj 100 mg/vial *Gliadel* wafer: 7.7 mg **SE:** ↓ BP, N/V, ↓ WBC & plt, phlebitis, facial flushing, hepatic/renal dysfunction, pulm fibrosis (may occur years after), optic neuroretinitis; heme tox may persist 4–6 wk after dose **Notes:** Do not give course more frequently than q6wk (cumulative tox) **Interactions:** ↑ Bleeding *W/* ASA, anticoagulants, NSAIDs; ↑ hepatic dysfunction *W/* etoposide; ↑ suppression of BM *W/* cimetidine, radiation or additional antineoplastics; ↓ effects *OF* phenytoin, digoxin; ↓ pulm Fxn **Labs:** ↑ AST, alk phos, bilirubin; ↑ HMG, Hct, WBC, RBC, plt counts; monitor PFTs **NIPE:** ⊘ PRG, breast-feeding, exposure to Infxns, ASA products; ✓ baseline PFTs, monitor pulm status

Carteolol (Ocupress, Carteolol Ophthalmic) [Beta-Blocker/ Glaucoma Agent] **Uses:** *↑ IOP, chronic open-angle glaucoma* **Action:** Blocks β-adrenergic receptors (β₁, β₂), mild ISA **Dose:** Ophthal 1 gtt in eye(s) bid **Caution:** [C, ?/–] Cardiac failure, asthma **CI:** Sinus bradycardia; heart block > 1st degree; bronchospasm **Disp:** Ophthal soln 1% **SE:** conjunctival hyperemia, anisocoria, keratitis, eye pain **NIPE:** Ophthal drug may cause photophobia & risk of burning; may ↑ cold sensitivity, mental confusion; no value in CHF; oral forms no longer available in US

Carvedilol (Coreg, Coreg CR) [Antihypertensive/Alpha-1- & Beta-Blocker] **Uses:** *HTN, mild–severe CHF, LVD post-MI* **Action:** Blocks adrenergic receptors, β₁, β₂, α₁ **Dose:** *HTN:* 6.25–12.5 mg bid or CR 20–80 mg PO daily *CHF:* 3.125–25 mg bid; w/ food to minimize ↓ BP **Caution:** [C (1st tri), D (2nd & 3rd tri), ?/–] asthma, DM **CI:** Decompensated CHF, 2nd-/3rd-degree heart block, SSS, severe bradycardia w/o pacemaker, asthma, severe hepatic impair **Disp:** Tabs 3.125, 6.25, 12.5, 25 mg; CR tabs 10, 20, 40, 80 mg **SE:** Dizziness, fatigue, hyperglycemia, may mask/potentiate hypoglycemia, bradycardia, edema, hypercholesterolemia **Interactions:** ↑ Effects *W/* cimetidine, clonidine, MAOIs, reserpine, verapamil, fluoxetine, paroxetine, EtOH; ↑ effects *OF* digoxin, hypoglycemics, cyclosporine, CCBs; ↓ effects *W/* rifampin, NSAIDs **Labs:** ↑ Digoxin levels; ↑ LFTs, K⁺, triglycerides, uric acid, BUN, Cr, alk phos, glucose; ↓ pt, INR, plts **NIPE:** Do not D/C abruptly; food slows absorption but reduces risk of dizziness; may cause dry eyes w/ contact lenses

Caspofungin (Cancidas) [Antifungal/Echinocandin] **Uses:** *Invasive aspergillosis refractory/intolerant to standard Rx, esophageal candidiasis* **Action:** Echinocandin; ↓ fungal cell wall synth; highest activity in regions of active cell growth **Dose:** 70 mg IV load day 1, 50 mg/d IV; ↓ in hepatic impair **Caution:** [C, ?/–] Do not use w/ cyclosporine; not studied as initial Rx **CI:** Allergy to any component **Disp:** Inj 50, 70 mg powder for recons **SE:** Fever, HA, N/V, thrombophlebitis at site **Interactions:** ↑ Effects *W/* cyclosporine; ↓ effects *W/* carbamazepine, dexamethasone, efavirenz, nelfinavir, nevirapine, phenytoin, rifampin; ↓ effect *OF* tacrolimus **Labs:** ↑ LFTs, serum alk phos; ↓ K⁺, Hgb, Hct **NIPE:**

Monitor during Inf; infuse slowly over 1 h & ⊘ mix w/ other drugs; limited experience beyond 2 wk of Rx

Cefaclor (Ceclor, Raniclor) [Antibiotic/Cephalosporin-2nd Generation] **Uses:** *Bacterial Infxns of the upper & lower resp tract, skin, bone, urinary tract, Abd* **Action:** 2nd-gen cephalosporin; ↓ cell wall synth *Spectrum:* More gram(−) activity than 1st-gen cephalosporins; effective against gram(+) (*Streptococcus* sp, *S aureus*); good gram(−) against *H influenzae, E coli, Klebsiella, Proteus* **Dose:** *Adults.* 250–500 mg PO tid; ER 375–500 mg bid *Peds.* 20–40 mg/kg/d PO ÷ 8–12 h; ↓ renal impair **Caution:** [B, +] antacids ↓ absorption **CI:** Cephalosporin/PCN allergy **Disp:** Caps 250, 500 mg; tabs ER 375, 500 mg; chew tabs *(Raniclor)* 250, 375 mg; susp 125, 187, 250, 375 mg/5 mL **SE:** N/D, rash, HA, rhinitis, vaginitis **Interactions:** ↑ Bleeding *W/* anticoagulants; ↑ nephrotox *W/* aminoglycosides, loop diuretics; ↑ effects *W/* probenecid; ↓ effects *W/* antacids, chloramphenicol **Labs:** ↑ LFTs, eosinophils; ↓ Hgb, Hct, plts, WBC; false(+) direct Coombs test **NIPE:** Take w/ food to < GI upset; monitor for super Infxn, ⊘ antacids w/in 2 h of XR tabs

Cefadroxil (Duricef) [Antibiotic/Cephalosporin-1st Generation] **Uses:** *Infxns of skin, bone, upper & lower resp tract, urinary tract* **Action:** 1st-gen cephalosporin; ↓ cell wall synth. *Spectrum:* Good gram(+) (group A β-hemolytic *Streptococcus, Staphylococcus*); gram(−) (*E coli, Proteus, Klebsiella*) **Dose:** *Adults.* 1–2 g/d PO, 2 ÷ doses *Peds.* 30 mg/kg/d ÷ bid; ↓ in renal impair **Caution:** [B, +] **CI:** Cephalosporin/PCN allergy **Disp:** Caps 500 mg; tabs 1 g; susp, 250, 500 mg/5 mL **SE:** N/V/D, rash **Interactions:** ↑ Nephrotox *W/* aminoglycosides, loop diuretics; ↑ effects *W/* probenecid **Labs:** LFTs, eosinophils, BUN, Cr; ↓ Hgb, Hct, plts, WBC false(+) direct Coombs test **NIPE:** Take w/ food to < GI upset; monitor for super Infxn

Cefazolin (Ancef, Kefzol) [Antibiotic/Cephalosporin-1st Generation] **Uses:** *Infxns of skin, bone, upper & lower resp tract, urinary tract* **Action:** 1st-gen cephalosporin; β-lactam ↓ cell wall synth *Spectrum:* Good gram(+) bacilli & cocci, (*Streptococcus, Staphylococcus* [except *Enterococcus*]); some gram(−) (*E coli, Proteus, Klebsiella*) **Dose:** *Adults.* 1–2 g IV q8h *Peds.* 25–100 mg/kg/d IV ÷ q6–8h; ↓ in renal impair **Caution:** [B, +] **CI:** Cephalosporin/PCN allergy **Disp:** Inj: 500 mg, 1, 10, 20 g **SE:** D, rash , Inj site pain **Notes:** Widely used for surgical prophylaxis **Interactions:** ↑ Bleeding *W/* anticoagulants; ↑ nephrotox *W/* aminoglycosides, loop diuretics; ↑ effects *W/* probenecid; ↓ effects *W/* antacids, chloramphenicol **Labs:** ↑ LFTs, eosinophils; false(+) direct Coombs test, Clinitest; monitor PT in pts w/ hepatic/renal impair, long-term use, or on anticoagulant therapy **NIPE:** Take w/ food to < GI upset; monitor for super Infxn; monitor renal Fxn

Cefdinir (Omnicef) [Antibiotic/Cephalosporin-3rd Generation] **Uses:** *Infxns of the resp tract, skin, bone, & urinary tract* **Action:** 3rd-gen cephalosporin; ↓ cell wall synth *Spectrum:* Many gram(+) & (−) organisms; more active than cefaclor & cephalexin against *Streptococcus, Staphylococcus*; some anaerobes

Dose: *Adults.* 300 mg PO bid or 600 mg/d PO *Peds.* 7 mg/kg PO bid or 14 mg/kg/d PO; ↓ in renal impair **Caution:** [B, +] w/ PCN-sensitive pts, serum sickness-like Rxns reported **CI:** Hypersensitivity to cephalosporins **Disp:** Caps 300 mg; susp 125, 250 mg/5 mL **SE:** Anaphylaxis, D, rare pseudomembranous colitis **Interactions:** ↑ Bleeding *W/* anticoagulants; ↑ nephrotox *W/* aminoglycosides, loop diuretics; ↑ effects *W/* probenecid; ↓ effects *W/* antacids, chloramphenicol; ↓ effects *W/* Fe supls **Labs:** ↑ LFTs, eosenophils; false(+) direct Coombs test & Clinitest **NIPE:** Take w/ food to < GI upset; monitor for super Infxn; stools may initially turn red in color; instruct pt to report persistent D; ⊘ antacids w/in 2 h of this drug; suspension contains sugar

Cefditoren (Spectracef) [Antibiotic/Cephalosporin-3rd Generation]
Uses: *Acute exacerbations of chronic bronchitis, pharyngitis, tonsillitis; skin Infxns* **Action:** 3rd-gen cephalosporin; ↓ cell wall synth *Spectrum:* Good gram(+) (*Streptococcus & Staphylococcus*); gram(−) (*H influenzae & M catarrhalis*) **Dose:** *Adults & Peds > 12 y. Skin:* 200 mg PO bid × 10 d *Chronic bronchitis ,pharyngitis, tonsillitis:* 400 mg PO bid × 10 d; avoid antacids w/in 2 h; take w/ meals; ↓ in renal impair **Caution:** [B, ?] Renal/hepatic impair **CI:** Cephalosporin/PCN allergy, milk protein, or carnitine deficiency **Disp:** 200-mg tabs **SE:** HA, N/V/D, colitis, nephrotox, hepatic dysfunction, SJS, toxic epidermal necrolysis, allergic Rxns **Notes:** Causes renal excretion of carnitine; tabs contain milk protein **Interactions:** ↑ Bleeding *W/* anticoagulants; ↑ nephrotox *W/* aminoglycosides, loop diuretics; ↑ effects *W/* probenecid; ↓ effects *W/* antacids, chloramphenicol **Labs:** ↑ LFTs; ↓ PT, monitor PT in renal or hepatic impair or poor nutritional state; false(+) direct Coombs test & Clinitest **NIPE:** High-fat meal will ↑ bioavailability; monitor for super Infxn; report persistent D; ⊘ antacids w/in 2 h of this drug

Cefepime (Maxipime) [Antibiotic/Cephalosporin-4th Generation] **Uses:** *Comp/uncomp UTI, pneumonia, empiric febrile neutropenia, skin/soft tissue Infxns, comp intra-Abd Infxns* **Action:** 4th-gen cephalosporin; ↓ cell wall synth *Spectrum:* Gram(+) *S pneumoniae, S aureus,* gram(−) *K pneumoniae, E coli, P aeruginosa,& Enterobacter* sp **Dose:** *Adults.* 1–2 g IV q8–12h *Peds.* 50 mg/kg q8h for febrile neutropenia; 50 mg/kg for skin/soft-tissue Infxns; ↓ in renal impair **Caution:** [B, +] **CI:** Cephalosporin/PCN allergy **Disp:** Inj 500 mg, 1, 2 g **SE:** Rash, pruritus, N/V/D, fever, HA **Interactions:** ↑ Nephrotox *W/* aminoglycosides, loop diuretics; ↓ effects *W/* probenecid **Labs:** ↑ LFTs; ↓ HMG, Hct, PT; (+) Coombs test w/o hemolysis **NIPE:** Monitor for super Infxn; report persistent D; monitor Inf site for inflammation; can give IM or IV; concern over ↑ death rates not confirmed by FDA

Cefixime (Suprax) [Antibiotic/Cephalosporin-3rd Generation]
Uses: *Resp tract, skin, bone, & UTI* **Action:** 3rd-gen cephalosporin; ↓ cell wall synth *Spectrum: S pneumoniae, S pyogenes, H influenzae,* & enterobacteria **Dose:** *Adults.* 400 mg PO ÷ daily–bid *Peds.* 8–20 mg/kg/d PO ÷ daily–bid; ↓ w/ renal impair **Caution:** [B, +] **CI:** Cephalosporin/PCN allergy **Disp:** Susp 100, 200 mg/5 mL

SE: N/V/D, flatulence, & Abd pain **Interactions:** ↑ Nephrotox W/ aminoglycosides, loop diuretics; ↑ effects W/ nifedipine, probenecid **Labs:** ↑ LFTs, eosinophils, BUN, Cr; monitor renal & hepatic Fxn; WBC; false(+) direct Coombs test **NIPE:** Monitor for super Infxn; after mixing susp it is stable for 14 d w/o refrigeration; use susp for otitis media

Cefoperazone (Cefobid) [Antibiotic/Cephalosporin-3rd Generation]

Uses: *Rx Infxns of the resp, skin, urinary tract, sepsis* **Action:** 3rd-gen cephalosporin; ↓ bacterial cell wall synth *Spectrum:* Gram(−) (eg, *E coli*, *Klebsiella*), *P aeruginosa* but < ceftazidime; gram(+) variable against *Streptococcus* & *Staphylococcus* sp **Dose:** *Adults.* 2–4 g/d IM/IV ÷ q8–12h (16 g/d max) *Peds.* (Not approved) 100–150 mg/kg/d IM/IV ÷ bid–tid (12 g/d max); ↓ in renal/hepatic impair **Caution:** [B, +] May ↑ bleeding risk **CI:** Cephalosporin/PCN allergy **Disp:** Powder for Inj 1, 2, 10 g **SE:** D, rash, hypoprothrombinemia, & bleeding (d/t MTT side chain) **Interactions:** ↑ Bleeding W/ anticoagulants; ↑ nephrotox W/ aminoglycosides, loop diuretics **Labs:** ↑ LFTs, eosinophils; monitor BUN, Cr; ↓ HMG, Hct, plts **NIPE:** Monitor for super Infxn; disulfiram-like Rxn w/ concurrent use of EtOH (tachycardia, N/V, sweating, flushing, HA, blurred vision, confusion)

Cefotaxime (Claforan) [Antibiotic/Cephalosporin-3rd Generation]

Uses: *Infxns of lower resp tract, skin, bone & Jt, urinary tract, meningitis, sepsis, PID, GC* **Action:** 3rd-gen cephalosporin; ↓ cell wall synth *Spectrum:* Most gram(−) (not *Pseudomonas*), some gram(+) cocci *S pneumoniae*, *S aureus* (penicillinase/nonpenicillinase producing), *H influenzae* (including ampicillin-resistant), not *Enterococcus*; many PCN-resistant pneumococci **Dose:** *Adults. Uncomp Infxn:* 2 g IV/IM q12h *Mod–severe Infxn* 1–2 g IV/IM; severe/septicemia 2 g IV/IM q4–8h *GC urethritis, cervicitis, rectal in female:* 0.5 g IM × 1; rectal GC men 1 g IM × 1 *Peds.* 50–200 mg/kg/d IV ÷ q6–8h; ↓ w/ renal/hepatic impair **Caution:** [B, +] Arrhythmia w/ rapid Inj; w/ colitis **CI:** Cephalosporin/PCN allergy **Disp:** Powder for Inj 500 mg, 1, 2, 10, 20 g, premixed Inf 20 mg/mL, 40 mg/mL **SE:** D, rash, pruritus, colitis **Interactions:** ↑ Nephrotox W/ aminoglycosides, loop diuretics; ↑ effects W/ probenecid **Labs:** ↑ LFTs, eosinophils, transaminases, BUN, Cr; ↓ HMG, Hct, plts, WBC **NIPE:** Monitor for super Infxn; IM Inj deep into large muscle mass; rotate Inf sites

Cefotetan (Cefotan) [Antibiotic/Cephalosporin-2nd Generation]

Uses: *Infxns of the upper & lower resp tract, skin, bone, urinary tract, Abd, & gynecologic system* **Action:** 2nd-gen cephalosporin; ↓ cell wall synth *Spectrum:* Less active against gram(+) anaerobes including *B fragilis*; gram(−), including *E coli*, *Klebsiella*, & *Proteus* **Dose:** *Adults.*1–3 g IV q12h *Peds.* 20–40 mg/kg/d IV ÷ q12h (6 g/d max) ↓ w/ renal impair **Caution:** [B, +] May ↑ bleeding risk; w/ h/o of PCN allergies, w/ other nephrotoxic drugs **CI:** Cephalosporin/PCN allergy **Disp:** Powder for Inj 1, 2, 10 g **SE:** D, rash, eosinophilia, ↑ transaminases, hypoprothrombinemia, & bleeding (d/t MTT side chain) **Interactions:** ↑ Bleeding W/ anticoagulants; ↑

nephrotox *W/* aminoglycosides, loop diuretics **Labs:** ↑ LFTs, eosinophils; ↓ HMG, Hct, plts **NIPE:** Monitor for super Infxn; rotate Inf sites; may interfere w/ warfarin

Cefoxitin (Mefoxin) [Antibiotic/Cephalosporin-2nd Generation]
Uses: *Infxns of the upper & lower resp tract, skin, bone, urinary tract, Abd, & gynecologic system* **Action:** 2nd-gen cephalosporin; ↓ cell wall synth *Spectrum:* Good gram(−) against enteric bacilli (ie, *E coli, Klebsiella,* & *Proteus*); anaerobic *B fragilis* **Dose:** *Adults.* 1–2 g IV q6–8h **Peds.** 80–160 mg/kg/d ÷ q4–6h (12 g/d max); ↓ w/ renal impair **Caution:** [B, +] **CI:** Cephalosporin/PCN allergy **Disp:** Powder for Inj 1, 2, 10 g **SE:** D, rash **Interactions:** ↑ Nephrotox *W/* aminoglycosides, loop diuretics; ↑ effects *W/* probenecid **Labs:** ↑ LFTs, eosinophils, transaminases, BUN, Cr; ↓ HMG, Hct, plts **NIPE:** Monitor for super Infxn, report persistent D

Cefpodoxime (Vantin) [Antibiotic/Cephalosporin-3rd Generation]
Uses: *Rx resp, skin, & UTI* **Action:** 3rd-gen cephalosporin; ↓ cell wall synth *Spectrum: S pneumoniae* or non-β-lactamase-producing *H influenzae;* acute uncomp *N gonorrhoeae;* some uncomp gram(−) (*E coli, Klebsiella, Proteus*) **Dose:** *Adults.* 100–400 mg PO q12h **Peds.** 10 mg/kg/d PO ÷ bid; ↓ in renal impair, w/ food **Caution:** [B, +] **CI:** Cephalosporin/PCN allergy **Disp:** Tabs 100, 200 mg; susp 50, 100 mg/5 mL **SE:** D, rash, HA **Interactions:** Drug interactions w/ agents that ↑ gastric pH; ↑ nephrotox *W/* aminoglycosides, loop diuretics; ↑ effects *W/* probenecid; ↓ effects *W/* antacids, chloramphenicol **Labs:** ↑ LFTs, eosinophils, transaminases; ↓ BUN, Cr; ↓ HMG, Hct, plts; (+) Coombs test **NIPE:** Food will ↑ absorption & < GI upset; monitor for super Infxn; ⊘ take w/in 2 h of antacids;

Cefprozil (Cefzil) [Antibiotic/Cephalosporin-2nd Generation]
Uses: *Rx resp tract, skin, & UTI* **Action:** 2nd-gen cephalosporin; ↓ cell wall synth *Spectrum:* Active against MSSA, *Streptococcus,* & gram(−) bacilli (*E coli, Klebsiella, P mirabilis, H influenzae, Moraxella*) **Dose:** *Adults.* 250–500 mg PO daily–bid **Peds.** 7.5–15 mg/kg/d PO ÷ bid; ↓ in renal impair **Caution:** [B, +] **CI:** Cephalosporin/PCN allergy **Disp:** Tabs 250, 500 mg; susp 125, 250 mg/5 mL **SE:** D, dizziness, rash **Interactions:** ↑ Nephrotox *W/* aminoglycosides, loop diuretics; ↑ effects *W/* probenecid; ↓ effects *W/* antacids, chloramphenicol **Labs:** ↑ LFTs, eosinophils, transaminases; ↓ HMG, Hct, plts **NIPE:** Food will ↑ absorption & < GI upset, monitor for super Infxn; ⊘ take w/in 2 h of antacids; stable after reconstitution for 14 d—keep refrigerated; use higher doses for otitis & pneumonia

Ceftaroline (Teflaro) [Cephalosporin] Uses: *Tx skin/skin structure Infxn & CAP* **Action:** Unclassified ("5th-gen") cephalosporin; ↓ cell wall synth *Spectrum:* Gram(+) *S aureus* (MSSA/MRSA), *S pyogenes, S agalactiae, S pneumoniae;* Gram(−) *E coli, K pneumoniae, K oxytoca, H influenza* **Dose:** *Adults.* 600 mg IV q12h; CrCl 30–50 mL/min, 400 mg IV q12h; CrCl 15–29 mL/min, 300 mg IV q12h; CrCl < 15 mL/min, 200 mg IV q12h; Inf over 1 h **Caution:** [B, ?/−] Monitor for *C difficile*–associated D **CI:** cephalsporin sensitivity **Disp:** Inj **SE:** Hypersensitivity Rxn, D/N, rash, constipation, phlebitis, **Labs:** ↑ LFTs, (+) Coombs test; ↓ K⁺

Ceftazidime (Fortaz, Tazicef) [Antibiotic/Cephalosporin-3rd Generation] Uses: *Rx resp tract, skin, bone, UTI, meningitis, & septicemia* Action: 3rd-gen cephalosporin; ↓ cell wall synth *Spectrum: P aeruginosa* sp, good gram(−) activity Dose: *Adults.* 500 mg−2 g IV/IM q8−12h *Peds.* 30−50 mg/kg/dose IV q8h; ↓ in renal impair Caution: [B, +] PCN sensitivity CI: Cephalosporin/PCN allergy Disp: Powder for Inj 500 mg, 1, 2, 6 g SE: D, rash Interactions: ↑ Nephrotox W/ aminoglycosides, loop diuretics; ↑ effects W/ probenecid; ↓ effects W/ antacids, chloramphenicol Labs: ↑ LFTs, eosinophils, transaminases; ↓ HMG, Hct, plts NIPE: Food will ↑ absorption & < GI upset, monitor for super Infxn; ⊘ take w/in 2 h of antacids; stable after reconstitution for 14 d—keep refrigerated; use only for proven or strongly suspected Infxn to ↓ development of drug resistance

Ceftibuten (Cedax) [Antibiotic/Cephalosporin-3rd Generation] Uses: *Rx resp tract, skin, UTI, & otitis media* Action: 3rd-gen cephalosporin; ↓ cell wall synth *Spectrum: H influenzae & M catarrhalis*; weak against *S pneumoniae* Dose: *Adults.* 400 mg/d PO *Peds.* 9 mg/kg/d PO; ↓ in renal impair; take on empty stomach (susp) Caution: [B, +] CI: Cephalosporin/PCN allergy Disp: Caps 400 mg; susp 90 mg/5 mL SE: D, rash Interactions: ↑ Nephrotox W/ aminoglycosides, loop diuretics; ↑ effects W/ probenecid; ↓ effects W/ antacids, chloramphenicol Labs: ↑ LFTs, eosinophils, transaminases; ↓ HMG, Hct, plts NIPE: Take oral suspension 1 h < or 2 h > a meal; monitor for super Infxn; stable after reconstitution for 14 d—keep refrigerated

Ceftizoxime (Cefizox) [Antibiotic/Cephalosporin-3rd Generation] Uses: *Rx resp tract, skin, bone, & UTI, meningitis, septicemia* Action: 3rd-gen cephalosporin; ↓ cell wall synth *Spectrum:* Good gram(−) bacilli (not *Pseudomonas*), some gram(+) cocci (not *Enterococcus*), & some anaerobes Dose: *Adults.* 1−4 g IV q8−12h *Peds.* 150−200 mg/kg/d IV ÷ q6−8h; ↓ in renal impair Caution: [B, +] CI: Cephalosporin/PCN allergy Disp: Inj 1, 2, 10 g SE: D, fever, rash, thrombocytosis Interactions: ↑ Nephrotox W/ aminoglycosides, loop diuretics; ↑ effects W/ probenecid Labs: ↑ LFTs, eosinophils, transaminases; ↓ HMG, Hct, plts NIPE: Monitor for super Infxn; stable after reconstitution for 1 d at room temperature & 4 d if refrigerated; IM Inj deep into large muscle mass

Ceftriaxone (Rocephin) [Antibiotic/Cephalosporin-3rd Generation] WARNING: Avoid in hyperbilirubinemic neonates or co-infused w/ calcium-containing products Uses: *Resp tract (pneumonia), skin, bone, Abd, UTI, meningitis, & septicemia* Action: 3rd-gen cephalosporin; ↓ cell wall synth *Spectrum:* Mod gram(+); excellent β-lactamase producers Dose: *Adults.* 1−2 g IV/IM q12−24h *Peds.* 50−100 mg/kg/d IV/IM ÷ q12−24h; ↓ w/ renal impair Caution: [B, +] CI: Cephalosporin allergy; hyperbilirubinemic neonates Disp: Powder for Inj 250 mg, 500 mg, 1, 2, 10 g; premixed 20, 40 mg/mL SE: D, rash, leukopenia, thrombocytosis Interactions: ↑ Nephrotox W/ aminoglycosides, loop diuretics; ↑ effects W/ probenecid Labs: ↑ LFTs, eosinophils, BUN, Cr; ↓ HMG, Hct, plts NIPE:

Monitor for super Infxn; solns are stable for 24 h at room temperature after dilution; IM Inj deep into large muscle mass

Cefuroxime (Ceftin [PO], Zinacef [Parenteral]) [Antibiotic/Cephalosporin-2nd Generation]
Uses: *Upper & lower resp tract, skin, bone, urinary tract, Abd, gynecologic Infxns* Action: ↓ cell wall synth Spectrum: Staphylococci, group B streptococci, H influenzae, E coli, Enterobacter, Salmonella,& Klebsiella Dose: Adults. 750 mg–1.5 g IV q6h or 250–500 mg PO bid Peds. 75–150 mg/kg/d IV ÷ q8h or 20–30 mg/kg/d PO ÷ bid; ↓ w/ renal impair; take PO w/ food Caution: [B, +] CI: Cephalosporin/PCN allergy Disp: Tabs 250, 500 mg; susp 125, 250 mg/5 mL; powder for Inj 750 mg, 1.5, 7.5 g SE: D, rash Notes: Cefuroxime film-coated tabs & susp not bioequivalent; do not substitute on a mg/mg basis; IV crosses blood–brain barrier Interactions: ↑ Nephrotox W/ aminoglycosides, loop diuretics; ↑ effects W/ probenecid; ↑ effects W/ Al & Mg antacids Labs: ↑ LFTs, eosinophils, BUN, Cr; ↓ HMG, Hct, plts NIPE: Monitor for super Infxn; high-fat meals ↑ drug bioavailability; give suspension w/ food; IM Inj deep into large muscle mass

Celecoxib (Celebrex) [Anti-Inflammatory/COX-2 Inhibitor]
WARNING: ↑ Risk of serious CV thrombotic events, MI, & stroke, can be fatal; ↑ risk of serious GI adverse events including bleeding, ulceration, & perforation of the stomach or intestines; can be fatal Uses: *OA, RA, ankylosing spondylitis acute pain, primary dysmenorrhea preventive in FAP* Action: NSAID; ↓ COX-2 pathway Dose: 100–200 mg/d or bid; FAP: 400 mg PO bid; ↓ w/ hepatic impair; take w/ food/milk Caution: [C/D (3rd tri), ?] w/ renal impair CI: Sulfonamide allergy, perioperative CABG Disp: Caps 100, 200, 400 mg SE: See Warning; GI upset, HTN, edema, renal failure, HA Interactions: ↑ Effects W/ fluconazole; ↑ effects OF Li; ↑ risks of GI upset and/or bleeding W/ ASA, NSAIDs, warfarin, EtOH; ↓ effects W/ Al- & Mg-containing antacids, ↑ effects OF thiazide diuretics, loop diuretics, ACEIs Labs: ↑ LFTs, BUN, Cr, CPK, alk phos; monitor for hypercholesterolemia, hyperglycemia, hypokalemia, hypophosphatemia, albuminuria, hematuria NIPE: Take w/ food if GI distress; watch for Sxs of GI bleed; no effect on plt/bleeding time; can affect drugs metabolized by P450 pathway

Cephalexin (Keflex, Panixine DisperDose) [Antibiotic/Cephalosporin-1st Generation]
Uses: *Skin, bone, upper/lower resp tract (streptococcal pharyngitis), otitis media, uncomp cystitis Infxns* Action: 1st-gen cephalosporin; ↓ cell wall synth Spectrum: Streptococcus (including β-hemolytic), Staphylococcus, E coli, Proteus, & Klebsiella Dose: Adults & Peds = 15 y. 250–1000 mg PO qid; Rx cystitis 7–14 d (4 g/d max) Peds < 15 y. 25–100 mg/kg/d PO ÷ bid–qid; ↓ in renal impair; on empty stomach Caution: [B, +] CI: Cephalosporin/PCN allergy Disp: Caps 250, 500 mg; (Panixine Disper-Dose) tabs for oral susp 100, 125, 250 mg; susp 125, 250 mg/5 mL SE: D, rash, gastritis, dyspepsia, C difficile colitis, vaginitis Interactions: ↑ Nephrotox W/ aminoglycosides, loop diuretics; ↑ effects W/ probenecid Labs: ↑ LFTs, eosinophils, alk phos, bilirubin,

LDH; ↓ HMG, Hct, plts **NIPE:** Food will ↑ absorption & < GI upset; monitor for super Infxn; oral susp stable for 14 d after reconstitution if refrigerated

Cephradine (Velosef) [Antibiotic/Cephalosporin-1st Generation] Uses: *Resp, GU, GI, skin, soft tissue, bone, & Jt Infxns* **Action:** 1st-gen cephalosporin; ↓ cell wall synth *Spectrum:* Gram(+) bacilli & cocci (not *Enterococcus*); some gram(−) (*E coli, Proteus, & Klebsiella*) **Dose: Adults.** 250–500 mg q6–12h (8 g/d max). *Peds > 9 mo.* 25–100 mg/kg/d ÷ bid–qid (4 g/d max); ↓ in renal impair **Caution:** [B, +] **CI:** Cephalosporin/PCN allergy **Disp:** Caps: 250, 500 mg; powder for susp 125, 250 mg/5 mL **SE:** Rash, , N/V/D **Interactions:** ↑ Nephrotox *W/* aminoglycosides, loop diuretics; ↑ effects *W/* probenecid **Labs:** ↑ LFTs, eosinophils, alk phos, bilirubin, LDH; ↓ HMG, Hct, plts **NIPE:** Food will ↑ absorption & < GI upset; monitor for super Infxn; oral suspension stable for 14 d after reconstitution if refrigerated

Certolizumab Pegol (Cimzia) [Tumor Necrosis Factor Blocker] **WARNING:** Serious Infxns (bacterial, fungal, TB, opportunistic) possible. D/C w/ severe Infxn/sepsis, test & monitor for TB w/ Tx; lymphoma/other CA possible in children/adolescents possible **Uses:** *Crohn Dz w/ inadequate response to conventional Tx; mod/severe RA* **Action:** TNF-α blocker **Dose:** *Crohn: Initial:* 400 mg SQ, repeat 2 & 4 wk after *Maint:* 400 mg SQ q4wk *RA: Initial:* 400 mg SQ, repeat 2 & 4 wk after *Maint:* 200 mg SQ qowk or 400 mg SQ q4wk **Caution:** [B, ?] Infxn, TB, autoimmune d/o, demyelinating CNS Dz, hep B reactivation **CI:** None **Disp:** Inj, powder for reconstitution 200 mg; Inj, soln 200 mg/mL (1 mL) **SE:** HA, N, URI, serious Infxns, TB, opportunistic Infxns, malignancies, demyelinating Dz, CHF, pancytopenia, lupus-like synd, new onset psoriasis **Interactions:** ↑ Risk of Infxn *W/* immunosuppressants **Labs:** May interfere w/ coagulation tests such as PTT **NIPE:** Do not give live/attenuated vaccines during therapy; avoid use w/ anakinra; 400 mg dose is 2 Inj of 200 mg each; monitor for Infxn

Cetirizine (Zyrtec, Zyrtec D) [Allergy/Antihistamine] [OTC] **Uses:** *Allergic rhinitis & other allergic Sxs including urticaria* **Action:** Nonsedating antihistamine; *ZyrtecD* contains decongestant **Dose:** *Adults & Children = 6 y.* 5–10 mg/d. *Zyrtec D:* 5/120 mg PO bid whole *Peds 6–11 mo.* 2.5 mg daily *12 mo–5 y.* 2.5 mg daily–bid; ↓ to qd in renal/hepatic impair **Caution:** [C, ?/−] w/ HTN, BPH, rare CNS stimulation, DM, heart Dz CI: Allergy to cetirizine, hydroxyzine, pseudoephedrine **Disp:** Tabs 5, 10 mg; chew tabs 5, 10 mg; syrup 1 mg/5 mL; *ZyrtecD:* Tabs 5/120 mg (cetirizine/pseudoephedrine) **SE:** HA, drowsiness, xerostomia **Interactions:** ↑ Effects *W/* anticholinergics, CNS depressants, theophylline, EtOH **Labs:** May cause false(−) w/ allergy skin tests **NIPE:** ⊘ Take w/ EtOH or CNS depressants can potentiate sedation; sun exposure can cause photosensitivity; swallow ER tabs whole

Cetuximab (Erbitux) [Antineoplastic/Recombinant Monoclonal Antibody] **WARNING:** Severe Inf Rxns including rapid onset of airway obst

(bronchospasm, stridor, hoarseness), urticaria, & ↓ BP; permanent D/C required; ↑ risk sudden death & cardiopulmonary arrest **Uses:** *EGFR + met colorectal CA w/ or w/o irinotecan, unresectable head/neck SCLC w/ RT; monotherapy in met head/neck CA* **Action:** Human/mouse recombinant MoAb; binds EGFR, ↓ tumor cell growth **Dose:** Per protocol; load 400 mg/m^2 IV over 2 h; 250 mg/m^2 given over 1 h 1 × wk **Caution:** [C, –] **Disp:** Inj 100 mg/50 mL **SE:** Acneform rash, asthenia/ malaise, N/V/D, Abd pain, alopecia, Inf Rxn, derm tox, interstitial lung Dz, fever, sepsis, dehydration, kidney failure, PE **Notes:** Assess tumor for EGFR before Rx; pretreatment w/ diphenhydramine **Interactions:** ⊘ Topical steroids; ↑ possibility of cardiotox **W/** radiation & cisplatin **Labs:** Monitor lytes, Mg^{2+}, Ca during & after drug therapy **NIPE:** Monitor for Inf Rxns for 1 h after Inf; during 1st 2 wk observe for skin tox; w/ mild SE ↓ Inf rate by 50%; limit sun exposure & UV light

Charcoal, Activated (Superchar, Actidose, Liqui-Char) [Adsorbent]
Uses: *Emergency poisoning by most drugs & chemicals (see CI)* **Action:** Adsorbent detoxicant **Dose:** Give w/ 70% sorbitol (2 mL/kg); repeated use of sorbitol not OK **Adults.** *Acute intoxication:* 25–100 g/dose *GI dialysis:* 20–50 g q6h for 1–2 d **Peds 1–12 y.** *Acute intoxication:* 1–2 g/kg/dose *GI dialysis:* 5–10 g/dose q4–8h **Caution:** [C, ?] May cause V (hazardous w/ petroleum & caustic ingestions); do not mix w/ dairy **CI:** Not effective for cyanide, mineral acids, caustic alkalis, organic solvents, Fe, EtOH, methanol poisoning, Li; do not use sorbitol in pts w/ fructose intolerance, intestinal obst, nonintact GI tract **Disp:** Powder, Liq, caps **SE:** Some Liq dosage forms in sorbitol base (a cathartic); V/D, black stools, constipation **Notes:** Charcoal w/ sorbitol not OK in children < 1 y; protect airway in lethargic/comatose pts **Interactions:** ↓ Effects if taken w/ ice cream, milk, sherbet; ↓ effects **OF** digoxin & absorption of other oral meds, ↓ effects **OF** syrup of ipecac **Labs:** Monitor for ↓ K$^+$ & Mg^{2+} **NIPE:** Most effective if given w/in 30 min of acute poisoning; only give to conscious pts

Chloral Hydrate (Aquachloral, Supprettes) [Sedative/Hypnotic/ CNS Depressant] [C-IV] **Uses:** *Short-term nocturnal & pre-op sedation* **Action:** Sedative hypnotic; active metabolite trichloroethanol **Dose:** **Adults.** *Hypnotic:* 500 mg–1 g PO or PR 30 min hs or before procedure *Sedative:* 250 mg PO or PR tid **Peds.** *Hypnotic:* 20–50 mg/kg/24 h PO or PR 30 min hs or before procedure *Sedative:* 5–15 mg/kg/dose q8h; avoid w/ CrCl < 50 mL/min or severe hepatic impair **Caution:** [C, +] Porphyria & in neonates, long-term care facility residents **CI:** Allergy to components; severe renal, hepatic, or cardiac Dz **Disp:** Caps 500 mg; syrup 500 mg/5 mL; supp 325, 500 mg **SE:** GI irritation, drowsiness, ataxia, dizziness, nightmares, rash **Interactions:** ↑ Effects **W/** antihistamines, barbiturates, paraldehyde, CNS depressants, opiate *analgesics,* EtOH; ↑ effects **OF** anticoagulants **Labs:** ↑ Eosinophils, BUN; ↓ WBCs **NIPE:** ⊘ Take w/ EtOH, CNS depressants; ⊘ chew or crush caps; may accumulate; tolerance may develop > 2 wk; taper dose; mix syrup in H$_2$O or fruit juice

Chlorambucil (Leukeran) [Antineoplastic/Alkylating Agent]
WARNING: Myelosuppressive, carcinogenic, teratogenic, associated w/ infertility
Uses: *CLL, Hodgkin Dz*, Waldenström macroglobulinemia **Action:** Alkylating agent (nitrogen mustard) **Dose:** (Per protocol) 0.1–0.2 mg/kg/d for 3–6 wk or 0.4 mg/kg/dose q2wk; ↓ w/ renal impair **Caution:** [D, ?] Sz disorder & BM suppression; affects human fertility **CI:** Previous resistance; alkylating agent allergy; w/ live vaccines **Disp:** Tabs 2 mg **SE:** ↓ BM, CNS stimulation, N/V, drug fever, rash, secondary leukemias, alveolar dysplasia, pulm fibrosis, hepatotoxic **Interactions:** ↑ BM suppression **W/** antineoplastic drugs & immunosuppressants; ↑ risk of bleeding **W/** ASA, anticoagulants **Labs:** ↑ Urine & serum uric acid, ALT, alk phos; ↓ HMG, Hct, neutrophil, plts, RBCs, WBCs; monitor LFTs, CBC, plts, serum uric acid **NIPE:** ⊘ PRG, breast-feeding, Infxn; ↑ fluids to 2–3 L/d; monitor lab work periodically & CBC w/ differential weekly during drug use; may cause hair loss; ↓ dose if pt has received radiation

Chlordiazepoxide (Librium, Mitran, Libritabs) [Anxiolytic, Sedative/Hypnotic/Benzodiazepine] [C-IV] **Uses:** *Anxiety, tension, EtOH withdrawal*, & pre-op apprehension **Action:** Benzodiazepine; antianxiety agent **Dose:** *Adults. Mild anxiety:* 5–10 mg PO tid–qid or PRN *Severe anxiety:* 25–50 mg IM, IV, or PO q6–8h or PRN *Peds > 6 y.* 0.5 mg/kg/24 h PO or IM ÷ q6–8h; ↓ in renal impair, elderly **Caution:** [D, ?] Resp depression, CNS impair, h/o of drug dependence; avoid in hepatic impair **CI:** Preexisting CNS depression, NAG **Disp:** Caps 5, 10, 25 mg; Inj 100 mg **SE:** Drowsiness, CP, rash, fatigue, memory impair, xerostomia, wgt gain **Interactions:** ↑ Effects **W/** antidepressants, antihistamines, anticonvulsants, barbiturates, general anesthetics, MAOIs, narcotics, phenothiazine cimetidine, disulfiram, fluconazole, itraconazole, ketoconazole, OCPs, INH, metoprolol, propoxyphene, propranolol, valproic acid, EtOH, grapefruit juice, kava kava, valerian; ↑ effects **OF** digoxin, phenytoin; ↓ effects **W/** aminophylline, antacids, carbamazepine, theophylline, rifampin, rifabutin, tobacco; ↓ effects **OF** levodopa **Labs:** ↑ LFTs, alk phos, bilirubin, triglycerides; ↓ granulocytes **NIPE:** ⊘ EtOH, PRG, breast-feeding; risk of photosensitivity—use sunscreen, orthostatic hypotension, tachycardia; erratic IM absorption

Chlorothiazide (Diuril) [Antihypertensive/Thiazide Diuretic] **Uses:** *HTN, edema* **Action:** Thiazide diuretic **Dose:** *Adults.* 500 mg–1 g PO daily–bid; 100–1000 mg/d IV (for edema only) *Peds > 6 mo.* 10–20 mg/kg/24 h PO ÷ bid; 4 mg/kg/d IV; OK w/ food **Caution:** [D, +] **CI:** Sensitivity to thiazides/sulfonamides, anuria **Disp:** Tabs 250, 500 mg; susp 250 mg/5 mL; Inj 500 mg/vial **SE:** dizziness, hyperglycemia, hyperuricemia, hyperlipidemia, photosensitivity **Interactions:** ↑ Effects **W/** ACEI, amphotericin B, corticosteroids; ↑ effects **OF** diazoxide, Li, MTX; ↓ effects **W/** colestipol, cholestyramine, NSAIDs; ↓ effects **OF** hypoglycemics **Labs:** ↓ K⁺, Na⁺; ↑ CPK, cholesterol, glucose, lytes, uric acid; monitor electrolytes **NIPE:** Do not use IM/SQ; take early in the day to avoid nocturia; monitor for gout, hyperglycemia, photosensitivity—use sunblock, I&O, wgt

Chlorpheniramine (Chlor-Trimeton, Others) [OTC] [Antihistamine/Propylamine]

WARNING: OTC meds w/ chlorpheniramine should not be used in peds < 2 y **Uses:** *Allergic rhinitis*, common cold **Action:** Antihistamine **Dose:** *Adults.* 4 mg PO q4–6h or 8–12 mg PO bid of SR *Peds.* 0.35 mg/kg/24 h PO ÷ q4–6h or 0.2 mg/kg/24 h SR **Caution:** [C, ?/–] BOO; NAG; hepatic Insuff **CI:** Allergy **Disp:** Tabs 4 mg; chew tabs 2 mg; SR tabs 8, 12 mg **SE:** Anticholinergic SE & sedation common, postural ↓ BP, QT changes, extrapyramidal Rxns, photosensitivity **Interactions:** ↑ Effects W/ other CNS depressants, EtOH, opioids, sedatives, MAOIs, atropine, haloperidol, phenothiazine, quinidine, disopyramide; ↑ effects OF epinephrine; ↓ effects OF heparin, sulfonylureas **Labs:** False(−) w/ allergy testing **NIPE:** D/C drug 4 d prior to allergy testing; take w/ food if GI distress; do not cut/crush/chew ER forms; recent deaths in pts < 2 y; associated w/ cough & cold meds [*MMWR* 2007 56(01):1–4]

Chlorpromazine (Thorazine) [Antipsychotic, Antiemetic/Phenothiazine]

Uses: *Psychotic disorders, N/V*, apprehension, intractable hiccups **Action:** Phenothiazine antipsychotic; antiemetic **Dose:** *Adults. Psychosis:* 10–25 mg PO bid–tid (usual 30–2000 mg/d in ÷ doses) *Severe Sxs:* 25 mg IM/IV initial; may repeat in 1–4 h; then 25–50 mg PO or PR tid *Hiccups:* 25–50 mg PO tid–qid *Children > 6 mo. Psychosis & N/V:* 0.5–1 mg/kg/dose PO q4–6h or IM/IV q6–8h **Caution:** [C, ?/–] Safety in children < 6 mo not established; Szs, avoid w/ hepatic impair, BM suppression **CI:** Sensitivity w/ phenothiazine; NAG **Disp:** Tabs 10, 25, 50, 100, 200 mg; soln 100 mg/mL; Inj 25 mg/mL **SE:** Extrapyramidal SE & sedation; α-adrenergic blocking properties; ↓ BP; ↑ QT interval **Interactions:** ↑ Effects W/ amodiaquine, chloroquine, sulfadoxine–pyrimethamine, antidepressants, narcotic analgesics, propranolol, quinidine, BBs, MAOIs, TCAs, EtOH, kava kava; ↑ effects OF anticholinergics, centrally acting antihypertensives, propranolol, valproic acid; ↓ effects W/ antacids, antidiarrheals, barbiturates, Li, tobacco; ↓ effects OF anticonvulsants, guanethidine, levodopa, Li, warfarin **Labs:** False(+) urine bilirubin; false(+) or (−) PRG test; ↑ alk phos, bilirubin, CK, GGT, eosinophil count; ↓ HMG, Hct, granulocytes, plts, WBC **NIPE:** Do not D/C abruptly; dilute PO conc in 2–4 oz of Liq; risk of photosensitivity—use sunscreen; risk of tardive dyskinesia; take w/ food if GI upset; may darken urine

Chlorpropamide (Diabinese) [Hypoglycemic/Sulfonylurea]

Uses: *Type 2 DM* **Action:** Sulfonylurea; ↑ pancreatic insulin release; ↑ peripheral insulin sensitivity; ↓ hepatic glucose output **Dose:** 100–500 mg/d; w/ food, ↓ hepatic impair **Caution:** [C, ?/–] CrCl < 50 mL/min; ↓ in hepatic impair **CI:** Cross-sensitivity w/ sulfonamides **Disp:** Tabs 100, 250 mg **SE:** HA, dizziness, rash, photosensitivity, hypoglycemia, SIADH **Interactions:** ↑ Effects W/ ASA, NSAIDs, anticoagulants, BBs, chloramphenicol, guanethidine, insulin, MAOIs, rifampin, sulfonamides, EtOH, juniper berries, ginseng, garlic, fenugreek, coriander, dandelion root, celery, bitter melon, ginkgo; ↓ effects W/ diazoxide, thiazide diuretics **Labs:** ↑ Alk phos, bilirubin, BUN, Cr, cholesterol; ↓ glucose HMG, Hct, plts, WBC **NIPE:** ⊘ EtOH (disulfiram-like Rxn)

Chlorthalidone (Hygroton, Others) [Antihypertensive/Thiazide Diuretic] Uses: *HTN* **Action:** Thiazide diuretic **Dose:** *Adults.* 25–100 mg PO daily *Peds.* (Not approved) 2 mg/kg/dose PO 3x/wk or 1–2 mg/kg/d PO; ↓ in renal impair; OK w/ food, milk **Caution:** [D, +] **CI:** Cross-sensitivity w/ thiazides or sulfonamides; anuria **Disp:** Tabs 15, 25, 50 mg **SE:** Dizziness, photosensitivity, hyperglycemia, hyperuricemia, sexual dysfunction **Interactions:** ↑ Effects W/ ACEIs, diazoxide; ↑ effects OF digoxin, Li, MTX; ↓ effects W/ cholestyramine, colestipol, NSAIDs; ↓ effects OF hypoglycemics; ↓ K+ W/ amphotericin B, carbenoxolone, corticosteroids **Labs:** ↑ Bilirubin, Ca²⁺, Cr, uric acid; ↑ glucose in DM; ↓ Mg²⁺, K+, Na+ **NIPE:** May take w/ food & milk, take early in day, use sunblock; ↑ K+-rich foods in diet

Chlorzoxazone (Paraflex, Parafon Forte DSC, Others) [Skeletal Muscle Relaxant/ANS Drug] Uses: *Adjunct to rest & physical therapy to relieve discomfort associated w/ acute, painful musculoskeletal conditions* **Action:** Centrally acting skeletal muscle relaxant **Dose:** *Adults.* 250–500 mg PO tid–qid *Peds.* 20 mg/kg/d in 3–4 ÷ doses **Caution:** [C, ?] Avoid EtOH & CNS depressants **CI:** Severe liver Dz **Disp:** Tabs 250, 500 mg **SE:** Drowsiness, tachycardia, dizziness, hepatotox, angioedema **Interactions:** ↑ Effects W/ antihistamines, CNS depressants, MAOIs, TCAs, opiates, EtOH, watercress **Labs:** ↑ Alk phos, bilirubin; monitor LFTs **NIPE:** Urine may turn reddish purple or orange

Cholecalciferol [Vitamin D₃] (Delta D) [Vitamin/Dietary Supplement] Uses: *Dietary supls to Rx vit D deficiency* **Action:** ↑ Intestinal Ca²⁺ absorption **Dose:** 400–1000 IU/d PO **Caution:** [A (D doses above the RDA), +] **CI:** ↑ Ca²⁺, hypervitaminosis, allergy **Disp:** Tabs 400, 1000 IU **SE:** Vit D tox (renal failure, HTN, psychosis) **Notes:** 1 mg cholecalciferol = 40,000 IU vit D activity **Interactions:** ↑ Risk of arrhythmias W/ cardiac glycosides; ↓ effects W/ cholestyramine, colestipol, mineral oil, orlistat, phenobarbital, phenytoin **Labs:** ↑ BUN, Ca, cholesterol, Cr, LFTs, urine urea **NIPE:** Vit D is fat-soluble; mineral oil interferes w/ vit D absorption; vit D is needed for Ca absorption

Cholestyramine (Questran, Questran Light, Prevalite) [Antilipemic, Bile Acid Sequestrant] Uses: *Hypercholesterolemia; hyperlipidemia, pruritus associated w/ partial biliary obst; D associated w/ excess fecal bile acids* pseudomembranous colitis, dig tox, hyperoxaluria **Action:** Binds intestinal bile acids, forms insoluble complexes **Dose:** *Adults.* Titrate: 4 g/d–bid ↑ to max 24 g/d ÷ 1–6 doses/d *Peds.* 240 mg/kg/d in 3 ÷ doses **Caution:** [C, ?] Constipation, PKU, may interfere w/ other drug absorption; consider supls w/ fat-soluble vits **CI:** Complete biliary or bowel obst; w/ mycophenolate hyperlipoproteinemia types III, IV, V **Disp:** *(Questran)* 4 g cholestyramine resin/9 g powder *(Prevalite)* w/ aspartame: 4 g resin/5.5 g powder *(Questran Light):* 4 g resin/6.4 g powder **SE:** Constipation, Abd pain, bloating, HA, rash, vit K deficiency **Interactions:** ↓ Effects OF APAP, amiodarone, anticoagulants, ASA, cardiac glycosides, clindamycin, corticosteroids, diclofenac, fat-soluble vits, gemfibrozil, glipizide, Fe salts, MTX, methyldopa, nicotinic acid, PCNs, phenobarbital, phenytoin, propranolol, thiazide diuretics, tetracyclines, thyroid drugs, troglitazone, warfarin if given w/ this drug **Labs:** ↑ Alk phos, PT; ↓ cholesterol, folic acid, vit A, D, K; ✓ lipids **NIPE:** ↑ Fluids, take other drugs 1–2 h before or 6 h after; OD may cause GI obst; mix 4 g in 2–6 oz of noncarbonated beverage

Ciclesonide, Inhalation (Alvesco) [Corticosteroid] Uses: *Asthma maint* **Action:** Inhaled steroid **Dose:** *Adults & Peds > 12 y.* On *bronchodilators alone:* 80 mcg bid (320 mcg/d max) *Inhaled corticosteroids:* 80 mcg bid (640 mcg/d max) *On oral corticosteroids:* 320 mcg bid, 640 mcg/d max **Caution:** [C, ?] **CI:** Status asthmaticus or other acute episodes of asthma, hypersensitivity **Disp:** Inh 80, 160 mcg/actuation **SE:** HA, nasopharyngitis, sinusitis, pharyngolaryngeal pain, URI, arthralgia, nasal congestion **Labs:** Monitor for ↓ BMD **NIPE:** Oral *Candida* risk, rinse mouth & spit after; taper systemic steroids slowly when transferring to ciclesonide; monitor growth in pediatric pts; counsel on use of device, clean mouthpiece weekly; monitor for changes in vision, ↑ IOP, cataracts

Ciclesonide, Nasal (Omnaris) [Corticosteroid] Uses: Allergic rhinitis **Action:** Nasal corticosteroid **Dose:** *Adults & Peds > 12 y.* 2 sprays each nostril 1×/d **Caution:** [C, ?/–]w/ ketoconazole **CI:** Component allergy **Disp:** Intranasal spray susp, 50 mcg/spray, 120 doses **SE:** adrenal suppression, delayed nasal wound healing, URI, HA, ear pain, epistaxis **Interactions:** ↑ Effects **W**/ ketoconazole **NIPE:** ↑ Risk viral Dz (eg, chickenpox), delayed growth in children; monitor for vision changes

Ciclopirox (Loprox, Penlac) [Antifungal/Antibiotic] Uses: *Tinea pedis, tinea cruris, tinea corporis, cutaneous candidiasis, tinea versicolor, tinea rubrum* **Action:** Antifungal antibiotic; cellular depletion of essential substrates and/or ions **Dose:** *Adults & Peds > 10 y.* Massage into affected area bid *Onychomycosis:* Apply to nails daily, w/ removal q7d **Caution:** [B, ?] **CI:** Component sensitivity **Disp:** Cream 0.77%, gel 0.77%, topical susp 0.77%, shampoo 1%, nail lacquer 8% **SE:** Pruritus, local irritation, burning **Interactions:** None noted **NIPE:** Nail lacquer may take 6 mo to see improvement; cream/gel/lotion see improvement by 4 wk; D/C w/ irritation; avoid dressings; gel best for athlete's foot

Cidofovir (Vistide) [Antiviral/Inhibits DNA Synthesis] WARNING: Renal impair is the major tox. Follow administration instructions; possible carcinogenic, teratogenic Uses: *CMV retinitis w/ HIV* **Action:** Selective inhibition of viral DNA synth **Dose:** *Rx:* 5 mg/kg IV over 1 h once/wk for 2 wk w/ probenecid *Maint:* 5 mg/kg IV once/2 wk w/ probenecid (2 g PO 3 h prior to cidofovir, then 1 g PO at 2 h & 8 h after cidofovir); ↓ in renal impair **Caution:** [C, −] SCr > 1.5 mg/dL or CrCl = 55 mL/min or urine protein > 100 mg/dL; w/ other nephrotoxic drugs **CI:** Probenecid or sulfa allergy **Disp:** Inj 75 mg/mL **SE:** Renal tox, chills, fever, HA, N/V/D, ↓ plt, neutropenia **Interactions:** ↑ Nephrotox **W**/ aminoglycosides, amphotericin B, foscarnet, IV pentamidine, NSAIDs, vancomycin; ↑ effects **W**/ zidovudine **Labs:** ↑ SCr, BUN, alk phos, LFTs, urine protein;

↓ Ca, HMG, Hct, neutrophils, plts; monitor for hematuria, glycosuria, hypocalcemia, hyperglycemia, hypokalemia, hyperlipidemia **NIPE:** Coadminister oral probenecid w/ each dose to < GI upset; possible hair loss; hydrate w/ NS prior to each Inf; use OCPs during & 1 mo after therapy; men should use barrier contraception during & 3 mo after therapy

Cilostazol (Pletal) [Antiplatelet, Arterial Vasodilator/Phosphodiesterase Inhibitor] Uses: *Reduce Sxs of intermittent claudication* **Action:** Phosphodiesterase III Inhib; ↑ cAMP in plts & blood vessels, vasodilation & inhibit plt aggregation **Dose:** 100 mg PO bid, 1/2 h before or 2 h after breakfast & dinner **Caution:** [C, +/–] ↓ Dose w/ drugs that inhibit CYP3A4 & CYP2C19 (Table 10) **CI:** CHF, hemostatic disorders, active pathologic bleeding **Disp:** Tabs 50, 100 mg **SE:** HA, palpitation, D **Interactions:** ↑ Effects **W/** diltiazem, macrolides, omeprazole, fluconazole, itraconazole, ketoconazole, sertraline, grapefruit juice; ↑ effects **OF** ASA; ↓ effects **W/** cigarette smoking **Labs:** ↑ HDL; ↓ triglycerides **NIPE:** Take on empty stomach; may take up to 12 wk to ↓ cramping pain; may cause dizziness

Cimetidine (Tagamet) (Tagamet HB, Tagamet DS OTC) [Antiulcerative/H₂-Receptor Antagonist] Uses: *Duodenal ulcer; ulcer prophylaxis in hypersecretory states (eg, trauma, burns); & GERD* **Action:** H₂-receptor antagonist **Dose:** *Adults. Active ulcer:* 2400 mg/d IV cont Inf or 300 mg IV q6h; 400 mg PO bid or 800 mg hs; maint 400 mg PO hs *GERD:* 300–600 mg PO q6h; maint 800 mg PO hs *Peds. Infants.* 10–20 mg/kg/24 h PO or IV ÷ q6–12h *Children.* 20–40 mg/kg/24 h PO or IV ÷ q6h; ↓ w/ renal Insuff & in elderly **Caution:** [B, +] Many drug interactions (P450 system) **CI:** Component sensitivity **Disp:** Tabs 200, 300, 400, 800 mg; Liq 300 mg/5 mL; Inj 300 mg/2 mL **SE:** Dizziness, HA, agitation, ↓ plt, gynecomastia **Interactions:** ↑ Effects **OF** benzodiazepines, disulfram, flecainide, INH, lidocaine, OCPs, sulfonylureas, warfarin, theophylline, phenytoin, metronidazole, triamterene, procainamide, quinidine, propranolol, diazepam, nifedipine, TCAs, procainamide, tacrine, carbamazepine, valproic acid, xanthines; ↓ effects **W/** antacids, tobacco; ↓ effects **OF** digoxin, ketoconazole, cefpodoxime, indomethacin, tetracyclines **Labs:** ↑ Cr, LFTs; ↓ HMG, Hct, neutrophils, plt counts **NIPE:** Take w/ meals; monitor for gynecomastia, breast pain, impotence; take 1 h before or 2 h after antacids; avoid EtOH

Cinacalcet (Sensipar) [Hyperparathyroidism Agent/Calcimimetics] Uses: *Secondary hyperparathyroidism in CRF; ↑ Ca²⁺ in parathyroid carcinoma* **Action:** ↓ PTH by ↑ calcium-sensing receptor sensitivity **Dose:** *Secondary hyperparathyroidism:* 30 mg PO daily *Parathyroid carcinoma:* 30 mg PO bid; titrate q2–4wk based on calcium & PTH levels; swallow whole; take w/ food **Caution:** [C, ?/–] w/ SZs, adjust w/ CYP3A4 Inhibs **Disp:** Tabs 30, 60, 90 mg **SE:** N/V/D, myalgia, dizziness **Interactions:** ↑ Effects **W/** CYP3A4 Inhibs such as ketoconazole, itraconazole, erythromycin; ↑ effects **OF** drugs metabolized at CYP2D6 such as TCA, thioridazine, flecainide, vinblastine **Labs:** ↓ Ca²⁺; monitor

Ca^{2+}, PO_4^{2-}, PTH **NIPE:** Must take drug w/ vit D and/or phosphate binders; ↑ conc of drug if taken w/ food

Ciprofloxacin (Cipro, Cipro XR, Proquin XR) [Antibiotic/Fluoro-quinolone] WARNING: ↑ Risk of tendonitis & tendon rupture ; ↑ risk w/ age > 60, transplant pts may worsen MG **Sxs Uses:** *Rx lower resp tract, sinuses, skin & skin structure, bone/Jts, complex intra Abd Infxn (w/ metronidazole), typhoid, infectious D, uncomp GC, Inh anthrax, & UT Infxns, including prostatitis* **Action:** Quinolone antibiotic; ↓ DNA gyrase *Spectrum:* Broad gram(+) & (−) aerobics; little *Streptococcus*; good *Pseudomonas, E coli, B fragilis, P mirabilis, K pneumoniae, C jejuni*, or *Shigella* **Dose: Adults.** 250–750 mg PO q12h; XR 500–1000 mg PO q24h; or 200–400 mg IV q12h; ↓ in renal impair **Caution:** [C, ?/−] Children < 18 y; avoid in MG **CI:** Component sensitivity; w/ tizanidine **Disp:** Tabs 100, 250, 500, 750 mg; tabs XR 500, 1000 mg; susp 5 g/100 mL, 10 g/100 mL; Inj 200, 400 mg; premixed piggyback 200, 400 mg/100 mL **SE:** Restlessness, N/V/D, rash, ruptured tendons **Interactions:** ↑ Effects *W/* probenecid; ↑ effects *OF* diazepam, theophylline, caffeine, metoprolol, propranolol, phenytoin, warfarin; ↓ effects *W/* antacids, didanosine, Fe salts, Mg, sucralfate, $NaHCO_3$, zinc **Labs:** ↑ LFTs, alk phos, serum bilirubin, LDH, BUN, SCr, K^+, PT, triglycerides; ↓ plts, WBC **NIPE:** N Give to children < 18 y; ↑ fluids to 2–3 L/d, may cause photosensitivity—use sunblock; avoid antacids; reduce/restrict caffeine intake; most tendon problems in Achilles, rare shoulder & hand

Ciprofloxacin, Ophthalmic (Ciloxan) [Antibiotic/Fluoroquinolone Opthalmic Agent] Uses: *Rx & prevention of ocular Infxns (conjunctivitis, blepharitis, corneal abrasions)* **Action:** Quinolone antibiotic; ↓ DNA gyrase **Dose:** 1–2 gtt in eye(s) q2h while awake for 2 d, then 1–2 gtt q4h while awake for 5 d, oint 1/2-in ribbon in eye tid × 2 d, then bid × 5 d **Caution:** [C, ?/−] **CI:** Component sensitivity **Disp:** Soln 3.5 mg/mL; oint 0.3%, 35 g **SE:** Local irritation **Interactions:** ↑ Theophylline levels; ↑ effects *OF* oral anticoagulants; ↑ renal tox *W/* cyclosporine **NIPE:** Limited systemic absorption

Ciprofloxacin, Otic (Cetraxal) [Antibiotic/Quinolone Otic Agent] Uses: *Otitis externa* **Acts:** Quinolone antibiotic; ↓ DNA gyrase *Spectrum: P aeruginosa, S aureus* **Dose: Adults & Peds > 1 y.** 0.25 mL in ear(s) q12h × 7 d **Caution:** [C,?/−] **CI:** Component sensitivity **Disp:** Soln 0.2% **SE:** Hypersensitivity Rxn, ear pruritus/pain, HA, fungal super Infxn **NIPE:** Limited systemic absorption

Ciprofloxacin & Dexamethasone, Otic (Ciprodex Otic) [Antibiotic/Fluoroquinolone Otic Agent] Uses: *Otitis externa, otitis media peds* **Action:** Quinolone antibiotic; ↓ DNA gyrase; w/ steroid **Dose: Adults.** 4 gtt in ear(s) bid × 7 d. **Peds > 6 mo.** 4 gtt in ear(s) bid for 7 d **Caution:** [C, ?/−] **CI:** Viral ear Infxns **Disp:** Susp ciprofloxacin 0.3% & dexamethasone 1% **SE:** Ear discomfort **NIPE:** OK w/ tympanostomy tubes; D/C if super Infxn or hypersensitivity; limited systemic absorption

Ciprofloxacin & Hydrocortisone, Otic (Cipro HC Otic) [Antibiotic/Fluoroquinolone Otic Agent] Uses: *Otitis externa* **Action:** Quinolone antibiotic; ↓ DNA gyrase; w/ steroid **Dose:** *Adults & Peds > 1 mo.* 1–2 gtt in ear(s) bid × 7 d **Caution:** [C, ?/–] **CI:** Perforated tympanic membrane, viral Infxns of the external canal **Disp:** Susp ciprofloxacin 0.2% & hydrocortisone 1% **SE:** HA, pruritus **NIPE:** D/C if hypersensitive Rxn; hold bottle in hand 1–2 min before use to warm susp & minimize dizziness

Cisplatin (Platinol, Platinol AQ) [Antineoplastic/Alkylating Agent]

WARNING: Anaphylactic-like Rxn, ototox, cumulative renal tox; doses > 100 mg/m² q3–4wk rarely used, do not confuse w/ carboplatin **Uses:** *Testicular, bladder, ovarian*, SCLC, NSCLC, breast, head & neck, & penile CAs; osteosarcoma; ped brain tumors **Action:** DNA-binding; denatures double helix; intrastrand cross-linking **Dose:** 10–20 mg/m²/d for 5 d q3wk; 50–120 mg/m² q3–4wk (per protocols); ↓ w/ renal impair **Caution:** [D, –] Cumulative renal tox may be severe; ↓ BM, hearing impair, preexisting renal Insuff **CI:** w/ Anthrax or live vaccines, platinum-containing compound allergy; w/ cidofovir **Disp:** Inj 1 mg/mL **SE:** Allergic Rxns, N/V, nephrotox (↑ w/ administration of other nephrotoxic drugs; minimize by NS Inf & mannitol diuresis), high-frequency hearing loss in 30%, peripheral "stocking glove"-type neuropathy, cardiotox (ST-, T-wave changes), ↓ Mg²⁺, mild ↓ BM, hepatotox; renal impair dose-related & cumulative **Notes:** Give taxanes before platinum derivatives **Interactions:** ↑ Effects *OF* antineoplastic drugs & radiation therapy; ↑ ototox *W/* loop diuretics; ↑ nephrotox *W/* aminoglycosides, amphotericin B, vancomycin; ↓ effects *W/* Na thiosulfate; ↓ effects *OF* phenytoin **Labs:** ✓ Mg²⁺, lytes before & w/in 48 h after cisplatin; ↑ BUN, Cr, serum bilirubin, AST, uric acid; ↓ Ca²⁺, Mg²⁺, phosphate, Na⁺, K⁺, RBC, WBC, plts **NIPE:** May cause infertility, ⊘ immunizations or products w/ ASA; instruct pt to report signs of Infxn & tinnitus

Citalopram (Celexa) [Antidepressant/SSRI]

WARNING: Closely monitor for worsening depression or emergence of suicidality, particularly in pts < 24 y **Uses:** *Depression* **Action:** SSRI **Dose:** Initial 20 mg/d, may ↑ to 40 mg/d; ↓ in elderly & hepatic/renal Insuff **Caution:** [C, +/–] h/o of mania, Szs & pts at risk for suicide **CI:** MAOI or w/in 14 d of MAOI use **Disp:** Tabs 10, 20, 40 mg; soln 10 mg/5 mL **SE:** Somnolence, insomnia, anxiety, xerostomia, N, diaphoresis, sexual dysfunction **Interactions:** ↑ Effects *W/* azole antifungals, cimetidine, Li, macrolides, EtOH; ↑ effects *OF* BBs, carbamazepine, CNS drugs, warfarin; ↓ effects *W/* carbamazepine; ↓ effects *OF* phenytoin; may cause fatal Rxn *W/* MAOIs **Labs:** ↓ LFTs; May cause ↓ Na⁺/SIADH; **NIPE:** ⊘ PRG, breast-feeding, use barrier contraception

Cladribine (Leustatin) [Antineoplastic Agent/Purine Nucleoside Analog]

WARNING: Dose-dependent reversible myelosuppression; neurotox, nephrotox, administer by physician w/ experience in chemotherapy regimens **Uses:** *HCL, CLL, NHLs, progressive MS* **Action:** Induces DNA strand breakage; interferes w/ DNA repair/synth; purine nucleoside analogue **Dose:** 0.09–0.1 mg/kg/d cont IV Inf for 1–7 d (per protocols); ↓ w/ renal impair **Caution:** [D, ?/–] Causes neutropenia & Infxn **CI:** Component sensitivity **Disp:** Inj 1 mg/mL **SE:**

BM, T-lymphocyte ↓ may be prolonged (26–34 wk), fever in 46%, tumor lysis synd, Infxns (esp lung & IV sites), rash (50%), HA, fatigue, N/V **Interactions:** ↑ Risk of bleeding *W/* anticoagulants, NSAIDs, salicylates, ↑ risk of nephrotox *W/* amphotericin B **Labs:** Monitor CBC, LFTs, SCr **NIPE:** ⊘ PRG, breast-feeding; consider prophylactic allopurinol

Clarithromycin (Biaxin, Biaxin XL) [Antibiotic/Macrolide] **Uses:** *Upper/lower resp tract, skin/skin structure Infxns, *H pylori* Infxns, & Infxns caused by nontuberculosis (atypical) *Mycobacterium*; prevention of MAC Infxns in HIV-Infxn* **Action:** Macrolide antibiotic, ↓ protein synth *Spectrum: H influenzae, M catarrhalis, S pneumoniae, M pneumoniae,* & *H pylori* **Dose:** *Adults.* 250–500 mg PO bid or 1000 mg (2 × 500 mg XL tab)/d *Mycobacterium:* 500 mg PO bid *Peds > 6 mo.* 7.5 mg/kg/dose PO bid; ↓ w/ renal impair **Caution:** [C, ?] Antibiotic-associated colitis; rare QT prolongation & ventricular arrhythmias, including torsades de pointes **CI:** Macrolide allergy; w/ ranitidine in pts w/ h/o of porphyria or CrCl < 25 mL/min **Disp:** Tabs 250, 500 mg; susp 125, 250 mg/5 mL; 500 mg XL tab **SE:** ↑ QT interval, causes metallic taste, N/D, Abd pain, HA, rash **Interactions:** ↑ Effects *W/* amprenavir, indinavir, nelfinavir, ritonavir; ↑ effects *OF* atorvastatin, buspirone, clozapine, colchicine, diazepam, felodipine, itraconazole, lovastatin, simvastatin, methylprednisolone, theophylline, phenytoin, quinidine, digoxin, carbamazepine, triazolam, warfarin, ergotamine, alprazolam, valproic acid; ↓ effects *W/* EtOH; ↓ effects *OF* PCN, zafirlukast **Labs:** ↑ Serum AST, ALT, GTT, alk phos, LDH, total bilirubin, BUN, Cr, PT, INR; ↓ WBC **NIPE:** May take w/ food; do not refrigerate susp & discard > 14 d

Clemastine Fumarate (Tavist, Dayhist, Antihist-1) [OTC] [Antihistamine] **Uses:** *Allergic rhinitis & Sxs of urticaria* **Action:** Antihistamine **Dose:** *Adults & Peds > 12 y.* 1.34 mg bid–2.68 mg tid; max 8.04 mg/d *< 6 y.* 0.335–0.67 mg/d ÷ into 2–3 doses (max 1.34 mg/d) *6–12 y.* 0.67–1.34 mg bid (max 4.02/d) **Caution:** [B, M] BOO; do not use w/ MAOI **CI:** NAG **Disp:** Tabs 1.34, 2.68 mg; syrup 0.67 mg/5 mL **SE:** Drowsiness, dyscoordination, epigastric distress, urinary retention **Interactions:** ↑ Effects *W/* CNS depressants, MAOIs, EtOH; ↓ effects *OF* heparin, sulfonylureas **NIPE:** Avoid EtOH

Clevidipine (Cleviprex) [Antihypertension/Calcium Channel Blocker] **Uses:** *HTN when PO not available/desirable* **Action:** Dihydropyridine CCB, potent arterial vasodilator **Dose:** 1–2 mg/h IV the maint 4–6 mg/h; 21 mg/h max (⊘ give > 1000 mL d/t ↑ lipid load) **Caution:** [C, ?] ↓ BP, syncope, and rebound HTN, reflex tachycardia, CHF **Contra:** *Hypersensitivity:* Component or formulation (soy, egg products); impaired lipid metabolism; severe AS **Disp:** Inj 0.5 mg/mL (50, 100 mL) **SE:** AF, fever, insomnia, N/V, HA, renal impair; **Interactions:** ↑ Risk of reflex tachycardia w/ BB **NIPE:** Monitor BP & pulse during Inf & until stabilized; monitor for rebound HTN at least 8 h after Inf ends

Clindamycin (Cleocin, Cleocin-T, Others) [Antibiotic/Lincomycin Derivative] **WARNING:** Pseudomembranous colitis may range from mild to life-threatening **Uses:** *Rx aerobic & anaerobic Infxns; topical for severe acne & Vag Infxns* **Action:** Bacteriostatic; interferes w/ protein synth **Spectrum:** Streptococci, pneumococci, staphylococci, & gram(+) & (−) anaerobes; no activity against gram(−) aerobes **Dose: Adults. PO:** 150–450 mg PO q6–8h **IV:** 300–600 mg IV q6h or 900 mg IV q8h **Vag:** 1 applicator hs for 7 d **Topical:** Apply 1% gel, lotion, or soln bid **Peds. Neonates.** (Avoid use; contains benzyl alcohol) 10–15 mg/kg/ 24 h ÷ q8–12h **Children > 1 mo.** 10–30 mg/kg/24 h ÷ q6–8h, to a max of 1.8 g/d PO or 4.8 g/d IV **Topical:** Apply 1%, gel, lotion, or soln bid; ↓ in severe hepatic impair **Caution:** [B, +] Can cause fatal colitis **CI:** h/o pseudomembranous colitis **Disp:** Caps 75, 150, 300 mg; susp 75 mg/5 mL; Inj 300 mg/2 mL; Vag cream 2%, topical soln 1%, gel 1%, lotion 1%, Vag supp 100 mg **SE:** D may be *C difficile* pseudomembranous colitis, rash **Interactions:** ↑ Effects of neuromuscular blockage **W/** tubocurarine, pancuronium; ↓ effects **W/** erythromycin, kaolin, foods **W/** Na cyclamate **Labs:** ↑ LFTs; monitor CBC, LFTs, BUN, Cr; ↓ WBC, plts **NIPE:** D/C drug w/ D, eval for *C difficile*; ⊘ intercourse, tampons, douches while using Vag cream; take oral meds w/ 8 oz H$_2$O

Clindamycin & Tretinoin (Veltin Gel) [Lincosamide + Retinoid]

Uses: *Acne vulgaris* **Action:** Lincosamide abx (↓ protein synth)w/a retinoid **Spectrum:** P acnes **Dose: Adults (> 12 y).** Apply pea size amount to area qd **Caution:** [C, ?/−] Do not use w/ erythromycin products **CI:** Hx regional enteritis/UC/ abx associated colitis **Disp:** Top Gel (clindamycin 1.2%/tretinoin 0.025%) **SE:** Dryness, irritation, erythema, pruritis, exfoliation, dermatitis, sunburn **Interaction:** May ↑ neuromuscular blockers **NIPE:** Avoid eyes, lips, mucous membranes; avoid erythromycin or additive irritation w/ topical products (eg, alcohol, drying agents); avoid sun & UV light

Clofarabine (Clolar) [Antineoplastic; Purine Nucleoside Antimetabolite]

Uses: Rx relapsed/refractory ALL after at least 2 regimens in children 1–21 y **Action:** Antimetabolite; ↓ ribonucleotide reductase w/ false nucleotide base-inhibiting DNA synth **Dose:** 52 mg/m² IV over 2 h daily × 5 d (repeat q2–6wk); per protocol **Caution:** [D, −] **Disp:** Inj 20 mg/20 mL **SE:** N/V/D, anemia, leukopenia, ↓ plt, neutropenia, Infxn **Interactions:** ↑ Additive risk w/ hepatotoxic or nephrotoxic drugs **Labs:** ↑ AST, ALT, Cr, HMG, Hct; monitor serum uric acid, phosphate, Ca & Cr bid for 2–3 d after starting chemotherapy **NIPE:** Monitor for tumor lysis synd & systemic inflammatory response synd (SIRS)/capillary leak synd; hydrate well

Clomiphene (Clomid) [Ovulatory stimulant.]

Uses: *Tx ovulatory dysfunction in women desiring PRG* **Action:** Nonsteroidal ovulatory stimulant; estrogen antagonist **Dose:** 50 mg × 5 d; if no ovulation ↑ to 100 mg × 5 d for 30 d later; ovulation usually 5–10 d post-course, time coitus w/ expected ovulation time **Caution:** [X; ?/−] R/O PRG & ovarian enlargement **CI:** Hypersensitivity, uterine bleed, PRG, ovarian cysts, liver dz, thyroid/adrenal dysfunction **Disp:** Tabs 50 mg **SE:** Ovarian enlargement, vasomotor flushes **NIPE:** D/C with visual changes

Clomipramine (Anafranil) [Tricyclic] WARNING: Closely monitor for suicidal thinking or unusual behavior changes **Uses:** *OCD,* depression, chronic pain, panic attacks **Action:** TCA; ↑ synaptic serotonin & norepinephrine **Dose:** **Adults.** Initial 25 mg/d PO in ÷ doses; ↑ over few wk 250 mg/d max qhs **Peds > 10 y.** Initial 25 mg/d PO in ÷ doses; ↑ over few wk 200 mg/d or 3 mg/kg/d max given hs **Caution:** [C; +/–] **CI:** W/ MAOIs, TCA allergy, during acute MI recovery **Disp:** Caps 25, 50, 75 mg **SE:** Anticholinergic [xerostomia, urinary retention, constipation], somnolence **Interactions:** ↑ Effects *OF* other CNS depressants, anticholinergics, sympathomimetics, other protein-bound drugs, EtOH; ↑ effects W/ CYP2D6 and/or CYP1A2 Inhibs; ↓ effects W/ barbiturates, carbamazepine, phenytoin, other CYP450 inducers; blocks guanethidine, clonidine **Labs:** Monitor plasma levels with cimetidine, SSRIs, phenothiazines **NIPE:** Take with food; do not take w/in 14 d of MAOI, do not abruptly D/C

Clonazepam (Klonopin) [C-IV] [Anticonvulsant/Benzodiazepine] **Uses:** *Lennox-Gastaut synd, akinetic & myoclonic Szs, absence Szs, panic attacks*, restless legs synd, neuralgia, parkinsonian dysarthria, bipolar disorder **Action:** Benzodiazepine; anticonvulsant **Dose:** **Adults.** 1.5 mg/d PO in 3 ÷ doses; ↑ by 0.5–1 mg/d q3d PRN up to 20 mg/d **Peds.** 0.01–0.03 mg/kg/24 h PO ÷ tid; ↑ to 0.1–0.2 mg/kg/24 h ÷ tid; avoid abrupt D/C **Caution:** [D, M] Elderly pts, resp Dz, CNS depression, severe hepatic impair, renal impair NAG **CI:** Severe liver Dz, acute NAG **Disp:** Tabs 0.5, 1, 2 mg, ODT 0.125, 0.25, 0.5, 1, 2 mg **SE:** CNS SE (drowsiness, dizziness, ataxia, memory impair) **Interactions:** ↑ CNS depression W/ antidepressants, antihistamines, opiates, benzodiazepines; ↑ effects W/ cimetidine, disulfiram, fluoxetine, INH, itraconazole, ketoconazole, metoprolol, valproic acid, EtOH, kava kava, valerian; ↓ effects W/ phenytoin **Labs:** ↑ LFTs, ↑ WBC, plts **NIPE:** ⊘ D/C abruptly; can cause retrograde amnesia; a CYP3A4 substrate

Clonidine, Oral (Catapres) [Antihypertensive/Centrally Acting Sympatholytic] Uses: *HTN*; opioid, EtOH, & tobacco withdrawal, ADHD **Action:** Centrally acting α-adrenergic stimulant **Dose:** **Adults.** 0.1 mg PO bid, adjust daily by 0.1–0.2-mg increments (max 2.4 mg/d) **Peds.** 5–10 mcg/kg/d ÷ q8–12h (max 0.9 mg/d); ↓ in renal impair **Caution:** [C, +/–] Avoid w/ BB, elderly, severe CV Dz, renal impair **CI:** Component sensitivity **Disp:** Tabs 0.1, 0.2, 0.3 mg **SE:** Drowsiness, orthostatic ↓ BP, xerostomia, constipation, bradycardia, dizziness **Interactions:** ↑ Sedation W/ CNS depressants; ↓ antihypertensive effects W/ amphetamines, BB, MAOIs TCA **Labs:** ↑ Glucose **NIPE:** More effective for HTN if combined w/ diuretics; withdraw slowly, rebound HTN w/ abrupt D/C of doses > 0.2 mg bid; ADHD use in peds; needs CV assessment before starting epidural clonidine (Duraclon) used for chronic CA pain

Clonidine, Oral, Extended Release (Kapvay, Jenloga) [Antihypertensive/Centrally Acting Sympatholytic] Uses: *ADHD alone or as adjunct (Kapvay)**HTN, alone or combo (Jenloga)* **Action:** Central α-adrenergic stimulant **Dose:** **Adults.** Jenloga: 0.1 mg PO qhs, titrate, Usual

0.2–0.6 mg/d; 0.6 mg/d max *Peds 6–17 y. Kapvay:* 0.1 mg PO qhs, adjust weekly per table to response; AM & hs doses may be ≠; max 0.4 mg/d; do not cut/crush/ chew tabs; ↓ in renal impair

Total Daily Dose	Morning Dose	Bedtime Dose
0.1 mg/d		0.1 mg
0.2 mg/d	0.1 mg	0.1 mg
0.3 mg/d	0.1 mg	0.2 mg
0.4 mg/d	0.2 mg	0.2 mg

Caution: [C, +/−] may cause severe ↓ HR & ↓ BP; w/ BP meds **CI:** Component sensitivity **Disp:** Tabs ER *Kapvay:* 0.1, 0.2 mg; *Jenloga:* 0.1 mg **SE:** Somnolence, fatigue, URI, irritability, sore throat, insomnia, nightmares, emotional disorder, constipation, congestion, ↑ temperature, dry mouth, ear pain **Interactions:** ↑ effects *OF* other CNS depressants, antihypertensives, EtOH; ↑ cardiac Sx (AV block, bradycardia) *W/* digitalis, CCB, BB; **NIPE:** On D/C, ↓ no more than 0.1 mg q3–7d; swallow whole; titrate by response

Clonidine, Transdermal (Catapres TTS) [Antihypertensive/ Centrally Acting Sympatholytic] Uses: *HTN* Action: Centrally acting α-adrenergic stimulant **Dose:** 1 patch q7d to hairless area (upper arm/torso); titrate to effect; ↓ w/ severe renal impair **Caution:** [C, +/−] Avoid w/ BB, withdraw slowly, in elderly, severe CV Dz & w/ renal impair **CI:** Component sensitivity **Disp:** TTS-1, TTS-2, TTS-3 (delivers 0.1, 0.2, 0.3 mg, respectively, of clonidine/d for 1 wk) **SE:** Drowsiness, orthostatic ↓ BP, xerostomia, constipation, bradycardia **Interactions:** ↑ Sedation *W/* CNS depressants; ↓ antihypertensive effects *W/* amphetamines, BB, MAOIs TCA **Labs:** ↑ Glucose, CK **NIPE:** Do not D/C abruptly (rebound HTN) doses > 2 TTS-3 usually not associated w/ ↑ efficacy; steady state in 2–3 d

Clopidogrel (Plavix) [Antiplatelet/Platelet Aggregation Inhibitor] Uses: *Reduce atherosclerotic events*, administer ASAP in ECC setting w/ high-risk ST depression or T-wave inversion **Action:** ↓ Plt aggregation **Dose:** 75 mg/d PO *ECC 2010:* ACS: 300–600 mg PO loading dose, then 75 mg/d PO; full effects take several d. **Caution:** [B, ?] Active bleeding; risk of bleeding from trauma & other; TTP; liver Dz; **CI:** Coagulation disorders, active/or intracranial bleeding; CABG planned w/in 5–7 d **Disp:** Tabs 75, 300 mg **SE:** ↑ bleeding time, GI intolerance, HA, dizziness, rash, ↓ plt **Interactions:** Do not use with PPI or other CYP2C19 (eg, fluconazole); OK with ranitidine, famotidine; ↑ risk of GI bleed *W/* ASA, NSAIDs, heparin, warfarin, feverfew, garlic, ginger, ginkgo; ↑ effects *OF* phenytoin, tamoxifen, tolbutamide **Labs:** ↑ LFTs; ↓ plts, WBC

NIPE: D/C drug 1 wk prior to surgery; plt aggregation to baseline 5 d after D/C; plt transfusion to reverse acutely; clinical response highly variable (?) genetic factors

Clorazepate (Tranxene) [Anxiolytic, Anticonvulsant, Sedative/ Hypnotic/Benzodiazepine] [C-IV] Uses: *Acute anxiety disorders, acute EtOH withdrawal Sxs, adjunctive Rx in partial Szs* **Action:** Benzodiazepine; anti-anxiety agent **Dose:** *Adults.* 15–60 mg/d PO single or ÷ doses *Elderly & debilitated pts.* Initial 7.5–15 mg/d in ÷ doses *EtOH withdrawal:* Day 1: Initial 30 mg; then 30–60 mg ÷ doses Day 2: 45–90 mg ÷ doses Day 3: 22.5–45 mg ÷ doses Day 4: 15–30 mg ÷ doses *Peds.* 3.75–7.5 mg/dose bid to 60 mg/d max ÷ bid **Caution:** [D, ?/–] Elderly; h/o depression **CI:** NAG; not OK < 9 y of age **Disp:** Tabs 3.75, 7.5, 15 mg; tabs-SD (daily) 11.25, 22.5 mg **SE:** CNS depressant effects (drowsiness, dizziness, ataxia, memory impair), ↓ BP **Interactions:** ↑ Effects *W/* antidepressants, antihistamines, barbiturates, MAOIs, opiates, phenothiazines, cimetidine, disulfiram, EtOH; ↓ effects *OF* levodopa; ↓ effects *W/* rifampin, ginkgo, tobacco **Labs:** ↓ Alk phos; monitor pts w/ renal/hepatic impair (drug may accumulate) **NIPE:** ⊘ D/C abruptly; may cause dependence

Clotrimazole (Lotrimin, Mycelex, Others) [Antifungal] [OTC] Uses: *Candidiasis & tinea Infxns* **Action:** Antifungal; alters cell wall permeability *Spectrum:* Oropharyngeal candidiasis, dermatophytoses, superficial mycoses, cutaneous candidiasis, & vulvovaginal candidiasis **Dose:** *PO: Prophylaxis:* One troche dissolved in mouth tid *Rx:* One troche dissolved in mouth 5 × /d for 14 d *Vag 1% cream:* 1 applicator-full hs for 7 d. *2% cream:* 1 applicator-full hs for 3 d *Tabs:* 100 mg vaginally hs for 7 d or 200 mg (2 tabs) vaginally hs for 3 d or 500-mg tabs vaginally hs once *Topical:* Apply bid 10–14 d **Caution:** [B (C if PO), ?] Not for systemic fungal Infxn; safety in children < 3 y not established **CI:** Component allergy **Disp:** 1% cream; soln; lotion; troche 10 mg; Vag tabs 100, 200, 500 mg; Vag cream 1%, 2% **SE:** *Topical:* Local irritation; *PO:* N/V **Interactions:** ↑ Effects *OF* cyclosporine, tacrolimus; ↓ effects *OF* spermicides **Labs:** ↑ LFTs **NIPE:** PO prophylaxis immunosuppressed pts

Clotrimazole & Betamethasone (Lotrisone) [Antifungal, Anti-Inflammatory] Uses: *Fungal skin Infxns* **Action:** Imidazole antifungal & anti-inflammatory. *Spectrum:* Tinea pedis, cruris, & corpora **Dose:** *Children = 17 y.* Apply & massage into area bid for 2–4 wk **Caution:** [C, ?] Varicella Infxn **CI:** Children < 12 y **Disp:** Cream 1% & 0.05% 15, 45 g; lotion 1% & 0.05%; 30 mL **SE:** Local irritation, rash **NIPE:** Not for diaper dermatitis or under occlusive dressings

Clozapine (Clozaril & FazaClo) [Antipsychotic/Dibenzodiazepine Derivative] **WARNING:** Myocarditis, agranulocytosis, Szs, & orthostatic ↓ BP associated w/ clozapine; ↑ mortality in elderly w/ dementia-related psychosis Uses: *Refractory severe schizophrenia*; childhood psychosis; obsessive-compulsive disorder; bipolar disorder **Action:** "Atypical" TCA **Dose:** 25 mg daily–bid initial; ↑ to 300–450 mg/d over 2 wk; maint lowest dose possible; do not D/C abruptly **Caution:** [B, +/−] Monitor for psychosis & cholinergic rebound **CI:** Uncontrolled epilepsy; comatose state; WBC < 3500 cells/mm³ & ANC < 2000 cells/mm³ before Rx or < 3000 cells/mm³ during Rx **Disp:** ODT 12.5, 25 ,100 mg; tabs 25, 100 mg **SE:** Sialorrhea, tachycardia, drowsiness, ↑ wgt, constipation, incontinence, rash, Szs, CNS stimulation, hyperglycemia **Interactions:** ↑ Effects W/ clarithromycin, cimetidine, erythromycin, fluoxetine, paroxetine, quinidine, sertraline; ↑ depressant effects W/ CNS depressants, EtOH; ↑ effects OF digoxin, warfarin; ↓ effects W/ carbamazepine, phenytoin, primidone, phenobarbital, valproic acid, St. John's wort, nutmeg, caffeine; ↓ effects OF phenytoin **Labs:** Monitor WBCs; weekly CBC mandatory 1st 6 mo, then qowk **NIPE:** ↑ Risk of developing agranulocytosis; avoid activities where sudden loss of consciousness could cause harm; benign temperature ↑ may occur during the 1st 3 wk of Rx

Cocaine [C-II] [Narcotic Analgesic] Uses: *Topical anesthetic for mucous membranes* **Action:** Narcotic analgesic, local vasoconstrictor **Dose:** Lowest topical amount that provides relief; 1 mg/kg max **Caution:** [C, ?] **CI:** PRG, ocular anesthesia **Disp:** Topical soln & viscous preps 4–10%; powder **SE:** CNS stimulation, nervousness, loss of taste/smell, chronic rhinitis, CV tox, abuse potential **Interactions:** ↑ Effects W/ MAOIs, ↑ risk of HTN & arrhythmias W/ epinephrine **NIPE:** Use only on PO, laryngeal, & nasal mucosa; do not use on extensive areas of broken skin

Codeine [C-II] [Analgesic, Antitussive/Opioid] Uses: *Mild–mod pain; symptomatic relief of cough* **Action:** Narcotic analgesic; ↓ cough reflex **Dose:** *Adults. Analgesic:* 15–20 mg PO or IM qid PRN *Antitussive:* 10–20 mg PO q4h PRN; max 120 mg/d *Peds. Analgesic:* 0.5–1 mg/kg/dose PO q4–6h PRN *Antitussive:* 1–1.5 mg/kg/24 h PO ÷ q4h; max 30 mg/24 h; ↓ in renal/hepatic impair **Caution:** [C (D if prolonged use or high dose at term), +] CNS depression, h/o drug abuse, severe hepatic impair **CI:** Component sensitivity **Disp:** Tabs 15, 30, 60 mg; soln 15 mg/5 mL; Inj 15, 30 mg/mL **SE:** Drowsiness, constipation, ↓ BP **Interactions:** ↑ CNS depression W/ CNS depressants, antidepressants, MAOIs, TCAs, barbiturates, benzodiazepines, muscle relaxants, phenothiazines, cimetidine, antihistamines, sedatives, EtOH; ↑ effects OF digitoxin, phenytoin, rifampin; ↓ effects W/ nalbuphine, pentazocine, tobacco **Labs:** ↑ Amylase, lipase, ↑ urine morphine **NIPE:** Usually combined w/ APAP for pain or w/ agents (eg, terpin hydrate) as an antitussive; 120 mg IM = 10 mg IM morphine

Colchicine (Colcrys) [Antigout Agent/Colchicum Alkaloid] Uses: *Acute gouty arthritis & prevention of recurrences; familial Mediterranean fever*; primary biliary cirrhosis **Action:** ↓ Migration of leukocytes; ↓ leukocyte lactic acid production **Dose:** *Initial:* PO: 0.6 mg/d and then 0.6 mg q1–2h until relief or GI SE develop (max 8 mg/d); do not repeat for 3 d *Prophylaxis:* PO: 0.6 mg/d or 3–4 d/wk; ↓ renal impair **Caution:** [D, +] w/ P-glycoprotein or CYP3A4 Inhib in pts w/ renal or hepatic impair; ↓ dose or avoid; Elderly **CI:** Serious renal, GI, hepatic, or cardiac disorders; blood dyscrasias **Disp:** Tabs 0.6 mg **SE:** N/V/D, Abd pain, BM suppression, hepatotox; local Rxn w/ SQ/IM **Notes:** IV no longer available **Interactions:** ↑ Risk of leukopenia *W/* phenylbutazone; ↓ effects *W/* loop diuretics; ↓ effects *OF* vit B_{12} **Labs:** ↑ Alk phos, ALT, AST; ↓ cholesterol, HMG, Hct, plts; false(+) urine Hgb & RBCs **NIPE:** ⊘ EtOH

Colesevelam (WelChol) [Antilipemic/Bile Acid Sequestrant] Uses:
Reduction of LDL & total cholesterol alone or in combo w/ a HMG-CoA reductase Inhib, improve glycemic control in Type 2 DM **Action:** Bile acid sequestrant **Dose:** 3 tabs PO bid or 6 tabs daily w/ meals **Caution:** [B, ?] Severe GI motility disorders; in pts w/ triglycerides > 300 mg/dL (may ↑ levels); use not established in peds **CI:** Bowel obst, serum triglycerides > 500; h/o hypertriglyceridemia-pancreatitis **Disp:** Tabs 625 mg; oral susp 1.875, 3.75 g **SE:** Constipation, dyspepsia, myalgia, weakness **Interactions:** ↓ Vit absorption **Labs:** Monitor lipids **NIPE:** Take w/ food & Liq; may ↓ absorption of fat-soluble vits

Colestipol (Colestid) [Antilipemic/Bile Acid Sequestrant] Uses:*
Adjunct to ↓ serum cholesterol in primary hypercholesterolemia, relieve pruritus associated w/ ↑ bile acids* **Action:** Binds intestinal bile acids to form insoluble complex **Dose:** Granules: 5–30 g/d ÷ 2–4 doses; tabs: 2–16 g/d ÷ daily–bid **Caution:** [C, ?] Avoid w/ high triglycerides; GI dysfunction **CI:** Bowel obst **Disp:** Tabs 1 g; granules 5, 7.5, 300, 450, 500 g **SE:** Constipation, Abd pain, bloating, HA, GI irritation & bleeding **Interactions:** ↓ Absorption *OF* numerous drugs esp anticoagulants, cardiac glycosides, digitoxin, digoxin, phenobarbital, PCN G, tetracycline, thiazide diuretics, thyroid drugs **Labs:** ↑ Alk phos; PT prolonged **NIPE:** Take other meds 1 h before or 4 h after colestipol; do not use dry powder; mix w/ beverages, cereals, etc; may ↓ absorption of other medications & fat-soluble vits

Conivaptan HCL (Vaprisol) [Hyponatremic Agent/Vasopressin Receptor Antagonist] Uses:
Euvolemic & hypervolemic hyponatremia **Action:** Dual arginine vasopressin V_{1A}/V_2 receptor antagonist **Dose:** 20 mg IV × 1 over 30 min, then 20 mg cont IV Inf over 24 h; 20 mg/d cont IV Inf for 1–3 more d; may ↑ to 40 mg/d if Na^+ not responding; 4 d max use; use large vein, change site q24h **Caution:** [C, ?/–] Rapid ↑ Na^+ (> 12 mEq/L/24 h) may cause osmotic demyelination synd; impaired renal/hepatic Fxn; may ↑ digoxin levels; CYP3A4 Inhib (Table 10) **CI:** Hypovolemic hyponatremia; w/ CYP3A4 Inhibs; anuria **Disp:** Amp 20 mg/4 mL **SE:** Inf site Rxns, HA, N/V/D, constipation, orthostatic ↓ BP, thirst, dry mouth, pyrexia, pollakiuria, polyuria, Infxn **Interactions:** ↑ Effects *OF* amlodipine, digoxin, midazolam, simvastatin, & CYP3A4 Inhibs such as clarithromycin, itraconazole, ketoconazole, ritonavir **Labs:** May ↑ digoxin level; ↓ K^+, Na^+, Mg^{2+}; monitor Na^+; D/C w/ very rapid ↑ Na^+ **NIPE:** Mix only w/ 5% dextrose; D/C w/ very rapid ↑ Na^+; monitor Na^+, vol, & neurologic status

Copper IUD Contraceptive (ParaGard T 380A) [Contraceptive]
Uses: *Contraception, long-term (up to 10 y)* **Action:** ?, Interfere w/ sperm survival/transport **Dose:** Insert any time during menstrual cycle; replace at 10 y max **Caution:** [C, ?] Remove w/ intrauterine PRG, ↑ risk of comps w/ PRG & device in place **CI:** Acute PID or in high-risk behavior; postpartum endometritis, cervicitis **Disp:** 52 mg IUD **SE:** PRG, ectopic PRG, pelvic Infxn w/ or w/o immunocompromised, embedment, perforation, expulsion, Wilson Dz, fainting w/ insert, Vag bleeding, expulsion **NIPE:** Counsel pt does not protect against STD/HIV; see package insert for detailed instructions; 99% effective

Cortisone, Systemic & Topical See Steroids & Tables 2 & 3

Cromolyn Sodium (Intal, NasalCrom, Opticrom, Others) [Antiasthmatic/Mast Cell Stabilizer] **Uses:** *Adjunct to the Rx of asthma; prevent exercise-induced asthma; allergic rhinitis; ophthal allergic manifestations*; food allergy, systemic mastocytosis, IBD **Action:** Antiasthmatic; mast cell stabilizer **Dose:** ***Adults & Children > 12 y.*** Inh: 20 mg (as powder in caps) inhaled qid or metered-dose inhaler 2 puffs qid *PO:* 200 mg qid 15–20 min ac, up to 400 mg qid *Nasal instillation:* Spray once in each nostril 2–6 × /d *Ophthal:* 1–2 gtt in each eye 4–6 × d *Peds.* Inh: 2 puffs qid of metered-dose inhaler *PO:* ***Infants < 2 y.*** (Not OK) 20 mg/kg/d in 4 ÷ doses *2–12 y.* 100 mg qid ac **Caution:** [B, ?] w/ renal/hepatic impair **CI:** Acute asthmatic attacks **Disp:** PO conc 100 mg/5 mL; soln for nebulizer 20 mg/2 mL; metered-dose inhaler; nasal soln 40 mg/mL; ophthal soln 4% **SE:** Unpleasant taste, hoarseness, coughing **Interactions:** None noted **Labs:** Monitor pulm Fxn tests **NIPE:** No benefit in acute Rx; 2–4 wk for max effect in perennial allergic disorders

Cyanocobalamin [Vitamin B$_{12}$] (Nascobal) [Vitamin B/Dietary Supplement] **Uses:** *Pernicious anemia & other w/ B$_{12}$ deficiency states;* ↑ requirements d/t PRG; thyrotoxicosis; liver or kidney Dz* **Action:** Dietary vit B$_{12}$ supls **Dose:** *Adults.* 30 mcg/d × 5–10 d 100 mcg IM or SQ daily; intranasal: 500 mcg once/wk for pts in remission, for 5–10 d, max 100 mcg IM 2 × /wk for 1 mo, then 100 mcg IM monthly *Peds.* Use 0.2 mcg/kg × 2 d test dose; if OK 30–50 mcg/d for 2 or more wk (total 10 mcg) then maint 100 mg/mo **Caution:** [A (C if dose exceeds RDA), +] **CI:** Allergy to cobalt; hereditary optic nerve atrophy; Leber Dz **Disp:** Tabs 50, 100, 250, 500, 1000, 2500, 5000 mcg; Inj 100, 1000 mcg/mL; intranasal (Nascobal) gel 500 mcg/0.1 mL **SE:** Itching, D, HA, anxiety **Interactions:** ↓ Effects d/t malabsorption of B$_{12}$ W/ aminosalicylic acid, aminoglycosides, chloramphenicol, EtOH **Labs:** ↓ K$^+$ levels **NIPE:** PO absorption erratic & not recommended; OK for use w/ hyperalimentation

Cyclobenzaprine (Flexeril) [Skeletal Muscle Relaxant/ANS Agent] **Uses:** *Relief of muscle spasm* **Action:** Centrally acting skeletal muscle relaxant; reduces tonic somatic motor activity **Dose:** 5–10 mg PO bid–qid (2–3 wk max) **Caution:** [B, ?] Shares the toxic potential of the TCAs; urinary hesitancy, NAG **CI:** Do not use concomitantly or w/in 14 d of MAOIs; hyperthyroidism; heart failure; arrhythmias **Disp:** Tabs 5, 10 mg **SE:** Sedation & anticholinergic effects **Interactions:** ↑ Effects of CNS depression **W/** CNS depressants, TCAs, barbiturates, EtOH; ↑ risk of HTN & convulsions **W/** MAOIs **NIPE:** ↑ Fluids & fiber for constipation; may inhibit mental alertness or physical coordination

Cyclobenzaprine, Extended Release (Amrix) [Skeletal Muscle Relaxant/ANS Agent] Uses: *Muscle spasm* **Action:** ? Centrally acting long-term muscle relaxant **Dose:** 15–30 mg PO daily 2–3 wk; 30 mg/d max **Caution:** [B, ?/–] w/ urinary retention, NAG, w/ EtOH/CNS depressant **CI:** MAOI w/in 14 d, elderly, arrhythmias, heart block, CHF, MI recovery phase, ↑ thyroid **Disp:** Caps 15, 30 ER **SE:** Dry mouth, drowsiness, dizziness, HA, N, blurred vision, dysgeusia **Interactions:** ↑ Effects of CNS depression **W/** CNS depressants, TCAs, barbiturates, EtOH; ↑ risk of HTN & convulsions **W/** MAOIs **NIPE:** ↑ Fluids & fiber constipation; may inhibit mental alertness or physical coordination; avoid abrupt D/C w/ long-term use

Cyclopentolate Ophthalmic (Cyclogyl, Cylate) [Anticholinergic/ Cycloplegic Mydriatic Agent] Uses: *Cycloplegia, mydriasis* **Action:** Cycloplegic mydriatic, anticholinergic inhibits iris sphincter & ciliary body **Dose:** *Adults.* 1 gtt in eye 40–50 min pre-procedure may repeat × 1 in 5–10 min **Peds.** As adult, children 0.5%; infants use 0.5% **Caution:** [C (may cause late-term fetal anoxia/bradycardia), +/–], premature infants HTN, Down synd, elderly **CI:** NAG **Disp:** Ophthal soln 0.5%, 1%, 2% **SE:** Tearing, HA, irritation, eye pain, photophobia, arrhythmia, tremor, ↑ IOP, confusion **Interactions:** ↓ Effects *OF* carbachol, cholinesterase Inhibs, pilocarpine **NIPE:** Burning sensation when instilled; compress lacrimal sac for several min after dose; heavily pigmented irises may require ↑ strength; peak 25–75 min, cycloplegia 6–24 h, mydriasis up to 24 h; 2% soln may result in psychotic Rxns & behavioral disturbances in peds

Cyclopentolate with Phenylephrine (Cyclomydril) [Anticholinergic/Cycloplegic Mydriatic, Alpha-Adrenergic Agonist] Uses: *Mydriasis greater than cyclopentolate alone* **Action:** Cycloplegic mydriatic, α-adrenergic agonist w/ anticholinergic to inhibit iris sphincter **Dose:** 1 gtt in eye q5–10 min (max 3 doses) 40–50 min pre-procedure **Caution:** (C [may cause late-term fetal anoxia/bradycardia], +/–] HTN, w/ elderly w/ CAD **CI:** NAG **Disp:** Ophthal soln cyclopentolate 0.2%/phenlephrine 1% (2, 5 mL) **SE:** Tearing, HA, irritation, eye pain, photophobia, arrhythmia, tremor **NIPE:** Compress lacrimal sac for several min after dose; heavily pigmented irises may require ↑ strength; peak 25–75 min, cycloplegia 6–24 h, mydriasis up to 24 h

Cyclophosphamide (Cytoxan, Neosar) [Antineoplastic/Alkylating Agent] Uses: *Hodgkin Dz & NHLs; multiple myeloma; SCLC, breast & ovarian CAs; mycosis fungoides; neuroblastoma; retinoblastoma; acute leukemias; allogeneic & ABMT w/ high doses; severe rheumatologic disorders (SLE, JRA)* **Action:** Alkylating agent **Dose:** *Adults.* (Per protocol) 500–1500 mg/m²; single dose at 2–4-wk intervals; 1.8 g/m² to 160 mg/kg (or at 12 g/m² in 75-kg individual) in the BMT setting (per protocols) **Peds.** *SLE:* 500–750 mg/m² qmo *JRA:* 10 mg/kg q2wk; ↓ w/ renal impair **Caution:** [D, ?] w/ BM suppression, hepatic Insuff **CI:** Component sensitivity **Disp:** Tabs 25, 50 mg; Inj 500 mg, 1, 2 g **SE:** ↓ BM; hemorrhagic cystitis, SIADH, alopecia, anorexia; N/V; hepatotox; rare interstitial pneumonitis; irreversible testicular atrophy possible; cardiotox rare; 2nd malignancies (bladder, ALL), risk 3.5% at 8 y, 10.7% at 12 y **Interactions:** ↑ Effects *W/* allopurinol, cimetidine, phenobarbital, rifampin; ↑ effects *OF* succinylcholine, warfarin; ↓ effects *OF* digoxin **Labs:** May ↓ uric acid level; ↓ HMG, Hct, plts, RBC, WBCs **NIPE:** May cause sterility, hair loss, ⊘ PRG, breast-feeding, immunizations; *hemorrhagic cystitis prophylaxis:* Cont bladder irrigation & MESNA uroprotection; encourage hydration, long-term bladder CA screening

Cyclosporine (Sandimmune, Neoral, Gengraf) [Immunosuppressant/ Polypeptide Antibiotic]   **WARNING:** ↑ Risk neoplasm, ↑ risk skin malignancies, ↑ risk HTN & nephrotox **Uses:** *Organ rejection in kidney, liver, heart, & BMT w/ steroids; RA; psoriasis* **Action:** Immunosuppressant; reversible inhibition of immunocompetent lymphocytes **Dose:** *Adults & Peds. PO:* 15 mg/kg/d 12 h pretransplant; after 2 wk, taper by 5 mg/wk to 5–10 mg/kg/d *IV:* If NPO, give 1/3 PO dose IV; ↓ in renal/hepatic impair **Caution:** [C, ?] Dose-related risk of nephrotox/hepatotox; live, attenuated vaccines may be less effective **CI:** Renal impair; uncontrolled HTN **Disp:** Caps 25, 100 mg; PO soln 100 mg/mL; Inj 50 mg/mL **SE:** May ↑ BUN & Cr & mimic transplant rejection; HTN; HA; hirsutism **Notes:** Levels: *Trough:* Just before next dose *Therapeutic:* Variable 150–300 ng/mL RIA **Interactions:** ↑ Effects *W/* azole antifungals, allopurinol, amiodarone, anabolic steroids, CCBs, cimetidine, chloroquine, clarithromycin, clonidine, diltiazem, macrolides, metoclopramide, nicardipine, NSAIDs, OCPs, ticlopidine, grapefruit juice; ↑ nephrotox *W/* aminoglycosides, amphotericin B, acyclovir, colchicine, enalapril, ranitidine, sulfonamides; ↑ risk of digoxin tox; ↑ risk of hyperkalemia *W/* diuretics, ACEIs; ↓ effects *W/* barbiturates, carbamazepine, INH, nafcillin, pyrazinamide, phenytoin, rifampin, sulfonamides, St. John's wort, alfalfa sprouts, astragalus, echinacea, licorice; ↓ effects *OF* immunizations **Labs:** ↑ SCr, BUN, LFTs, LDL, glucose; ↓ HMG, plts, WBCs; monitor Cr, CBC, LFTs **NIPE:** Monitor BP & ✓ for hyperglycemia, hyperkalemia, hyperuricemia; risk of photosensitivity—use sunscreen; administer in glass container; Neoral & Sandimmune not interchangeable

Cyclosporine Ophthalmic (Restasis) [Immunosuppressant/Anti-Inflammatory] **Uses:** *↑ Tear production suppressed d/t ocular inflammation* **Action:** Immune modulator, anti-inflammatory **Dose:** 1 gtt bid each eye 12 h apart; OK w/ artificial tears, allow 15 min between **Caution:** [C, –] **CI:** Ocular Infxn, component allergy **Disp:** Single-use vial 0.05% **SE:** Ocular burning/hyperemia **NIPE:** ⊘ Children < 16 y; may insert contact lenses 15 min after installation; mix vial well

Cyproheptadine (Periactin) [Antihistamine, Antipruritic] Uses: *Allergic Rxns; itching* **Action:** Phenothiazine antihistamine; serotonin antagonist **Dose:** **Adults.** 4–20 mg PO ÷ q8h; max 0.5 mg/kg/d **Peds 2–6 y.** 2 mg bid–tid (max 12 mg/24 h) **7–14 y.** 4 mg bid–tid; ↓ in hepatic impair **Caution:** [B, ?] Elderly, CV Dz, asthma, thyroid Dz, BPH **CI:** Neonates or < 2 y; NAG; BOO; acute asthma; GI obst; w/ MAOI **Disp:** Tabs 4 mg; syrup 2 mg/5 mL **SE:** Anticholinergic, drowsiness **Interactions:** ↑ Effects **W/** CNS depressants, MAOIs, EtOH; ↓ effects **OF** epinephrine, fluoxetine **Labs:** False(−) allergy skin testing **NIPE:** ↑ Risk photosensitivity—use sunscreen, take w/ food if GI distress; may stimulate appetite

Cytarabine [ARA-C] (Cytosar-U) [Antineoplastic/Antimetabolite] WARNING: Administration by experienced physician in properly equipped facility; potent myelosuppressive agent Uses: *Acute leukemias, CML, NHL; IT for leukemic meningitis or prophylaxis* **Action:** Antimetabolite; interferes w/ DNA synth **Dose:** 100–150 mg/m^2/d for 5–10 d (low dose); 3 g/m^2 q12h for 6–12 doses (high dose); 1 mg/kg 1–2/wk (SQ maint); 5–70 mg/m^2 up to 3/wk IT (per protocols); ↓ in renal/ hepatic impair **Caution:** [D, ?] In elderly, w/ marked BM suppression, ↓ dosage by ↓ the number of d of administration **CI:** Component sensitivity **Disp:** Inj 100, 500, 1, 2 g, also 20, 100 mg/mL **SE:** ↓ BM, N/V/D, stomatitis, flu-like synd, rash on palms/soles, hepatic/cerebellar dysfunction w/ high doses, noncardiogenic pulm edema, neuropathy, fever **Interactions:** ↓ Effects **OF** digoxin, flucytosine **Labs:** ↑ Uric acid, ↓ HMG, Hct, plts, RBCs, WBCs **NIPE:** ⊘ EtOH, NSAIDs, ASA, PRG, breast-feeding, immunizations; little use in solid tumors; high-dose tox limited by corticosteroid ophth soln

Cytarabine Liposome (DepoCyt) [Antineoplastic/Antimetabolite] WARNING: Can cause chemical arachnoiditis (N/V/HA, fever) ↓ severity w/ dexamethasone. Administer by experienced physician in properly equipped facility Uses: *Lymphomatous meningitis* **Action:** Antimetabolite; interferes w/ DNA synth **Dose:** 50 mg IT q14d for 5 doses, then 50 mg IT q28d × 4 doses; use dexamethasone prophylaxis **Caution:** [D, ?] May cause neurotox; blockage to CSF flow may ↑ the risk of neurotox; use in peds not established **CI:** Active meningeal Infxn **Disp:** IT Inj 50 mg/5 mL **SE:** Neck pain/rigidity, HA, confusion, somnolence, fever, back pain, N/V, edema, neutropenia, ↓ plt, anemia **Interactions:** ↓ Effects **OF** digoxin, flucytosine **Labs:** ↑ Uric acid, ↓ HMG, Hct, plts, RBCs, WBCs **NIPE:** ⊘ EtOH, NSAIDs, ASA, PRG, breast-feeding, immunizations; cytarabine liposomes are similar in microscopic appearance to WBCs; caution in interpreting CSF studies

Cytomegalovirus Immune Globulin [CMV-IG IV] (CytoGam) [Immune Globulin] Uses: *Prophylaxis/attenuation CMV Dz associated w/ transplantation* **Action:** IgG antibodies to CMV **Dose:** 150 mg/kg/dose w/in 72 h of transplant & wks 2, 4, 6, 8, & 100 mg/kg/dose wks 12, 16 posttransplant; see package insert **Caution:** [C, ?] Anaphylactic Rxns; renal dysfunction **CI:** Allergy to immunoglobulins; IgA deficiency **Disp:** Inj 50 mg/mL **SE:** Flushing, N/V, muscle cramps, wheezing, HA, fever **Interactions:** ↓ Effects *OF* live virus vaccines **NIPE:** IV only; administer by separate line; do not shake

Dabigatran (Pradaxa) [Direct Thrombin Inhibitor] **Uses:** *↓ risk stroke/ systemic embolism w/ non-valvular AF* **Action:** Thrombin Inhib **Dose:** *Adults.* CrCl > 30 mL/min: 150 mg PObid; CrCl 15–30 mL/min: 75mg PO bid **Caution:** [C, ?/–] avoid w/ P-gp inducers (ie, rifampin) **CI:** Active bleeding **Disp:** Caps 75, 150 mg **SE:** Bleeding, gastritis, dyspepsia **Interactions:** ↑ Effects *W/* ketoconazole, amiodarone, quinidine, clopidogrel, verapamil; ↑ risk of bleeding *W/* fibrinolytics, heparin, NSAIDs, plt Inhibs; ↓ effects *W/* rifampin **Labs:** Monitor aPTT **NIPE:** Do not chew/break/open caps; see label to convert between other anticoagulants; do not undergo surgery or dental procedures while using dabigatran

Dacarbazine (DTIC) [Antineoplastic/Alkylating Agent] **WARNING:** Causes hematopoietic depression, hepatic necrosis, may be carcinogenic, teratogenic **Uses:** *Melanoma, Hodgkin Dz, sarcoma* **Action:** Alkylating agent; antimetabolite as a purine precursor; ↓ protein synth, RNA, & esp DNA **Dose:** 2–4.5 mg/kg/d for 10 consecutive d or 250 mg/m²/d for 5 d (per protocols); ↓ in renal impair **Caution:** [C, ?] in BM suppression; renal/hepatic impair **CI:** Component sensitivity **Disp:** Inj 100, 200 mg **SE:** ↓ BM, N/V, hepatotox, flu-like synd, ↓ BP, photosensitivity, alopecia, facial flushing, facial paresthesias, urticaria, phlebitis at Inj site **Interactions:** ↑ Risk of bleeding *W/* anticoagulants, ASA; ↓ effects *W/* phenobarbital, phenytoin **Labs:** ↑ AST, ALT; ↓ plts, RBCs, WBCs; monitor CBC, plt **NIPE:** Risk of photosensitivity—use sunscreen; hair loss; Infxn; avoid extrav

Daclizumab (Zenapax) [Immunosuppressant/Immunomodulator] **WARNING:** Administration under skilled supervision in equipped facility **Uses:** *Prevent acute organ rejection* **Action:** IL-2 receptor antagonist **Dose:** 1 mg/kg/dose IV; 1st dose pretransplant, then 1 mg/kg q14d × 4 doses **Caution:** [C, ?] **CI:** Component sensitivity **Disp:** Inj 5 mg/mL **SE:** Hyperglycemia, edema, HTN, ↑ BP, constipation, HA, dizziness, anxiety, nephrotox, pulm edema, pain, anaphylaxis/hypersensitivity **Interactions:** ↑ Risk of mortality *W/* corticosteroids, cyclosporine, mycophenolate mofetil **NIPE:** ⊘ Immunizations; Infxns; ↑ fluid intake; administration w/in 4 h of prep

Dactinomycin (Cosmegen) [Antineoplastic/Antibiotic] **WARNING:** Administration under skilled supervision in equipped facility; powder & soln toxic, corrosive, mutagenic, carcinogenic, & teratogenic; avoid exposure & use precautions **Uses:** *Choriocarcinoma, Wilms tumor, Kaposi & Ewing sarcomas, rhabdomyosarcoma, uterine & testicular CA* **Action:** DNA intercalating agent **Dose:** *Adults.* 0.5 mg/d for 5 d; 2 mg/wk for 3 consecutive wk; 15 mcg/kg or 0.45 mg/m²/d (max 0.5 mg) for 5 d q3–8wk *Peds. Sarcoma* (per protocols); ↓ in renal impair **Caution:** [C, ?] **CI:** Concurrent/recent chickenpox or herpes zoster; infants < 6 mo **Disp:** Inj 0.5 mg **SE:** Myelo-/immunosuppression, severe N/V/D, alopecia, acne, hyperpigmentation, radiation recall phenomenon, tissue damage w/ extrav, hepato-tox **Interactions:** ↑ Effects *OF* BM suppressants, radiation therapy; ↓ effects *OF* vit K **Labs:** Monitor CBC; ↓ HMG, Hct, plts, RBCs, WBCs **NIPE:** ⊘ PRG, breast-feeding; risk of irreversible infertility; reversible hair loss; ↑ fluids to 2–3 L/d; classified as antibiotic but not used as antimicrobial

Dalfampridine (Ampyra) [Potassium Channel Blocker] Uses: *Improve walking w/ MS* **Action:** K+ channel blocker **Dose:** 10 mg PO q12h **Caution:** [C,?/–] not w/ other 4-aminopyridines **CI:** Hx Sz;w/ CrCl ≤ 50 mL/min **Disp:** Tab ER 10 mg **SE:** HA, N, constipation, dyspepsia, dizziness, insomnia, UTI, nasopharyngitis, back pain, pharyngolaryngeal pain, asthenia, balance disor-der, MS relapse, paresthesia, Sz **NIPE:** Do not cut/chew/crush/dissolve tab; dis-tributed through specialty pharmacies, call (888) 881-1918.

Dalteparin (Fragmin) [Anticoagulant/Low-Molecular-Weight Heparin] WARNING: ↑ Risk of spinal/epidural hematoma w/ LP **Uses:** *Unstable angina, non-Q-wave MI, prevent & Rx DVT following surgery (hip, Abd), pt w/ restricted mobility, extended Rx for PE DVT in CA pt* **Action:** LMW heparin **Dose:** *Angina/MI:* 120 units/kg (max 10,000 units) SQ q12h w/ ASA *DVT prophylaxis:* 2500–5000 units SQ 1–2 h pre-op, then daily for 5–10 d *Systemic anticoagulation:* 200 units/kg/d SQ or 100 units/kg bid SQ *CA:* 200 IU/kg (max 18,000 IU) SQ q24h × 30 d, mo 2–6 150 IU/kg SQ q24h (max 18,000 IU) **Cau-tion:** [B, ?] In renal/hepatic impair, active hemorrhage, cerebrovascular Dz, cere-bral aneurysm, severe HTN **CI:** HIT; pork product allergy; w/ mifepristone **Disp:** *Inj:* 2500 units (16 mg/0.2 mL), 5000 units (32 mg/0.2 mL), 7500 units (48 mg/0.3 mL), 10,000 units (64 mg/mL), 25,000 units (3.8 mL) *Prefilled vials:* 10,000 units/mL (9.5 mL) **SE:** Bleeding, pain at site, ↓ plt **Interactions:** ↑ Bleeding *W/* oral anticoagulants, plt Inhibs, warfarin, garlic, ginger, ginkgo, ginseng, chamomile **Labs:** ↑ AST, ALT; monitor CBC & plts **NIPE:** ⊘ Give IM or IV; administration SQ route only; predictable effects eliminate lab monitoring of drug's effect

Dantrolene (Dantrium) [Skeletal Muscle Relaxant/Hydantoin Derivative] WARNING: Hepatotox reported; D/C after 45 d if no benefit observed **Uses:** *Rx spasticity d/t upper motor neuron disorders (eg, spinal cord injuries, stroke, CP, MS), malignant hyperthermia* **Action:** Skeletal muscle relax-ant **Dose:** *Adults. Spasticity:* 25 mg PO daily; ↑ 25 mg to affect to 100 mg max PO qid PRN *Peds.* 0.5 mg/kg/dose bid; ↑ by 0.5 mg/kg to effect, to 3 mg/kg/dose max qid PRN *Adults & Peds. Malignant hyperthermia: Rx:* Cont rapid IV, start 1 mg/kg until Sxs subside or 10 mg/kg is reached *Postcrisis followup:* 4–8 mg/kg/d in 3–4 ÷ doses for 1–3 d to prevent recurrence **Caution:** [C, ?] Impaired cardiac/pulm/hepatic Fxn **CI:** Active hepatic Dz; where spasticity needed to maint posture or balance **Disp:** Caps 25, 50, 100 mg; powder for Inj 20 mg/vial **SE:** Hepatotox, drowsiness, dizziness, rash, muscle weakness, D/N/V PE w/ pericarditis, D, blurred vision, hep **Interactions:** ↑ Effects *W/* CNS depressants, antihistamines, opiates, EtOH; ↑ risk of hepatotox *W/* estrogens; ↑ risk of CV collapse & VF *W/* CCBs;

↓ plasma protein binding **W/** clofibrate, warfarin **Labs:** ↑ LFTs—monitor **NIPE:** ↑ Risk of photosensitivity—use sunblock; ⊘ EtOH, CNS depressants, sunlight

Dapsone, Oral [Antileprotic, Antimalarial] Uses: *Rx & prevent PCP; toxoplasmosis prophylaxis; leprosy* **Action:** Unknown; bactericidal Dose: **Adults.** PCP prophylaxis 50–100 mg/d PO; Rx PCP 100 mg/d PO w/ TMP 15–20 mg/kg/d for 21 d **Peds.** *PCP prophylaxis alternated* Dose: (> 1 mo) 4 mg/kg/dose once/wk (max 200 mg) *Prophylaxis of PCP:* 1–2 mg/kg/24 h PO daily; max 100 mg/d **Caution:** [C, +] G6PD deficiency; severe anemia **CI:** Component sensitivity **Disp:** Tabs 25, 100 mg **SE:** Hemolysis, methemoglobinemia, agranulocytosis, rash, cholestatic jaundice **Interactions:** ↑ Effects **W/** probenecid, TMP; ↓ effects **W/** activated charcoal, rifampin **Labs:** Monitor CBC, LFTs **NIPE:** ↑ Risk of photosensitivity—use sunblock; absorption ↑ by an acidic environment; for leprosy, combine w/ rifampin & other agents

Dapsone, Topical (Aczone) [Antileprotic, Antimalarial] Uses: *Topical for acne vulgaris* **Action:** Unknown; bactericidal **Dose:** Apply pea-size amount & rub into areas bid; wash hands after **Caution:** [C, +] G6PD deficiency; severe anemia **CI:** Component sensitivity **Disp:** 5% gel **SE:** Skin oiliness/peeling, dryness, erythema **Labs:** Check G6PD levels before use; follow CBC if G6PD deficient **NIPE:** Not for oral, ophthalmic, or intravag use

Daptomycin (Cubicin) [Antibiotic/Cyclic Lipopeptide Antibacterial] Uses: *Comp skin/skin structure Infxns d/t gram(+) organisms* S aureus, bacteremia, MRSA endocarditis **Action:** Cyclic lipopeptide; rapid membrane depolarization & bacterial death. Spectrum: *S aureus* (including MRSA), *S pyogenes, S agalactiae, S dysgalactiae* subsp *Equisimilis,* & *E faecalis* (vancomycin-susceptible strains only) **Dose:** *Skin:* 4 mg/kg IV daily × 7–14 d (over 2 min) *Bacteremia & endocarditis:* 6 mg/kg q48h; ↓ w/ CrCl < 30 mL/min or dialysis: q48h **Caution:** [B, ?] w/ HMG-CoA Inhibs **Disp:** Inj 250, 500 mg/10 mL **SE:** Anemia, constipation, N/V/D, HA, rash, site Rxn, muscle pain/weakness, edema, cellulitis, hypo-/hyperglycemia, , cough, back pain, Abd pain, anxiety, CP, sore throat, cardiac failure, confusion, *Candida* Infxns **Interactions:** ↑ Effects **OF** anticoagulants; ↓ effects **OF** tobramycin; ↓ effects **W/** tobramycin **Labs:** Monitor CPK baseline & weekly, LFTs, PT, INR; ↑ alk phos, CPK, LFTs; ↓ HMG, Hct, K⁺ **NIPE:** Safety & efficacy not established in pts < 18 y; consider D/C HMG-CoA reductase Inhibs to ↓ myopathy risk; not for Rx PNA

Darbepoetin Alfa (Aranesp) [Antianemic/Hematopoietic] **WARNING:** Associated w/ ↑ CV, thromboembolic events and/or mortality; D/C if Hgb > 12 g/dL; may ↑ tumor progression & death in CA pts Uses: *Anemia associated w/ CRF*, anemia in nonmyeloid malignancy w/ concurrent chemotherapy **Action:** Erythropoiesis, recombinant erythropoietin variant Dose: 0.45 mcg/kg single IV or SQ qwk; titrate, do not exceed target Hgb of 12 g/dL; use lowest doses possible, see package insert to convert from Epogen **Caution:** [C, ?] May ↑ risk of CV and/or neurologic SE in renal failure; HTN; w/ h/o Szs **CI:** Uncontrolled HTN, component allergy **Disp:** 25, 40, 60, 100, 200, 300 mcg/mL; 150 mcg/0.075 mL in polysorbate or albumin excipient **SE:** May ↑ cardiac risk, CP, hypo-/hypertension, N/V/D, myalgia, arthralgia, dizziness, edema, fatigue, fever, ↑ risk Infxn **Interactions:** None noted **Labs:** Monitor weekly CBC until stable **NIPE:** Longer 1/2-life than Epogen; monitor BP & for Sz activity, shaking vial inactivates drug

Darifenacin (Enablex) [Antispasmodic/Anticholinergic] Uses: *OAB* Urinary antispasmodic **Action:** Muscarinic receptor antagonist **Dose:** 7.5 mg/d PO; 15 mg/d max (7.5 mg/d w/ mod hepatic impair or w/ CYP3A4 Inhibs); w/ drugs metabolized by CYP2D (Table 10); swallow whole **Caution:** [C, ?/–] w/ hepatic impair **CI:** Urinary/gastric retention, uncontrolled NAG, paralytic ileus **Disp:** Tabs ER 7.5, 15 mg **SE:** Xerostomia/eyes, constipation, dyspepsia, Abd pain, retention, abnormal vision, dizziness, asthenia; **Interactions:** ↑ clarithromycin, itraconazole, ketoconazole, ritonavir, nelfinavir, ↑ effects **OF** digoxin, flecainide, TCAs, thioridazine **Labs:** Monitor LFTs **NIPE:** Take w/ or w/o food & swallow whole; drug will relieve Sxs but not treat cause; may cause heat prostration d/t < sweating

Darunavir (Prezista) [Antiretroviral/Protease Inhibitor] Uses: *Rx HIV w/ resistance to multiple protease Inhibs* **Action:** HIV-1 protease Inhib **Dose:** *Adult.* Rx-naïve & w/o darunavir-resistance substitutions: 800 mg w/ ritonavir 100 mg qd. *Rx experienced w/ one darunavir resistance:* 600 mg w/ ritonavir 100 mg bid w/ food. *Peds (6–18 y & > 20 kg).* Dose based on body wgt (see label); do not exceed the Rx experienced adult dose. Do not use qd dosing in peds; w/ food **Caution:** [B, ?/–] h/o allergy, CYP3A4 substrate, changes levels of many meds (see Interactions) **CI:** w/ Astemizole, terfenadine, dihydroergotamine, ergonovine, ergotamine, methylergonovine, pimozide, midazolam, triazolam **Disp:** Tabs 75, 150, 400, 600 mg **SE:** Central redistribution of fat (metabolic synd), N **Interactions:** ↑ Effects **OF** amiodarone, atorvastatin, bepridil, clarithromycin, cyclosporine, dihydropyridine, felodipine, HMG-CoA reductase Inhibs (statins), itraconazole, ketoconazole, lidocaine, nifedipine, pravastatin, quinidine, sildenafil, tacrolimus, trazodone, vardenafil; ↓ effects **W/** carbamazepine, phenobarbital, phenytoin, rifabutin, rifampin, efavirenz, St. John's wort; ↓ effects **OF** methadone, rifampin, SSRI, trazodone, warfarin **Labs:** ↑ Amylase, glucose; cholesterol, triglycerides, LFTs, uric acid; ↓ WBCs, neutrophils **NIPE:** Administer w/ ritonavir & food; do not use w/ salmeterol, colchicine (w/ renal impair) do not use w/ severe hepatic impair); adjust dose w/ bosentan, tadalafil for PAH

Dasatinib (Sprycel) [Antineoplastic/Protein-Tyrosin Kinase Inhibitor] Uses: CML, Ph⁺, ALL **Action:** Multi TKI **Dose:** 70 mg PO bid; adjust w/ CYP3A4 Inhibs/inducers (Table 10) **Caution:** [D, ?/–] **CI:** None **Disp:** Tabs 20, 50, 70 mg **SE:** ↓ BM, edema, fluid retention, PEs, N/V/D, Abd pain, bleeding, fever, ↑ QT **Interactions:** ↑ Effects **W/** atazanavir, clarithromycin, erythromycin, indinavir, itraconazole, ketoconazole, nefazodone, nelfinavir, ritonavir, saquinavir, telithromycin; ↓ effects W/ antacids, carbamazepine, dexamethasone, phenobarbital, phenytoin, rifampicin, St. John's wort **Labs:** ↑ LFTs, Cr, uric acid, troponin levels; ↓ plts, RBC, neutrophils; monitor CBC weekly for 2 mo, then monthly **NIPE:** ⊘ Chew or crush tabs; replace K^+, Mg before Rx

Daunorubicin (Daunomycin, Cerubidine) [Antineoplastic/Anthracycline]
WARNING: Cardiac Fxn should be monitored risk for potential risk for cardiac tox & CHF, renal/hepatic dysfunction **Uses:** *Acute leukemias* **Action:** DNA intercalating agent; ↓ topoisomerase II; generates oxygen free radicals **Dose:** 45–60 mg/m^2/d for 3 consecutive d; 25 mg/m^2/wk (per protocols); ↓ in renal/hepatic impair **Caution:** [D, ?] **CI:** Component sensitivity **Disp:** Inj 20, 50 mg **SE:** ↓ BM, mucositis, N/V, orange urine, alopecia, radiation recall phenomenon, hepatotox (hyperbilirubinemia), tissue necrosis w/ extrav, cardiotox (1–2% CHF w/ 550 mg/m^2 cumulative dose) **Interactions:** ↑ Risk of cardiotox W/ cyclophosphamide; ↑ myelosuppression W/ antineoplastic agents; ↓ response to live virus vaccines **Labs:** ↓ Neutrophils, plts **NIPE:** ⊘ ASA, NSAIDs, EtOH, PRG; breast-feeding, immunizations; risk of hair loss; prevent cardiotox w/ dexrazoxane (w/ > 300 mg/m^2 daunorubicin cum dose); IV use only; allopurinol prior to ↓ hyperuricemia

Decitabine (Dacogen) [Nucleoside Analogue]
Uses: *MDS* **Action:** Inhibits DNA methyltransferase **Dose:** 15 mg/m^2 cont Inf over 3 h; repeat q8h × 3 d; repeat cycle q6wk, min 4 cycles; delay Tx & ↓ dose if inadequate hematologic recovery at 6 wk (see label protocol); delay Tx w/ Cr > 2 mg/dL or bilirubin > 2 × ULN **Caution:** [D, ?/–] Avoid PRG; males should not father a child during or 2 mo after; renal/hepatic impair **Disp:** Powder 50 mg/vial **SE:** Febrile neutropenia, edema, petechiae, N/V/D, constipation, stomatitis, dyspepsia, cough, fever, fatigue, hyperglycemia, Infxn, HA **Labs:** ↑ LFTs, bilirubin, glucose; {doubleup} WBC, ↓ Hgb, ↓ plt; check CBC & plt before each cycle & PRN **NIPE:** May premedicate w/ antiemetic; ⊘ PRG; males should not father a child during or 2 mo after use; use appropriate contraception

Deferasirox (Exjade) [Iron-Chelating Agent]
Uses: *Chronic Fe overload d/t transfusion in pts > 2 y* **Action:** Oral Fe chelator **Dose:** *Initial:* 20 mg/kg PO/d; adjust by 5–10 mg/kg q3–6mo based on monthly ferritin; 30 mg/kg/d max; on empty stomach 30 min before food; hold dose if ferritin < 500 mcg/L, dissolve in H_2O, OJ/apple juice (< 1 g/3.5 oz; > 1 g in 7 oz) drink stat; resuspend residue & swallow; do not chew, swallow whole tabs or take w/ Al-containing antacids **Caution:** [B, ?/–] Elderly, renal impair, heme disorders; ↑ MDS in pt 60 y **Disp:** Tabs for oral susp 125, 250, 500 mg **SE:** N/V/D, Abd pain, skin rash, HA, fever, cough, Infxn, hearing loss, dizziness, cataracts, retinal disorders, ↑ IOP, lens opacities, dizziness **Interactions:** ⊘ Combine W/ other Fe-chelator therapies **Labs:** ↑ Cr & LFTs; ✓ Cr weekly 1st mo then qmo, ✓ CBC, urine protein, LFTs; monitor monthly Cr, urine protein, LFTs **NIPE:** ARF, cytopenias possible; dose to nearest whole tab; auditory/ophthal testing initially & q12mo

Degarelix (Firmagon) [GnRH Receptor Antagonist] Uses: *Advanced PCa* **Action:** Reversible LHRH antagonist, ↓ LH & testosterone w/o flare seen w/ LHRH agonists **Dose:** Initial 240 mg SQ in two 120 mg doses (40 mg/mL) maint 80 mg SQ (20 mg/mL) q28d **Caution:** [Not for women] **CI:** Use in women **Disp:** Inj vial 120 mg (initial); 80 mg (maint) **SE:** Inj site Rxns, hot flashes, ↑ wgt **Notes:** Requires 2 Inj (vol); 44% testosterone castrate (< 50 ng/dL) at day 1, 96% day 3 **Interactions:** Caution W/ Class Ia (eg, quinidine, procainamide) or Class III (amiodarone, sotalol) antiarrhythmics; ↑ risk of QT prolongation **Labs:** Monitor PSA; ↑ serum GGT **NIPE:** Give SQ Inj in abdomen—avoid waist & rib areas

Delavirdine (Rescriptor) [Antiretroviral/NNRTI] Uses: *HIV Infxn* **Action:** NNRTI **Dose:** 400 mg PO tid **Caution:** [C, ?] CDC recs HIV-infected mothers not to breast-feed (transmission risk); w/ renal/hepatic impair **CI:** Use w/ drugs dependent on CYP3A for clearance (Table 10) **Disp:** Tabs 100, 200 mg **SE:** Fat redistribution, immune reconstitution synd, HA, fatigue, rash, ↑ transaminases, N/V/D **Interactions:** Numerous drug interactions; ↑ Effects W/ fluoxetine; ↑ effects OF benzodiazepines, cisapride, clarithromycin, dapsone, ergotamine, indinavir, lovastatin, midazolam, nifedipine, quinidine, ritonavir, simvastatin, terfenadine, triazolam, warfarin; ↑ CYP; ↓ effects W/ antacids, barbiturates, carbamazepine, cimetidine, famotidine, lansoprazole, nizatidine, phenobarbital, phenytoin, ranitidine, rifabutin, rifampin; ↓ effects OF didanosine **Labs:** Monitor LFTs, ↑ AST, ALT, ↓ HMG, Hct, plts, neutrophil counts, WBC **NIPE:** Take w/o regard to food; avoid antacids

Demeclocycline (Declomycin) [Antibiotic] Uses: *SIADH* **Action:** Antibiotic, antagonizes ADH action on renal tubules **Dose:** 300–600 mg PO q12h on empty stomach; ↓ in renal failure; avoid antacids **Caution:** [D, +] Avoid in hepatic/renal impair & children **CI:** Tetracycline allergy **Disp:** Tabs 150, 300 mg **SE:** D, Abd cramps, photosensitivity, DI **Interactions:** ↑ Effects OF digoxin, anticoagulants; ↓ effects W/ antacids, Bi salts, Fe, NaHCO₃, barbiturates, carbamazepine, hydantoins, food; ↓ effects OF OCPs, PCN **Labs:** False(−) urine glucose; monitor CBC, LFTs, BUN, Cr **NIPE:** Risk of photosensitivity—use sunblock & avoid sunlight; not for peds < 8 y

Denosumab (Prolia, Xgeva) [Osteoclast Inhibitor (RANKL Inhibitor)] Uses: *Tx osteoporosis postmenopausal women (Prolia); prevent skeletal events w/ bone mets from solid tumors (Xgeva)* **Action:** RANK ligand (RANKL) Inhib (human IgG2 MoAb); inhibits osteoclasts **Dose:** *Prolia:* 60 mg SQ q6mo *Xgeva:* 120 mg SQ q4w; in upper arm, thigh, Abd **Caution:** [C,?/–] **CI:** Hypocalcemia **Disp:** Inj **SE:** Hypophosphatemia, serious Infxns, dermatitis, rashes, eczema, jaw osteonecrosis, pancreatitis, pain (musculoskeletal, back), fatigue, asthenia, dyspnea, N, Abd pain, flatulence, hypercholesterolemia, anemia, cystitis **Interactions:** ↑ risk of Infxn W/ immunosuppressants; ↑ risk of jaw osteonecrosis W/ corticosteroids **Labs:** ↓ Ca²⁺ **NIPE:** Give Ca 1000 mg & vit D 400 IU/d; w/ D/C BMD levels return to baseline at 1 y

Desipramine (Norpramin) [Antidepressant/TCA] **WARNING:** Closely monitor for worsening depression or emergence of suicidality **Uses:** *Endogenous depression*, chronic pain, peripheral neuropathy **Action:** TCA; ↑ synaptic serotonin or norepinephrine in CNS **Dose:** *Adults.* 100–200 mg/d single or ÷ dose; usually single hs dose (max 300 mg/d) *Peds 6–12 y.* 1–3 mg/kg/d ÷ dose, 5 mg/kg/d max; ↓ dose in elderly **Caution:** [C, ?/–] CV Dz, Sz disorder, hypothyroidism, elderly, liver impair **CI:** MAOIs w/in 14 d; during AMI recovery phase **Disp:** Tabs 10, 25, 50, 75, 100, 150 mg; caps 25, 50 mg **SE:** Anticholinergic (blurred vision, urinary retention, xerostomia); orthostatic ↓ BP; ↑ QT interval, arrhythmias **Interactions:** ↑ Effects *W/* cimetidine, diltiazem, fluoxetine, indinavir, MAOIs, paroxetine, propoxyphene, quinidine, ritonavir ranitidine, EtOH, grapefruit juice; ↑ effects *OF* Li, sulfonylureas; ↓ effects *W/* barbiturates, carbamazepine rifampin, tobacco **NIPE:** Full effect of drug may take 4 wk; blue-green urine; risk of photosensitivity—use sunblock & avoid sunlight

Desirudin (Iprivask) [Direct Thrombin Inhibitor (Recombinant Hirudin)] **WARNING:** Recent/planned epidural/spinal anesthesia, ↑ epidural/spinal hematoma risk w/ paralysis; consider risk vs benefit before neuraxial intervention **Uses:** *DVT Px in hip replacement* **Action:** Thrombin Inhib **Dose:** *Adults.* 15 mg SQ q12h, initial 5–15 min prior to surgery *CrCl 31-60 mL/min:* 5 mg SQ q12h; CrCl < 31 mL/min: 1.7 mg SQ q12h; v aPTT & SCr daily for dosage mod **Caution:** [C, ?/–] Active bleeding, irreversible coags, hypersens to hirudins **Disp:** Inj **SE:** Hemorrhage, N/V, Inj site mass, wound secretion, anemia, thrombophlebitis, ↓ BP, dizziness, anaphylactic Rxn, fever **Interactons:** ↑ risk of bleeding *W/* anticoagulants, NSAIDs, plt Inhibs **NIPE:** Monitor for neurologic impair—may indicate spinal/epidural hematoma

Desloratadine (Clarinex) [Antihistamine/Selective H₁-Receptor Antagonist] **Uses:** *Seasonal & perennial allergic rhinitis; chronic idiopathic urticaria* **Action:** Active metabolite of Claritin, ↑ H₁-antihistamine, blocks inflammatory mediators **Dose:** *Adults & Peds >12 y.* 5 mg PO daily; 5 mg PO qod w/ hepatic/renal impair **Caution:** [C, ?/–] RediTabs contain phenylalanine **Disp:** Tabs & RediTabs (rapid dissolving) 5 mg, syrup 0.5 mg/mL **SE:** Allergy, anaphylaxis, somnolence, HA, dizziness, fatigue, pharyngitis, xerostomia, N, dyspepsia, myalgia **Labs:** ↑ LFTs, bilirubin **NIPE:** Take w/o regard to food

Desmopressin (DDAVP, Stimate) [Antidiuretic Hormone] **WARNING:** Not for hemophilia B or w/ factor VIII Ab; not for hemophilia A w/ factor VIII levels = 5% **Uses:** *DI (intranasal & parenteral); bleeding d/t uremia, hemophilia A, & type I von Willebrand Dz (parenteral), nocturnal enuresis* **Action:** Synthetic analogue of vasopressin (human ADH); ↑ factor VIII **Dose:** *DI: Intranasal: Adults.* 0.1–0.4 mL (10–40 mcg/d in 1–3 ÷ doses) *Peds 3 mo–12 y.* 0.05–0.3 mL/d in 1 or 2 doses *Parenteral: Adults.* 0.5–1 mL (2–4 mcg/d in 2 ÷ doses); converting from nasal to parenteral, use 1/10 nasal dose *PO: Adults.* 0.05 mg bid; ↑ to max of 1.2 mg *Hemophilia A & von Willebrand Dz (type I): Adults & Peds > 10 kg.*

0.3 mcg/kg in 50 mL NS, Inf over 15–30 min *Peds < 10 kg.* As above w/ dilution to 10 mL w/ NS *Nocturnal enuresis: Peds > 6 y.* 20 mcg intranasally hs **Caution:** [B, M] Avoid overhydration **CI:** Hemophilia B; CrCl < 50 mL/min, severe classic von Willebrand Dz; pts w/ factor VIII antibodies; hyponatremia **Disp:** Tabs 0.1, 0.2 mg; Inj 4, 15 mcg/mL; nasal soln 0.1, 1.5 mg/mL **SE:** Facial flushing, HA, dizziness, vulval pain, nasal congestion, pain at Inj site, H_2O intoxication **Interactions:** ↑ Antidiuretic effects *W/* carbamazepine, chlorpropamide, clofibrate; ↑ effects *OF* vasopressors; ↓ antidiuretic effects *W/* demeclocycline, Li, norepinephrine **Labs:** ↓ Na^+ **NIPE:** Monitor I&O, ⊘ EtOH, overhydration; in very young & old pts, ↓ fluid intake to avoid H_2O intoxication & ↓ Na^+

Desvenlafaxine (Pristiq) [Serotonin-Norepinephrine Reuptake Inhibitor (SNRI)]
WARNING: Monitor for worsening or emergence of suicidality, particularly in ped, adolescent, & young adult pts **Uses:** *MDD* **Action:** Selective SNRI **Dose:** 50 mg PO daily, ↓ w/ renal impair **Caution:** [C, ±/M] **CI:** Hypersensitivity, MAOI w/ or w/in 14 d of stopping MAOI **Disp:** Tabs 50, 100 mg **SE:** N, dizziness, insomnia, hyperhidrosis, constipation, somnolence, ↓ appetite, anxiety, & specific male sexual Fxn disorders **Interactions:** ↑ Effects *W/* CYP3A4 Inhibs; ↑ effects *OF* anticoagulants; ↓ effects *OF* CYP3A4 substrates **NIPE:** Tabs should be taken whole, allow 7 d after stopping before starting an MAOI; ⊘ ETOH; caution w/ other serotonergics & CNS active drugs

Dexmedetomidine (Precedex) [Sedative/Selective Alpha-2-Agonist]
Uses: *Sedation in intubated & non-intubated pts* **Action:** Sedative; selective α_2-agonist **Dose:** *Adults.* **ICU sedation:** 1 mcg/kg IV over 10 min, then 0.2–0.7 mcg/kg/h *Procedural sedation:* 0.5–1 mcg/kg IV over 10 min, then 0.2–1 mcg/kg/h; ↓ in elderly, liver Dz **Caution:** [C; ?/–] **CI:** None **Disp:** Inj 200 mcg/2 mL **SE:** Hypotension, bradycardia **NIPE:** Tachyphylaxis & tolerance associated w/ exposure > 24 h

Dexamethasone, Nasal (Dexacort Phosphate Turbinaire) [Anti-Inflammatory, Immunosuppressant/Glucocorticoid]
Uses: *Chronic nasal inflammation or allergic rhinitis* **Action:** Anti-inflammatory corticosteroid **Dose:** *Adults & Peds > 12 y.* 2 sprays/nostril bid–tid, max 12 sprays/d *Peds 6–12 y.* 1–2 sprays/nostril bid, max 8 sprays/d **Caution:** [C, ?] **CI:** Untreated Infxn **Disp:** Aerosol, 84 mcg/activation **SE:** Local irritation **NIPE:** Use decongestant nose gtt 1st if nasal congestion

Dexamethasone, Ophthalmic (AK-Dex Ophthalmic, Decadron Ophthalmic) [Anti-Inflammatory, Immunosuppressant/Glucocorticoid]
Uses: *Inflammatory or allergic conjunctivitis* **Action:** Anti-inflammatory corticosteroid **Dose:** Instill 1–2 gtt tid–qid **Caution:** [C, ?/–] **CI:** Active untreated bacterial, viral, & fungal eye Infxns **Disp:** Susp & soln 0.1%; oint 0.05% **SE:** Long-term use associated w/ cataracts **NIPE:** Eval IOP & lens if prolonged use

Dexamethasone Systemic, Topical (Decadron) [Anti-Inflammatory, Immunosuppressant/Glucocorticoid]
See Steroids, Systemic; Tables 2 & 3

Dexlansoprazole (Dexilant) [Proton Pump Inhibitor] Uses: *Healing and maint of all grades of erosive esophagitis, Tx of heartburn associated w/ nonerosive GERD* **Action:** PPI **Dose:** *Adults. Esophagitis:* 60 mg PO daily × 8 wk; maint 30 mg PO daily × 6 mo *GERD:* 30 mg PO daily × 4 wk; w/ mod hepatic impair; max 30 mg/d **Caution:** [B, ?/–] Do not use w/ drugs w/ pH-based absorption (eg, ampicillin, Fe salts, ketoconazole) **CI:** None **Disp:** Caps 30 mg, 60 mg, DR **SE:** N/V/D, Abd pain, flatulence, URI **Interactions:** Avoid w/ atazanavir; ↓ effects *OF* atazanavir; ↓ absorption *OF* ketoconazole, digoxin, Fe, ampicillin **Labs:** Monitor INR if on warfarin **NIPE:** w or w/o food; swallow whole or open caps, sprinkle on applesauce & swallow stat; clinical response does not R/O gastric malignancy? ↑ Risk of fxs w/ all PPI; risk of hypomagnesemia w/ long-term use, monitor

Dexmethylphenidate (Focalin, Focalin XR) [C-II] [Stimulant]
WARNING: Caution w/ Hx drug dependence/alcoholism. Chronic abuse may lead to tolerance, psychological dependence & abnormal behavior; monitor closely during withdrawal Uses: *ADHD* **Action:** CNS stimulant, blocks reuptake of norepinephrine & DA **Dose:** *Adults. Focalin:* 2.5 mg PO bid, ↑ by 2.5–5 mg weekly; max 20 mg/d *Focalin XR:* 10 mg PO daily, ↑ 10 mg weekly; max 40 mg/d *Peds ≥ 6 y. Focalin:* 2.5 mg PO bid, ↑ 2.5–5 mg weekly; max 20 mg/d *Focalin XR:* 5 mg PO daily, ↑ 5 mg weekly; max 30 mg/d; if already on methylphenidate, start w/ 1/2 current total daily dose **Caution:** [C, ?/–] Avoid w/ known cardiac abnormality; may ↓ metabolism of warfarin/anticonvulsants/antidepressants **CI:** Agitation, anxiety, tension, glaucoma, Hx motor tic, family Hx/dx Tourette w/ or w/in 14 d of MAOI; hypersensitivity to methylphenidate **Disp:** Tabs 2.5, 5, 10 mg; caps ER 5, 10, 15, 20, 30, 40 mg **SE:** HA, anxiety, dyspepsia, ↓ appetite, Wgt loss, dry mouth, visual disturbances, ↑ HR, HTN, MI, stroke, sudden death, Szs, growth suppression, aggression, mania, psychosis **Interactions:** ↑ Effects *OF* anticonvulsants, oral anticoagulants, TCA, SSRIs, phenylbutazone; ↓ effects *OF* guanethidine, antihypertensives **Labs:** ✓ CBC w/ prolonged use **NIPE:** Swallow ER caps whole or sprinkle contents on applesauce (do not crush/chew); do not give w/in 14 d of MAOI

Dexpanthenol (Ilopan-Choline Oral, Ilopan) [Cholinergic] Uses: *Minimize paralytic ileus, Rx post-op distention* **Action:** Cholinergic agent **Dose:** *Adults. Relief of gas:* 2–3 tabs PO tid. *Prevent post-op ileus:* 250–500 mg IM stat, repeat in 2 h, then q6h PRN *Ileus:* 500 mg IM stat, repeat in 2 h, then q6h, PRN **Caution:** [C, ?] **CI:** Hemophilia, mechanical bowel obst **Disp:** Inj 250 mg/mL; tabs 50 mg; cream 2% **SE:** GI cramps **NIPE:** Monitor BP during IV administration

Dexrazoxane (Zinecard, Totect) [Chelating Agent] Uses: *Prevent anthracycline-induced (eg, doxorubicin) cardiomyopathy (Zinecard), extrav of anthracycline chemotherapy (Totect)* **Action:** Chelates heavy metals; binds intracellular Fe & prevents anthracycline-induced free radicals **Dose:** *Systemic (cardiomyopathy, Zinecard):* 10:1 ratio dexrazoxane:doxorubicin 30 min before each dose, 5:1 ratio w/ CrCl < 40 mL/min *Extrav (Totect):* IV Inf over 1–2 h qd × 3 d, w/in 6 h of extrav *Day 1:* 1000 mg/m^2 (max 2000 mg) *Day 2:* 1000 mg/m^2 (max 2000 mg) *Day 3:* 500 mg/m^2 (max: 1000 mg) w/ CrCl < 40 mL/min, ↓ dose by 50% **Caution:** [D, –] **CI:** Component sensitivity **Disp:** Inj powder 250, 500 mg (10 mg/mL) **SE:** ↓ BM, fever, Infxns, stomatitis, alopecia, N/V/D **Interactions:** ↑ Length of muscle relaxation *W/* succinylcholine **Labs:** ↑ LFTs **NIPE:** Inj site pain

Dextran 40 (Gentran 40, Rheomacrodex) [Plasma Volume Expander, Glucose Polymer] **Uses:** *Shock, prophylaxis of DVT & thromboembolism, adjunct in peripheral vascular surgery* **Action:** Expands plasma vol; ↓ blood viscosity **Dose:** *Shock:* 10 mL/kg Inf rapidly; 20 mL/kg max 1st 24 h; beyond 24 h 10 mL/kg max; D/C after 5 d *Prophylaxis of DVT & thromboembolism:* 10 mL/kg IV day of surgery, then 500 mL/d IV for 2–3 d, then 500 mL IV q2–3d based on risk for up to 2 wk **Caution:** [C, ?] Inf Rxns; w/ corticosteroids **CI:** Major hemostatic defects; cardiac decompensation; renal Dz w/ severe oliguria/ anuria **Disp:** 10% dextran 40 in 0.9% NaCl or 5% dextrose **SE:** Allergy/anaphylactoid Rxn (observe during 1st min of Inf), arthralgia, cutaneous Rxns, ↓ BP, fever **Interactions:** ↑ Bleeding times *W/* antiplt agents or anticoagulants **Labs:** Monitor Cr & lytes; ↑ ALT, AST **NIPE:** Draw blood before administration of drug; pt should be well hydrated prior to Inf

Dextroamphetamine (Dexedrine) [C-II] [Amphetamine] **WARNING:** Amphetamines have a high potential for abuse. Long-term use may lead to dependence **Uses:** *ADHD, narcolepsy* **Action:** CNS stimulant; ↑ DA & norepinephrine release **Dose:** *ADHD ≥ 6 y:* 5 mg daily–bid, ↑ by 5 mg/d weekly PRN, max 60 mg/d ÷ bid–tid *Peds 3–5 y:* 2.5 mg PO daily, ↑ 2.5 mg/d weekly PRN to response *Peds < 3 y:* Not recommended *Narcolepsy 6–12 y:* 5 mg daily, ↑ by 5 mg/d weekly PRN max 60 mg/d ÷ bid–tid *≥ 12 y:* 10–60 mg/d ÷ bid–tid; ER caps once daily **Caution:** [C; +/–] Hx drug abuse; separate 14 d from MAOIs **CI:** Advanced arteriosclerosis, CVD, mod–severe HTN, hyperthyroidism, glaucoma **Disp:** Tabs 5,10 mg; ER caps 5, 10, 15 mg **SE:** HTN, ↓ appetite, insomnia **Interactions:** ↑ Risk of hypertensive crisis *W/* MAOIs; ↑ effects *W/* thiazides, TCAs; ↓ effects *OF* meperidine, norepinephrine, phenobarbital, phenytoin; ↓ effects *W/* Li, psychotropics; ↓ effects *OF* adrenergic blockers, sedatives, antihypertensives **Labs:** Interferes *W/* urinary steroid tests **NIPE:** May open ER caps, do not crush beads

Dextromethorphan (Benylin DM, Delsym, Mediquell, PediaCare 1, others) [OTC] [Antitussive] **Uses:** *Control nonproductive cough* **Action:** Suppresses medullary cough center **Dose:** *Adults.* 10–30 mg PO q4h PRN (max 120 mg/24 h) *Peds 2–6 y.* 2.5–7.5 mg q4–8h (max 30 mg/24 h) *7–12 y.* 5–10 mg q4–8h (max 60 mg/24 h) **Caution:** [C, ?/–] Not for persistent or chronic cough **CI:** 2 y **Disp:** Caps 30 mg; lozenges 2.5, 5, 7.5, 15 mg; syrup 15 mg/15 mL, 10 mg/5 mL; Liq 10 mg/15 mL, 3.5, 7.5, 15 mg/5 mL; sustained-action Liq 30 mg/5 mL **SE:** GI disturbances **Interactions:** ↑ Effects *W/* amiodarone, fluoxetine, quinidine, terbinafine; ↑ risk of serotonin synd *W/* sibutramine, MAOIs; ↑ CNS depression *W/* antihistamines, antidepressants, sedative, opioids, EtOH **NIPE:** ↑ Fluids, humidity to environment, D/C MAOIs for 14 d before administering drug; found in combo OTC products w/ guaifenesin; deaths reported in pts < 2 y; abuse potential; efficacy in children debated

Dextrose 50%/25% Uses: Hypoglycemia, insulin OD **Action:** Sugar source in the form of d-glucose **Dose:** *Adults.* 1 50 mL amp of 50% soln IV *Peds. ECC 2010: Hypoglycemia:* 0.5–1 g/kg (25% max IV/IO conc); 50% dextrose (0.5 g/mL): 1–2 mL/kg; 25% dextrose (0.25 g/mL): 2–5 mL/kg; 10% dextrose (0.1 g/mL): 5–10 mL/kg; 5 % dextrose (0.95 g/mL): 10–20 mL/kg if vol tolerated **Caution:** [C, M] w/ suspected intracranial bleeding can ↑ ICP **CI:** None if given to pt w/ documented hypoglycemia **Disp:** Injectable forms **SE:** Burning at IV site, local tissue necrosis w/ extrav; neurologic Sxs (Wernicke encephalopathy) if pt thiamine deficient **NIPE:** If pt is mentating well enough to protect airway, use oral glucose first; lower concs used in IV fluids

Diazepam (Valium, Diastat) [C-IV] [Anxiolytic, Skeletal Muscle Relaxant, Anticonvulsant, Sedative/Hypnotic/Benzodiazepine] Uses: *Anxiety, EtOH withdrawal, muscle spasm, status epilepticus, panic disorders, amnesia, pre-op sedation* **Action:** Benzodiazepine **Dose:** *Adults. Status epilepticus:* 5–10 mg q10–20min to 30 mg max in 8-h period *Anxiety, muscle spasm:* 2–10 mg PO bid–qid or IM/IV q3–4h PRN *Pre-op:* 5–10 mg PO or IM 20–30 min or IV just prior to procedure *EtOH withdrawal:* Initial 2–5 mg IV, then 5–10 mg q5–10min, 100 mg in 1 h max. May require up to 1000 mg/24 h for severe withdrawal; titrate to agitation; avoid excessive sedation; may lead to aspiration or resp arrest *Peds. Status epilepticus:* **< 5 y.** 0.05–0.3 mg/kg/dose IV q15–30min up to a max of 5 mg **> 5 y.** To max of 10 mg *Sedation, muscle relaxation:* 0.04–0.3 mg/kg/dose q2–4h IM or IV to max of 0.6 mg/kg in 8 h, or 0.12–0.8 mg/kg/24 h PO ÷ tid–qid; ↓ w/ hepatic impair **Caution:** [D, ?/–] **CI:** Coma, CNS depression, resp depression, NAG, severe uncontrolled pain; ↓ BP, rash, ↓ resp rate **Disp:** Tabs 2, 5, 10 mg; soln 1, 5 mg/mL; Inj 5 mg/mL; rectal gel 2.5, 5, 10, 20 mg/mL **SE:** Sedation, amnesia, bradycardia, ↓ BP, rash, ↓ resp rate **Notes:** 5 mg/min IV max in adults or 1–2 mg/min in peds (resp arrest possible) **Interactions:** ↑ Effects *W/* antihistamines, azole antifungals, BBs, CNS depressants, cimetidine, ciprofloxin, disulfiram, INH, OCP, omeprazole, phenytoin, valproic acid, verapamil, EtOH, kava kava, valerian; ↑ effects *OF* digoxin, diuretics; ↓ effects *W/* barbiturates, carbamazepine, theophylline, ranitidine, tobacco; ↓ effects *OF* haloperidol, levodopa **Labs:** Monitor LFTs, BUN, Cr, CBC w/ long-term drug use **NIPE:** Risk ↑ Sz activity; IM absorption erratic; avoid abrupt D/C

Diazoxide (Proglycem) [Antihypertensive/Peripheral Vasodilator] Uses: *Hypoglycemia d/t hyperinsulinism (Proglycem); hypertensive crisis (Hyperstat)* **Action:** ↓ Pancreatic insulin release; antihypertensive **Dose:** Repeat in 5–15 min until BP controlled; repeat q4–24h; monitor BP closely. *Hypoglycemia: Adults & Peds.* 3–8 mg/kg/24 h PO ÷ q8–12h *Neonates.* 8–15 mg/kg/24 h ÷ in 3 equal doses; maint 8–10 mg/kg/24 h PO in 2–3 equal doses **Caution:** [C, ?] ↓ Effect w/ phenytoin; ↑ effect w/ diuretics, warfarin **CI:** Allergy to thiazides or other sulfonamide-containing products; HTN associated w/ aortic coarctation, AV shunt, or Pheo **Disp:** Caps 50 mg; PO susp 50 mg/mL; IV 15 mg/mL **SE:** Hyperglycemia, ↓ BP, dizziness, Na+ & H₂O retention, N/V, weakness **Interactions:** ↑ Effects **W/** carboplatin, cisplatin, diuretics, phenothiazines; ↑ effects **OF** anticoagulants; ↓ effects **W/** sulfonylureas; ↓ effects **OF** phenytoin, sulfonylureas **Labs:** ↑ Serum uric acid, glucose; can give false(−) insulin response to glucagons; ↓ neutrophil count, HMG, Hct, WBC **NIPE:** Daily wgt, ↑ reversible body hair growth; Rx extra v w/ warm compress

Dibucaine (Nupercainal) [Topical Anesthetic] Uses: *Hemorrhoids & minor skin conditions* **Action:** Topical anesthetic **Dose:** Insert PR w/ applicator bid & after each BM; apply sparingly to skin **Caution:** [C, ?] topical use only **CI:** Component sensitivity **Disp:** 1% oint w/ rectal applicator; 0.5% cream **SE:** Local irritation, rash **Interactions:** None noted

Diclofenac, Oral (Cataflam, Voltaren, Voltaren XR,) [Antiarthritic, Anti-Inflammatory/NSAID] WARNING: May ↑ risk of CV events & GI bleeding; CI in post-op CABG Uses: *Arthritis & pain, oral & topical, actinic keratosis* **Action:** NSAID **Dose:** 50–75 mg PO bid; w/ food or milk **Caution:** [C (avoid after 30 wk), ?] CHF, HTN, renal/hepatic dysfunction, & h/o PUD, asthma **CI:** NSAID/ASA allergy; porphyria; following CABG **Disp:** Tabs 50 mg; tabs DR 25, 50, 75, 100 mg; XR tabs 100 mg **SE:** *Oral:* Abd cramps, heartburn, GI ulceration, rash, interstitial nephritis **Interactions:** ↑ Risk of bleeding **W/** feverfew, garlic, ginger, ginkgo; ↑ effects **OF** digoxin, MTX, cyclosporine, Li, insulin, sulfonylureas, K⁺-sparing diuretics, warfarin; ↓ effects **W/** ASA; ↓ effects **OF** thiazide diuretics, furosemide, BBs **Labs:** ↑ LFTs, serum glucose & cortisol; ↓ serum uric acid; monitor LFTs, CBC, BUN, Cr **NIPE:** Risk of photosensitivity—use sunblock; take w/ food; ⊘ crush tabs; watch for GI bleed

Diclofenac, Topical (Flector Patch, Pennsaid, Solaraze, Voltaren Gel) [Antiarthritic, Anti-Inflammatory/NSAID+ Prostaglandin E₁ Analogue] WARNING: May ↑ risk of CV events & GI bleeding; CI in post-op CABG Uses: *Arthritis of the knee (Pennsaid); arthritis of knee/hands (Voltaren Gel) pain d/t strain, sprain, & contusions (Flector patch), actinic keratosis (Solaraze)* **Action:** NSAID **Dose:** *Flector Patch:* 1 patch to painful area *Pennsaid:* 10 gtt spread around knee; repeat until 40 gtt applied *Usual dose:* 40 gtt/knee qid; wash hands; wait until it dries before dressing *Solaraze:* 0.5 g to each 5 × 5 cm lesion 60–90 d *Voltaren Gel:* Upper extremity 2 g qid (max 8 g/d); lower extremity 4 g qid (max 16 g/d) **Caution:** [C (avoid after 30 wk), ?] avoid nonintact skin; CV events possible w/ CHF, ↑ BP, renal/hepatic dysfunction, w/ Hx PUD, asthma; avoid w/ PO NSAID **CI:** NSAID/ASA allergy; following CABG; component allergy **Disp:** *Flector Patch:* 180 mg (10 × 14 cm); *Voltaren Gel 1%; Solaraze 3%* **SE:** Pruritus, dermatitis, burning, dry skin, N, HA **Interactions:** ↑ Risk of bleeding **W/** feverfew, garlic, ginger, ginkgo; ↑ effects **OF** digoxin, MTX, cyclosporine, Li, insulin, sulfonylureas, K⁺-sparing diuretics, warfarin; ↓ effects

W/ ASA; ↓ effects *OF* thiazide diuretics, furosemide, BBs **Labs:** ✓ CBC, LFTs periodically **NIPE:** Do not apply patch/gel to damaged skin or while bathing; no box warning on *Solaraze*

Diclofenac Ophthalmic (Voltaren Ophthalmic) [NSAID] **Uses:** *Inflammation postcataract or pain/photophobia postcorneal refractive surgery* **Action:** NSAID **Dose:** *Post-op cataract:* 1 gtt qid, start 24 h post-op × 2 wk *Post-op refractive:* 1–2 gtts w/in 1 h pre-op & w/in 15 min post-op then qid up to 3 d **Caution:** [C, ?] May ↑ bleed risk in ocular tissues **CI:** NSAID/ASA allergy **Disp:** Ophthal soln 0.1% 2.5, 5 mL bottle **SE:** Burning/stinging/itching, keratitis, ↑ IOP, lacrimation, abnormal vision, conjunctivitis, lid swelling, discharge, iritis **Interactions:** ↑ Effects *OF* oral anticoagulants **NIPE:** ⊘ Wear soft contact lenses; may delay wound healing

Diclofenac & Misoprostol (Arthrotec) [Antiarthritic, Anti-Inflammatory/NSAIDs + Prostaglandin E$_1$ (PGE$_1$) Analogue] **WARNING:** May induce abortion, birth defects; do not take if PRG; may ↑ risk of CV events & GI bleeding; CI in post-op CABG **Uses:** *OA & RA w/* ↑ risk GI bleed* **Action:** NSAID w/ GI protective PGE$_1$ **Dose:** *OA:* 50–75 mg PO bid–tid; RA 50 mg bid–qid or 75 mg bid; w/ food or milk **Caution:** [X, ?] CHF, HTN, renal/hepatic dysfunction, & Hx PUD, asthma; avoid w/ porphyria **CI:** PRG; GI bleed; renal/hepatic failure; severe CHF; NSAID/ASA allergy; following CABG **Disp:** Tabs *Arthrotec 50:* 50 mg diclofenac w/ 200 mcg misoprostol *Arthrotec 75:* 75 mg diclofenac w/ 200 mcg misoprostol **SE:** *Oral:* Abd cramps, heartburn, GI ulcers, rash, interstitial nephritis **Interactions:** ↑ Risk of GI bleed *W/* oral corticosteroids, anticoagulants, prolonged NSAID use, EtOH, smoking; ↓ effects *OF* ACE Inhibs, diuretics, digoxin, methotrexate, cyclosporine, Li, warfarin **Labs:** ✓ CBC, LFTs **NIPE:** Do not crush tabs; watch for GI bleed; PRG test females before use

Dicloxacillin (Dynapen, Dycill) [Antibiotic/Penicillin] **Uses:** *Rx of pneumonia, skin, & soft-tissue Infxns, & osteomyelitis caused by penicillinase-producing staphylococci* **Action:** Bactericidal; ↓ cell wall synth **Spectrum:** *S aureus & Streptococcus* **Dose:** *Adults.* 150–500 mg qid (2 g/d max) *Peds < 40 kg.* 12.5–100 mg/kg/d ÷ qid; take on empty stomach **Caution:** [B, ?] **CI:** Component or PCN sensitivity **Disp:** Caps 125, 250, 500 mg; soln 62.5 mg/5 mL **SE:** N/D, Abd pain **Interactions:** ↑ Effects *W/* disulfiram, probenecid; ↓ effects *OF* MTX; ↓ effects *W/* macrolides, tetracyclines, food; ↓ effects *OF* OCPs, warfarin **Labs:** False ↑ urine glucose; ↓ eosinophils; ↓ HMG, Hct, plts, WBC; monitor PTT if pt on warfarin **NIPE:** Take w/ H$_2$O

Dicyclomine (Bentyl) [Antimuscarinic, GI Antispasmodic/Anticholinergic] **Uses:** *Functional IBS* **Action:** Smooth-muscle relaxant **Dose:** *Adults.* 20 mg PO qid; ↑ to 160 mg/d max or 20 mg IM q6h, 80 mg/d ÷ qid then ↑ to 160 mg/d, max 2 wk *Peds Infants > 6 mo.* 5 mg/dose tid–qid *Children.* 10 mg/dose tid–qid **Caution:** [B, −] **CI:** Infants < 6 mo, NAG, MyG, severe UC, BOO, GI obst, reflux esophagitis **Disp:** Caps 10, 20 mg; tabs 20 mg; syrup 10 mg/5 mL; Inj

10 mg/mL **SE:** Anticholinergic SEs may limit dose **Interactions:** ↑ Anticholinergic effects **W/** anticholinergics, antihistamines, amantadine, MAOIs, TCAs, phenothiazides; ↑ effects **OF** atenolol, digoxin; ↓ effects **W/** antacids; ↓ effects **OF** haloperidol, ketoconazole, levodopa, phenothiazines **NIPE:** Do not administer IV; ⊘ EtOH, CNS depressant; adequate hydration; take 30–60 min ac

Didanosine [ddI] (Videx) [Antiretroviral, NRTI]   WARNING: Allergy manifested as fever, rash, fatigue, GI/resp Sxs reported; D/C drug stat & do not rechallenge; lactic acidosis & hepatomegaly/steatosis reported **Uses:** *HIV Infxn in zidovudine-intolerant pts* **Action:** NRTI **Dose:** *Adults.* > 60 kg: 400 mg/d PO or 200 mg PO bid < 60 kg: 250 mg/d PO or 125 mg PO bid; adults should take 2 tabs/ administration **Peds.** 2 wk–8 mo: 100 mg/m² PO bid > 8 mo: 120 mg/m² PO bid; on empty stomach; ↓ w/ renal impair **Caution:** [B, −] CDC rec HIV-infected mothers not breast-feed **CI:** Component sensitivity **Disp:** Chew tabs 25, 50, 100, 150, 200 mg; powder packets 100, 167, 250, 375 mg; powder for soln 2, 4 g **SE:** Pancreatitis, peripheral neuropathy, D, HA **Interactions:** ↑ Effects **W/** allopurinol, ganciclovir; ↓ effects **W/** methadone, food; ↑ risk of pancreatitis **W/** thiazide diuretics, IV pentamidine, EtOH; ↓ effects **W/** azole antifungals, dapsone, delavirdine, ganciclovir, indinavir, quinolone, ranitidine, tetracycline **Labs:** ↑ LFTs, uric acid, amylase, lipase, triglycerides **NIPE:** May cause hyperglycemia; do not take w/ meals; thoroughly chew tabs, do not mix w/ fruit juice or acidic beverages; reconstitute powder w/ H₂O

Diflunisal (Dolobid) [Analgesic, Antipyretic, Anti-Inflammatory/ NSAID]   WARNING: May ↑ risk of CV events & GI bleeding; CI in post-op CABG **Uses:** *Mild–mod pain; OA* **Action:** NSAID **Dose:** *Pain:* 500 mg PO bid *OA:* 500–1500 mg PO in 2–3 ÷ doses; ↓ in renal impair, take w/ food/milk **Caution:** [C (D 3rd tri or near delivery), ?] CHF, HTN, renal/hepatic dysfunction, & h/o PUD **CI:** Allergy to NSAIDs or ASA, active GI bleed, post-CABG **Disp:** Tabs 250, 500 mg **SE:** May ↑ bleeding time; HA, Abd cramps, heartburn, GI ulceration, rash, interstitial nephritis, fluid retention **Interactions:** ↑ Effects **W/** probenecid; ↑ effects **OF** APAP, anticoagulants, digoxin, HCTZ, indomethacin, Li, MTX, phenytoin, sulfonamides, sulfonylureas; ↓ effects **W/** antacids, ASA; ↓ effects **OF** furosemide **Labs:** ↑ Salicylate levels **NIPE:** Take w/ food; ⊘ chew or crush tabs

Digoxin (Lanoxin, Lanoxicaps, Digitek) [Antiarrhythmic/Cardiac Glycoside]   Uses: *CHF, AF & A flutter, & PAT* **Action:** Positive inotrope; ↑ AV node refractory period **Dose:** *Adults. PO digitalization:* 0.5–0.75 mg PO, then 0.25 mg PO q6–8h to total 1–1.5 mg *IV or IM digitalization:* 0.25–0.5 mg IM or IV, then 0.25 mg q4–6h to total 0.125–0.5 mg/d PO, IM, or IV (average daily dose 0.125–0.25 mg) *Peds Preterm Infants. Digitalization:* 30 mcg/kg PO or 25 mcg/kg IV; give 1/2 of dose initial, then 1/4 of dose at 8–12-h intervals for 2 doses *Maint:* 5–7.5 mcg/kg/24 h PO or 4–6 mcg/kg/24 h IV ÷ q12h *Term Infants. Digitalization:* 25–35 mcg/kg PO or 20–30 mcg/kg IV; give 1/2 the initial dose, then 1/3 of dose at 8–12 h *Maint:* 6–10 mcg/kg/24 h PO or 5–8 mcg/kg/24 h ÷ q12h *1 mo–2 y. Digitalization:* 35–60 mcg/kg PO or 30–50 mcg/kg IV; give 1/2 the initial dose, then 1/3 dose at 8–12-h intervals for 2 doses *Maint:* 10–15 mcg/kg/24 h PO or 7.5–15 mcg/kg/24 h IV ÷ q12h *2–10 y. Digitalization:* 30–40 mcg/kg PO or 25 mcg/kg IV; give 1/2 initial dose, then 1/3 of the dose at 8–12-h intervals for 2 doses *Maint:* 8–10 mcg/kg/24 h PO or 6–8 mcg/kg/24 h IV ÷ q12h *7–10 y.* Same as for adults; ↓ in renal impair **Caution:** [C, +] w/ ↓ K⁺, Mg²⁺, renal failure **CI:** AV block; IHSS; constrictive pericarditis **Disp:** Caps 0.05, 0.1, 0.2 mg; tabs 0.125, 0.25, 0.5 mg; elixir 0.05 mg/mL; Inj 0.1, 0.25 mg/mL **SE:** Can cause heart block; ↓ K⁺ potentiates tox; N/V, HA, fatigue, visual disturbances (yellow-green halos around lights), cardiac arrhythmias **Notes:** *Levels: Trough:* Just before next dose *Therapeutic:* 0.8–2.0 ng/mL *Toxic* > 2 ng/mL *1/2-life:* 36 h **Interactions:** ↑ Effects *W/* alprazolam, amiodarone, azole antifungals, BBs, carvedilol, cyclosporine, corticosteroids, diltiazem, diuretics, erythromycin, NSAIDs, quinidine, spironolactone, tetracyclines, verapamil, goldenseal, hawthorn, licorice, quinine, Siberian ginseng; ↓ effects *W/* charcoal, cholestyramine, cisapride, neomycin, rifampin, sucralfate, thyroid hormones, psyllium, St. John's wort **Labs:** Monitor serum electrolytes **NIPE:** Different bioavailability in various brands; IM Inj painful, has erratic absorption & should not be used

Digoxin Immune Fab (Digibind, DigiFab) [Cardiac Glycoside Antidote/Antibody Fragment]   Uses: *Life-threatening digoxin intoxication* **Action:** Antigen-binding fragments bind & inactivate digoxin **Dose:** *Adults & Peds.* Based on serum level & pt's wgt; see charts provided w/ drug **Caution:** [C, ?] **CI:** Sheep product allergy **Disp:** Inj 38 mg/vial **SE:** Worsening of cardiac output or CHF, ↓ K⁺, facial swelling, & redness **Notes:** Each vial binds ≈ 0.6 mg of digoxin **Interactions:** ↓ Effects *OF* cardiac glycosides **Labs:** ↓ K⁺ level **NIPE:** Will take up to 1 wk for accurate serum digoxin levels after use of Digibind; renal failure may require redosing on several days

Diltiazem (Cardizem, Cardizem CD, Cardizem LA, Cardizem SR, Cartia XT, Dilacor XR, Diltia XT, Taztia XT, Tiamate, Tiazac) [Antianginal/CCB]   Uses: *Angina, prevention of reinfarction, HTN, AF or flutter, & PAT* **Action:** CCB **Dose:** *Stable angina PO:* Initial, 30 mg PO qid; ↑ to 180–360 mg/d in 3–4 ÷ doses PRN; XR 120 mg/d (540 mg/d max) *LA:* 180–360 mg/d *HTN:* SR: 60–120 mg PO bid; ↑ to 360 mg/d max *CD or XR:* 120–360 mg/d (max 540 mg/d) or LA 180–360 mg/d *IV:* 0.25 mg/kg IV bolus over 2 min; may repeat in 15 min at 0.35 mg/kg; begin Inf of 5–15 mg/h *ECC 2010:* **Acute rate control:** 0.25 mg/kg (15–20 mg) over 2 min followed in 15 min by 0.35 mg/kg (20–25 mg) over 2 min maint Inf 5–15 mg/h **Caution:** [C, +] **CI:** SSS, AV block, ↓ BP, AMI, pulm congestion **Disp:** *Cardizem CD:* Caps 120, 180, 240, 300, 360 mg *Cardizem LA:* XR tabs 120, 180, 240, 300, 360, 420 mg *Cardizem SR:* Caps 60, 90, 120 mg *Cardizem:* Tabs 30, 60, 90, 120 mg *Cartia XT:* Caps 120, 180, 240, 300 mg *Dilacor XR:* Caps 180, 240 mg *Diltia XT:* Caps 120, 180, 240 mg *Tiazac:* Caps 120, 180, 240, 300, 360, 420 mg *Tiamate (XR):* Tabs 120, 180, 240 mg; Inj 5 mg/mL *Taztia XT:* XR caps 120, 180, 240, 300, 360 mg **SE:** Gingival hyperplasia,

bradycardia, AV block, ECG abnormalities, edema, dizziness, HA **Interactions:** ↑ Effects W/ α-blockers, amiodarone, azole antifungals, BBs, cimetidine, cyclosporine, digoxin, erythromycin, fentanyl, H_2-receptor antagonists, Li, nitroprusside, quinidine, theophylline, EtOH, grapefruit juice; ↑ effects OF carbamazepine, cyclosporine, digitalis glycosides, quinidine, phenytoin, prazosin, theophylline, TCAs; ↓ effects W/ NSAIDs, phenobarbital, rifampin **Labs:** ↑ LFTs **NIPE:** ⊘ Chew or crush SR or ER preps; risk of photosensitivity—use sunblock; Cardizem CD, Dilacor XR, & Tiazac not interchangeable

Dimenhydrinate (Dramamine, Others) [Antiemetic/Antivertigo/Anticholinergic]
Uses: *Prevention & Rx of N/V, dizziness, or vertigo of motion sickness* **Action:** Antiemetic, action unknown **Dose:** *Adults.* 50–100 mg PO q4–6h, max 400 mg/d; 50 mg IM/IV PRN *Peds 2–6 y.* 12.5–25 mg q6–8h max 75 mg/d *6–12 y.* 25–50 mg q6–8h max 150 mg/d **Caution:** [B, ?] **CI:** Component sensitivity **Disp:** Tabs 50 mg; chew tabs 50 mg; Liq 12.5 mg/4 mL, 12.5, 15.62 mg/5 mL **SE:** Anticholinergic SE **Interactions:** ↑ Effects W/ CNS depressants, antihistamines, opioids, quinidine, TCAs, EtOH; prolonged anticholinergic effects W/ MAOIs **Labs:** False allergy skin tests **NIPE:** ⊘ Drug 72 h prior to allergy skin testing; take 30 min before travel for motion sickness

Dimethyl Sulfoxide [DMSO] (Rimso-50) [GU Agent]
Uses: *Interstitial cystitis* **Action:** Unknown **Dose:** Intravesical, 50 mL, retain for 15 min; repeat q2wk until relief **Caution:** [C, ?] **CI:** Component sensitivity **Disp:** 50% & 100% soln **SE:** Cystitis, eosinophilia, GI, & taste disturbance **Interactions:** ↓ Effects OF sulindac **Labs:** Monitor CBC, LFTs, BUN, Cr levels **NIPE:** ↑ Taste & smell of garlic

Dinoprostone (Cervidil Vag Insert, Prepidil Vag Gel, Prostin E2) [Prostaglandin/Abortifacient]
WARNING: Should only be used by trained personnel in an appropriate hospital setting **Uses:** *Induce labor; terminate PRG (12–20 wk); evacuate uterus in missed abortion or fetal death* **Action:** Prostaglandin, changes consistency, dilatation, & effacement of the cervix; induces uterine contraction **Dose:** *Gel:* 0.5 mg; if no cervical/uterine response, repeat 0.5 mg q6h (max 24-h dose 1.5 mg) *Vag insert:* 1 insert (10 mg = 0.3 mg dinoprostone/h over 12 h); remove w/ onset of labor or 12 h after insertion *Vag supp:* 20 mg repeated q3–5h; adjust *PRN supp:* 1 high in vagina, repeat at 3–5-h intervals until abortion (240 mg max) **Caution:** [X, ?] **CI:** Ruptured membranes, allergy to prostaglandins, placenta previa or AUB, when oxytocic drugs CI or if prolonged uterine contractions are inappropriate (h/o C-section, cephalopelvic disproportion, etc) **Disp:** *Endocervical gel:* 0.5 mg in 3-g syringes (w/ 10- & 20-mm shielded catheter) *Vag gel:* 0.5 mg/3 g *Vag supp:* 20 mg *Vag insert, CR:* 10 mg **SE:** N/V/D, dizziness, flushing, HA, fever, abnormal uterine contractions **Interactions:** ↑ Effects of oxytocics, ↓ effects W/ large amts EtOH **NIPE:** Pt supine after insertion of supp or gel up to 1/2 h

Diphenhydramine (Benadryl) [Antihistamine/Antitussive/Antiemetic] [OTC]
Uses: *Rx & prevent allergic Rxns, motion sickness, potentiate

narcotics, sedation, cough suppression, & Rx of extrapyramidal Rxns* **Action:** Antihistamine, antiemetic **Dose:** *Adults.* 25–50 mg PO, IV, or IM bid–tid *Peds > 2 y.* 5 mg/kg/24 h PO or IM ÷ q6h (max 300 mg/d); ↑ dosing interval w/ mod–severe renal Insuff **Caution:** [B, –] elderly, NAG, BPH, w/ MAOI **CI:** Acute asthma **Disp:** Tabs, caps 25, 50 mg; elixir 12.5 mg/5 mL; syrup 12.5 mg/5 mL; Liq 6.25, 12.5 mg/5 mL; Inj 50 mg/mL, cream 2% **SE:** Anticholinergic (xerostomia, urinary retention, sedation) **Interactions:** ↑ Effects *W/* CNS depressants, antihistamines, opioids, MAOIs, TCAs, EtOH **Labs:** ↓ Response to allergy skin testing; ↓ HMG, Hct, plts **NIPE:** ↑ Risk of photosensitivity—use sunblock; may cause drowsiness

Diphenoxylate + Atropine (Lomotil, Lonox) [C-V] [Opioid Antidiarrheal] Uses: *D* Action: Constipating meperidine congener, ↓ GI motility

Dose: *Adults.* Initial, 5 mg PO tid–qid until controlled, then 2.5–5 mg PO bid; 20 mg/d max *Peds > 2 y.* 0.3–0.4 mg/kg/24 h (of diphenoxylate) bid–qid, 10 mg/d max **Caution:** [C, +] elderly, w/ renal impair **CI:** Obstructive jaundice, D d/t bacterial Infxn; children < 2 y **Disp:** Tabs 2.5 mg diphenoxylate/0.025 mg atropine; Liq 2.5 mg diphenoxylate/0.025 mg atropine/5 mL **SE:** Drowsiness, dizziness, xerostomia, blurred vision, urinary retention, constipation **Interactions:** ↑ Effects *W/* CNS depressants, opioids, EtOH, ↑ risk HTN crisis *W/* MAOIs **NIPE:** ↓ Effectiveness w/ D caused by antibiotics

Diphtheria & Tetanus Toxoids (Td) (Decavac—for > 7 y) [Td Vaccine]

Uses: Primary immunization, booster (peds 7–9 y; peds 11–12 y if 5 y since last shot then q10y); tetanus protection after wound **Actions:** Active immunization **Dose:** 0.5 mL IM × 1; **Caution:** [C, ?/–] **CI:** Component sensitivity **Disp:** Single-dose syringes 0.5 mL **SE:** Inj site pain, redness, swelling; fever, fatigue, HA, malaise, neuro disorders rare **Interactions:** ↑ Risk of suboptimal response *W/* concomitant vaccines, radiation, chemotherapy, high-dose steroids **NIPE:** If IM, use only preservative-free Inj; use DTaP (Adacel) rather than TT or Td all adults 19–64 y who have not previously received one dose of DTaP (protection adult pertussis) & Tdap for ages 10–18 y (Boostrix); **do not confuse** Td (for adults) w/ DT (for children < 7 y)

Diphtheria & Tetanus Toxoids (DT) (Generic Only—for < 7 y) [Tetanus Vaccine] Uses: Primary immunization ages < 7 y (DTaP is recom-

mended vaccine) **Actions:** Active immunization **Dose:** 0.5 mL IM × 1 **Caution:** [C, N/A] **CI:** Component sensitivity **Disp:** Single-dose syringes 0.5 mL **SE:** Inj site pain, redness, swelling; fever, fatigue, myalgias/arthralgias, N/V, Szs, other neurological disorders rare **Interactions:** ↑ Risk of suboptimal response *W/* chemotherapy, high-dose corticosteroids > 2 wk, radiation **NIPE:** If IM, use only preservative-free Inj. **Do not confuse** DT (for children < 7 y) w/ Td (for adults); DTaP is recommended for primary immunization

Diphtheria, Tetanus Toxoids, & Acellular Pertussis Adsorbed (DTaP) (Ages < 7 y) (Daptacel, Infanrix, Tripedia) Uses: Primary vaccination;

5 Inj at 2, 4, 6, 15–18 mo, & 4–6 y **Actions:** Active immunization **Dose:** 0.5 mL IM × 1 as in previous **Caution:** [C, N/A] **CI:** Component sensitivity; if previous

pertussis vaccine caused progressive neurologic disorder/encephalopathy w/in 7 d of shot **Disp:** SDV 0.5 mL **SE:** Inj site nodule/pain/swelling/redness; drowsiness, fatigue, fever, fussiness, irritability, lethargy, V, prolonged crying; rare ITP & neurologic disorders **Interactions:** ↑ Risk of suboptimal response *W/* chemotherapy, high-dose corticosteroids > 2 wk, radiation **NIPE:** If IM, use only preservative-free Inj; DTaP recommended for primary immunization age < 7 y, if age 7–9 y use Td, ages > 10–11 y use Tdap; if encephalopathy or other neurologic disorder w/in 7 d of previous dose. **Do not use** DTaP use DT or Td depending on age

Diphtheria, Tetanus Toxoids, & Acellular Pertussis Adsorbed (Tdap) (Ages > 10–11 y) (Boosters: Adacel, Boostrix) **Uses:** *Catch-up" vaccination if 1 or more of the 5 childhood doses of DTP or DTaP missed; all adults 19–64 y who have not received one dose previously (adult pertussis protection) or if around infants < 12 mo; booster q10y; tetanus protection after wound **Actions:** Active immunization **Dose:** 0.5 mL IM × 1 **Caution:** [C, ?/–] **CI:** Component sensitivity;if previous pertussis vaccine caused progressive neurologic disorder/encephalopathy w/in 7 d of shot **Disp:** SDV 0.5 mL **SE:** Inj site pain, redness, swelling; Abd pain, arthralgias/myalgias, fatigue, fever, HA, N/V/D, rash, tiredness **Interactions:** ↑ Risk of suboptimal response *W/* chemotherapy, high-dose corticosteroids > 2 wk, radiation **NIPE:** If IM, use only preservative-free Inj; ACIP rec: Tdap for ages 10–18 y (*Boostrix*) or 11–64 y (*Adacel*); Td should be used in children 7–9 y

Diphtheria, Tetanus Toxoids, & Acellular Pertussis Adsorbed, Hep B (Recombinant), & Inactivated Poliovirus Vaccine [IPV] Combined (Pediarix) [Vaccine, Inactivated] **Uses:** *Vaccine against diphtheria, tetanus, pertussis, HBV, polio (types 1, 2, 3) as a 3-dose primary series in infants & children < 7 y, born to HBsAg(–) mothers* **Actions:** Active immunization **Dose:** *Infants:* Three 0.5-mL doses IM, at 6–8-wk intervals, start at 2 mo; child given 1 dose of hep B vaccine, same; previously vaccinated w/ 1 or more doses inactivated poliovirus vaccine, use to complete series **Caution:** [C, N/A] **CI:** HBsAg(+) mother, adults, children > 7 y, immunosuppressed, allergy to yeast, neomycin, polymyxin B, or any component, encephalopathy, or progressive neurologic disorders; caution in bleeding disorders **Disp:** SDV 0.5 mL **SE:** Drowsiness, restlessness, fever, fussiness, ↓ appetite, nodule redness, Inj site pain/swelling **Interactions:** ↓ Effects *W/* immunosuppressants, corticosteroids **NIPE:** If IM use only preservative-free Inj

Dipivefrin (Propine) [Alpha-Adrenergic Agonist/Glaucoma Agent] **Uses:** *Open-angle glaucoma* **Action:** α-Adrenergic agonist **Dose:** 1 gtt in eye q12h **Caution:** [B, ?] **CI:** NAG **Disp:** 0.1% soln **SE:** HA, local irritation, blurred vision, photophobia, HTN **Interactions:** ↑ Effects *W/* BBs, ophthal anhydrase Inhibs, osmotic drugs, sympathomimetics, ↑ risk of cardiac arrhythmias *W/* digoxin, TCAs **NIPE:** Discard discolored solns

Dipyridamole (Persantine) [Coronary Vasodilator/Platelet Aggregation Inhibitor] **Uses:** *Prevent post-op thromboembolic disorders, often in combo w/ ASA or warfarin (eg, CABG, vascular graft); w/ warfarin after artificial heart valve; chronic angina; w/ ASA to prevent coronary artery thrombosis; dipyridamole IV used in place of exercise stress test for CAD* **Action:** Antiplt activity; coronary vasodilator **Dose:** *Adults.* 75–100 mg PO tid–qid; stress test 0.14 mg/kg/min (max 60 mg over 4 min) *Peds > 12 y.* 3–6 mg/kg/d ÷ tid (safety/efficacy not established) **Caution:** [B, ?/–] w/ other drugs that affect coagulation **CI:** Component sensitivity **Disp:** Tabs 25, 50, 75 mg; Inj 5 mg/mL **SE:** HA, ↓ BP, N, Abd distress, flushing rash, dizziness, dyspnea **Interactions:** ↑ Effects *W/* anticoagulants, heparin, evening primrose oil, feverfew, garlic, ginger, ginkgo, ginseng, grapeseed extract; ↑ effects *OF* adenosine; ↑ bradycardia *W/* BBs; ↓ effects *W/* aminophylline **NIPE:** IV use can worsen angina; ⊘ EtOH or tobacco because of vasoconstriction effects; + effects may take several mo

Dipyridamole & Aspirin (Aggrenox) [Platelet Aggregation Inhibitor] **Uses:** *↓ Reinfarction after MI; prevent occlusion after CABG; ↓ risk of stroke* **Action:** ↓ Plt aggregation (both agents) **Dose:** 1 cap PO bid **Caution:** [C, ?] **CI:** Ulcers, bleeding diathesis **Disp:** Dipyridamole (XR) 200 mg/ASA 25 mg **SE:** *ASA component:* Allergic Rxns, skin Rxns, ulcers/GI bleed, bronchospasm *Dipyridamole component:* Dizziness, HA, rash **Interactions:** ↑ Risk of GI bleed *W/* EtOH, NSAIDs; ↑ effects *OF* acetazolamide, adenosine, anticoagulants, methotrexate, oral hypoglycemics; ↓ effects *OF* ACEIs, BB, cholinesterase Inhibs, diuretics **NIPE:** Swallow caps whole

Disopyramide (Norpace, Norpace CR, NAPAmide, Rythmodan) [Antiarrhythmic/Pyridine Derivative] **WARNING:** Excessive mortality or nonfatal cardiac arrest rate w/ use in asymptomatic non-life-threatening ventricular arrhythmias w/ MI 6 d to 2 y prior. Restrict use to life-threatening arrhythmias only **Uses:** *Suppression & prevention of VT* **Action:** Class Ia antiarrhythmic; stabilizes membranes, depresses action potential **Dose:** *Adults.* Immediate < 50 kg 200 mg, > 50 kg 300 mg, maint 400–800 mg/d ÷ q6h or q12h for CR, max 1600 mg/d *Peds < 1 y.* 10–30 mg/kg/24 h PO (÷ qid) *1–4 y.* 10–20 mg/kg/24 h PO (÷ qid) *4–12 y.* 10–15 mg/kg/24 h PO (÷ qid) *12–18 y.* 6–15 mg/kg/24 h PO (÷ qid); ↓ in renal/hepatic impair **Caution:** [C, +] Elderly, w/ abnormal ECG, lytes, liver/renal impair, NAG **CI:** AV block, cardiogenic shock, ↓ BP, CHF **Disp:** Caps 100, 150 mg; CR caps 100, 150 mg **SE:** Anticholinergic SEs; negative inotrope, may induce CHF **Notes:** *Levels: Trough:* Just before next dose *Therapeutic:* 2–5 mcg/mL *Toxic* > 5 mcg/mL *1/2-life:* 4–10 h **Interactions:** ↑ Effects *W/* cimetidine, clarithromycin, erythromycin, quinidine; ↑ effects *OF* digoxin, hypoglycemics, insulin, warfarin; ↑ risk of arrhythmias *W/* pimozide; ↓ effects *W/* barbiturates, phenytoin, phenobarbital, rifampin **Labs:** ↑ LFTs, lipids, BUN, Cr; ↓ serum glucose, HMG, Hct **NIPE:** Risk of photosensitivity—use sunblock; daily wgt

Dobutamine (Dobutrex) [Inotropic/Adrenergic, Beta-1 Agonist] **Uses:** *Short-term in cardiac decompensation secondary to ↓ contractility* **Action:** Positive inotrope **Dose:** *Adults.* *ECC 2010:* 2–20 mcg/kg/min; titrate to HR not

> 10% of baseline **Peds. ECC 2010:** Shock w/ high SVR: 2–20 mcg/kg/min; titrate **Caution:** [C, ?] w/ arrhythmia, MI, severe CAD, ↓ vol **CI:** Sensitivity to sulfites, IHSS **Disp:** Inj 250 mg/20 mL, 12.5/mL **SE:** CP, HTN, dyspnea **Interactions:** ↑ Effects *W*/ furazolidone, methyldopa, MAOIs, TCAs; ↓ effects *W*/ BBs, NaHCO₃; ↓ effects *OF* guanethidine **Labs:** ↓ K⁺ **NIPE:** Eval for adequate hydration; monitor I&O; monitor PWP & cardiac output if possible; monitor ECG for ↑ HR or ectopic activity; monitor BP

Docetaxel (Taxotere) [Antineoplastic/Antimitotic Agent] WARNING:
Do not administer if neutrophil count < 1500 cell/mm³; severe Rxns possible in hepatic dysfunction **Uses:** *Breast (anthracycline-resistant), ovarian, lung, & prostate CA* **Action:** Antimitotic agent; promotes microtubular aggregation; semisynthetic taxoid **Dose:** 100 mg/m² over 1 h IV q3wk (per protocols); dexamethasone 8 mg bid prior & continue for 3–4 d; ↓ dose w/ ↑ bilirubin levels **Caution:** [D, –] Sensitivity to meds w/ polysorbate 80, component sensitivity **Disp:** Inj 20 mg/0.5 mL, 80 mg/2 mL **SE:** ↓ BM, neuropathy, N/V, alopecia, fluid retention synd; cumulative doses of 300–400 mg/m² w/o steroid prep & post-Tx & 600–800 mg/m² w/ steroid prep; allergy possible (rare w/ steroid prep) **Interactions:** ↑ Effects *W*/ cyclosporine, ketoconazole, erythromycin, terfenadine **Labs:** ↑ AST, ALT, alk phos, bilirubin; ↓ plts, WBCs; frequent CBC during therapy; ✓ bilirubin, AST and ALT prior to each cycle **NIPE:** ↑ Fluids to 2–3 L/d, ↑ risk of hair loss, ↑ susceptibility to Infxn; urine may become reddish-brown

Docusate Calcium (Surfak)/Docusate Potassium (Dialose)/Docusate Sodium (DOSS, Colace) [Emollient Laxative/Fecal Softener] Uses:
Constipation; adjunct to painful anorectal conditions (hemorrhoids) **Action:** Stool softener **Dose:** *Adults.* 50–500 mg PO ÷ daily–qid *Peds Infants–3 y.* 10–40 mg/24 h ÷ daily–qid *3–6 y.* 20–60 mg/24 h ÷ daily–qid. *6–12 y.* 40–120 mg/24 h ÷ daily–qid **Caution:** [C, ?] **CI:** Use w/ mineral oil; intestinal obst, acute Abd pain, N/V **Disp:** *Ca:* Caps 50, 240 mg *K⁺:* Caps 100, 240 mg *Na:* Caps 50, 100 mg; syrup 50, 60 mg/15 mL; Liq 150 mg/15 mL; soln 50 mg/mL **SE:** Rare Abd cramping, D **Interactions:** ↑ Absorption of mineral oil **NIPE:** Take w/ full glass of H₂O; no laxative action; do not use > 1 wk; short-term use

Dofetilide (Tikosyn) [Antiarrhythmic] WARNING:
To minimize the risk of induced arrhythmia, hospitalize for minimum of 3 d to provide calculations of CrCl, cont ECG monitoring, & cardiac resuscitation **Uses:** *Maint nl sinus rhythm in AF/A flutter after conversion* **Action:** Class III antiarrhythmic, prolongs action potential duration **Dose:** Based on CrCl & QTc; CrCl > 60 mL/min 500 mcg PO q12h, ✓ QTc 2–3 h after, if QTc > 15% over baseline or > 500 msec, ↓ to 250 mcg q12h, ✓ after each dose; if CrCl < 60 mL/min, see package insert; D/C if QTc > 500 msec after dosing adjustments **Caution:** [C, –] w/ AV block, renal Dz, lytes imbalance **CI:** Baseline QTc > 440 msec, CrCl < 20 mL/min; w/ verapamil, cimetidine, TMP, ketoconazole, quinolones, ACE Inhibs/HCTZ combo **Disp:** Caps 125, 250, 500 mcg **SE:** Ventricular arrhythmias, QT ↑, torsades de pointes, rash, HA, CP,

dizziness **Interactions:** ↑ Effects *W/* amiloride, amiodarone, azole antifungals, cimetidine, diltiazem, macrolides, metformin, megestrol, nefazodone, norfloxacin, SSRIs, TCAs, triamterene, TMP, verapamil, zafirlukast, quinine, grapefruit juice **Labs:** Correct K⁺ & Mg²⁺ before use; monitor LFTs, BUN, Cr **NIPE:** Take w/o regard to food; avoid w/ other drugs that ↑ QT interval; hold Class I/III antiarrhythmics for 3 1/2-lives prior to dosing; amiodarone level should be < 0.3 mg/L before use; do not initiate if HR < 60 BPM; restricted to participating prescribers

Dolasetron (Anzemet) [Antiemetic/Selective Serotonin 5-HT₃ Receptor Antagonist] **Uses:** *Prevent chemotherapy & post-op associated N/V* **Action:** 5-HT₃ receptor antagonist **Dose:** *Adults. PO:* 100 mg PO as a single dose 1 h prior to chemotherapy *Post-op:* 12.5 mg IV, 100 mg PO 2 h pre-op *Peds 2–16 y.* 1.8 mg/kg PO (max 100 mg) as single dose *Post-op:* 0.35 mg/kg IV or 1.2 mg/kg PO **Caution:** [B, ?] w/ cardiac conduction problems **CI:** IV use with chemotherapy; component sensitivity **Disp:** Tabs 50, 100 mg; Inj 20 mg/mL **SE:** ↑ QT interval, D, HTN, HA, Abd pain, urinary retention **Interactions:** ↑ Effects *W/* cimetidine; ↑ risk of arrhythmias *W/* diuretics; ↓ effects *W/* rifampin **Labs:** Transient ↑ LFTs **NIPE:** Monitor ECG for prolonged QT interval; frequently causes HA; IV form no longer approved for chemotherapy-induced N&V d/t heart rhythm abnormailties

Donepezil (Aricept) [Reversible Acetylcholinesterase Inhibitor] **Uses:** *Severe Alzheimer dementia* ADHD; behavioral synds in dementia; dementia w/ Parkinson Dz; Lewy-body dementia **Action:** ACH Inhib **Dose:** *Adults.* 5 mg qhs, ↑ to 10 mg PO qhs after 4–6 wk *Peds. ADHD:* 5 mg/d **Caution:** [C, ?] Risk for bradycardia w/ preexisting conduction abnormalities, may exaggerate succinylcholine-type muscle relaxation w/ anesthesia, ↑ gastric acid secretion **CI:** Hypersensitivity **Disp:** Tabs 5, 10, 23 mg; ODT 5, 10 mg **SE:** N/V/D, insomnia, Infxn, muscle cramp, fatigue, anorexia **Interactions:** Drugs that affect CYP2D6 & CYP3A4 may affect rate of elimination; ↑ effects *OF* succinylcholine-type muscle relaxants, other cholinesterase Inhibs, cholinergic agonists (eg, bethanechol); ↓ effects *OF* anticholinergic drugs; concomitant NSAIDs may ↑ risk of GI bleed **NIPE:** N/V/D dose-related & resolves in 1–3 wk

Dopamine (Intropin) [Vasopressor/Adrenergic] **WARNING:** Vesicant, give phentolamine w/ extrav **Uses:** *Short-term use in cardiac decompensation secondary to ↓ contractility; ↑ organ perfusion (at low dose)* **Action:** Positive inotropic agent w/ dose response: 1–10 mcg/kg/min β effects (↑ CO & renal perfusion); 10–20 mcg/kg/min β effects (peripheral vasoconstriction, pressor); > 20 mcg/kg/min peripheral & renal vasoconstriction **Dose:** *Adults.* 5 mcg/kg/min by cont Inf, ↑ by 5 mcg/kg/min to 50 mcg/kg/min max to effect *ECC 2010:* 2–20 mcg/kg/min **Peds.** *ECC 2010:* Shock w/ adequate intravascular vol & stable rhythm: 2–20 mcg/kg/min; titrate, if > 20 mcg/kg/min needed, consider alternative adrenergic **Caution:** [C, ?] ↓ Dose w/ MAOI **CI:** Pheo, VF, sulfite sensitivity **Disp:** Inj 40, 80, 160 mg/mL, premixed 0.8, 1.6, 3.2 mg/mL **SE:** Tachycardia, vasoconstriction, ↓ BP,

HA, N/V, dyspnea **Notes:** > 10 mcg/kg/min ↓ renal perfusion **Interactions:** ↑ Effects W/ α-blockers, diuretics, ergot alkaloids, MAOIs, BBs, anesthetics, phenytoin; ↓ effects W/ guanethidine **Labs:** ↑ Glucose, urea levels **NIPE:** Maint adequate hydration; monitor urinary output & ECG for ↑ HR, BP, ectopy; monitor PCWP & cardiac output if possible; phentolamine used for extrav 10–15 mL NS w/ 5–10 mg of phentolamine

Doripenem (Doribax) [Carbapenem] Uses: *Comp intra-Abd & UTI including pyelo* **Action:** Carbapenem, ↓ cell wall synth, a β-lactam *Spectrum:* Excellent gram(+) (except MRSA & *Enterococcus* sp), excellent gram(−) coverage including β-lactamase producers, good anaerobic **Dose:** 500 mg IV q8h, ↓ w/ renal impair **Caution:** [B, ?] **CI:** Carbapenems β-lactams hypersensitivity **Disp:** 500 mg single-use vial **SE:** HA, N/D, rash, phlebitis **Interactions:** ↑ Effects W/ probenecid; may ↓ valproic acid levels; overuse may ↑ bacterial resistance **NIPE:** Monitor for *C difficile*–associated D

Dornase Alfa (Pulmozyme, DNase) [Respiratory Inhalant/ Enzyme/Recombinant Human DNAse] Uses: *↓ Frequency of resp Infxns in CF* **Action:** Enzyme cleaves extracellular DNA, ↓ mucous viscosity **Dose: Adults.** Inh 2.5 mg/d dosing w/ FVC > 85% w/ OK nebulizer *Peds > 5 y.* Inh 2.5 mg/daily, bid if FVC > 85% **Caution:** [B, ?] **CI:** Chinese hamster product allergy **Disp:** Soln for Inh 1 mg/mL **SE:** Pharyngitis, voice alteration, CP, rash **NIPE:** Teach pt to use nebulizer; do not mix w/ other drugs in nebulizer

Dorzolamide (Trusopt) [Carbonic Anhydrase Inhibitor, Sulfon-amide/Glaucoma Agent] Uses: *Open-angle glaucoma, ocular HTN* **Action:** Carbonic anhydrase Inhib **Dose:** 1 gtt in eye(s) tid **Caution:** [C, ?] w/ NAG, CrCl < 30 mL/min **CI:** Component sensitivity **Disp:** 2% soln **SE:** Irritation, bitter taste, punctate keratitis, ocular allergic Rxn **Interactions:** ↑ Effects W/ oral carbonic anhydrase Inhibs, salicylates **NIPE:** ⊘ Wear soft contact lenses

Dorzolamide & Timolol (Cosopt) [Carbonic Anhydrase Inhibitor/ Beta-Adrenergic Blocker] Uses: *Open-angle glaucoma, ocular HTN* **Action:** Carbonic anhydrase Inhib w/ β-adrenergic blocker **Dose:** 1 gtt in eye(s) bid **Caution:** [C, ?] CrCl < 30mL/min **CI:** Component sensitivity, asthma, severe COPD, sinus bradycardia, AV block **Disp:** Soln dorzolamide 2% & timolol 0.5% **SE:** Irritation, bitter taste, superficial keratitis, ocular allergic Rxn **NIPE:** ⊘ Wear soft contact lenses

Doxazosin (Cardura, Cardura XL) [Antihypertensive/Alpha-Blocker] Uses: *HTN & symptomatic BPH* **Action:** α₁-Adrenergic blocker; relaxes bladder neck smooth muscle **Dose:** *HTN:* Initial 1 mg/d PO; may be ↑ to 16 mg/d PO *BPH:* Initial 1 mg PO, may ↑ to 8 mg/d; XL 2–8 mg qAM **Caution:** [B, ?] w/ Liver impair **CI:** Component sensitivity; use w/ PDE5 Inhib (eg, sildenafil), can ↓ BP **Disp:** Tabs 1, 2, 4, 8 mg; XL 4, 8 mg **SE:** Dizziness, HA, drowsiness, fatigue, malaise, sexual dysfunction, doses > 4 mg ↑ postural ↓ BP risk; IFIS **Interactions:** ↑ Effects W/ nitrates, antihypertensives, EtOH; ↓ effects W/ NSAIDs, butcher's broom; ↓ effects *OF* clonidine **NIPE:** May be taken w/ food; 1st dose hs; syncope may occur w/in 90 min of initial dose

Doxepin (Adapin) [Antidepressant/TCA] **WARNING:** Closely monitor for worsening depression or emergence of suicidality **Uses:** *Depression, anxiety, chronic pain* **Action:** TCA; ↑ synaptic CNS serotonin or norepinephrine **Dose:** 25–150 mg/d PO, usually hs but can ÷ doses; up to 300 mg/d for depression; ↓ in hepatic impair **Caution:** [C, ?/–] w/ EtOH abuse, elderly, w/ MAOI **CI:** NAG, urinary retention, MAOI use w/in 14 d, in recovery phase of MI **Disp:** Caps 10, 25, 50, 75, 100, 150 mg; PO conc 10 mg/mL **SE:** Anticholinergic SEs, ↓ BP, tachycardia, drowsiness, photosensitivity **Interactions:** ↑ Effects *W/* fluoxetine, MAOIs, albuterol, CNS depressants, anticholinergics, propoxyphene, quinidine, EtOH, grapefruit juice; ↑ effects *OF* carbamazepine, anticoagulants, amphetamines, thyroid drugs, sympathomimetics; effects *W/* ascorbic acid, cholestyramine, tobacco; ↓ effects *OF* bretylium, guanethidine, levodopa **Labs:** ↑ Serum bilirubin, alk phos, glucose **NIPE:** Risk of photosensitivity—use sunblock, urine may turn blue-green, may take 4–6 wk for full effect

Doxepin (Silenor) [H₁-Receptor Antagonist] **Uses:** *Insomnia* **Action:** TCA **Dose:** Take w/in 30 min hs 6 mg qd; 3 mg in elderly; 6 mg/d max; not w/in 3 h of a meal. **Caution:** [C, ?/–] w/ EtOH abuse/elderly/sleep apnea/CNS depressants; may cause abnormal thinking & hallucinations; may worsen depression **CI:** NAG, urinary retention, MAOI w/in 14 d **Disp:** Tabs 3, 6 mg **SE:** Somnolence/sedation, N, URI **Interactions:** ↑ Effects *W/* CNS depressants, antihistamines, cimetidine, EtOH; ↑ risk of hypoglycemia *W/* tolazamide **NIPE:** Monitor for new onset behavioral changes

Doxepin, Topical (Zonalon, Prudoxin) [Antipruritic] **Uses:** *Short-term Rx pruritus (atopic dermatitis or lichen simplex chronicus)* **Action:** Antipruritic; H₁- & H₂-receptor antagonism **Dose:** Apply thin coating qid, 8 d max **Caution:** [C, ?/–] **CI:** Component sensitivity **Disp:** 5% cream **SE:** ↓ BP, tachycardia, drowsiness **NIPE:** Limit application area to avoid systemic tox; photosensitivity—use sunblock

Doxorubicin (Adriamycin, Rubex) [Antineoplastic/Anthracycline Antibiotic] **Uses:** *Acute leukemias; Hodgkin Dz & NHLs; soft tissue, osteo- & Ewing sarcoma; Wilms tumor; neuroblastoma; bladder, breast, ovarian, gastric, thyroid, & lung CAs* **Action:** Intercalates DNA; ↓ DNA topoisomerases I & II **Dose:** 60–75 mg/m² q3wk; ↓ w/ hepatic impair; IV use only ↓ cardiotox w/ weekly (20 mg/m²/wk) or cont INF (60–90 mg/m² over 96 h); (per protocols) **Caution:** [D, ?] **CI:** Severe CHF, cardiomyopathy, preexisting ↓ BM, previous Rx w/ total cumulative doses of doxorubicin, idarubicin, daunorubicin **Disp:** Inj 10, 20, 50, 75, 150, 200 mg **SE:** ↓ BM, venous streaking & phlebitis, N/V/D, mucositis, radiation recall phenomenon, cardiomyopathy rare (dose-related) **Notes:** Limit of 550 mg/m² cumulative dose (400 mg/m² w/ prior mediastinal irradiation); dexrazoxane may limit cardiac tox **Interactions:** ↑ Effects *W/* streptozocin, verapamil, green tea;

↑ BM depression *W/* antineoplastic drugs & radiation; ↓ effects *W/* phenobarbital; ↓ effects *OF* digoxin, phenytoin, live virus vaccines **Labs:** ↑ Bilirubin, glucose, urine, & plasma uric acid levels; ↓ Ca, HMG, Hct, plts, WBCs **NIPE:** ⊘ PRG, use contraception at least 4 mo after drug Rx; red/orange urine; tissue damage w/ extrav; vesicant w/ extrav; Rx w/ dexrazoxane

Doxycycline (Adoxa, Periostat, Oracea, Vibramycin, Vibra-Tabs) [Antibiotic/Tetracycline] Uses: *Broad-spectrum antibiotic*acne vulgaris, uncomp GC, *Chlamydia,* PID, Lyme Dz, skin Infxns, anthrax, malaria prophylaxis **Action:** Tetracycline; bacteriostatic; ↓ protein synth *Spectrum:* Limited gram(+) & (−), *Rickettsia* sp, *Chlamydia, M pneumoniae, B anthracis* **Dose:** *Adults.* 100 mg PO q12h on 1st d, then 100 mg PO daily–bid or 100 mg IV q12h *Acne:* qd *Chlamydia:* × 7 d *Lyme:* × 21 d *PID:* × 14 d *Peds > 8 y.* 5 mg/kg/24 h PO, 200 mg/d max ÷ daily–bid **Caution:** [D, +] Hepatic impair **CI:** Children < 8 y, severe hepatic dysfunction **Disp:** Tabs 20, 50, 75, 100, 150 mg; caps 50, 100 mg; Oracea 40 mg caps (30 mg timed release, 10 mg DR); syrup 50 mg/5 mL; susp 25 mg/5 mL; Inj 100, 200 mg/vial **SE:** D, GI disturbance, photosensitivity **Interactions:** ↑ Effects *OF* digoxin, warfarin; ↓ effects *W/* antacids, Fe, barbiturates, carbamazepine, phenytoins, food; ↓ effects *OF* PCN **Labs:** ↑ LFTs, BUN, eosinophils; ↓ HMG, Hct, plts, neutrophils, WBC **NIPE:** ↑ Risk of super Infxn, ⊘ PRG, use barrier contraception; tetracycline of choice w/ renal impair; for inhalational anthrax use w/ 1–2 additional antibiotics, not for CNS anthrax

Dronabinol (Marinol) [C-II] [Antiemetic, Appetite Stimulant/Antivertigo] Uses: *N/V associated w/ CA chemotherapy; appetite stimulant* **Action:** Antiemetic; ↓ V center in the medulla **Dose:** *Adults & Peds. Antiemetic:* 5–15 mg/m²/dose q4–6h *PRN: Adults. Appetite stimulant:* 2.5 mg PO before lunch & dinner; max 20 mg/d **Caution:** [C, ?] elderly, h/o psychological disorder, Sz disorder, substance abuse **CI:** h/o schizophrenia, sesame oil hypersensitivity **Disp:** Caps 2.5, 5, 10 mg **SE:** Drowsiness, dizziness, anxiety, mood change, hallucinations, depersonalization, orthostatic ↓ BP, tachycardia **Interactions:** ↑ Effects *W/* anticholinergics, CNS depressants, EtOH; ↓ effects *OF* theophylline **NIPE:** Principal psychoactive substance present in marijuana

Dronedarone (Multaq) [Antiarrhythmic/Benzofurans] WARNING: CI w/ NYHA Class IV HF or NYHA Class II–III HF w/ decompensation **Uses:** *AF/A flutter* **Action:** Antiarrhythmic **Dose:** 400 mg PO bid w/ AM & PM meal **Caution:** [X, −] w/ Other drugs (see drug labeling) **CI:** See Warning 2nd-/3rd-degree AV block or SSS (unless w/ pacemaker), HR < 50 BPM, w/ strong CYP3A Inhib, w/ drugs/herbals that ↑ QT interval, QTc interval = 500 ms, severe hepatic impair, PRG **Disp:** Tabs 400 mg **SE:** N/V/D, Abd pain, asthenia, HF, ↑ QTc, bradycardia, rash **Interactions:** ↑ Risk of prolonged QT Interval *W/* antidepressants, antipsychotics, macrolides, phenothiazine, TCA; ↑ risk of CV Rxns *W/* amiodarone, BB, CCB, disopyramide, dofetilide, flecainide, propafenone, quinidine, sotalol, grapefruit juice; ↑ effects *OF* SSRIs, statins, TCA ↓ effects *W/* carbamazepine, phenobarbital, phenytoin, rifampin, St. John's wort **Labs:** ↑ serum crea; {doubleup} K+, ↑ Mg2+**NIPE:** Avoid grapefruit juice

Droperidol (Inapsine) [General Anesthetic/Butyrophenone]
WARNING: Cases of QT interval prolongation & torsades de pointes (some fatal) reported **Uses:** *N/V; anesthetic premedication* **Action:** Tranquilizer, sedation, antiemetic **Dose:** *Adults. N:* Initial max 2.5 mg IV/IM, may repeat 1.25 mg based on response *Premedicate:* 2.5–10 mg IV, 30–60 min pre-op *Peds. Premedicate:* 0.1–0.15 mg/kg/dose **Caution:** [C, ?] w/ hepatic/renal impair **CI:** Component sensitivity **Disp:** Inj 2.5 mg/mL **SE:** Drowsiness, ↓ BP, occasional tachycardia & extrapyramidal Rxns, ↑ QT interval, arrhythmias **Interactions:** ↑ Effects *W/* CNS depressants, fentanyl, EtOH; ↑ hypotension *W/* antihypertensives, nitrates **NIPE:** Give IV push slowly over 2–5 min

Drospirenone/Ethinyl Estradiol (YAZ) [Estrogen & Progestin Supls) WARNING: Cigarette smoking & use of estrogen-based OCPs have ↑ risk of serious CV SEs; risk ↑ w/ age (esp > 35 y) & smoking > 15 cigarette/d
Uses: OCPs; PMDD **Action:** Suppresses ovulation by imitating the feedback inhibition of endogenous estrogen & progesterone on the pituitary & hypothalamus **Dose:** 1 tab PO OD × 28 d, repeat **Caution:** [X, –], Has antimineralocorticoid activity w/ potential hyperkalemia in renal, adrenal, & hepatic Insuff **CI:** Pts w/ renal Insuff, hepatic impair, adrenal Insuff, DVT, PE, CVD, CAD, estrogen-dependent neoplasms, AUB, PRG, heavy smokers > 35 y **Disp:** Drospirenone (3 mg)/ethinyl estradiol (20 mcg), 28-d pack has 24 active tabs & 4 inert tabs **SE:** Hyperkalemia, HTN, N, V, HA, breakthrough bleeding, amenorrhea, mastodynia, ↑ risk of gallbladder Dz & thromboembolic disorders **Interactions:** ↑ Risk of hyperkalemia *W/* ACEIs, ARBs, aldosterone antagonists, heparin, NSAIDs, spirolactone, K+-sparing diuretics, K+ supls, ↑ effects *OF* cyclosporine, prednisolone, theophylline; ↓ effects *W/* barbiturates, carbamazepine, griseofulvin, modafinil, phenobarbital, phenylbutazone, phenytoin, pioglitazone, rifabutin, rifampin, ritonavir, topiramate, St. John's wort **Labs:** ↑ Uptake of T3, ↓ T4 sex hormone-binding globulin levels; triglycerides **NIPE:** Antimineralocorticoid activity comparable to spirolactone 25 mg; in pts taking meds that ↑ K+, monitor serum K+ during 1st Tx cycle; Sunday start regimen or postpartum use requires additional contraceptive methods during 1st cycle; use barrier contraception if taking anticonvulsants; may cause vision changes or ↓ contact lens tolerability; ∅ protection against HIV or STDs; ∅ smoke cigarettes

Drotrecogin Alfa (Xigris) [Antithrombotic/Activated Protein C (Recombinant)]
Uses: *↓ Mortality in adults w/ severe sepsis (w/ acute organ dysfunction) at high risk of death (eg, determined by APACHE II score [www.ncemi.org])* **Action:** Recombinant human-activated protein C; antithrombotic & anti-inflammatory, unclear mechanism **Dose:** 24 mcg/kg/h, total of 96 h **Caution:** [C, ?] w/ anticoagulation, INR > 3, plt < 30,000 cells/mm³, GI bleed w/in 6 wk **CI:**

Active bleeding, recent stroke/CNS surgery, head trauma/CNS lesion w/ herniation risk, trauma w/ ↑ bleeding risk, epidural catheter, mifepristone **Disp:** 5-, 20-mg vials **SE:** Bleeding **Notes:** Single-organ dysfunction & recent surgery may not be at high risk of death irrespective of APACHE II score & therefore not indicated *Percutaneous procedures:* D/C Inf 2 h before & resume 1 h after *Major surgery:* D/C Inf 2 h before & resume 12 h after in absence of bleeding **Interactions:** ↑ Risk of bleeding *W/* plt Inhibs, anticoagulants **Labs:** ↑ aPTT **NIPE:** D/C drug 2 h before invasive procedures

Duloxetine (Cymbalta) [Antidepressant/SSNRI] **WARNING:** Antidepressants may ↑ risk of suicidality; consider risks/benefits of use. Closely monitor for clinical worsening, suicidality, or behavior changes **Uses:** *Depression, DM peripheral neuropathic pain, GAD fibromyalgia, chronic OA, & back pain * **Action:** Selective serotonin & norepinephrine reuptake Inhib (SSNRI) **Dose:** *Depres*sion: 40–60 mg/d PO ÷ bid *DM neuropathy:* 60 mg/d PO *GAD:*60 mg/d, max 120 mg/d *Fibromyalgia, OA/back pain:* 30–60 mg/d, 60 mg/d max **Caution:** [C, ?/–] Use in 3rd tri; avoid if CrCl < 30 mL/min, NAG, w/ fluvoxamine, Inhibs of CYP2D6 (Table 10), TCAs, phenothiazines, Class Ic antiarrhythmics (Table 9) **CI:** MAOI use w/in 14 d, w/ thioridazine, NAG, hepatic Insuff **Disp:** Caps DR 20, 30, 60 mg **SE:** N, dry mouth, somnolence, fatigue, constipation, ↓ appetite, hyperhydrosis **Interactions:** ↑ Effects *OF* flecainide, propafenone, phenothiazines, TCAs; ↑ effects *W/* cimetidine, fluvoxamine, quinolones; ↑ risk *OF* hypertensive crisis *W/* MAOIs w/in 14 d of taking duloxetine **Labs:**? ↑ LFTs **NIPE:** ↑ Risk of liver damage *W/* EtOH use; N D/C drug abruptly; swallow whole; monitor BP

Dutasteride (Avodart) [Androgen Hormone Inhibitor/BPH Agent] **Uses:** *Symptomatic BPH to improve Sxs, ↓ risk of retention & BPH surgery alone or in combo w/ tamsulosin* **Action:** 5α-Reductase Inhib; ↓ intracellular dihydrotestosterone (DHT) **Dose:** *Monotherapy:* 0.5 mg PO/d *Combo:* 0.5 mg PO qd w/ tamsulosin 0.4 mg qd **Caution:** [X, –] Hepatic impair; pregnant women should not handle pills **CI:** Women, peds **Disp:** Caps 0.5 mg **SE:** ↑ testosterone, ↑ TSH, impotence, ↓ libido, gynecomastia, ejaculatory disturbance **Interactions:** ↑ Effects *W/* cimetidine, ciprofloxacin, diltiazem, ketoconazole, ritonavir, verapamil **Labs:** ↓ PSA levels; ✓ new baseline PSA at 6 mo (corrected PSA × 2); any PSA rise on dutasteride suspicious for CA **NIPE:** ⊘ Handling by PRG women; take w/o regard to food; no blood donation until 6 mo after D/C; under FDA review for PCa chemotherapy prevention; now available in fixed dose combo w/ tamsulosin (see *Jalyn)*

Dutasteride & Tamsulosin (Jalyn) [BPH Agent/Type I & II 5 Alpha-Reductase Inhibitor + Alpha-1A-Blocker] **Uses:** *Symptomatic BPH to improve Sxs * **Action:** 5α-Reductase Inhib (↓ intracellular DHT) w/ α-blocker **Dose:** 1 cap daily after same meal **Caution:** [X, –] IFIS (tamsulosin) discuss w/ ophthalmologist before cataract surgery; rare priapism; w/ warfarin **CI:** Women, peds, component sensitivity **Disp:** Caps 0.5 mg dutasteride w/ 0.4 mg tamsulosin **SE:** Impotence, ↓ libido, ejaculation disorders, & breast disorders **Interactions:** ↑ Effects *W/* cimetidine, diltiazem, erythromycin, terbinatine **Labs:** ↓ PSA, ✓ new baseline PSA at 6 mo **NIPE:** No blood donation until 6 mo after D/C therapy; any PSA rise on dutasteride suspiciousfor CA (see also Dutasteride & Tamsulosin); wait at least 6 mo after last dose to donate blood.

Ecallantide (Kalbitor) [Plasma Kallikrein Inhibitor] WARNING: Anaphylaxis reported, administer in a settingable to manage anaphylaxis & HAE, monitor closely **Uses:** *Acute attacks of hereditary angioedema (HAE)* **Action:** Plasma kallikrein Inhib **Dose: Adult & ≥ 16 y.** 30 mg SC in three 10 mg Injs; if attack persists may repeat 30 mg dose w/in 24 h **Caution:** [C, ?/–] Hypersensitivity Rxns **CI:** Hypersensitivity to ecallantide **Disp:** Inj10 mg/mL **SE:** HA, N/V/D, pyrexia, Inj site Rxn, nasopharyngitis, fatigue, Abd pain

Echothiophate Iodine (Phospholine Ophthalmic) [Cholinesterase Inhibitor/Glaucoma Agent] **Uses:** *Glaucoma* **Action:** Cholinesterase Inhib **Dose:** 1 gtt eye(s) bid w/ 1 dose hs **Caution:** [C, ?] **CI:** Active uveal inflammation, inflammatory Dz of iris/ciliary body, glaucoma iridocyclitis **Disp:** Powder, reconstitute 1.5 mg/0.03%; 3 mg/0.06%; 6.25 mg/0.125%; 12.5 mg/0.25% **SE:** Local irritation, myopia, blurred vision, ↓ BP, bradycardia **Interactions:** ↑ Effects *W/* cholinesterase Inhibs, pilocarpine, succinylcholine, carbamate, or organophosphate insecticides; ↑ effects *OF* cocaine; ↓ effects *W/* anticholinergics, atropine, cyclopentolate, ophthal adrenocorticoids **NIPE:** ⊘ Drug 2 wk before surgery if succinylcholine to be administered; keep drug refrigerated; monitor for lens opacities

Econazole (Spectazole) [Topical Antifungal] **Uses:** *Tinea, cutaneous Candida,* & tinea versicolor Infxns* **Action:** Topical antifungal **Dose:** Apply to areas bid (daily for tinea versicolor) for 2–4 wk **Caution:** [C, ?] **CI:** Component sensitivity **Disp:** Topical cream 1% **SE:** Local irritation, pruritus, erythema **Interactions:** ↓ Effects *W/* corticosteroids **NIPE:** Topical use only; ⊘ eye area; early Sx/clinical improvement; complete course to avoid recurrence

Eculizumab (Soliris) [Complement Inhibitor]   WARNING: ↑ Risk of meningococcal Infxns (give meningococcal vaccine 2 wk prior to 1st dose & revaccinate per guidelines) **Uses:** *Rx paroxysmal nocturnal hemoglobinuria* **Action:** Complement Inhib **Dose:** 600 mg IV q7d × 4 wk, then 900 mg IV 5th dose 7 d later, then 900 mg IV q14d **Caution:** [C, ?] **CI:** Active *N meningitidis* Infxn; if not vaccinated w/ meningococcal vaccine against *N meningitidis* **Disp:** 300 mg vial **SE:** Meningococcal Infxn, HA, nasopharyngitis, N, back pain, Infxns, fatigue, severe hemolysis on D/C **NIPE:** IV over 35 min (2-h max Inf time); monitor for 1 h for S/Sx of Inf Rxn

Edrophonium (Tensilon, Reversol) [Cholinergic Muscle Stimulant/Anticholinesterase] **Uses:** *Diagnosis of MyG; acute MyG crisis; curare antagonist, reverse of nondepolarizing neuromuscular blockers* **Action:** Anticholinesterase **Dose: Adults.** *Test for MyG:* 2 mg IV in 1 min; if tolerated, give 8 mg IV; (+) test is brief ↑ in strength **Peds.** *Test for MyG:* Total dose 0.2 mg/kg; 0.04 mg/kg test dose; if no Rxn, give remainder in 1-mg increments to 10 mg max;

↓ in renal impair **Caution:** [C, ?] **CI:** GI or GU obst; allergy to sulfite **Disp:** Inj 10 mg/mL **SE:** N/V/D, excessive salivation, stomach cramps, ↑ aminotransferases **Interactions:** ↑ Effects W/ tacrine; ↑ cardiac effects W/ digoxin; ↑ effects OF neo-stigmine, pyridostigmine, succinylcholine, jaborandi tree, pill-bearing spurge; ↓ effects W/ corticosteroids, procainamide, quinidine **Labs:** ↑ AST, ALT, serum amylase **NIPE:** ↑ Risk uterine irritability & premature labor in PRG pts near term; can cause severe cholinergic effects; keep atropine available

Efavirenz (Sustiva) [Antiretroviral/NNRTI] Uses: *HIV Infxns* **Action:** Antiretroviral; NNRTI **Dose:** *Adults.* 600 mg/d PO qhs *Peds = 3 y 10–< 15 kg.* 200 mg PO qd *15–< 20 kg.* 250 mg PO qd *20–< 25 kg.* 300 mg PO qd *25–< 32.5 kg.* 350 mg PO qd *32.5–< 40 kg.* 400 mg PO qd *= 40 kg.* 600 mg PO qd; on empty stomach **Caution:** [D, ?] CDC rec HIV-infected mothers not breast-feed **CI:** w/ Astemizole, bepridil, cisapride, midazolam, pimozide, triazolam, ergot derivatives, vori-conazole **Disp:** Caps 50, 100, 200; Tabs 600 mg **SE:** Somnolence, vivid dreams, depres-sion, CNS Sxs, dizziness, rash, N/V/D **Interactions:** ↑ Effects W/ ritonavir; ↓ effects OF CNS depressants, ergot derivatives, midazolam, ritonavir, simvastatin, triazolam, warfarin; ↓ effects W/ carbamazepine, phenobarbital, rifabutin, rifampin, saquinavir, St. John's wort; ↓ effects OF amprenavir, carbamazepine, clarithromy-cin, indinavir, phenobarbital, saquinavir, warfarin; may alter effectiveness of OCPs **Labs:** ↑ LFTs, cholesterol; monitor LFT, cholesterol; ✓ LFTs (esp w/ underlying liver Dz), cholesterol **NIPE:** ⊘ High-fat foods; take w/o regard to food; use barrier contraception; not for monotherapy

Efavirenz, Emtricitabine, Tenofovir (Atripla) [Combination Anti-Retroviral] **WARNING:** Lactic acidosis & severe hepatomegaly w/ steatosis, including fatal cases, reported w/ nucleoside analogues alone or combo w/ other antiretrovirals **Uses:** *HIV Infxns* **Action:** Triple fixed-dose combo NNRTI/ nucleoside analogue **Dose:** *Adults.* 1 tab PO on empty stomach; hs dose may ↓ CNS SE **Caution:** [D, ?] CDC rec HIV-infected mothers not breast-feed, w/ obe-sity **CI:** < 18 y, w/ astemizole, midazolam, triazolam, or ergot derivatives (CYP3A4 competition by efavirenz could cause serious/life-threatening SE) **Disp:** Tab efa-virenz 600 mg/emtricitabine 200 mg/tenofovir 300 mg **SE:** Somnolence, vivid dreams, HA, dizziness, rash, N/V/D, ↓ BMD **Interactions:** ↑ Effects OF ritonavir, tenofovir, ethinyl estradiol levels ↓ effects W/ phenobarbital, rifampin, rifabutin, saquinavir; ↓ effects OF indinavir, amprenavir, clarithromycin, methadone, rifabu-tin, sertraline, statins, saquinavir; monitor warfarin levels **Labs:** Monitor LFT, cho-lesterol **NIPE:** ⊘ EtOH; ⊘ PRG & breast-feeding; do not use in HIV & hep B coinfection; see individual agents for additional info

Eletriptan (Relpax) [Analgesic/Antimigraine Agent] Uses: *Acute Rx of migraine* **Action:** Selective serotonin receptor (5-HT$_{1B/1D}$) agonist **Dose:** 20–40 mg PO, may repeat in 2 h; 80 mg/24 h max **Caution:** [C, +] **CI:** h/o isch-emic heart Dz, coronary artery spasm, stroke or TIA, peripheral vascular Dz, IBD, uncontrolled HTN, hemiplegic or basilar migraine, severe hepatic impair, w/in 24 h of another 5-HT$_1$ agonist or ergot, w/in 72 h of CYP3A4 Inhibs **Disp:** Tabs 20, 40 mg **SE:** Dizziness, somnolence, N, asthenia, xerostomia, paresthesias; pain, pressure, or tightness in chest, jaw, or neck; serious cardiac events **Interactions:** ↑ Risk of serotonin synd *W/* SSRIs; ↑ risks of prolonged vasospasms *W/* ergot-containing medications **Labs:** None known **NIPE:** Not for migraine prevention; ⊘ EtOH; ⊘ use for more than 3 migraine attacks/mo

Eltrombopag (Promacta) [Thrombopoietin Receptor Agonist]
WARNING: May cause hepatotox ✓ baseline ALT/AST/bilirubin, q2wk w/ dosage adjustment, then monthly. D/C if ALT is > 3× ULN w/ ↑ bilirubin, or Sx of liver injury **Uses:** *Tx plt in idiopathic ↓ plt refractory to steroids, immune globulins, splenectomy* **Action:** Thrombopoietin receptor agonist **Dose:** 50 mg PO daily, adjust to keep plt = 50,000 cells/mm^3; 75 mg/d max; start 25 mg/d if East-Asian or w/ hepatic impair; on an empty stomach; not w/in 4 h of product w/ polyvalent cations **Caution:** [C, ?/–] Risk for BM reticulin fiber deposition, heme malignancies, rebound ↓ plt on D/C, thromboembolism **CI:** None **Disp:** Tabs 25, 50 mg **SE:** Rash, bruising, menorrhagia, N/V, dyspepsia, limb pain, myalgia, paresthesia, cataract, conjunctival hemorrhage **Interactions:** ↑ Effects *W/* ciprofloxacin, fluvoxamine, gemfibrozil, TMP; ↑ effects *OF* benzylpenicillin, most statins, methotrexate, nateglinide, repaglinide, rifampine **Labs:** ↓ plt, ↑ ALT/AST **NIPE:** D/C If no ↑ plt count after 4 wk; restricted distribution PROMACTA® Cares (1-877-9-PROMACTA)

Emedastine (Emadine) [Antihistamine] **Uses:** *Allergic conjunctivitis* **Action:** Antihistamine; selective H$_1$-antagonist **Dose:** 1 gtt in eye(s) up to qid **Caution:** [B, ?] **CI:** Allergy to ingredients (preservatives benzalkonium, tromethamine) **Disp:** 0.05% soln **SE:** HA, blurred vision, burning/stinging, corneal infiltrates/staining, dry eyes, foreign body sensation, hyperemia, keratitis, tearing, pruritus, rhinitis, sinusitis, asthenia, bad taste, dermatitis, discomfort **NIPE:** Do not use contact lenses if eyes are red; may reinsert contact lenses 10 min after administration if eyes not red

Emtricitabine (Emtriva) [Antiretroviral/NRTI] **WARNING:** Lactic acidosis, & severe hepatomegaly w/ steatosis reported; not for HBV Infxn **Uses:** HIV-1 Infxn **Action:** NRTI **Dose:** 200 mg caps or 240 mg soln PO daily; ↓ w/ renal impair **Caution:** [B, –] risk of liver Dz **CI:** Component sensitivity **Disp:** Soln 10 mg/mL, caps 200 mg **SE:** HA, N/D, rash, rare hyperpigmentation of feet & hands, post-Tx exacerbation of hep **Interactions:** None noted *W/* additional NRTIs **Labs:** ↑ LFTs, bilirubin, triglycerides, glucose **NIPE:** Take w/o regard to food; causes redistribution & accumulation of body fat; take w/ other antiretrovirals; not a cure for HIV or prevention of opportunistic Infxns; 1st one-daily NRTI; caps/soln not equivalent; not recommended as monotherapy; screen for hep B, do not use w/ HIV & HBV coinfection

Enalapril (Vasotec) [Antihypertensive/ACEI] **WARNING:** ACE Inhibits used during PRG can cause fetal injury & death **Uses:** *HTN, CHF, LVD* **DN Action:** ACE Inhib **Dose:** *Adults.* 2.5–40 mg/d PO; 1.25 mg IV q6h *Peds.* 0.05–0.08 mg/kg/d PO q12–24h; ↓ w/ renal impair **Caution:** [C (1st tri), D (2nd & 3rd tri), +] D/C stat w/ PRG, w/ NSAIDs, K$^+$ supls **CI:** Bilateral RAS, angioedema

Disp: Tabs 2.5, 5, 10, 20 mg; IV 1.25 mg/mL (1, 2 mL) **SE:** ↓ BP w/ initial dose (esp w/ diuretics), nonproductive cough, angioedema **Interactions:** ↑ Effects W/ loop diuretics; ↑ risk of cough W/ capsaicin; ↑ effects OF α-blockers, insulin, Li; ↑ risk of hyperkalemia W/ K⁺ supls, K⁺-sparing diuretics, salt substitutes, TMP; ↓ effects W/ ASA, NSAIDs, rifampin **Labs:** May cause ↑ K⁺, ↑ Cr—monitor levels **NIPE:** Several wk needed for full hypotensive effect; D/C diuretic for 2–3 d prior to start

Enfuvirtide (Fuzeon) [Antiretroviral/Fusion Inhibitor] WARNING: Rarely causes allergy; never rechallenge **Uses:** *w/ Antiretroviral agents for HIV-1 in Tx-experienced pts w/ viral replication despite ongoing therapy* **Action:** Viral fusion Inhib **Dose: Adults.** 90 mg (1 mL) SQ bid in upper arm, anterior thigh, or abdomen; rotate site **Peds.** See package insert **Caution:** [B, –] **CI:** Previous allergy to drug **Disp:** 90 mg/mL recons; pt kit w/ supplies × 1 mo **SE:** Inj site Rxns; pneumonia, D, N, fatigue, insomnia, peripheral neuropathy **Interactions:** None noted W/ other antiretrovirals **Labs:** ↑ LFTs, triglycerides; ↓ HMG, Hct, eosinophils **NIPE:** Does not cure HIV; does not ↓ risk of transmission or prevent opportunistic Infxns; take w/o regard to food; available via restricted distribution system; use stat on recons or refrigerate (24 h max)

Enoxaparin (Lovenox) [Anticoagulant/Low-Molecular-Weight Heparin Derivative] WARNING: Recent or anticipated epidural/spinal anesthesia ↑ risk of spinal/epidural hematoma w/ subsequent paralysis **Uses:** *Prevention & Rx of DVT; Rx PE; unstable angina & non-Q-wave MI* **Action:** LMW heparin; inhibit thrombin by complexing w/ antithrombin III **Dose: Adults.** *Prevention:* 30 mg SQ bid or 40 mg SQ q24h *DVT/PE Rx:* 1 mg/kg SQ q12h or 1.5 mg/kg SQ q24h *Angina:* 1 mg/kg SQ q12h *Ancillary to AMI fibrinolysis:* 30 mg IV bolus, then 1 mg/kg SQ bid *(ECC 2005)* CrCl < 30 mL/min ↓ to 1 mg/kg SQ qd **Peds.** *Prevention:* 0.5 mg/kg SQ q12h *DVT/PE Rx:* 1 mg/kg SQ q12h; ↓ dose w/ CrCl < 30 mL/min **Caution:** [B, ?] Not for prophylaxis in prosthetic heart valves **CI:** Active bleeding, HIT Ab **Disp:** Inj 10 mg/0.1 mL (30-, 40-, 60-, 80-, 100-, 120-, 150-mg syringes); 300-mg/mL multidose vial **SE:** Bleeding, hemorrhage, bruising, ↓ plt, fever, pain/hematoma at site **Interactions:** ↑ Bleeding effects W/ ASA, anticoagulants, cephalosporins, NSAIDs, PCN, chamomile, garlic, ginger, ginkgo, feverfew, horse chestnut **Labs:** ↑ AST, ALT; no effect on bleeding time, plt Fxn, PT, or aPTT; monitor plt for HIT, clinical bleeding; may monitor antifactor Xa **NIPE:** Administer deep SQ; ⊘ IM

Entacapone (Comtan) [Antiparkinsonian Agent/COMT Inhibitor] **Uses:** *Parkinson Dz* **Action:** Selective & reversible carboxymethyl transferase Inhib **Dose:** 200 mg w/ each levodopa/carbidopa dose; max 1600 mg/d; ↓ levodopa/carbidopa dose 25%/w/ levodopa dose > 800 mg **Caution:** [C, ?] Hepatic impair **CI:** Use w/ MAOI **Disp:** Tabs 200 mg **SE:** Dyskinesia, hyperkinesia, N, D, dizziness, hallucinations, orthostatic ↓ BP **Interactions:** ↑ Effects W/ ampicillin, chloramphenicol cholestyramine, erythromycin, MAOIs, probenecid, rifampin

↑ risk of arrhythmias & HTN *W/* bitolterol, DA, dobutamine, epinephrine, isoetharine, methyldopa, norepinephrine **Labs:** Monitor LFTs **NIPE:** ⊘ D/C abruptly, breast-feed; brownish-orange urine

Ephedrine [Vasopressor/Decongestant/Bronchodilator] Uses: *Acute bronchospasm, bronchial asthma, nasal congestion*, ↓ BP, narcolepsy, enuresis, & MyG **Action:** Sympathomimetic; stimulates α & β receptors; bronchodilator **Dose:** *Adults.* *Congestion:* 25–50 mg PO q6h PRN; ↓ *BP:* 25–50 mg IV q5–10min, 150 mg/d max *Peds.* 0.2–0.3 mg/kg/dose IV q4–6h PRN **Caution:** [C, ?/–] **CI:** Arrhythmias; NAG **Disp:** Nasal soln 0.48%, 0.5%; caps 25 mg; Inj 50 mg/mL; nasal spray 0.25% **SE:** CNS stimulation (nervousness, anxiety, trembling), tachycardia, arrhythmia, HTN, xerostomia, dysuria **Interactions:** ↑ Effects *W/* acetazolamide, antacids, MAOIs, TCAs, urinary alkalinizers; ↑ effects *OF* sympathomimetics; ↓ response *W/* diuretics, methyldopa, reserpine, urinary acidifiers; ↓ effects *OF* antihypertensives, BBs, dexamethasone, guanethidine **Labs:** False ↑ urine amino acids; can cause false(+) amphetamine EMIT **NIPE:** ⊘ EtOH; store away from light/heat; protect from light; monitor BP, HR, urinary output; take last dose 4–6 h before hs; abuse potential, OTC sales mostly banned/restricted

Epinephrine (Adrenalin, Sus-Phrine, EpiPen, EpiPen Jr, Others) [Vasopressor/Bronchodilator/Cardiac Stimulant, Local Anesthetic] Uses: *Cardiac arrest, anaphylactic Rxn, bronchospasm, open-angle glaucoma* **Action:** β-Adrenergic agonist, some α effects **Dose:** *Adults.* *ECC 2010:* 1-mg (10 mL of 1:10,000 soln) IV/IO push, repeat q3–5min (0.2 mg/kg max) if 1 mg dose fails *Inf:* 0.1–0.5 mcg/kg/min, titrate. ET 2–2.5 mg in 20 mL NS **Profound bradycardia/hypotension:** 2–10 mcg/min (1 mg in 250 mL D₅W) **Allergic Rxn:** 0.3–0.5 mg (0.3–0.5 mL of 1:1000 soln) SQ **Anaphylaxis:** 0.3–0.5 (3–5 mL of 1:10,000 soln) IV *Asthma:* 0.1–0.5 mL SQ of 1:1000 dilution, repeat q20min–4h, or 1 Inh (metered-dose) repeat in 1–2 min, or susp 0.1–0.3 mL SQ for extended effect *Peds.* *ECC 2010:* **Pulseless arrest:** 0.01 mg/kg (0.1 mL/kg 1:10,000) IV/IO q3–5 min; max dose 1 mg; OK via ET tube 0.1 mg/kg (0.1 mL/kg 1:1000) until IV/IO access **Symptomatic Bradycardia:** 0.01 mg/kg (0.1 mL/kg 1:10,000) cont Inf: Typical 0.1–1 mcg/kg/min, titrate **Anaphylaxis/Status Asthmaticus:** 0.01 mg/kg (0.01 mL/kg 1:1000) IM, repeat PRN; max single dose 0.3 mg **Caution:** [C, ?] ↓ Bronchodilation w/ BBs **CI:** Cardiac arrhythmias, NAG **Disp:** Inj 1:1000; 1:2000; 1:10,000; 1:100,000; susp for Inj 1:200; aerosol 220 mcg/spray; 1% Inh soln; EpiPen Autoinjector 1 dose = 0.30 mg; EpiPen Jr 1 dose = 0.15 mg **SE:** CV (tachycardia, HTN, vasoconstriction), CNS stimulation (nervousness, anxiety, trembling), ↓ renal blood flow **Interactions:** ↑ HTN effects *W/* α-blockers, BBs, ergot alkaloids, furazolidone, MAOIs; ↑ cardiac effects *W/* antihistamines, cardiac glycosides, levodopa, thyroid hormones, TCAs; ↑ effects *OF* sympathomimetics; ↓ effects *OF* diuretics, guanethidine, hypoglycemics, methyldopa **Labs:** ↑ BUN, glucose, & lactic acid w/ prolonged use **NIPE:** ⊘ OTC Inh drugs; can give via ET tube if no central line (use 2–2.5 × IV dose); EpiPen for pt self-use (www.EpiPen.com)

Epinastine (Elestat) [Antihistamine/Mast Cell Stabilizer] Uses: Itching w/ allergic conjunctivitis **Action:** Antihistamine **Dose:** 1 gtt bid **Caution:** [C, ?/–] **Disp:** Soln 0.05% **SE:** Burning, folliculosis, hyperemia, pruritus, URI, HA, rhinitis, sinusitis, cough, pharyngitis **NIPE:** Remove contacts before, reinsert in 10 min

Epirubicin (Ellence) [Antineoplastic/Anthracycline] **WARNING:** Do not give IM or SQ. Extrav causes tissue necrosis; potential cardiotox; severe myelosuppression; ↓ dose w/ hepatic impair **Uses:** *Adjuvant therapy for + axillary nodes after resection of primary breast CA* **Actions:** Anthracycline cytotoxic agent **Dose:** Per protocols; ↓ dose w/ hepatic impair **Caution:** [D, –] **CI:** Baseline neutrophil count < 1500 cells/mm³, severe cardiac Insuff, recent MI, severe arrhythmias, severe hepatic dysfunction, previous anthracyclines @ max cumulative dose **Disp:** Inj 50 mg/25 mL, 200 mg/100 mL **SE:** Mucositis, N/V/D, alopecia, ↓ BM, cardiotox, secondary AML, tissue necrosis w/ extrav (see Adriamycin for Rx), lethargy **Interactions:** ↑ Effects OF cimetidine; ↑ effects OF cytotoxic drugs, radiation therapy; ↑ risk of HF W/ CCBs, trastuzumab; incompatible chemically W/ 5-FU, heparin **Labs:** ✓ CBC, bilirubin, AST, Cr, cardiac Fxn before/during each cycle; ✓ HMG, Hct, neutrophils, plts, WBC **NIPE:** ⊘ Handle if PRG breast-feeding; urine reddish up to 2 d after Tx, use contraception during Tx, burning at Inj site indicates infiltration; menstruation may cease permanently

Eplerenone (Inspra) [Antihypertensive/Selective Aldosterone Receptor Antagonist] **Uses:** *HTN* **Action:** Selective aldosterone antagonist **Dose:** *Adults.* 50 mg PO daily–bid, doses > 100 mg/d no benefit w/ ↑ K⁺; ↓ to 25 mg PO daily if giving w/ CYP3A4 Inhibs **Caution:** [B, +/–] w/ CYP3A4 Inhibs (Table 10); monitor K⁺ w/ ACE Inhib, ARBs, NSAIDs, K⁺-sparing diuretics, grapefruit juice, St. John's wort **CI:** K⁺ > 5.5 mEq/L; NIDDM w/ microalbuminuria; SCr > 2 mg/dL (males), > 1.8 mg/dL (females); CrCl < 30 mL/min; w/ K⁺ supls/K⁺-sparing diuretics, ketoconazole **Disp:** Tabs 25, 50 mg **SE:** HA, dizziness, gynecomastia, D, orthostatic ↓ BP **Interactions:** ↑ Risk hyperkalemia W/ ACEIs; ↑ risk of toxic effects W/ azole antifungals, erythromycin, saquinavir, verapamil, ↑ effects OF Li; ↓ effects W/ NSAIDs **Labs:** ↑ K⁺, cholesterol, triglycerides **NIPE:** ⊘ High-K⁺ foods; may cause reversible breast pain or enlargement w/ use; may take 4 wk for full effect

Epoetin Alfa [Erythropoietin, EPO] (Epogen, Procrit) [Recombinant Human Erythropoietin] **WARNING:** ↑ Mortality, serious CV/thromboembolic events, & tumor progression. Renal failure pts experienced ↑ greater risks (death/CV events) on ESAs to target higher Hgb levels. Maint Hgb 10–12 g/dL. In CA pt, ESAs ↓ survival/time to progression in some CAs when dosed Hgb > 12 g/dL. Use lowest dose needed. Use only for myelosuppressive chemotherapy. D/C following chemotherapy. Pre-op ESA ↑ DVT. Consider DVT prophylaxis **Uses:** *CRF-associated anemia, zidovudine Rx in HIV-infected pts, CA chemotherapy; ↓ transfusions associated w/ surgery* **Action:** Induces erythropoiesis **Dose:** *Adults & Peds.* 50–150 units/kg IV/SQ 3 × /wk; adjust dose q4–6wk

PRN *Surgery:* 300 units/kg/d × 10 d before to 4 d after; ↓ dose if Hct ~ 36% or Hgb, ↑ > (12 g/dL or Hgb ↑ > 1 g/dL in 2-wk period; hold dose if Hgb > 12 g/dL **Caution:** [C, +] **CI:** Uncontrolled HTN **Disp:** Inj 2000, 3000, 4000, 10,000, 20,000, 40,000 units/mL **SE:** HTN, HA, fatigue, fever, tachycardia, N/V **Interactions:** None noted **Labs:** ↑ WBCs, plts; monitor baseline & posttreatment Hct/Hgb, ferritin **NIPE:** Monitor for access line clotting; ⊘ shake vial; refrigerate; monitor posttreatment BP

Epoprostenol (Flolan) [Antihypertensive] **Uses:** *Pulm HTN* **Action:** Dilates pulm/systemic arterial vascular beds; ↓ plt aggregation **Dose:** Initial 2 ng/kg/min; ↑ by 2 ng/kg/min q15min until dose-limiting SE (CP, dizziness, N/V, HA, ↓ BP, flushing); IV cont Inf 4 ng/kg/min < max tolerated rate; adjust based on response; see package insert **Caution:** [B, ?] ↑ Tox w/ diuretics, vasodilators, acetate in dialysis fluids, anticoagulants **CI:** Chronic use in CHF 2nd degree, if pt develops pulm edema w/ dose initiation, severe LVSD **Disp:** Inj 0.5, 1.5 mg **SE:** Flushing, tachycardia, CHF, fever, chills, nervousness, HA, N/V/D, jaw pain, flu-like Sxs **Interactions:** ↑ Risk of bleeding W/ anticoagulants, antiplts; ↑ effects OF digoxin; ↓ BP W/ antihypertensives, diuretics, vasodilators **NIPE:** ⊘ Mix or administre w/ other drugs; abrupt D/C can cause rebound pulm HTN; monitor bleeding w/ other antiplt/anticoagulants; watch ↓ BP W/ other vasodilators/diuretics

Eprosartan (Teveten) [Antihypertensive/ARB] **Uses:** *HTN*, DN, CHF **Action:** ARB **Dose:** 400–800 mg/d single dose or bid **Caution:** [C (1st tri), D (2nd & 3rd tri), D/C stat when PRG detected) w/ Li, ↑ K+ w/ K+-sparing diuretics/supls/high-dose TMP **CI:** Bilateral RAS, 1st-degree aldosteronism **Disp:** Tabs 400, 600 mg **SE:** Fatigue, depression, URI, UTI, Abd pain, rhinitis/pharyngitis/cough, hypertriglyceridemia **Interactions:** ↑ Risk of hyperkalemia W/ K+-sparing diuretics, K+ supls, TMP; ↑ effects OF Li **Labs:** ↑ BUN, triglycerides; ↓ HMG, Hct, neutrophils **NIPE:** Monitor CBC & differential, renal Fxn; ⊘ PRG, breast-feeding

Eptifibatide (Integrilin) [Antiplatelet Agent] **Uses:** *ACS, PCI* **Action:** Glycoprotein IIb/IIIa Inhib **Dose:** 180 mcg/kg IV bolus, then 2 mcg/kg/min cont Inf; ↓ in renal impair (SCr > 2 mg/dL, < 4 mg/dL: 135 mcg/kg bolus & 0.5 mcg/kg/min Inf) *PCI:* 135 mcg/kg IV bolus, then 0.5 mcg/kg/min; bolus again in 10 min *ECC 2010:* ACS: 180 mcg/kg/min IV bolus over 1–2 min, then 2 mcg/kg/min, then repeat bolus in 10 min; continue Inf 18–24 h post PCI **Caution:** [B, ?] Monitor bleeding w/ other anticoagulants **CI:** Other glycoprotein IIb/IIIa Inhibs, h/o abnormal bleeding, hemorrhagic stroke (w/in 30 d), severe HTN, major surgery (w/in 6 wk), plt count < 100,000 cells/mm³, renal dialysis **Disp:** Inj 0.75, 2 mg/mL **SE:** Bleeding, ↓ BP, Inj site Rxn, ↓ plt **Interactions:** ↑ Bleeding W/ ASA, cephalosporins, clopidogrel, heparin, NSAIDs, thrombolytics, ticlopidine, warfarin, evening primrose oil, feverfew, garlic, ginger, ginkgo, ginseng **Labs:** ↓ Plts; monitor bleeding, coagulants, plts, SCr, ACT w/ prothrombin consumption index (keep ACT 200–300 s)

Eribulin (Halaven) [Non-Taxane Microtubule Dynamics Inhibitor] Uses: *Met breast CA after 2 chemotherapy regimens (including anthracycline & taxane)* Action: Microtubule Inhib Dose: *Adults.* 1.4 mg/m² IV (over 2–5 min) days 1 & 8 of 21-d cycle; ↓ dose w/ hepatic & mod renal impair; delay/↓ for tox (see label) Caution : [D, –] Disp: Inj SE: fatigue/asthenia, neuropathy, N/V/D, constipation, pyrexia, alopecia, ↑ QT, arthralgia/myalgia, back pain, cough, dyspnea, UTI Labs: ↓ WBC/Hct/plt; ✓ CBC & monitor NIPE: Monitor for neuropathy prior to dosing

Erlotinib (Tarceva) [Antineoplastic] Uses: *NSCLC after failing 1 chemotherapy; CA pancreas* Action: HER2/EGFR TKI Dose: *CA Pancreas:* 100 mg *Others:* 150 mg/d PO 1 h ac or 2 h pc; ↓ (in 50-mg decrements) w/ severe Rxn or w/ CYP3A4 Inhibs (Table 10); per protocols Caution: [D, ?/–]; w/ CYP3A4 (Table 10) Inhibs Disp: Tabs 25, 100, 150 mg SE: Rash, N/V/D, anorexia, Abd pain, fatigue, cough, dyspnea, edema, stomatitis, conjunctivitis, pruritus, skin/nail changes, Infxn, interstitial lung Dz Interactions: ↑ Drug plasma levels W/ CYP3A4 Inhibs (clarithromycin, ritonavir, ketoconazole); ↓ drug plasma levels W/ CYP3A4 inducers (carbamazepine, phenytoin, phenobarbital, St. John's wort); ↑ risk of bleeding W/ anticoagulants, NSAIDs (Table 10) Labs: ↑ LFTs; monitor LFTs, PT, INR; may ↑ INR w/ warfarin NIPE: ⊘ PRG or lactation; use adequate contraception; ↑ drug metabolism in smokers

Ertapenem (Invanz) [Anti-Infective/Carbapenem] Uses: *Comp intra-Abd, acute pelvic, & skin Infxns, pyelo, CAP* Action: A carbapenem; β-lactam antibiotic, ↓ cell wall synth Spectrum: Good gram(+/–) & anaerobic coverage, not *Pseudomonas,* PCN-resistant pneumococci, MRSA, *Enterococcus,* β-lactamase (+) *H influenzae, Mycoplasma, Chlamydia* Dose: *Adults.* 1 g IM/IV daily; 500 mg/d in CrCl < 30 mL/min *Peds 3 mo–12 y.* 15 mg/kg bid IM/IV, max 1 g/d Caution: [B, ?/–] Sz h/o, CNS disorders, β-lactam & multiple allergies, probenecid ↓ renal clearance CI: Component hypersensitivity or amide anesthetics Disp: Inj 1 g/vial SE: HA, N/V/D, Inj site Rxns, thrombocytosis Notes: Can give IM × 7 d, IV × 14 d; 137 mg Na⁺ (6 mEq)/g ertapenem Interactions: ↑ Effects W/ probenecid Labs: ↑ LFTs, glucose, K⁺, Cr, PT, PTT, RBCs, urine WBCs NIPE: Monitor for super Infxn

Erythromycin (E-Mycin, E.E.S., Ery-Tab, EryPed, Ilotycin) [Antibiotic/Macrolide] Uses: *Bacterial Infxns; bowel prep*; ↑ GI motility (*prokinetic*); *acne vulgaris* Action: Bacteriostatic; interferes w/ protein synth Spectrum: Group A streptococci (*S pyogenes*), *S pneumoniae, N meningitidis, N gonorrhoeae* (if PCN-allergic), *Legionella, M pneumoniae* Dose: *Adults.* Base 250–500 mg PO q6–12h or ethylsuccinate 400–800 mg q6–12h; 500 mg–1 g IV q6h *Prokinetic:* 250 mg PO tid 30 min ac *Peds.* 30–50 mg/kg/d PO ÷ q6–8h or 20–40 mg/kg/d IV ÷ q6h, max 2 g/d Caution: [B, +] ↑ Tox for carbamazepine, cyclosporine, digoxin, methylprednisolone, theophylline, felodipine, warfarin, simvastatin/lovastatin; ↓ sildenafil dose w/ use CI: Hepatic impair, preexisting liver

Dz (estolate), use w/ pimozide **Disp:** *Lactobionate (Ilotycin):* Powder for Inj 500 mg, 1 g *Base:* Tabs 250, 333, 500 mg; caps 250 mg *Estolate (Ilosone):* Susp 125, 250 mg/5 mL *Stearate (Erythrocin):* Tabs 250, 500 mg *Ethylsuccinate (EES, EryPed):* Tabs 250 mg; tabs 400 mg; susp 200, 400 mg/5 mL **SE:** HA, Abd pain, N/V/D; [QT prolongation, torsades de pointes, ventricular arrhythmias/VT (rarely)]; cholestatic jaundice (estolate) **Notes:** 400 mg ethylsuccinate = 250 mg base/estolate **Interactions:** ↑ Effects W/ amprenavir, indinavir, ritonavir, saquinavir, grapefruit juice; ↑ effects *OF* alprazolam, benzodiazepines, buspirone, carbamazepine, clozapine, colchicines, cyclosporine, digoxin, felodipine, lovastatin, midazolam, quinidine, sildenafil, simvastatin, tacrolimus, theophylline, triazolam, valproic acid; ↑ QT W/ astemizole, cisapride; ↓ effects *OF* PCN, zafirlukast **Labs:** ↑ LFTs, eosinophils, neutrophils, plts; ↓ bicarbonate levels **NIPE:** Take w/ food to minimize GI upset, monitor for super Infxn & ototox; lactobionate contains benzyl alcohol (caution in neonates)

Erythromycin & Benzoyl Peroxide (Benzamycin) [Anti-Infective, Macrolide/Keratolytic]
Uses: *Topical for acne vulgaris* **Action:** Macrolide antibiotic w/ keratolytic **Dose:** Apply bid (AM & PM) **Caution:** [C, ?] **CI:** Component sensitivity **Disp:** Gel erythromycin 30 mg/benzoyl peroxide 50 mg/g **SE:** Local irritation, dryness **Interactions:** ↑ irritation W/ other topical agents; ↑ transient skin discoloration W/ PABA sunscreen **NIPE:** May cause super Infxn; D/C if irritation or dryness occurs; may bleach hair or fabrics

Erythromycin & Sulfisoxazole (Eryzole, Pediazole) [Anti-Infective, Macrolide/Sulfonamide]
Uses: *Upper & lower resp tract; bacterial Infxns; H influenzae otitis media in children*; Infxns in PCN-allergic pts **Action:** Macrolide antibiotic w/ sulfonamide **Dose:** *Adults.* Based on erythromycin content; 400 mg erythromycin/1200 mg sulfisoxazole PO q6h *Peds > 2 mo.* 40–50 mg/kg/d erythromycin & 150 mg/kg/d sulfisoxazole PO ÷ q6h; max 2 g/d erythromycin or 6 g/d sulfisoxazole × 10 d; ↓ in renal impair **Caution:** [C (D if near term), +] w/ PO anticoagulants, hypoglycemics, phenytoin, cyclosporine **CI:** Infants < 2 mo **Disp:** Susp erythromycin ethylsuccinate 200 mg/sulfisoxazole 600 mg/5 mL (100, 150, 200 mL) **SE:** GI upset **Interactions:** ↑ Effects of sulfonamides W/ ASA, diuretics, NSAIDs, probenecid **Labs:** False(+) urine protein **NIPE:** ↑ Risk of photosensitivity—use sunblock, ↑ fluid intake

Erythromycin, Ophthalmic (Ilotycin Ophthalmic) [Anti-Infective, Macrolide, Opthalmic Agent]
Uses: *Conjunctival/corneal Infxns* **Action:** Macrolide antibiotic **Dose:** 1/2 in 2–6 × /d Caution: [B, +] **CI:** Erythromycin hypersensitivity **Disp:** 0.5% oint **SE:** Local irritation **NIPE:** May cause burning, stinging, blurred vision

Erythromycin, Topical (A/T/S, Eryderm, Erycette, T-Stat) [Topical Anti-Infective, Macrolide]
Uses: *Acne vulgaris* **Action:** Macrolide antibiotic **Dose:** Wash & dry area, apply 2% product over area bid **Caution:** [B, +] **CI:** Component sensitivity **Disp:** Soln 1.5%, 2%; gel 2%; pads & swabs 2% **SE:** Local irritation

Escitalopram (Lexapro) [Antidepressant/SSRI] WARNING: Closely monitor for worsening depression or emergence of suicidality, particularly in ped pts **Uses:** Depression, anxiety **Action:** SSRI **Dose:** *Adults.* 10–20 mg PO daily; 10 mg/d in elderly & hepatic impair **Caution:** [C, +/–] Serotonin synd (Table 11); use w/ escitalopram, NSAID, ASA, or other drugs affecting coagulation associated w/ ↑ bleeding risk **CI:** w/ or w/in 14 d of MAOI **Disp:** Tabs 5, 10, 20 mg; soln 1 mg/mL **SE:** N/V/D, sweating, insomnia, dizziness, xerostomia, sexual dysfunction **Interactions:** ↑ Risk of serotonin synd *W/* linezolid; ↑ risk of bleeding *W/* anticoagulants, ASA, NSAIDs; may ↑ CNS effects *W/* CNS depressants **NIPE:** Do not D/C abruptly; full effects may take 3 wk; take w/o regard to food; may cause ↑ appetite & wgt gain

Esmolol (Brevibloc) [Antiarrhythmic/Beta-Blocker] Uses: *SVT & noncompensatory sinus tachycardia, AF/A flutter* **Action:** β_1-Adrenergic blocker; Class II antiarrhythmic **Dose:** *Adults & Peds. ECC 2010:* 0.5 mg/kg (500 mcg/kg) over 1 min, then 0.05 mg/kg/min (50 mcg/kg/min) Inf; if inadequate response after 5 min, repeat 0.5 mg/kg bolus then titrate Inf up to 0.2 mg/kg/min (200 mcg/kg/min); max 0.3 mg/kg/min (300 mcg/kg/min) **Caution:** [C (1st tri), D (2nd or 3rd tri), ?] **CI:** Sinus bradycardia, heart block, uncompensated CHF, cardiogenic shock, ↓ BP **Disp:** Inj 10, 20, 250 mg/mL; premix Inf 10 mg/mL **SE:** ↓ BP; bradycardia, diaphoresis, dizziness **Interaction:** ↑ Effects *W/* verapamil; ↑ effects *OF* digoxin, antihypertensives, nitrates; ↑ HTN *W/* amphetamines, cocaine, ephedrine, epinephrine, MAOIs, norepinephrine, phenylephrine, pseudoephedrine; ↓ effects *OF* glucagons, insulin, hypoglycemics, theophylline; ↓ effects *W/* NSAIDs, thyroid hormones **Labs:** ↑ Glucose, cholesterol **NIPE:** Monitor BS of pts w/ DM; pain on Inj; hemodynamic effects back to baseline w/in 30 min after D/C Inf

Esomeprazole (Nexium) [Gastric Acid Inhibitor/Proton Pump Inhibitor] Uses: *Short-term (4–8 wk) for erosive esophagitis/GERD; H pylori Infxn in combo w/ antibiotics* **Action:** PPI, ↓ gastric acid **Dose:** *Adults. GERD/erosive gastritis:* 20–40 mg/d PO × 4–8 wk; 20–40 mg IV 10–30 min Inf or > 3 min IV push, 10 d max *Maint:* 20 mg/d PO *H pylori Infxn:* 40 mg/d PO, plus clarithromycin 500 mg PO bid & amoxicillin 1000 mg/bid for 10 d *Peds < 1 y.* Not recommended *GERD:* 1–11 y *< 20 kg:* 10 mg *> 20 kg:* 10 or 20 mg *12–17 y > 20 kg:* 20 or 40 mg; for all peds give once daily for up to 8 wk **Caution:** [B, ?/–] **CI:** Component sensitivity **Disp:** Caps 20, 40 mg; IV 20, 40 mg **SE:** HA, D, Abd pain, Inj site Rxns **Interactions:** ↑ Effects *W/* amoxicillin, clarithromycin; ↑ effects *OF* benzodiazepines, saquinavir, warfarin; ↓ effects *OF* digoxin, ketoconazole, Fe salts; may affect drugs metabolized by CYP2C19 **Labs:** ↑ SCr, uric acid, LFTs, HMG, WBCs, plts, K+, thyroxine levels; risk of hypomagnesemia w/ long-term use, monitor **NIPE:** Take drug 1 h before food; ⊘ EtOH; do not chew; may open caps & sprinkle on applesauce; ↑ risk of fxs w/ all PPIs; may give antacids concomitantly

Estazolam (ProSom) [Hypnotic/Benzodiazepine] [C-IV] Uses: *Short-term management of insomnia* **Action:** Benzodiazepine **Dose:** 1–2 mg PO qhs PRN;

↓ in hepatic impair/elderly/debilitated **Caution:** [X, –] ↑ Effects w/ CNS depressants; cross-sensitivity w/ other benzodiazepines **CI:** PRG, component hypersensitivity, w/ itraconazole or ketoconazole **Disp:** Tabs 1, 2 mg **SE:** Somnolence, weakness, palpitations, anaphylaxis, angioedema, amnesia **Interactions:** ↑ Effects W/ amoxicillin, clarithromycin; ↑ effects OF diazepam, phenytoin, warfarin; ↓ effects W/ food; ↓ effects OF azole antifungals, digoxin **Labs:** ↑ LFTs **NIPE:** Take at least 1 h ac; may cause psychological/physical dependence; avoid abrupt D/C after prolonged use

Esterified Estrogens (Estratab, Menest) [Estrogen Supplement]
WARNING: ↑ Risk endometrial CA. Do not use in the prevention of CV Dz or dementia; ↑ risk of MI, stroke, breast CA, PE, & DVT, in postmenopausal women **Uses:** *Vasomotor Sxs or vulvar/Vag atrophy w/ menopause*; female hypogonadism, PCa, prevent osteoporosis **Action:** Estrogen supls **Dose:** *Menopausal vasomotor Sx:* 0.3–1.25 mg/d, cyclically 3 wk on, 1 wk off; add progestin 10–14 d w/ 28-d cycle w/ uterus intact *Vulvovaginal atrophy:* Same regimen except use 0.3–1.25 mg *Hypogonadism:* 2.5–7.5 mg/d PO × 20 d, off × 10 d; add progestin 10–14 d w/ 28-d cycle w/ uterus intact **Caution:** [X, –] **CI:** Undiagnosed genital bleeding, breast CA, estrogen-dependent tumors, thromboembolic disorders, thrombophlebitis, recent MI, PRG, severe hepatic Dz **Disp:** Tabs 0.3, 0.625, 1.25, 2.5 mg **SE:** N, HA, bloating, breast enlargement/tenderness, edema, venous thromboembolism, hypertriglyceridemia, gallbladder Dz **Interactions:** ↑ Effects OF corticosteroids, cyclosporine, TCAs, theophylline, caffeine, tobacco; ↓ effects W/ barbiturates, phenytoin, rifampin; ↓ effects OF anticoagulants, hypoglycemics, insulin, tamoxifen **Labs:** ↑ Prothrombin & factors VII, VIII, IX, X, plt aggregation, thyroid-binding globulin, T₄, triglycerides; ↓ antithrombin III, folate **NIPE:** ⊘ PRG, breast-feeding; use lowest dose for shortest time (see WHI data [www.whi.org])

Esterified Estrogens + Methyltestosterone (Estratest, Estratest HS, Syntest DS, HS) [Estrogen & Androgen Supplement] **WARNING:** ↑ Risk endometrial CA. Avoid in PRG. Do not use in the prevention of CV Dz or dementia; ↑ risk of MI, stroke, breast CA, PE, & DVT, in postmenopausal women **Uses:** *Vasomotor Sxs*; postpartum breast engorgement **Action:** Estrogen & androgen supls **Dose:** 1 tab/d × 3 wk, 1 wk off **Caution:** [X, –] **CI:** Genital bleeding of unknown cause, breast CA, estrogen-dependent tumors, thromboembolic disorders, thrombophlebitis, recent MI, PRG **Disp:** Tabs (estrogen mg/methyltestosterone mg) 0.625/1.25, 1.25/2.5 **SE:** N, HA, bloating, breast enlargement/tenderness, edema, ↑ triglycerides, venous thromboembolism, gallbladder Dz **Interactions:** ↑ Effects OF insulin; ↓ effects OF oral anticoagulants **NIPE:** Use lowest dose for shortest time; (see WHI data [www.whi.org])

Estradiol, Gel (Divigel) [Estrogen Supplement] **WARNING:** ↑ Risk of endometrial CA. Do not use in the prevention of CV Dz or dementia; ↑ risk MI, stroke, breast CA, PE, & DVT in postmenopausal women (50–79 y). ↑ Dementia risk in postmenopausal women (= 65 y) **Uses:** *Vasomotor Sx in menopause* **Action:** Estrogen **Dose:** 0.25 g qd on right or left upper thigh **Caution:** [X, +/–]

May ↑ PT/PTT/plt aggregation w/ thyroid Dz **CI:** Undiagnosed genital bleeding, breast CA, estrogen-dependent tumors, thromboembolic disorders, thrombophlebitis, recent MI, PRG, severe hepatic Dz **Disp:** 0.1% gel 0.25/0.5/1 g single-dose foil packets w/ 0.25, 0.5, 1 mg estradiol, respectively **SE:** N, HA, bloating, breast enlargement/tenderness, edema, venous thromboembolism, ↑ BP, hypertriglyceridemia, gallbladder Dz **NIPE:** If person other than pt applies, glove should be used, keep dry stat after, rotate site; contains alcohol, caution around flames until dry, not for Vag use

Estradiol, Gel (Elestrin) [Estrogen Supplement]   WARNING: Do not use in the prevention of CV Dz or dementia; ↑ risk MI, stroke, breast CA, PE, & DVT in postmenopausal women **Uses:** *Postmenopausal vasomotor Sxs* **Action:** Estrogen **Dose:** Apply 0.87–1.7 g to skin qd; add progestin × 10–14 d/28-d cycle w/ intact uterus; use lowest effective estrogen dose **Caution:** [X, ?] **CI:** AUB, breast CA, estrogen-dependent tumors, thromboembolic disorders, recent MI, PRG, severe hepatic Dz **Disp:** Gel 0.06% **SE:** Thromboembolic events, MI, stroke, ↑ BP, breast/ovarian/endometrial CA, site Rxns, Vag spotting, breast changes, Abd bloating, cramps, HA, fluid retention **NIPE:** Apply to upper arm, wait > 25 min before sunscreen; avoid concomitant use for > 7 d; ✓ BP, breast exams

Estradiol, Oral (Estrace, Delestrogen, Femtrace) [Estrogen Supplement]   WARNING:↑ Risk of endometrial CA; avoid in PRG **Uses:** *Atrophic vaginitis, menopausal vasomotor Sxs, ↑ low estrogen levels, palliation breast & PCa* **Action:** Estrogen **Dose:** *PO:* 1–2 mg/d, adjust PRN to control Sxs *Vag cream:* 2–4 g/d × 2 wk, then 1 g 1–3×/wk *Vasomotor Sx/Vag atrophy:* 10–20 mg IM q4wk, D/C or taper at 3–6-mo intervals *Hypoestrogenism:* 10–20 mg IM q4wk *PCa:* 30 mg IM q12wk **Caution:** [X, –] **CI:** Genital bleeding of unknown cause, breast CA, porphyria, estrogen-dependent tumors, thromboembolic disorders, thrombophlebitis; recent MI; hepatic impair **Disp:** Ring, 0.05, 0.1, 2 mg; gel 0.061%; tabs 0.5, 1, 2 mg; Vag cream 0.1 mg/g, depot Inj (Delestrogen) 10, 20, 40 mg/mL **SE:** N, HA, bloating, breast enlargement/tenderness, edema, ↑ triglycerides, venous thromboembolism, gallbladder Dz **Interactions:** ↑ Effects *W/* grapefruit juice; ↑ effects *OF* corticosteroids, cyclosporine, TCAs, theophylline, caffeine, tobacco; ↓ effects *W/* barbiturates, carbamazepine, phenytoin, primidone, rifampin; ↓ effects *OF* clofibrate, hypoglycemics, insulin, tamoxifen, warfarin **Labs:** ↑ Prothrombin & factors VII, VIII, IX, X, plt aggregation, thyroid-binding globulin, T₄, triglycerides; ↓ antithrombin III, folate **NIPE:** ⊘ PRG, breast-feeding

Estradiol, Spray (Evamist) [Estrogen Supplement]   WARNING: ↑ Risk of endometrial CA. Do not use in the prevention of CV Dz or dementia; ↑ risk MI, stroke, breast CA, PE, & DVT in postmenopausal women (50–79 y). ↑ Dementia risk in postmenopausal women (= 65 y) **Uses:** *Vasomotor Sx in menopause* **Action:** Estrogen **Dose:** 1 spray on inner surface of forearm **Caution:** [X, +/–] May ↑ PT/PTT/plt aggregation w/ thyroid Dz **CI:** Undiagnosed genital bleeding, breast CA, estrogen-dependent tumors, thromboembolic disorders, thrombophlebitis, recent

MI, PRG, severe hepatic Dz **Disp:** 1.53 mg/spray (56-spray container) **SE:** N, HA, bloating, breast enlargement/tenderness, edema, venous thromboembolism, ↑ BP, hypertriglyceridemia, gallbladder Dz **NIPE:** Contains alcohol, caution around flames until dry; not for Vag use

Estradiol, Transdermal (Estraderm, Climara, Vivelle, Vivelle Dot) [Estrogen Supplement] **WARNING:** ↑ Risk of endometrial CA. Do not use in the prevention of CV Dz or dementia; ↑ risk MI, stroke, breast CA, PE, & DVT in postmenopausal women (50–79 y). ↑ Dementia risk in postmenopausal women (= 65 y) **Uses:** *Severe menopausal vasomotor Sxs; female hypogonadism* **Action:** Estrogen supls **Dose:** Start 0.0375–0.05 mg/d patch 2 × /wk based on product; adjust PRN to control Sxs; w/ intact uterus cycle 3 wk on 1 wk off or use cyclic progestin 10–14 d **Caution:** [X, –] See Estradiol **CI:** PRG, AUB, porphyria, breast CA, estrogen-dependent tumors, h/o thrombophlebitis, thrombosis **Disp:** Transdermal patches (mg/24 h) 0.025, 0.0375, 0.05, 0.06, 0.075, 0.1 **SE:** N, bloating, breast enlargement/tenderness, edema, HA, hypertriglyceridemia, gallbladder Dz; see Estradiol **NIPE:** Do not apply to breasts, place on trunk, rotate sites

Estradiol, Vaginal (Estring, Femring, Vagifem) [Estrogen Supplement] **WARNING:** ↑ Risk of endometrial CA. Do not use in the prevention of CV Dz or dementia; ↑ risk MI, stroke, breast CA, PE, & DVT in postmenopausal women (50–79 y) **Uses:** *Postmenopausal Vag atrophy (Estring), vasomotor Sxs & vulvar/Vag atrophy associated w/ menopause (Femring), atrophic vaginitis (Vagifem)* **Action:** Estrogen **Dose:** *Estring:* Insert ring into upper 3rd of Vag vault; remove & replace after 90 d; reassess 3–6 mo *Femring:* Use lowest effective dose, insert vaginally, replace q3mo *Vagifem:* 1 tab vaginally qd × 2 wk, then maint 1 tab 2 × /wk, D/C or taper at 3–6 mo **Caution:** [X, –] Tox shock reported **CI:** Undiagnosed genital bleeding, breast CA, estrogen-dependent tumors, thromboembolic disorders, thrombophlebitis, recent MI, PRG, severe hepatic Dz **Disp:** *Estring* ring: 0.0075 mg/24 h *Femring* 0.05 & 0.1 mg/d *Vagifem* tabs (Vag): 25 mcg **SE:** HA, leukorrhea, back pain, candidiasis, vaginitis, Vag discomfort/hemorrhage, arthralgia, insomnia, Abd pain **Labs:** May ↑ PT/PTT/plt aggregation w/ thyroid Dz **NIPE:** Remove during Vag Infxn Tx & during Tx w/ other vaginally administered preps

Estradiol Cypionate & Medroxyprogesterone Acetate (Lunelle) [Estrogen & Progestin Supplement] **WARNING:** Cigarette smoking ↑ risk of serious CV SE from contraceptives w/ estrogen. This risk ↑ w/ age & w/ heavy smoking (> 15 cigarette/d) & is marked in women > 35 y. Women who use Lunelle should not smoke **Uses:** *Contraceptive* **Action:** Estrogen & progestin **Dose:** 0.5 mL IM (deltoid, anterior thigh, buttock) monthly, do not exceed 33 d **Caution:** [X, M] HTN, gallbladder Dz, ↑ lipids, migraines, sudden HA, valvular heart Dz w/ comps **CI:** PRG, heavy smokers > 35 y, DVT, PE, cerebrovascular/CV Dz, estrogen-dependent neoplasm, undiagnosed AUB, porphyria, hepatic tumors, cholestatic jaundice **Disp:** Estradiol cypionate (5 mg), medroxyprogesterone acetate (25 mg) SDV or syringe (0.5 mL) **SE:** Arterial thromboembolism, HTN, cerebral hemorrhage, MI, amenorrhea, acne, breast tenderness; see Estradiol **Interactions:** ↓ Effects *W*/ aminoglutethimide **Labs:** Monitor lipids **NIPE:** Start w/in 5 d of menstruation

Estradiol/Levonorgestrel Transdermal (Climara Pro) [Estrogen & Progesterone Supplement] WARNING: ↑ Risk of endometrial CA. Do not use in the prevention of CV Dz or dementia; ↑ risk MI, stroke, breast CA, PE, & DVT in postmenopausal women (50–79 y). ↑ Dementia risk in postmenopausal women (= 65 y) **Uses:** *Menopausal vasomotor Sx; prevent postmenopausal osteoporosis* **Action:** Estrogen & progesterone **Dose:** 1 patch 1 × /wk **Caution:** [X, –] w/ ↓ thyroid **CI:** AUB,estrogen-sensitive tumors, h/o thromboembolism, liver impair, PRG, hysterectomy **Disp:** Estradiol 0.045 mg/levonorgestrel 0.015/mg d patch **SE:** Site Rxn, Vag bleed/spotting, breast changes, Abd bloating/cramps, HA, retention fluid, edema, ↑ BP **NIPE:** Apply lower Abd; for osteoporosis give CA²⁺/ vit D supls; follow breast exams; intolerance to contact lenses; D/C use at least 2 wk before surgery

Estradiol/Norethindrone Acetate (Femhrt, Activella) [Estrogen & Progesterone Supplement] WARNING: ↑ Risk of endometrial CA. Do not use in the prevention of CV Dz or dementia; ↑ risk MI, stroke, breast CA, PE, & DVT in postmenopausal women (50–79 y). ↑ Dementia risk in postmenopausal women (= 65 y) **Action:** *Menopause vasomotor Sxs; prevent osteoporosis* **Action:** Estrogen/progestin; plant derived **Dose:** 1 tab/d start w/ lowest dose combo **Caution:** [X, –] w/ ↓ CA²⁺/thyroid **CI:** PRG; h/o breast CA; estrogen-dependent tumor; abnormal genital bleeding; h/o DVT, PE, or related disorders; recent (w/in past y) arterial thromboembolic Dz (CVA, MI) **Disp:** *Femhrt* tabs (mcg/mg) 2.5/0.5, 5/1; *Activella* tabs (mg/mg) 1.0/0.5, 0.5/0.1 **SE:** Thrombosis, dizziness, HA, libido changes, insomnia, emotional stability, breast pain **Interactions:** ↑ Effects *W*/ vit C, APAP, atorvastatin; ↓ effects *W*/ rifampin, troglitazone, anticonvulsants; ↓ effects *OF* temazepam, morphine, clofibrate; monitor use of theophylline, cyclosporine **Labs:** Monitor serum lipids **NIPE:** Use in women w/ intact uterus; caution in heavy smokers; intolerance to contact lenses; D/C 2 wk before surgery

Estramustine Phosphate (Emcyt) [Antimicrotubule Agent] **Uses:** *Advanced PCa* **Action:** Estradiol w/ nornitrogen mustard; exact mechanism unknown **Dose:** 14 mg/kg/d in 3–4 ÷ doses; on empty stomach, no dairy products **Caution:** [NA, not used in females] **CI:** Active thrombophlebitis or thromboembolic disorders **Disp:** Caps 140 mg **SE:** N/V, exacerbation of preexisting CHF, edema, hepatic disturbances, thrombophlebitis, MI, PE, gynecomastia in 20–100% **Interactions:** ↓ Absorption & effects *W*/ antacids, Ca supls, Ca-containing foods; ↓ effects *OF* anticoagulants **Labs:** Monitor bilirubin & LFTs during & 2 mo after Tx is D/C **NIPE:** Take on empty stomach, several wk may be needed for full effects, store in refrigerator; low-dose breast irradiation before may ↓ gynecomastia; use effective contraception

Estrogen, Conjugated (Premarin) [Estrogen/Hormone] WARNING: ↑ Risk of endometrial CA. Do not use in the prevention of CV Dz or dementia; ↑

risk MI, stroke, breast CA, PE, & DVT in postmenopausal women (50–79 y). ↑ Dementia risk in postmenopausal women (= 65 y) **Uses:** *Mod–severe menopausal vasomotor Sxs; atrophic vaginitis; dyspareunia; palliative advanced CAP; prevention & Tx of estrogen-deficiency osteoporosis* **Action:** Estrogen hormonal replacement **Dose:** 0.3–1.25 mg/d PO; intravag cream 0.5–2g × 21 d, then off × 7 d or 0.5 mg twice weekly **Caution:** [X, –] **CI:** Severe hepatic impair, genital bleeding of unknown cause, breast CA, estrogen-dependent tumors, thromboembolic disorders, thrombosis, thrombophlebitis, recent MI **Disp:** Tabs 0.3, 0.45, 0.625, 0.9, 1.25, 2.5 mg; Vag cream 0.625 mg/g **SE:** ↑ Risk of endometrial CA, gallbladder Dz, thromboembolism, HA, & possibly breast CA **Interactions:** ↑ Effects *OF* corticosteroids, cyclosporine, TCAs, theophylline, tobacco; ↓ effects *OF* anticoagulants, clofibrate; ↓ effects *W/* barbiturates, carbamazepine, phenytoin, rifampin **Labs:** ↑ Prothrombin & factors VII, VIII, IX, X, plt aggregation, thyroid-binding globulin, T_4, triglycerides; ↓ antithrombin III, folate **NIPE:** ⊘ PRG, breast-feeding; generic products not equivalent

Estrogen, Conjugated Synthetic (Cenestin, Enjuvia) [Estrogen/ Hormone] WARNING: ↑ Risk of endometrial CA. Do not use in the prevention of CV Dz or dementia; ↑ risk MI, stroke, breast CA, PE, & DVT in postmenopausal women (50–79 y). ↑ Dementia risk in postmenopausal women (= 65 y) **Uses:** *Vasomotor menopausal Sxs, vulvovaginal atrophy, prevent postmenopausal osteoporosis* **Action:** Multiple estrogen hormonal replacement **Dose:** For all w/ intact uterus progestin × 10–14 d/28-d cycle *Vasomotor:* 0.3–1.25 mg (Enjuvia) 0.625–1.25 mg (Cenestin) PO daily *Vag atrophy:* 0.3 mg/d (Enjuvia) *Osteoporosis:* (Cenestin) 0.625 mg/d **Caution:** [X, –] **CI:** See Estrogen, Conjugated **Disp:** Tabs Cenestin 0.3, 0.45, 0.625, 0.9; Enjuvia XR 0.3, 0.45, 0.625, 1.25 mg **SE:** ↑ Risk endometrial/breast CA, gallbladder Dz, thromboembolism **NIPE:** D/C if jaundice occurs & 2 wk before surgery

Estrogen, Conjugated + Medroxyprogesterone (Prempro, Premphase) [Estrogen/Progestin Hormones] WARNING: Should not be used for the prevention of CV Dz or dementia; ↑ risk of MI, stroke, breast CA, PE, & DVT; ↑ risk of dementia in postmenopausal women **Uses:** *Mod–severe menopausal vasomotor Sxs; atrophic vaginitis; prevent postmenopausal osteoporosis* **Action:** Hormonal replacement **Dose:** *Prempro:* 1 tab PO daily *Premphase:* 1 tab PO daily **Caution:** [X, –] **CI:** Severe hepatic impair, genital bleeding of unknown cause, breast CA, estrogen-dependent tumors, thromboembolic disorders, thrombosis, thrombophlebitis **Disp:** (As estrogen/medroxyprogesterone) *Prempro:* Tabs 0.3/1.5, 0.45/1.5, 0.625/2.5, 0.625/5 mg *Premphase:* Tabs 0.625/0 mg (d 1–14) & 0.625/5 mg (d 15–28) **SE:** Gallbladder Dz, thromboembolism, HA, breast tenderness **NIPE:** Intolerance to contact lenses; see WHI (www.whi.org); use lowest dose/shortest time possible

Estrogen, Conjugated + Methylprogesterone (Premarin + Methylprogesterone) [Estrogen & Androgen Hormones] WARNING:

Do not use in the prevention of CV Dz or dementia; ↑ risk of endometrial CA **Uses:** *Menopausal vasomotor Sxs; osteoporosis* **Action:** Estrogen & androgen combo **Dose:** 1 tab/d **Caution:** [X, –] **CI:** Severe hepatic impair, AUB, breast CA, estrogen-dependent tumors, thromboembolic disorders, thrombosis, thrombophlebitis **Disp:** Tabs 0.625 mg estrogen, conjugated, & 2.5 or 5 mg of methylprogesterone **SE:** N, bloating, breast enlargement/tenderness, edema, HA, hypertriglyceridemia, gallbladder Dz **NIPE:** Intolerance to contact lenses; D/C if jaundice occurs & 2 wk before surgery

Estrogen, Conjugated + Methyltestosterone (Premarin + Methyltestosterone) [Estrogen & Androgen Hormones] WARNING: Do not use in the prevention of CV Dz or dementia; ↑ risk of endometrial CA

Uses: *Mod–severe menopausal vasomotor Sxs*; postpartum breast engorgement **Action:** Estrogen & androgen combo **Dose:** 1 tab/d × 3 wk, then 1 wk off **Caution:** [X, –] **CI:** Severe hepatic impair, genital bleeding of unknown cause, breast CA, estrogen-dependent tumors, thromboembolic disorders, thrombophlebitis **Disp:** Tabs (estrogen mg/methyltestosterone mg) 0.625/5, 1.25/10 **SE:** N, bloating, breast enlargement/tenderness, edema, HA, hypertriglyceridemia, gallbladder Dz **NIPE:** Intolerance to contact lenses; D/C if jaundice occurs & 2 wk before surgery

Eszopiclone (Lunesta) [Hypnotic/Nonbenzodiazepine] [C-IV]

Uses: *Insomnia* **Action:** Nonbenzodiazepine hypnotic **Dose:** 2–3 mg/d hs **Elderly:** 1–2 mg/d hs; w/ hepatic impair use w/ CYP3A4 Inhib (Table 10); 1 mg/d hs **Caution:** [C, ?/–] **Disp:** Tabs 1, 2, 3 mg **SE:** HA, xerostomia, dizziness, somnolence, hallucinations, rash, Infxn, unpleasant taste, anaphylaxis, angioedema **Interactions:** ↑ Effects *W/* itraconazole, ketoconazole, ritonavir; ↑ CNS effects *W/* CNS depressants; ↓ effects *W/* rifampin **NIPE:** High-fat meals ↓ absorption

Etanercept (Enbrel) [Antirheumatic/TNF Blocker] WARNING: Serious Infxns (bacterial sepsis, TB, reported); D/C w/ severe Infxn. Eval for TB risk; test for TB before use; lymphoma/other CA possible in children/adolescents possible

Uses: *↓ Sxs of RA in pts who fail other DMARD*, Crohn Dz **Action:** TNF receptor blocker **Dose:** *Adults.* RA 50 mg SQ weekly or 25 mg SQ 2 × /wk (separated by at least 72–96 h) *Peds 4–17 y.* 0.8 mg/kg/wk (max 50 mg/wk) or 0.4 mg/kg (max 25 mg/dose) 2 × /wk 72–96 h apart **Caution:** [B, ?] w/ predisposition to Infxn (ie, DM); may ↑ risk of malignancy in peds & young adults **CI:** Active Infxn **Disp:** 25 mg/vial, 50 mg/mL syringe **SE:** HA, rhinitis, Inj site Rxn, URI, new onset psoriasis **Interactions:** ↓ Response to live virus vaccine **NIPE:** Rotate Inj sites; ⊘ live vaccines

Ethambutol (Myambutol) [Antitubercular Agent]

Uses: *Pulm TB* & other mycobacterial Infxns, MAC **Action:** ↓ RNA synth **Dose:** *Adults & Peds > 12 y.* 15–25 mg/kg/d PO single dose; ↓ in renal impair, take w/ food, avoid antacids **Caution:** [C, +] **CI:** Unconscious pts, optic neuritis **Disp:** Tabs 100, 400 mg **SE:** HA, hyperuricemia, acute gout, Abd pain, optic neuritis, GI upset **Interactions:** ↑ Neurotox *W/* neurotoxic drugs; ↓ effects *W/* Al salts **Labs:** ↑ LFTs **NIPE:** Monitor visual acuity

Ethinyl Estradiol (Estinyl, Feminone) [Estrogen Supplement]
WARNING: ↑ Risk endometrial CA. Avoid in PRG. Do not use in the prevention of CV Dz or dementia; ↑ risk of MI, stroke, breast CA, PE, DVT, in postmenopausal women **Uses:** *Menopausal vasomotor Sxs; female hypogonadism* **Action:** Estrogen supls **Dose:** 0.02–1.5 mg/d ÷ daily–tid **Caution:** [X, –] **CI:** Severe hepatic impair; genital bleeding of unknown cause, breast CA, estrogen-dependent tumors, thromboembolic disorders, thrombophlebitis **Disp:** Tabs 0.02, 0.05, 0.5 mg **SE:** N, bloating, breast enlargement/tenderness, edema, HA, hypertriglyceridemia, gallbladder Dz **Interactions:** ↑ Effects *OF* corticosteroids; ↓ effects *W/* barbiturates, carbamazepine, hypoglycemics, insulin, phenytoin, primidone, rifampin, ↓ effects *OF* anticoagulants, tamoxifen **Labs:** ↑ Prothrombin & factors VII, VIII, IX, X, plt aggregation, thyroid-binding globulin, T₄, triglycerides; ↓ antithrombin III, folate **NIPE:** ⊘ PRG, breast-feeding

Ethinyl Estradiol & Drospirenone (YAZ) [Estrogen & Progestin Supplement] **WARNING:** Cigarette smoking & use of estrogen-based OCPs have ↑ risk of serious CV SE; risk ↑ w/ age (esp > 35 y) & smoking > 15 cigarette/d **Uses:** OCP; PMDD **Action:** Suppresses ovulation by imitating the feedback inhibition of endogenous estrogen & progesterone on the pituitary & hypothalamus **Dose:** 1 tab PO OD × 28 d, repeat **Caution:** [X, –] Has antimineralocorticoid activity w/ potential hyperkalemia in renal Insuff, adrenal Insuff, hepatic Insuff **CI:** Pts w/ renal Insuff, hepatic impair, adrenal Insuff, DVT, PE, CVD, CAD, estrogen-dependent neoplasms, AUB, PRG, heavy smokers > 35 y **Disp:** Ethinyl estradiol (20 mcg), drospirenone (3 mg) 28-d pack has 24 active tabs & 4 inert tabs **SE:** Hyperkalemia, HTN, N, V, HA, breakthrough bleeding, amenorrhea, mastodynia, ↑ risk of gallbladder Dz & thromboembolic disorders **Interactions:** ↑ Risk of hyperkalemia *W/* ACEIs, ARBs, aldosterone antagonists, heparin, NSAIDs, spironolactone, K⁺-sparing diuretics, K⁺ supls, ↑ effects *OF* cyclosporine, prednisolone, theophylline; ↓ effects *W/* barbiturates, carbamazepine, griseofulvin, modafinil, phenobarbital, phenylbutazone, phenytoin, pioglitazone, rifabutin, rifampin, ritonavir, topiramate, St. John's wort **Labs:** ↑ Uptake of T₃, ↓ T₄ sex hormone-binding globulin levels; triglycerides **NIPE:** Antimineralocorticoid activity comparable to spironolactone 25 mg; in pts taking meds that ↑ K⁺ monitor serum K⁺ during 1st Rx cycle; Sunday start regimen or postpartum use requires additional contraceptive methods during 1st cycle; use barrier contraception if taking anticonvulsants; may cause vision changes or ↓ contact lens tolerability; ⊘ protection against HIV or STDs; ⊘ smoke cigarettes

Ethinyl Estradiol/Levonorgestrel (Seasonale) [Estrogen & Progestin Supplement] **WARNING:** Cigarette smoking & use of estrogen-based OCPs have ↑ risk of serious CV SE; risk ↑ w/ age (esp> 35 y) & smoking > 15 cigarette/d **Uses:** OCP **Action:** Suppresses ovulation by imitating the feedback inhibition of endogenous estrogen & progesterone on the pituitary & hypothalamus **Dose:** 1 tab PO OD for 91 d; repeat. Use Sunday start for 1st cycle **Caution:** [X, –] **CI:** Pts w/ DVT, PE, CVD, CAD, estrogen-dependent neoplasms, AUB, PRG, hepatic impair

Disp: Tabs levonorgestrel 0.15 mg & ethinyl estradiol 30 mcg; 91-d pack has 84 active tabs & 7 inert tabs **SE:** HTN, N, V, HA, breakthrough bleeding, amenorrhea, mastodynia, ↑ risk of gallbladder Dz & thromboembolic disorders **Interactions:** ↓ Effects W/ barbiturates, carbamazepine, griseofulvin, modafinil, phenobarbital, phenytoin, pioglitazone, rifabutin, rifampin, ritonavir, topiramate, St. John's wort **Labs:** ↑ Uptake of T_3, ↓ T_4 sex hormone-binding globulin levels **NIPE:** Sunday start regimen requires additional contraceptive methods during 1st cycle; use barrier contraception if taking anticonvulsants; may cause vision changes or ↓ contact lens tolerability; ⊘ protection against HIV or STDs; ⊘ smoke cigarettes

Ethinyl Estradiol & Norelgestromin (Ortho Evra) [Estrogen & Progestin Hormones] **Uses:** *Contraceptive patch* **Action:** Estrogen & progestin **Dose:** Apply patch to abdomen, buttocks, upper torso (not breasts), or upper outer arm at the beginning of the menstrual cycle; new patch is applied weekly for 3 wk; wk 4 is patch-free **Caution:** [X, M] **CI:** PRG, h/o or current DVT/PE, stroke, MI, CV Dz, CAD; SBP > 160 mm Hg or DBP> 100 mm Hg; severe HA w/ focal neurological Sx; breast/endometrial CA; estrogen-dependent neoplasms; hepatic dysfunction; jaundice; major surgery w/ prolonged immobilization; heavy smoking if > 35 y **Disp:** 20 cm² patch (6 mg norelgestromin [active metabolite norgestimate] & 0.75 mg of ethinyl estradiol) **SE:** Breast discomfort, HA, site Rxns, N, menstrual cramps; thrombosis risks similar to OCP; ↓ effects W/ hepatic enzyme inducing drugs such as griseofulvin, rifampin, St. John's wort **Labs:** ↑ Serum amylase, Na, Ca, protein **NIPE:** Less effective in women > 90 kg; instruct pt does not protect against STD/HIV; discourage smoking

Ethosuximide (Zarontin) [Anticonvulsant] **Uses:** *Absence (petit mal) Szs* **Action:** Anticonvulsant; ↑ Sz threshold **Dose:** *Adults & Peds > 6 y.* Initial: 500 mg PO ÷ bid; ↑ by 250 mg/d q4–7d PRN (max 1500 mg/d) usual maint 20–30 mg/kg *Peds 3–6 y.* Initial: 15 mg/kg/d PO ÷ bid Maint: 15–40 mg/kg/d ÷ bid, max 1500 mg/d **Caution:** [D, +] in renal/hepatic impair; antiepileptics may ↑ risk of suicidal behavior or ideation **CI:** Component sensitivity **Disp:** Caps 250 mg; syrup 250 mg/5 mL **SE:** Blood dyscrasias, GI upset, drowsiness, dizziness, irritability **Notes:** *Levels: Trough:* Just before next dose *Therapeutic: Peak:* 40–100 mcg/mL *Toxic trough:* > 100 mcg/mL *1/2-life:* 25–60 h **Interactions:** ↑ Effects W/ INH, phenobarbital, EtOH; ↑ effects OF CNS depressants, phenytoin; ↓ effects W/ carbamazepine, valproic acid, ginkgo; ↓ effects OF phenobarbital **Labs:** Monitor BUN, Cr, LFTs **NIPE:** Take w/ food; ⊘ EtOH

Etidronate Disodium (Didronel) [Hormone/Bisphosphonates] **Uses:** * ↑ Ca²⁺ of malignancy, Paget Dz, & heterotopic ossification* **Action:** ↓ Nl & abnormal bone resorption **Dose:** *Paget Dz:* 5–10 mg/kg/d PO ÷ doses (for 3–6 mo). ↑ Ca²⁺: 7.5 mg/kg/d IV Inf over 2 h × 3 d, then 20 mg/kg/d PO on last day of Inf × 1–3 mo **Caution:** [B PO (C parenteral), ?] bisphosphonates may cause severe musculoskeletal pain **CI:** Overt osteomalacia, SCr > 5 mg/dL **Disp:** Tabs 200, 400 mg; Inj 50 mg/mL **SE:** GI intolerance (↓ by ÷ daily doses); hyperphosphatemia, hypomagnesemia, bone pain, abnormal taste, fever, convulsions, nephrotox **Interactions:** ↓ Effects W/ antacids, foods that contain Ca; monitor warfarin **NIPE:** Take PO on empty stomach 2 h before or 2 h pc

Etodolac [Antiarthritic/NSAID] WARNING: May ↑ risk of CV events & GI bleeding; may worsen ↑ BP **Uses:** *OA & pain*, RA **Action:** NSAID **Dose:** 200–400 mg PO bid–qid (max 1200 mg/d) **Caution:** [C (D 3rd tri), ?] ↑ Bleeding risk w/ ASA, warfarin; ↑ nephrotox w/ cyclosporine; h/o CHF, HTN, renal/hepatic impair, PUD **CI:** Active GI ulcer **Disp:** Tabs 400, 500 mg; ER tabs 400, 500, 600 mg; caps 200, 300 mg **SE:** N/V/D, gastritis, Abd cramps, dizziness, HA, depression, edema, renal impair **Interactions:** ↑ Risk of bleeding W/ anticoagulants, antiplts; ↑ effects OF Li, MTX, digoxin, cyclosporine; ↓ effects W/ ASA; ↓ effects OF antihypertensives **Labs:** ↑ LFTs, BUN, Cr; ↓ HMG, Hct, plts, WBC, uric acid **NIPE:** Take w/ food; do not crush tabs

Etomidate (Amidate) [Hypnotic] **Uses:** *Induce general or short-procedure anesthesia* **Action:** Short-acting hypnotic **Dose:** *Adults & Peds > 10 y.* Induce anesthesia 0.2–0.6 mg/kg IV over 30–60 s; Peds < 10 y. Not recommended **Peds. ECC 2010:** **Rapid sedation:** 0.2–0.4 mg/kg IV/IO over 30–60; max dose 20 mg **Caution:** [C; ?] **CI:** Hypersensitivity **Disp:** Inj 2 mg/mL **SE:** Inj site pain, myoclonus **NIPE:** May induce cardiac depression in elderly

Etonogestrel/Ethinyl Estradiol Vaginal Insert (NuvaRing) [Estrogen & Progestin Hormones] **Uses:** *Contraceptive* **Action:** Estrogen & progestin combo **Dose:** Rule out PRG 1st; insert ring vaginally for 3 wk, remove for 1 wk; insert new ring 7 d after last removed (even if bleeding) at same time of d ring removed. 1st d of menses is d 1, insert before d 5 even if bleeding. Use other contraception for 1st 7 d of starting therapy. See package insert if converting from other contraceptive; after delivery or PRG not breastfeeding, start 4 wk postpartum (if not breastfeeding) **Caution:** [X, ?/–] HTN, gallbladder Dz, ↑ lipids, migraines, sudden HA **CI:** PRG, heavy smokers > 35 y, DVT, PE, cerebrovascular/CV Dz, estrogen-dependent neoplasm, undiagnosed abnormal genital bleeding, hepatic tumors, cholestatic jaundice **Disp:** Intravag ring: Ethinyl estradiol 0.015 mg/d & etonogestrel 0.12 mg/d **NIPE:** If ring removed, rinse w/ cool/lukewarm H₂O (not hot) & reinsert ASAP; if not reinserted w/in 3 h, effectiveness ↓; do not use w/ diaphragm

Etonogestrel Implant (Implanon) [Hormone] **Uses:** *Contraception* **Action:** Transforms endometrium from proliferative to secretory **Dose:** 1 implant subdermally q3y **Caution:** [X, +] Exclude PRG before implant **CI:** PRG, hormonally responsive tumors, breast CA, AUB, hepatic tumor, active liver Dz, h/o thromboembolic Dz **Disp:** 68-mg implant **SE:** Spotting, irregular periods, amenorrhea, dysmenorrhea, HA, tender breasts, N, wgt gain, acne, ectopic PRG, PE, ovarian cysts, stroke, ↑ BP **Interactions:** ↑ Effects W/ ketoconazole, itraconazole, other hepatic enzyme Inhibs **Labs:** Monitor LFTs **NIPE:** 99% Effective; remove implant & replace; restricted distribution; healthcare provider must register & train; does not protect against STDs

Etoposide [VP-16] (VePesid, Toposar) [Antineoplastic] Uses: *Testicular, NSCLC, Hodgkin Dz, & NHLs, peds ALL, & allogeneic/autologous BMT in high doses* **Action:** Topoisomerase II Inhib **Dose:** 50 mg/m²/d IV for 3–5 d; 50 mg/m²/d PO for 21 d (PO availability = 50% of IV); 2–6 g/m² or 25–70 mg/kg in BMT (per protocols); ↓ in renal/hepatic impair **Caution:** [D, –] **CI:** IT administration **Disp:** Caps 50 mg; Inj 20 mg/mL **SE:** N/V (emesis in 10–30%), ↓ BM, alopecia, ↓ BP w/ rapid IV, anorexia, anemia, leukopenia, ↑ risk secondary leukemias **Interactions:** ↑ Bleeding *W/* ASA, NSAIDs, warfarin; ↑ BM suppression *W/* antineoplastics & radiation; ↑ effects *OF* cisplatin; ↓ effects *OF* live vaccines **Labs:** ↑ Uric acid; ↓ HMG, Hct, plts, RBC, WBC **NIPE:** N, EtOH, immunizations, PRG, breast-feeding; use contraception; 2–3 L/d fluids

Etravirine (Intelence) [Nonnucleoside Reverse Transcriptase Inhibitor] Uses: *HIV* **Action:** NNRTI **Dose:** 200 mg PO bid following a meal **Caution:** [B, ±] **CI:** None **Disp:** Tabs 100 mg **SE:** N/V/D, rash, severe/potentially life-threatening skin Rxns, fat redistribution **Interactions:** Many interactions: substrate/inducer (CYP3A4), substrate/Inhib (CYP2C9, CYP2C19); do not use w/ tipranavir/ritonavir, fosamprenavir/ritonavir, atazanavir/ritonavir, protease Inhibs w/o ritonavir, & non-NRTIs; ↑ effects *OF* warfarin, diazepam; ↑ effects *W/* lopinavir, ritonavir **Labs:** Monitor BS & LFTs **NIPE:** Take after meals

Everolimus (Afinitor) [mTOR Kinase Inhibitor] Uses: *Advanced RCC w/ sunitinib or sorafenib failure,* subependymal giant cell astrocytoma in nonsurgical candidates w/ tuberous sclerosis* **Action:** mTOR Inhib (mammalian rapamycin target) **Dose:** 10 mg PO qd ↓ to 5 mg w/ SE or hepatic impair **Caution:** [D, –] Avoid w/ or if received live vaccines; w/ CYP3A4 Inhibs **Disp:** Tabs 5, 10 mg **SE:** Noninfectious pneumonia, Infxn risk, oral ulcers, asthenia, cough, fatigue, D **Interactions:** ↑ Effects *W/* mod–strong CYP3A4 Inhibs: amprenavir, aprepitant, atazanavir, clarithromycin, delavirdine, diltiazem, erythromycin, fluconazole, fosamprenavir, indinavir, itraconazole, ketoconazole, nefazodone, nelfinavir, ritonavir, saquinavir, telithromycin, verapamil, voriconazole, grapefruit juice; ↓ effects *W/* strong CYP3A4 inducers: carbamazepine, dexamethasone, phenobarbital, phenytoin, rifabutin, rifampin **Labs:** ↑ Glucose/SCr/lipids; ↓ Hgb/WBC/plt; monitor CBC, LFT, glucose, lipids **NIPE:** ⊘ Live vaccines; swallow whole w/ H₂O; monitor for pneumonitis—reduce dose and/or manage w/ corticosteroids; monitor for Infxn & D/C if fungal Infxn occurs; monitor for stomatitis—treat w/ nonalcoholic, non-peroxide mouthwash; see also Everolimus (Zortress)

Everolimus (Zortress) [Immunosuppressant (Macrolide)] Uses: *Prevent renal transplant rejection; combo w/ basiliximab w/ ↓ dose of steroids & cyclosporine* **Action:** mTOR Inhib (mammalian rapamycin target) **Dose:** 7.5 mg PO bid, adjust to trough levels 3–8 ng/mL **Caution:** [D, ?] **CI:** Compound/rapamycin-derivative hypersensitivity **Disp:** Tabs 0.25, 0.5, 0.75 mg **SE:** Peripheral edema, constipation, ↑ BP, N, UTI **Interactions:** Avoid live vaccines, simvastatin, lovastatin; ↑ risk of angioedema *W/* ACEI; ↑ effects *W/* ketoconazole, itraconazole, voriconazole, clarithromycin, telithromycin, ritonavir, grapefruit juice, digoxin; ↓ effects W/ carbamazepine, phenobarbital, phenytoin, rifampin, rifabulin, efavirenz, nevirapine, St. Johns wort **Labs:** ↑ Lipids; ↓ Hct; follow CBC, LFT, glucose, lipids **NIPE:** Trough level 3–8 ng/mL w/ cyclosporine; see also Everolimus (Afinitor); avoid sunlight & UV light

Exemestane (Aromasin) [Antineoplastic] Uses: *Advanced breast CA in postmenopausal women w/ progression after tamoxifen* **Action:** Irreversible, steroidal aromatase Inhib; ↓ estrogens **Dose:** 25 mg PO daily after a meal **Caution:** [D, ?/–] **CI:** PRG, component sensitivity **Disp:** Tabs 25 mg **SE:** Hot flashes, N, fatigue, ↑ alk phos **Interactions:** ↓ Effects W/ erythromycin, ketoconazole, phenobarbital, rifampin, other drugs that inhibit P4503A4, St. John's wort, black cohosh, dong quai **Labs:** ↑ Alk phos, bilirubin, alk phos **NIPE:** ⊘ PRG, breast-feeding; take pc & same time each d; monitor BP

Exenatide (Byetta) [Hypoglycemic/Incretin] Uses: Type 2 DM combined w/ metformin and/or sulfonylurea **Action:** An incretin mimetic: ↑ insulin release, ↓ glucagon secretion, ↓ gastric emptying, promotes satiety **Dose:** 5 mcg SQ bid w/in 60 min before AM & PM meals; ↑ to 10 mcg SQ bid after 1 mo PRN; do not give pc **Caution:** [C, ?/–] **CI:** CrCl < 30 mL/min **Disp:** Soln 5, 10 mcg/dose in pre-filled pen **SE:** Hypoglycemia, N/V/D, dizziness, HA, dyspepsia, ↓ appetite, jittery; acute pancreatitis **Interactions:** May ↓ absorption of oral drugs (take antibiotics/contraceptives 1 h before) **Labs:** Monitor Cr, warfarin **NIPE:** Consider ↓ sulfonylurea & insulin to ↓ risk of hypoglycemia; discard pen 30 d after 1st use

Ezetimibe (Zetia) [Antilipemic/Selective Cholesterol Absorption Inhibitor] Uses: *Hypercholesterolemia alone or w/ a HMG-CoA reductase Inhib* **Action:** ↓ Cholesterol & phytosterol absorption **Dose:** *Adults & Peds > 10 y.* 10 mg/d PO **Caution:** [C, +/–] Bile acid sequestrants ↓ bioavailability **CI:** Hepatic impair **Disp:** Tabs 10 mg **SE:** HA, D, Abd pain, ↑ transaminases w/ HMG-CoA reductase Inhib, erythema multiforme **Notes:** See Ezetimibe/Simvastatin **Interactions:** ↑ Effects W/ cyclosporine; ↓ effects W/ cholestyramine, fenofibrate, gemfibrozil **Labs:** ↑ LFTs **NIPE:** If used w/ fibrates ↑ risk of cholelithiasis

Ezetimibe/Simvastatin (Vytorin) [Antilipemic/HMG-CoA Reductase Inhibitor] Uses: *Hypercholesterolemia* **Action:** ↓ Absorption of cholesterol & phytosterol w/ HMG-CoA-reductase Inhib **Dose:** 10/10–10/80 mg/d PO; w/ cyclosporine/danazol: 10/10 mg/d max; w/ amiodarone/verapamil: 10/20 mg/d max; ↓ w/ severe renal Insuff; give 2 h before or 4 h after bile acid sequestrants **Caution:** [X, –]; w/ CYP3A4 Inhibs (Table 10), gemfibrozil, niacin > 1 g/d, danazol, amiodarone, verapamil **CI:** PRG/lactation; liver Dz, ↑ LFTs **Disp:** Tabs (ezetimibe mg/simvastatin mg) 10/10, 10/20, 10/40, 10/80 **SE:** HA, GI upset, myalgia, myopathy (muscle pain, weakness, or tenderness w/ CK 10 × ULN, rhabdomyolysis), hep, Infxn **Interactions:** ↑ Risk of myopathy W/ clarithromycin, erythromycin, itraconazole, ketoconazole **Labs:** Monitor LFTs, lipids **NIPE:** ⊘ PRG or lactation; use adequate contraception; ⊘ EtOH; ezetimibe/simvastatin combo lowered LDL more than simvastatin alone in ENHANCE study, but there was no difference in carotid-intima media thickness

Famciclovir (Famvir) [Antiviral/Synthetic Nucleoside] Uses: *Acute herpes zoster (shingles) & genital herpes* Action: ↓ Viral DNA synth Dose: *Zoster:* 500 mg PO q8h × 7 d *Simplex:* 125–250 mg PO bid; ↓ w/ renal impair Caution: [B, –] CI: Component sensitivity Disp: Tabs 125, 250, 500 mg SE: Fatigue, dizziness, HA, pruritus, N/D Interactions: ↑ Effects W/ cimetidine, probenecid, theophylline; ↑ effects OF digoxin NIPE: Not affected by food, therapy most effective if taken w/in 72 h of initial lesion

Famotidine (Pepcid, Pepcid AC) [OTC] [Antisecretory/H$_2$-Receptor Antagonist] Uses: *Short-term Tx of duodenal ulcer & benign gastric ulcer; maint for duodenal ulcer, hypersecretory conditions, GERD, & heartburn* Action: H$_2$-antagonist; ↓ gastric acid Dose: *Adults. Ulcer:* 20 mg IV q12h or 20–40 mg PO qhs × 4–8 wk *Hypersecretion:* 20–160 mg PO q6h *GERD:* 20 mg PO bid × 6 wk; maint: 20 mg PO hs *Heartburn:* 10 mg PO PRN q12h *Peds.* 0.5–1 mg/kg/d; ↓ in severe renal Insuff Caution: [B, M] CI: Component sensitivity Disp: Tabs 10, 20, 40 mg; chew tabs 10 mg; susp 40 mg/5 mL; gelatin caps 10 mg, Inj 10 mg/2 mL SE: Dizziness, HA, constipation, D, ↓ plt Interactions: ↑ GI irritation W/ caffeinated foods, EtOH, nicotine Labs: ↓ BUN, Cr, LFTs NIPE: ⊘ ASA, EtOH, tobacco, caffeine—d/t ↑ SEs; take hs; chew tabs contain phenylalanine

Febuxostat (Uloric) [Antigout/Xanthine oxidase Inhibitor] Uses: *Chronic management of hyperuricemia w/ gout* Action: Xanthine oxidase Inhib (enzyme that converts hypoxanthine to xanthine to uric acid) Dose: 40 mg PO 1 × daily, 80 mg if uric acid not < 6 mg/dL after 2 wk Caution: [C, ?/–] CI: Use w/ azathioprine, mercaptopurine, theophylline Disp: Tabs 40, 80 mg SE: LFTs, rash, myalgia Interactions: ↑ Effects OF xanthine oxidase substrate drugs: Azathioprine, mercaptopurine, theophylline Labs: Monitor uric acid < & 2 wk > start of therapy; monitor LFTs 2 & 4 mo > initiation & periodically; ↑ LFTs, ↑ or ↓ WBC NIPE: OK to continue drug w/ gouty flare or use w/ NSAIDs/colchicine on initiation of therapy for up to 6 mo; chronic management of hyperuricemia w/ gout. Not for use in asymptomatic pts

Felodipine (Plendil) [Antihypertensive/CCB] Uses: *HTN & CHF* Action: CCB Dose: 2.5–10 mg PO daily; swallow whole; ↓ in hepatic impair Caution: [C, ?] ↑ Effect w/ azole antifungals, erythromycin, grapefruit juice CI: Component sensitivity Disp: XR tabs 2.5, 5, 10 mg SE: Peripheral edema, flushing, tachycardia, HA, gingival hyperplasia Interactions: ↑ Effects W/ azole antifungals, cimetidine, cyclosporine, ranitidine, propranolol, EtOH, grapefruit juice; ↑ effects OF digoxin, erythromycin; ↓ effects W/ barbiturates, carbamazepine, nafcillin, NSAIDS, oxcarbazepine, phenytoin, rifampin; ↓ effects OF theophylline NIPE: ⊘ D/C abruptly; follow BP in elderly & w/ hepatic impair

Fenofibrate (TriCor, Antara, Lofibra, Lipofen, Triglide) [Antilipemic/Fibric Acid Derivative] Uses: *Hypertriglyceridemia, hypercholesteremia* Action: ↓ Triglyceride synth Dose: 43–160 mg/d; ↓ w/ renal impair; take w/ meals

Caution: [C, ?] **CI:** Hepatic/severe renal Insuff, primary biliary cirrhosis, unexplained ↑ LFTs, gallbladder Dz **Disp:** Caps 50, 100, 150 mg; caps (micronized): (Lofibra) 67, 134, 200 mg, (Antara) 43, 130 mg; tabs 54, 160 mg **SE:** GI disturbances, cholecystitis, arthralgia, myalgia, dizziness **Interactions:** ↑ Effects *OF* anticoagulants; ↑ risk of rhabdomyolysis & ARF *W/* statins; ↑ risk of renal dysfunction *W/* immunosuppressants, nephrotoxic agents; ↓ effects *W/* bile acid sequestrants **Labs:** ↑ LFTs, BUN, Cr; ↓ Hgb, Hct, WBCs, uric acid; monitor LFTs **NIPE:** Food ↑ drug absorption; EtOH ↑ triglycerides; may take up to 2 mo to modify lipids

Fenofibric Acid (Trilipix) [Antilipemic/Fibrate] Uses: *Adjunct to diet for triglycerides, to ↓ LDL-C, cholesterol, triglycerides, & apo B, to –HDL-C in hypercholesterolemia/mixed dyslipidemia; adjunct to diet w/ a statin to ↑ triglycerides & –HDL-C w/ CHD or w/ CHD risk* **Action:** Agonist of peroxisome a proliferator-activated receptor-α (PPAR-α), causes VLDL catabolism, fatty acid oxidation, and clearing of triglyceride-rich particles w/ ↓ VLDL, triglycerides; HDL in some **Dose:** Mixed dyslipidemia w/ a statin 135 mg PO 1× daily *Hypertriglyceridemia:* 45–135 mg 1× daily; maint based on response *Primary hypercholesterolemia/mixed dyslipidemia:* 135 mg PO 1× daily; 135 mg/d max; titrate at 4–8 wk intervals **Caution:** [C, –], Multiple interactions, embolic phenomenon **CI:** Severe renal impair, pt on dialysis, active liver/gall bladder Dz, nursing **Disp:** DR caps 45, 135 mg **SE:** HA, back pain, nasopharyngitis, URI, N/D, myalgia, gall stones, rare myositis/rhabdomyolysis **Interactions:** ↑ Effects *OF* HMG-CoA reductase Inhibits, warfarin; ↑ risk of nephrotox w/ cyclosporine; ↓ effects *W/* bile acid sequestrants **Labs:** ↑ CBC (usually stabilizes), ✓ CBC, lipid panel, LFTs; D/C if LFTs > 3 × ULN **NIPE:** Avoid w/ max dose of a statin—↑ risk of myopathy; give 1h < or 4–6 h > bile acid sequestrants; use w/ low-fat/low-cholesterol diet & w/ a statin

Fenoldopam (Corlopam) [Antihypertensive/Vasodilator] Uses: *Hypertensive emergency* **Action:** Rapid vasodilator **Dose:** Initial 0.03–0.1 mcg/kg/min IV Inf, titrate q15min by 1.6 mcg/kg/min to max 0.05–0.1 mcg/kg/min **Caution:** [B, ?] w/ BBs **CI:** Allergy to sulfites **Disp:** Inj 10 mg/mL **SE:** ↓ BP, edema, facial flushing, N/V/D, atrial flutter/AF, ↑ IOP **Interactions:** ↑ Effects *W/* APAP ↑ hypotension *W/* BBs; ↓ effects *W/* DA antagonists, metoclopramide **Labs:** ↑ Serum urea nitrogen, Cr, LFTs, LDH, K+ **NIPE:** Avoid concurrent BBs; asthmatics have ↑ risk of sulfite sensitivity

Fenoprofen (Nalfon) [Analgesic/NSAID] WARNING: May ↑ risk of CV events & GI bleeding Uses: *Arthritis & pain* **Action:** NSAID **Dose:** 200–600 mg q4–8h, to 3200 mg/d max; w/ food **Caution:** [B (D 3rd tri), +/–] CHF, HTN, renal/hepatic impair, h/o PUD **CI:** NSAID sensitivity **Disp:** Caps 200, 300, 600 mg **SE:** GI disturbance, dizziness, HA, rash, edema, renal impair, hep **Interactions:** ↑ Effects *W/* ASA, anticoagulants; ↑ hyperkalemia *W/* K+-sparing diuretics; ↑ effects *OF* anticoagulants, MTX; ↓ effects *W/* phenobarbital; ↓ effects *W/* antihypertensives **Labs:** False ↑ free & total T_3 levels **NIPE:** ∅ ASA, EtOH, OTC drugs; swallow whole

Fentanyl (Sublimaze) [C-II] [Opioid Analgesic] Uses: *Short-acting analgesic* in anesthesia & PCA **Action:** Narcotic analgesic **Dose:** *Adults.* 25–100 mcg/kg/ dose IV/IM titrated *Anesthesia:* 5–15 mcg/kg *Pain:* 200 mcg over 15 min, titrate to effect *Peds.* 1–2 mcg/kg IV/IM q1–4h titrate; ↓ in renal impair **Caution:** [B, +] **CI:** Paralytic ileus ↑ ICP, resp depression, severe renal/hepatic impair **Disp:** Inj 0.05 mg/mL **SE:** Sedation, ↓ BP, bradycardia, constipation, N, resp depression, miosis **Interactions:** ↑ Effects W/ CNS depressants, cimetidine, erythromycin, ketoconazole, phenothiazine, ritonavir, TCAs, EtOH, grapefruit juice; ↑ risks of HTN crisis W/ MAOIs; ↑ risk of CNS & resp depression W/ protease Inhibs; ↓ effects W/ buprenorphine, dezocine, nalbuphine, pentazocine **Labs:** ↑ Serum amylase, lipase; ↓ HMG, Hct, plts, WBCs **NIPE:** 0.1 mg fentanyl = 10 mg morphine IM

Fentanyl Iontophoretic Transdermal System (Ionsys) [Opioid Analgesic] WARNING: Use only w/ hospitalized pts, D/C on discharge; fentanyl may result in potentially life-threatening resp depression & death Uses: *Short-term in-hospital analgesia* **Action:** Opioid narcotic, iontophoretic transdermal **Dose:** 40 mcg/activation by pt; dose given over 10 min; max over 24 h 3.2 mg (80 doses) **Caution:** [C, –] **CI:** See Fentanyl **Disp:** Battery-operated self-contained transdermal system, 40 mcg/activation, 80 doses **SE:** See Fentanyl, site Rxn **Interactions:** ↑ Effects W/ CNS depressants, cimetidine, erythromycin, ketoconazole, phenothiazine, ritonavir, TCAs, EtOH, grapefruit juice; ↑ risks of HTN crisis W/ MAOIs; ↑ risk of CNS & resp depression W/ protease Inhibs; ↓ effects W/ buprenorphine, dezocine, nalbuphine, pentazocine **Labs:** ↑ Serum amylase, lipase; ↓ HMG, Hct, plts, WBCs **NIPE:** Choose nl skin site chest or upper outer arm; pts must have access to supplemental analgesia; instruct in device use; dispose properly at discharge

Fentanyl, Transdermal (Duragesic) [C-II] [Opioid Analgesic] WARNING: Potential for abuse & fatal OD Uses: *Persistent mod–severe chronic pain in pts already tolerant to opioids* **Action:** Narcotic **Dose:** Apply patch to upper torso q72h; dose based on narcotic requirements in previous 24 h; start 25 mcg/h patch q72h; ↑ fentanyl effect, w/ h/o substance abuse **CI:** Not opioid tolerant, short-term pain management, post-op pain in outpatient surgery, mild pain, PRN use ↑ ICP, resp depression, severe renal/hepatic impair, peds < 2 y **Disp:** Patches 12.5, 25, 50, 75, 100 mcg/h **SE:** Resp depression (fatal), sedation, ↓ BP, bradycardia, constipation, N, miosis **Interactions:** ↑ Effects W/ CNS depressants, cimetidine, erythromycin, ketoconazole, phenothiazine, ritonavir, TCAs, EtOH, grapefruit juice; ↑ risks of HTN crisis W/ MAOIs; ↑ risk of CNS & resp depression W/ protease Inhibs; ↓ effects W/ buprenorphine, dezocine, nalbuphine, pentazocine **Labs:** ↑ Serum amylase, lipase; ↓ HMG, Hct, plts, WBCs **NIPE:** 0.1 mg fentanyl = 10 mg morphine IM; do not cut patch; peak level 24–72 h; ↑ risk of ↑ absorption w/ elevated temperature; cleanse skin only w/ H_2O; ⊘ soap, lotions, or EtOH because they may ↑ absorption; ⊘ use in children < 110 lb

Fentanyl, Transmucosal (Abstral, Actiq, Fentora, Onsolis) [C-II] [Opioid Analgesic] **WARNING:** Potential for abuse & fatal OD; use only in pts w/ chronic pain who are opioid tolerant; CI in acute/post-op pain; do not substitute for other fentanyl products; fentanyl can be fatal to children, keep away; use w/ strong CYP3A4 Inhib; may ↑ fentanyl levels. *Abstral, Onsolis* restricted distribution **Uses:** *Breakthrough CA pain w/ tolerance to opioids* **Action:** Narcotic analgesic, transmucosal absorption **Dose:** Titrate to effect *Abstral*: Start 100 mcg SL, 2 doses max per pain breakthrough episode; wait 2 h for next breakthrough dose; limit to < 4 breakthrough doses w/ successful baseline dosing *Actiq*: Start 200 mcg PO × 1, may repeat × 1 after 30 min *Fentora*: Start 100 mcg buccal tab × 1, may repeat in 30 min, 4 tabs/dose max *Onsolis*: Start 200 mcg film, ↑ 200 mcg increments to max four 200 mcg films or single 1200 mcg film **Caution:** [B, +] Resp/CNS depression possible; CNS depressants/CYP3A4 Inhib may ↑ effect; may impair tasks (driving, machinery); w/ severe renal/hepatic impair **CI:** Opioid intolerant pts, acute/post-op pain **Disp:** *Abstral*: SL tab 100, 200, 300, 400, 600, 800 mcg *Actiq*: Lozenges on stick 200, 400, 600, 800, 1200, 1600 mcg *Fentora*: Buccal tabs 100, 200, 300, 400, 600, 800 mcg *Onsolis*: Buccal soluble film 200, 400, 600, 800, 1200 mcg **SE:** Sedation, ↓ BP, ↓ HR, constipation, N/V, ↓ resp, dyspnea, HA, miosis, anxiety, confusion, depression, rash dizziness **Interactions:** ↑ Effects **W/** CNS depressants, cimetidine, erythromycin, ketoconazole, phenothiazine, ritonavir, TCAs, EtOH, grapefruit juice; ↑ risks of HTN crisis **W/** MAOIs; ↑ risk of CNS & resp depression **W/** protease Inhibs; ↓ effects **W/** buprenorphine, dezocine, nalbuphine, pentazocine **Labs:** ↑ Serum amylase, lipase; ↓ HMG, Hct, plts, WBCs **NIPE:** 0.1 mg fentanyl = 10 mg IM morphine; for use in pts already tolerant to opioid therapy; ○ use w/in 14 d of MAOI

Ferrous Gluconate (Fergon [OTC], Others) [Oral Iron Supplement] **WARNING:** Accidental OD of Fe-containing products is a leading cause of fatal poisoning in children < 6. Keep out of reach of children **Uses:** *Fe-deficiency anemia* & *Fe supls* **Action:** Dietary supls **Dose:** *Adults.* 100–200 mg of elemental Fe/d ÷ doses **Peds.** 4–6 mg/kg/d ÷ doses; on empty stomach (OK w/ meals if GI upset occurs); avoid antacids **Caution:** [A, ?] **CI:** Hemochromatosis, hemolytic anemia **Disp:** Tabs Fergon 240 mg (27 mg Fe), 246 mg (28 mg Fe), 300 mg (34 mg Fe), 325 mg (36 mg Fe) **SE:** GI upset, constipation, dark stools, discoloration of urine, may stain teeth **Interactions:** ↑ Effects **W/** chloramphenicol, citrus fruits or juices, vit C; ↓ effects **W/** antacids, levodopa, black cohosh, chamomile, feverfew, gossypol, hawthorn, nettle, plantain, St. John's wort, whole-grain breads, cheese, eggs, milk, coffee, tea, yogurt; ↓ effects **OF** fluoroquinolones, tetracycline **Labs:** False(+) stool guaiac test **NIPE:** ○ Antacids, tetracyclines, take Liq form in Liq & through a straw to prevent teeth staining; 12% elemental Fe; keep away from children; severe tox in OD

Ferrous Gluconate Complex (Ferrlecit) [Iron Supplement] **Uses:** *Fe-deficiency anemia or supls to erythropoietin therapy* **Action:** Fe supls **Dose:**

Test **Dose:** 2 mL (25 mg Fe) IV over 1 h, if OK, 125 mg (10 mL) IV over 1 h *Usual cumulative* **Dose:** 1 g Fe over 8 sessions (until favorable Hct) **Caution:** [B, ?] **CI:** Non–Fe-deficiency anemia; CHF; Fe overload **Disp:** Inj 12.5 mg/mL Fe **SE:** ↓ BP, serious allergic Rxns, GI disturbance, Inj site Rxn **Interactions:** ↑ Effects *W/* chloramphenicol, citrus fruits or juices, vit C; ↓ effects *W/* antacids, levodopa, black cohosh, chamomile, feverfew, gossypol, hawthorn, nettle, plantain, St. John's wort, whole-grain breads, cheese, eggs, milk, coffee, tea, yogurt; ↓ effects *OF* fluoroquinolones, tetracycline **Labs:** False(+) stool guaiac test **NIPE:** Dose expressed as mg Fe; may infuse during dialysis

Ferrous Sulfate (OTC) [Iron Supplement]
Uses: *Fe-deficiency anemia & Fe supls* **Action:** Dietary supls **Dose:** *Adults.* 100–200 mg elemental Fe/d in ÷ doses *Peds.* 1–6 mg/kg/d ÷ daily–tid; on empty stomach (OK w/ meals if GI upset occurs); avoid antacids **Caution:** [A, ?] ↑ Absorption w/ vit C; ↓ absorption w/ tetracycline, fluoroquinolones, antacids, H₂-blockers, PPI **CI:** Hemochromatosis, hemolytic anemia **Disp:** Tabs 187 mg (60 mg Fe), 200 mg (65 mg Fe), 324 mg (65 mg Fe), 325 mg (65 mg Fe); SR caplets & tabs 160 mg (50 mg Fe), 200 mg (65 mg Fe); gtt 75 mg/0.6 mL (15 mg Fe/0.6 mL); elixir 220 mg/5 mL (44 mg Fe/5 mL); syrup 90 mg/5 mL (18 mg Fe/5 mL) **SE:** GI upset, constipation, dark stools, discolored urine **Interactions:** ↑ Effects *W/* chloramphenicol, citrus fruits or juices, vit C; ↓ effects *W/* antacids, levodopa, black cohosh, chamomile, feverfew, gossypol, hawthorn, nettle, plantain, St. John's wort, whole-grain breads, cheese, eggs, milk, coffee, tea, yogurt; ↓ effects *OF* fluoroquinolones, tetracycline **Labs:** False(+) stool guaiac test **NIPE:** Take w/ meals if GI upset; can cause severe tox

Ferumoxytol (Feraheme) [Hematinic]
Uses: *Fe-deficiency anemia in chronic kidney Dz* **Action:** Fe replacement **Dose:** *Adults.* 510 mg IV × 1, then 510 mg IV × 1 3–8 later; give 1 mL/s **Caution:** [C, ?/–] Monitor for hypersensitivity & ↓ BP for 30 min after dose **CI:** Fe overload; hypersensitivity to ferumoxytol **Disp:** IV soln 30 mg/mL (510 mg elemental Fe/17 mL) **SE:** N/D, constipation, dizziness, hypotension, peripheral edema, hypersensitivity Rxn **Interactions:** May ↓ absorption *OF* oral Fe Prep **Labs:** May transiently (up to 3 mo) affect diagnostic ability of MRI **NIPE:** ✓ Hematologic response 1 mo after 2nd dose

Fesoterodine Fumarate (Toviaz) [Muscarinic Receptor Antagonist]
Uses: *OAB w/ urge urinary incontinence, urgency, frequency* **Action:** Competitive muscarinic receptor antagonist, ↓ bladder muscle contractions **Dose:** 4 mg PO qd, to 8 mg PO daily PRN **Caution:** [C, –] Avoid > 4 mg w/ severe renal Insuff or w/ CYP3A4 Inhibs (eg, ketoconazole, clarithromycin); w/ BOO, ↓ GI motility/constipation, NAG, MyG **CI:** Urinary/gastric retention, or uncontrolled NAG, hypersensitivity to class **Disp:** Tabs 5, 10 mg **SE:** Dry mouth, constipation, ↓ sweating can cause heat prostration **Interactions:** ↑ Effects *W/* CYP3A4 Inhibs: Amiodarone, amprenavir, atazanavir, ciprofloxacin, cisapride, clarithromycin, diltiazem, erythromycin, fluconazole, fluvoxamine, indinavir, itraconazole, ketoconazole, nefazodone, nelfinavir, norfloxacin, ritonavir, telithromycin, troleandomycin, verapamil

voriconazole, grapefruit juice; ↑ CNS depression W/ EtOH, other CNS depressants
NIPE: Swallow whole, in elderly (> 75 y)—↑ risk of anticholinergic SEs

Fexofenadine (Allegra, Allegra-D) [Antihistamine/H₁-Receptor Antagonist] Uses: *Allergic rhinitis chronic idiopathic urticaria* Action: Selective antihistamine, antagonizes H₁-receptors; Allegra D contains pseudoephedrine Dose: *Adults & Peds > 12 y.* 60 mg PO bid or 180 mg/d; 12-h ER form bid, 24-h ER form qd *Peds 6–11 y.* 30 mg PO bid; ↓ in renal impair Caution: [C, ?] W/ Nevirapine CI: Component sensitivity Disp: Tabs 30, 60, 180 mg; Susp 6 mg/mL; Allegra-D 12-h ER tab (60 mg fexofenadine/120 mg pseudoephedrine), Allegra-D 24-h ER tab (180 mg fexofenadine/240 mg pseudoephedrine) SE: Drowsiness (rare), HA Interactions: ↑ Effects W/ erythromycin, ketoconazole; ↓ absorption & effects W/ antacids, apples, OJ, grapefruit juice NIPE: ⊘ EtOH or CNS depressants

Fidaxomicin (Dificid) [Macrolide/Antibiotic] Uses: *C difficile–associated D* Action: Macrolide antibiotic Dose: 200 mg PO bid × 10 d Caution: [B, +/–] Not for systemic Infxn or < 18 y; to ↓ resistance, use only when diagnosis suspected/proven Disp: Tabs 200 mg SE: N/V, Abd pain, GI bleed, anemia, neutropenia NIPE: Minimal systemic absorption

Filgrastim [G-CSF] (Neupogen) [Hematopoietic/Colony-Stimulating Factor] Uses: *↑ Incidence of Infxn in febrile neutropenic pts; Rx chronic neutropenia* Action: Recombinant G-CSF Dose: *Adults & Peds.* 5 mcg/kg/d SQ or IV single daily dose; D/C when ANC > 10,000 cells/mm³ Caution: [C, ?] w/ drugs that potentiate release of neutrophils (eg, Li) CI: Allergy to *E coli*–derived proteins or G-CSF Disp: Inj 300, 600 mcg/mL SE: Fever, alopecia, N/V/D, splenomegaly, bone pain, HA, rash Interactions: ↑ Interference W/ cytotoxic drugs; ↑ release of neutrophils W/ Li Labs: Monitor CBC & plts NIPE: Monitor for cardiac events; no benefit W/ ANC > 10,000 cells/mm³

Finasteride (Proscar, Propecia) [Androgen Hormone Inhibitor/Steroid] Uses: *BPH & androgenetic alopecia* Action: ↓ 5α-Reductase Dose: *BPH:* 5 mg/d PO *Alopecia:* 1 mg/d PO; food ↓ absorption Caution: [X, –] Hepatic impair CI: Pregnant women should avoid handling pills, teratogen to male fetus Disp: Tabs 1 mg (*Propecia*), 5 mg (*Proscar*) SE: ↓ Libido, vol ejaculate, ED, gynecomastia Interactions: ↑ Effects W/ saw palmetto; ↓ effects W/ anticholinergics, adrenergic bronchodilators, theophylline Labs: ↓ PSA by 50%; reestablish PSA baseline 6 mo (double PSA for "true" reading) NIPE: 3–6 mo for effect on urinary Sxs; continue to maint new hair, not for use in women; potential chemoprevention for PCa; no role in diagnosed PCa

Fingolimod (Gilenya) [Sphingosine 1-Phosphate Receptor Modulator] Uses: *Relapsing MS* Action: Sphingosine 1-phosphate receptor modulator; ↓ lymphocyte migration into CNS Dose: *Adults.* 0.5 mg PO once/d; monitor for 6 h after 1st dose for bradycardia; monitor Caution: [C, –] Monitor w/ severe hepatic impair ; avoid live vaccines during & 2 mo after D/C Disp: Caps

0.5 mg **SE:** HA, D, back pain, dizziness, bradycardia, AV block, HTN, Infxns, macular edema, cough, dyspnea **Interactions:** ↑ Risk of rhythm disturbances W/ Class Ia or III ;↑ levels W/ ketoconazole **Labs:** ↑ LFTs; obtain baseline CBC, LFTs **NIPE:** Obtain baseline ECG, & eye exam; women of childbearing potential should use contraception during & 2 mo after D/C

Flavoxate (Urispas) [Antispasmodic] Uses: *Relief of Sx of dysuria, urgency, nocturia, suprapubic pain, urinary frequency, incontinence* **Action:** Antispasmodic **Dose:** 100–200 mg PO tid–qid **Caution:** [B, ?] **CI:** GI obst, GI hemorrhage, ileus, achalasia, BPH **Disp:** Tabs 100 mg **SE:** Drowsiness, blurred vision, xerostomia **Interactions:** ↑ Effects OF CNS depressants **NIPE:** ↑ Risk of heat stroke w/ exercise & in hot weather

Flecainide (Tambocor) [Antiarrhythmic/Benzamide Anesthetic] **WARNING:** ↑ Mortality in pts w/ ventricular arrhythmias & recent MI; pulm effects reported; ventricular proarrhythmic effects in AF/A flutter, not recommended for chronic AF Uses: Prevent AF/A flutter & PSVT, *prevent/suppress life-threatening ventricular arrhythmias* **Action:** Class Ic antiarrhythmic **Dose:** *Adults.* 100 mg PO q12h; ↑ by 50 mg q12h q4d to max 400 mg/d **Peds.** 3–6 mg/kg/d in 3 ÷ doses; ↓ w/ renal impair **Caution:** [C, +] Monitor w/ hepatic impair; ↑ conc w/ amiodarone, digoxin, quinidine, ritonavir/amprenavir, BBs, verapamil; may worsen arrhythmias **CI:** 2nd-/3rd-degree AV block, right BBB w/ bifascicular or trifascicular block, cardiogenic shock, CAD, ritonavir/amprenavir, alkalinizing agents **Disp:** Tabs 50, 100, 150 mg **SE:** Dizziness, visual disturbances, dyspnea, palpitations, edema, CP, tachycardia, CHF, HA, fatigue, rash, N **Notes:** *Levels: Trough:* Just before next dose; *Therapeutic:* 0.2–1 mcg/mL; *Toxic:* > 1 mcg/mL; *1/2-life:* 11–14 h **Interactions:** ↑ Effects W/ alkalinizing drugs, amiodarone, cimetidine, propranolol, quinidine; ↑ effects OF digoxin; ↑ risk of arrhythmias W/ CCBs, antiarrhythmics, disopyramide; ↓ effects W/ acidifying drugs, tobacco **Labs:** ↑ Alk phos **NIPE:** Initiate Rx in hospital; dose q8h if pt is intolerant/uncontrolled at q12h; full effects may take 3–5 d

Floxuridine (FUDR) [Pyrimidine Antimetabolite] **WARNING:** Administration by experienced physician only; pts should be hospitalized for 1st course d/t risk for severe Rxn Uses: *GI adenoma, liver, renal CAs*; colon & pancreatic CAs **Action:** Converted to 5-FU; inhibits thymidylate synthase; ↓ DNA synthase (S-phase specific) **Dose:** 0.1–0.6 mg/kg/d for 1–6 wk (per protocols) usually intra-arterial for liver mets **Caution:** [D, –] Interaction w/ vaccines **CI:** BM suppression, poor nutritional status, serious Infxn, PRG, component sensitivity **Disp:** Inj 500 mg **SE:** ↓ BM, anorexia, Abd cramps, N/V/D, mucositis, alopecia, skin rash, & hyperpigmentation; rare neurotox (blurred vision, depression, nystagmus, vertigo, & lethargy); intra-arterial catheter-related problems (ischemia, thrombosis, bleeding, & Infxn) **Interactions:** ↑ Effects W/ metronidazole **Labs:** ↑ LFTs, 5-HIAA urine excretion; ↓ plasma albumin **NIPE:** Need effective birth control; palliative Rx for inoperable/incurable pts; ↑ risk of photosensitivity—use sunscreen

Fluconazole (Diflucan) [Antifungal/Synthetic Azole] Uses: *Candidiasis (esophageal, oropharyngeal, urinary tract, Vag prophylaxis); cryptococcal meningitis, prophylaxis w/ BMT* Action: Antifungal; ↓ cytochrome P-450 sterol demethylation *Spectrum:* All *Candida* sp except *C krusei* Dose: *Adults.* 100–400 mg/d PO or IV *Vaginitis:* 150 mg PO daily *Crypto:* Doses up to 800 mg/d reported: 400 mg d 1, then 200 mg × 10–12 wk after CSF(−) Peds. 3–6 mg/kg/d PO or IV; 12 mg/kg/d/systemic Infxn; ↓ in renal impair Caution: [C, −] CI: None Disp: Tabs 50, 100, 150, 200 mg; susp 10, 40 mg/mL; Inj 2 mg/mL SE: HA, rash, GI upset Interactions: ↑ Effects *W/* HCTZ, anticoagulants; ↑ effects *OF* amitriptyline, benzodiazepines, carbamazepine, cyclosporine, hypoglycemics, losartan, methadone, phenytoin, quinidine, tacrolimus, TCAs, theophylline, caffeine, zidovudine; ↓ effects *W/* cimetidine, rifampin Labs: ↑ LFTs; ↓ K⁺ NIPE: PO (preferred) = IV levels; monitor ECG for hypokalemia (flattened T waves)

Fludarabine Phosphate (Flamp, Fludara) [Antineoplastic] WARNING: Administration only under supervision of qualified physician experienced in chemotherapy. Can ↓ BM & cause severe CNS effects (blindness, coma, & death). Severe/fatal autoimmune hemolytic anemia reported; monitor for hemolysis. Use w/ pentostatin not recommended (fatal pulm tox) Uses: *Autoimmune hemolytic anemia, CLL, cold agglutinin hemolysis*, low-grade lymphoma, mycosis fungoides Action: ↓ Ribonucleotide reductase; blocks DNA polymerase-induced DNA repair Dose: 18–30 mg/m²/d for 5 d, as a 30-min Inf (per protocols); ↓ w/ renal impair Caution: [D, −] Give cytarabine before fludarabine (↓ its metabolism) CI: w/ Pentostatin, severe Infxns, CrCl < 30 mL/min, hemolytic anemia Disp: Inj 50 mg SE: ↓ BM, N/V/D, edema, CHF, fever, chills, fatigue, dyspnea, nonproductive cough, pneumonitis, severe CNS tox rare in leukemia, autoimmune hemolytic anemia Interactions: ↑ Effects *W/* other myelosuppressive drugs; ↑ risk of pulm effects *W/* pentostatin Labs: ↑ LFTs NIPE: May take several wk for full effect, use barrier contraception

Fludrocortisone Acetate (Florinef) [Steroid/Mineralocorticoid] Uses: *Adrenocortical Insuff, Addison Dz, salt-wasting synd* Action: Mineralocorticoid Dose: *Adults.* 0.1–0.2 mg/d PO Peds. 0.05–0.1 mg/d PO Caution: [C, ?] CI: Systemic fungal Infxns; known allergy Disp: Tabs 0.1 mg SE: HTN, edema, CHF, HA, dizziness, convulsions, acne, rash, bruising, hyperglycemia, hypothalamic-pituitary-adrenal suppression, cataracts Interactions: ↑ Risk of hypokalemia *W/* amphotericin B, thiazide diuretics, loop diuretics; ↓ effects *W/* rifampin, barbiturates, hydantoins; ↓ effects *OF* ASA, INH Labs: ↓ Serum K⁺ NIPE: Eval for fluid retention; for adrenal Insuff, use w/ glucocorticoid; dose changes based on plasma renin activity; monitor ECG for hypokalemia (flattened T waves)

Flumazenil (Romazicon) [Antidote/Antibenzodiazepine] Uses: *Reverse sedative effects of benzodiazepines & general anesthesia* Action: Benzodiazepine receptor antagonist Dose: *Adults.* 0.2 mg IV over 15 s; repeat PRN, to 1 mg max (5 mg max in benzodiazepine OD) Peds. 0.01 mg/kg (0.2 mg/dose max) IV over 15 s;

repeat 0.005 mg/kg at 1-min intervals to max 1 mg total; ↓ in hepatic impair **Caution:** [C, ?] **CI:** TCA OD; if pts given benzodiazepines to control life-threatening conditions (ICP/status epilepticus) **Disp:** Inj 0.1 mg/mL **SE:** N/V, palpitations, HA, anxiety, nervousness, hot flashes, tremor, blurred vision, dyspnea, hyperventilation, withdrawal synd **Interactions:** ↑ Risk of Szs & arrhythmias when benzodiazepine action is reduced **NIPE:** Food given during IV administration will reduce drug serum level; does not reverse narcotic Sx or amnesia; use associated w/ Szs

Flunisolide (AeroBid, Aerospan, Nasarel) [Corticosteroid] Uses: *Asthma in pts requiring chronic steroid therapy; relieve seasonal/perennial allergic rhinitis* **Action:** Topical steroid **Dose:** *Adults. Metered-dose Inh:* 2 Inh bid (max 8/d) *Nasal:* 2 sprays/nostril bid (max 8/d) *Peds > 6 y. Metered-dose Inh:* 2 Inh bid (max 4/d) *Nasal:* 1–2 sprays/nostril bid (max 4/d) **Caution:** [C, ?] w/ Adrenal Insuff **CI:** Status asthmaticus, viral, TB, fungal, bacterial Infxn **Disp:** AeroBid 0.25 mg/Inh; Nasarel 29 mcg/spray; Aerospan 80 mcg/Inh (CFC-Free) **SE:** Tachycardia, bitter taste, local effects, oral candidiasis **NIPE:** Shake well before use; not for acute asthma

Fluorouracil [5-FU] (Adrucil) [Antineoplastic/Antimetabolite] **WARNING:** Administration by experienced chemotherapy physician only; pts should be hospitalized for 1st course d/t risk for severe Rxn Uses: *Colorectal, gastric, pancreatic, breast, basal cell*, head, neck, bladder, Ca **Action:** Inhibits thymidylate synthetase (↓ DNA synth, S-phase specific) **Dose:** 370–1000 mg/m²/d × 1–5 d IV push to 24-h cont Inf; protracted venous Inf of 200–300 mg/m²/d (per protocol); 800 mg/d max **Caution:** [D, ?] ↑ Tox w/ allopurinol; do not give *Moraxella catarrhalis* vaccine (MRX) before 5-FU **CI:** Poor nutritional status, depressed BM Fxn, not for use in asymptomatic patients, major surgery w/in past mo, G6PD enzyme deficiency, PRG, serious Infxn, bilirubin > 5 mg/dL **Disp:** Inj 50 mg/mL **SE:** Stomatitis, esophagopharyngitis, N/V/D, anorexia, ↓ BM, rash/dry skin/photosensitivity, tingling in hands/feet w/ pain (palmar–plantar erythrodysesthesia), phlebitis/discoloration at Inj sites **Interactions:** ↑ Effects W/ leucovorin Ca **Labs:** ↑ LFTs **NIPE:** ↑ Thiamine intake; ⊘ EtOH, ↑ risk of photosensitivity—use sunscreen, ↑ fluids 2–3 L/d, use barrier contraception

Fluorouracil, Topical [5-FU] (Efudex) [Antineoplastic/Antimetabolite] Uses: *Basal cell carcinoma; actinic/solar keratosis* **Action:** Inhibits thymidylate synthetase (↓ DNA synth, S-phase specific) **Dose:** 5% cream bid × 2–6 wk **Caution:** [D, ?] Irritant chemotherapy **CI:** Component sensitivity **Disp:** Cream 0.5%, 1%, 5%; soln 1%, 2%, 5% **SE:** Rash, dry skin, photosensitivity **NIPE:** Healing may not be evident for 1–2 mo; wash hands thoroughly; avoid occlusive dressings; do not overuse

Fluoxetine (Prozac, Sarafem) [Antidepressant/SSRI] **WARNING:** Closely monitor for worsening depression or emergence of suicidality, particularly in ped pts Uses: *Depression, obsessive-compulsive disorder (OCD), panic disorder, bulimia (Prozac)**PMDD (Sarafem)* **Action:** SSRI **Dose:** 20 mg/d PO (max

80 mg/d ÷ dose); weekly 90 mg/wk after 1–2 wk of standard dose *Bulimia:* 60 mg qAM *Panic disorder:* 20 mg/d *OCD:* 20–80 mg/d *PMDD:* 20 mg/d or 20 mg intermittently, start 14 d prior to menses, repeat w/ each cycle; ↓ in hepatic failure **Caution:** [C, ?/–] Serotonin synd w/ MAOI, SSRI, serotonin agonists; linezolid; QT prolongation w/ phenothiazines **CI:** MAOI/thioridazine (wait 5 wk after D/C before w/ MAOI) **Disp:** *Prozac:* Caps 10, 20, 40 mg; scored tabs 10, 20 mg; SR caps 90 mg; soln 20 mg/5 mL *Sarafem:* Caps 10, 20 mg **SE:** N, nervousness, wgt loss, HA, insomnia **Interactions:** ↑ Effects *W/* CNS depressants, MAOIs, EtOH, St. John's wort; ↑ effects *OF* alprazolam, BBs, carbamazepine, clozapine, cardiac glycosides, diazepam, dextromethorphan, loop diuretics, haloperidol, phenytoin, Li, ritonavir, thioridazine, tryptophan, warfarin, sympathomimetic drugs; ↓ effects *W/* cyproheptadine; ↓ effects *OF* buspirone, statins **Labs:** ↑ LFTs, BUN, Cr, urine albumin **NIPE:** ↑ Risk of serotonin synd *W/* St. John's wort; may take > 4 wk for full effects

Fluoxymesterone (Halotestin, Androxy) [CIII] [Hormone]
Uses: Androgen-responsive met *breast CA, hypogonadism* **Action:** ↓ Secretion of LH & FSH (feedback inhibition) **Dose:** *Breast CA:* 10–40 mg/d ÷ × 1–3 mo *Hypogonadism:* 5–20 mg/d **Caution:** [X, ?/–] ↑ Effect w/ anticoagulants, cyclosporine, insulin, Li, narcotics **CI:** Serious cardiac, liver, or kidney Dz; PRG **Disp:** Tabs 10 mg **SE:** Priapism, edema, virilization, amenorrhea & menstrual irregularities, hirsutism, alopecia, acne, N, cholestasis; suppression of factors II, V, VII, & X, & polycythemia; ↑ libido, HA, anxiety **Interactions:** ↑ Effects *W/* narcotics, EtOH, echinacea; ↑ effects *OF* anticoagulants, cyclosporine, insulin, hypoglycemics, tacrolimus; ↓ effects *W/* anticholinergics, barbiturates **Labs:** ↑ Cr, CrCl; ↓ thyroxine-binding globulin, ↓ serum total T_4 **NIPE:** Radiographic exam of hand/wrist q6mo in prepubertal children

Fluphenazine (Prolixin, Permitil) [Antipsychotic/Phenothiazine]
Uses: *Schizophrenia* **Action:** Phenothiazine antipsychotic; blocks postsynaptic mesolimbic dopaminergic brain receptors **Dose:** 0.5–10 mg/d in ⅓ doses PO q6–8h, average maint 5 mg/d; or 1.25 mg IM, then 2.5–10 mg/d in ⅓ doses q6–8h PRN; ↓ in elderly **Caution:** [C, ?/–] **CI:** Severe CNS depression, coma, subcortical brain damage, blood dyscrasias, hepatic Dz, w/ caffeine, tannic acid, or pectin-containing products **Disp:** Tabs 1, 2.5, 5, 10 mg; elixir 2.5 mg/5 mL; Inj 2.5 mg/mL; depot Inj 25 mg/mL **SE:** Drowsiness, extrapyramidal effects **Interactions:** ↑ Effects *W/* antimalarials, BBs, CNS depressants, EtOH, kava kava; ↑ effects *OF* anticholinergics, BBs, nitrates; ↓ effects *W/* antacids, caffeine, tobacco; ↓ effects *OF* anticonvulsants, guanethidine, levodopa, sympathomimetics **Labs:** ↑ LFTs, ↓ HMG, Hct, plts, WBC **NIPE:** ↑ Risk of photosensitivity—use sunblock; urine may turn pink or red, ↑ risk of heatstroke in hot weather; less sedative/hypotensive than chlorpromazine; may cause over sedation w/ anticholinergics

Flurazepam (Dalmane) [C-IV] [Sedative/Hypnotic/Benzodiazepine]
Uses: *Insomnia* **Action:** Benzodiazepine **Dose:** *Adults & Peds > 15 y.* 15–30 mg PO qhs PRN; ↓ in elderly **Caution:** [X, ?/–] Elderly, low albumin, hepatic

impair **CI:** NAG; PRG **Disp:** Caps 15, 30 mg **SE:** "Hangover" d/t accumulation of metabolites, apnea, anaphylaxis, angioedema, amnesia **Interactions:** ↑ CNS depression W/ antidepressants, antihistamines, opioids, EtOH; ↑ effects OF digoxin, phenytoin; ↑ effects W/ cimetidine, disulfiram, fluoxetine, INH, ketoconazole, metoprolol, OCPs, propranolol, SSRIs, valproic acid, chamomile, kava kava, passion flower, valerian; ↓ effects OF levodopa; ↓ effects W/ barbiturates, rifampin, theophylline, nicotine **Labs:** ↑ LFTs **NIPE:** ⊘ In PRG or lactation; use adequate contraception; ⊘ EtOH; ⊘ D/C abruptly w/ long-term use; may cause dependency

Flurbiprofen (Ansaid, Ocufen) [Analgesic/NSAID] WARNING: May ↑ risk of CV events & GI bleeding **Uses:** *Arthritis, ocular surgery* **Action:** NSAID **Dose:** 50–300 mg/d ÷ bid–qid, max 300 mg/d w/ food, ocular 1 gtt q30 min × 4, beginning 2 h pre-op **Caution:** [B (D in 3rd tri), +] **CI:** PRG (3rd tri); ASA allergy **Disp:** Tabs 50, 100 mg **SE:** Dizziness, GI upset, PUD, ocular irritation **Interactions:** ↑ Effects W/ amprenavir, anticonvulsants, azole antifungals, BBs, CNS depressants, cimetidine, ciprofloxin, clozapine, digoxin, disulfiram, diltiazem, INH, levodopa, macrolides, OCPs, rifampin, ritonavir, SSRIs, valproic acid, verapamil, EtOH, grapefruit juice, kava kava, valerian; ↓ effects W/ aminophylline, carbamazepine, rifampin, rifabutin, theophylline; ↓ effects OF levodopa **Labs:** ↑ LFTs **NIPE:** ⊘ PRG, breast-feeding; take w/ food to ↓ GI upset

Flutamide (Eulexin) [Antineoplastic/Antiandrogen] WARNING: Liver failure & death reported. Measure LFTs before, monthly, & periodically after; D/C stat if ALT 2 × ULN or jaundice develops **Uses:** Advanced *PCa* (w/ LHRH agonists, eg, leuprolide or goserelin); w/ radiation & GnRH for localized CAP **Action:** Nonsteroidal antiandrogen **Dose:** 250 mg PO tid (750 mg total) **Caution:** [D, ?] **CI:** Severe hepatic impair **Disp:** Caps 125 mg **SE:** Hot flashes, loss of libido, impotence, N/V/D, gynecomastia, hepatic failure **Interactions:** ↑ Effects W/ anticoagulants **Labs:** ↑ LFTs (monitor) **NIPE:** ⊘ EtOH; urine amber/yellow-green in color

Fluticasone Furoate (Veramyst) [Steroid] **Uses:** *Seasonal allergic rhinitis* **Action:** Topical steroid **Dose:** *Adults & Peds > 12 y.* 2 sprays/nostril/d, then 1 spray/d maint *Peds 2–11 y.* 1–2 sprays/nostril/d **Caution:** [C, M] Avoid w/ ritonavir, other steroids, recent nasal surgery/trauma **CI:** None **Disp:** Nasal spray 27.5 mcg/actuation **SE:** HA, epistaxis, nasopharyngitis, pyrexia, pharyngolaryngeal pain, cough, nasal ulcers, back pain, anaphylaxis **Interactions:** ⊘ Ritonavir & caution w/ potent CYP3A4 Inhib (Table 10) **NIPE:** Monitor for growth suppression in children; ↑ risk of *Candida* Infxns

Fluticasone Propionate, Nasal (Flonase) [Anti-Inflammatory/ Corticosteroid] **Uses:** *Seasonal allergic rhinitis* **Action:** Topical steroid **Dose:** *Adults & Peds > 12 y.* 2 sprays/nostril/d **Peds 4–11 y.** 1–2 sprays/nostril/d **Caution:** [C, M] **CI:** Primary Rx of status asthmaticus **Disp:** Nasal spray 50 mcg/actuation **SE:** HA, dysphonia, oral candidiasis **Interactions:** ↑ Effects W/ ketoconazole **Labs:** ↑ Glucose **NIPE:** Clear nares of exudate before use

Fluticasone Propionate, Inhalation (Flovent HFA, Flovent Diskus) [Anti-Inflammatory/Corticosteroid] Uses: *Chronic asthma* Action: Topical steroid Dose: *Adults & Peds > 12 y.* 2–4 puffs bid *Peds 4–11 y.* 50 or 44 mcg bid Caution: [C, M] CI: Status asthmaticus Disp: *Diskus* dry powder: 50, 100, 250 mcg/action; *HFA*; MDI 44/110/220 mcg/Inh SE: HA, dysphonia, oral candidiasis Interactions: ↑ Effects W/ ketoconazole Labs: ↑ Cholesterol NIPE: Risk of thrush, rinse mouth after; consult use of devices

Fluticasone Propionate & Salmeterol Xinafoate (Advair Diskus, Advair HFA, 45/21, 115/21, 230/21 Inhaled Aerosol) [Anti-Inflammatory/Corticosteroid] WARNING: ↑ Risk of worsening wheezing or asthma-related death w/ LA β₂-adrenergic agonists Uses: *Maint therapy for asthma* Action: Corticosteroid w/ LA bronchodilator β₂ agonist Dose: *Adults & Peds > 12 y.* 1 Inh bid q12h; titrate to lowest effective dose (4 Inh or 920/84 mcg/d max) Caution: [C, M] CI: Acute asthma attack; conversion from PO steroids; w/ phenothiazines Disp: Diskus = metered-dose Inh powder (fluticasone mcg /salmeterol mcg) 100/50, 250/50, 500/50; HFA = aerosol 45/21, 115/21, 230/21 mg SE: URI, pharyngitis, HA Interactions: ↑ Bronchospasm W/ BBs; ↑ hypokalemia W/ loop & thiazide diuretics; ↑ effects W/ ketoconazole, MAOIs, TCAs Labs: ↑ Cholesterol NIPE: Combo of Flovent & Serevent; do not wash mouthpiece, do not exhale into device; Advair HFA for pts not controlled on other meds (eg, low-medium dose Inh steroids) or whose Dz severity warrants 2 maint therapies; rinse mouth after use

Fluvastatin (Lescol) [Antilipemic/HMG-CoA Reductase Inhibitor] Uses: *Atherosclerosis, primary hypercholesterolemia, heterozygous familial hypercholesterolemia hypertriglyceridemia* Action: HMG-CoA reductase Inhib Dose: 20–40 mg bid PO or XL 80 mg/d ↓ w/ hepatic impair Caution: [X, −] CI: Active liver Dz, ↑ LFTs, PRG, breast-feeding Disp: Caps 20, 40 mg; XL 80 mg SE: HA, dyspepsia, N/D, Abd pain Interactions: ↑ Effects W/ azole antifungals, cimetidine, danazol, glyburide, macrolides, phenytoin, ritonavir, EtOH; ↑ effects OF diclofenac, glyburide, phenytoin, warfarin; ↓ effects W/ cholestyramine, colestipol, isradipine, rifampin Labs: ↑ LFTs, (monitor) NIPE: Dose no longer limited to hs; ↑ photosensitivity—use sunblock; OK w/ grapefruit

Fluvoxamine (Luvox, Luvox CR) [Antidepressant/SSRI] WARNING: Closely monitor for worsening depression or emergence of suicidality, particularly in ped pts Uses: *Obsessive-compulsive disorder (OCD)*, seasonal affective disorder (SAD) Action: SSRI Dose: Initial 50-mg single qhs dose, ↑ to 300 mg/d in ÷ doses; CR: 100–300 mg PO qhs, may ↑ by 50 mg/d qwk, max 300 mg/d; ↓ in elderly/ hepatic impair, titrate slowly; ÷ doses > 100 mg Caution: [C, ?/−] Interactions (MAOIs, phenothiazines, SSRIs, serotonin agonists, others) CI: MAOI w/in 14 d; w/ alosetron, tizanidine, thioridazine, pimozide Disp: Tabs 25, 50, 100 mg; caps ER 100, 150 mg SE: HA, N/D, somnolence, insomnia Interactions: ↑ Effects W/ melatonin, MAOIs; ↑ effects OF BBs, benzodiazepines, methadone, carbamazepine, haloperidol, Li, phenytoin, TCAs, theophylline, warfarin, St. John's wort; ↑ risks of serotonin synd *W/* buspirone, dexfenfluramine, fenfluramine, tramadol, nefazodone, sibutramine, tryptophan; ↓ effects *W/* buspirone, cyproheptadine, tobacco; ↓ effects *OF* buspirone, HMG-CoA reductase Inhibs **Labs:** ↓ Na⁺ **NIPE:** ⊘ MAOIs for 14 d before start of drug; ⊘ EtOH; gradual taper to D/C

Folic Acid [Vitamin Supplement] **Uses:** *Megaloblastic anemia; folate deficiency* **Action:** Dietary supls **Dose:** *Adults. Supls:* 0.4 mg/d PO *PRG:* 0.8 mg/d PO *Folate deficiency:* 1 mg PO daily–tid *Peds. Supls:* 0.04–0.4 mg/24 h PO, IM, IV, or SQ *Folate deficiency:* 0.5–1 mg/24 h PO, IM, IV, or SQ **Caution:** [A, +] **CI:** Pernicious, aplastic, normocytic anemias **Disp:** Tabs 0.4, 0.8, 1 mg; Inj 5 mg/mL **SE:** Well tolerated **Interactions:** ↓ Effects *W/* anticonvulsants, sulfasalazine, aminosalicyclic acid, chloramphenicol, MTX, OCPs, pyrimethamine, triamterene, TMP; ↓ effects *OF* phenobarbital, phenytoin **NIPE:** OK for all women of childbearing age; ↓ fetal neural tube defects by 50%; no effect on normocytic anemias

Fondaparinux (Arixtra) [Anticoagulant/Factor X Inhibitor] **WARNING:** When epidural/spinal anesthesia or spinal puncture is used, pts anticoagulated or scheduled to be anticoagulated w/ LMW heparins, heparinoids, or fondaparinux are at risk for epidural or spinal hematoma, which can result in long-term or permanent paralysis **Uses:** *DVT prophylaxis* w/ hip fx, hip or knee replacement, Abd surgery; w/ DVT or PE in combo w/ warfarin **Action:** Synth Inhib of activated factor X; a pentasaccharide **Dose:** 2.5 mg SQ daily, up to 5–9 d; start > 6 h post-op; ↓ w/ renal impair **Caution:** [B, ?] ↑ Bleeding risk w/ anticoagulants, antiplts, drotrecogin alfa, NSAIDs **CI:** wgt < 50 kg, CrCl < 30 mL/min, active bleeding, SBE ↓ plt w/ antiplt Ab **Disp:** Prefilled syringes w/ 27-gauge needle: 2.5/0.5, 5/0.4, 7.5/0.6, 10/0.8 mg/mL **SE:** ↑ Plt, anemia, fever, N **Interactions:** ↑ Effects *W/* anticoagulants, cephalosporins, NSAIDs, PCNs, salicylates **Labs:** ↓ LFTs; ↑ HMG, Hct, glucose **NIPE:** D/C if plts < 100,000 cells/mm³; only give SQ; may monitor antifactor Xa levels

Formoterol Fumarate (Foradil, Perforomist) [Bronchodilator/Beta-2-Adrenergic Agonist] **WARNING:** May ↑ risk of asthma-related death **Uses:** *Long-term Rx of bronchoconstriction in COPD, EIB (only Foradil)* **Action:** LA β₂ agonist **Dose:** *Adults. Performist:* 20-mcg Inh q12h *Foradil:* 12-mcg Inh q12h, 24 mcg/d max *EIB:* 12 mcg 15 min before exercise *Peds > 5 y. Foradil:* See Adult dosage **Caution:** [C, M] Not for acute Sx, w/ CV Dz, w/ adrenergic meds, xanthine derivatives meds that ↑ QT; BBs may ↓ effect, D/C w/ ECG change **CI:** None **Disp:** Foradil caps 12 mcg for aerolizer inhaler (12 & 60 doses) **SE:** N/D, nasopharyngitis, dry mouth, angina, HTN, ↓ BP, tachycardia, arrhythmias, nervousness, HA, tremor, muscle cramps, palpitations, dizziness **Interactions:** ↑ Effects *W/* adrenergics; ↓ effects *OF* BBs; ↑ risk of hypokalemia *W/* corticosteroids, diuretics, xanthins; ↑ risk of arrhythmias *W/* MAOIs, TCAs **Labs:** ↑ Glucose; ↓ K⁺ **NIPE:** Do not swallow caps; only use w/ inhaler; do not start w/ worsening or acutely deteriorating asthma; excess use may ↑ CV risks; not for oral use

Fosamprenavir (Lexiva) [Antiretroviral/Protease Inhibitor]
WARNING: Do not use w/ severe liver dysfunction, reduce dose w/ mild–mod liver impair (fosamprenavir 700 mg bid w/o ritonavir) **Uses:** HIV Infxn **Action:** Protease Inhib **Dose:** 1400 mg bid w/o ritonavir; w/ ritonavir, fosamprenavir 1400 mg + ritonavir 200 mg daily or fosamprenavir 700 mg + ritonavir 100 mg bid; w/ efavirenz & ritonavir: fosamprenavir 1400 mg + ritonavir 300 mg daily **Caution:** [C, ?/–] **CI:** w/ Drugs that use CYPA4 for clearance (Table 10) such as w/ rifampin, lovastatin, simvastatin, delaviridine, ergot alkaloids, midazolam, triazolam, or pimozide; sulfa allergy **Disp:** Tabs 700 mg **SE:** N/V/D, HA, fatigue, rash **Interactions:** ↑ Effects W/ indinavir, nelfinavir; ↑ effects OF antiarrhythmics, amitriptyline, atorvastatin, benzodiazepine, bepridil, CCBs, cyclosporine, ergotamine, ethinyl estradiol, imipramine, itraconazole, ketoconazole, midazolam, norethindrone, rapamycin, rifabutin, sildenafil, tacrolimus, TCA, vardenafil, warfarin; ↓ effects W/ antacids, carbamazepine, dexamethasone, didanosine, efavirenz, H₂-receptor antagonists, nevirapine, phenobarbital, phenytoin, PPIs, rifampin St. John's wort; ↓ effects OF methadone **Labs:** ↑ LFTs; triglycerides, lipase; ↓ neutrophils **NIPE:** Take w/o regard to food; use barrier contraception; monitor for opportunistic Infxn; inform about fat redistribution/accumulation; replaced amprenavir

Fosaprepitant (Emend, Injection) [Substance P/Neurokinin-1 Receptor Antagonist] **Uses:** *Prevent chemotherapy-associated N/V* **Action:** Substance P/neurokinin-1 receptor antagonist **Dose:** *Chemotherapy:* 115 mg IV 30 min before chemotherapy on d 1 (followed by aprepitant [Emend, Oral] 80 mg PO d 2 & 3) in combo w/ other antiemetics **Caution:** [B, ?/–] Potential for drug interactions, substrate & mod CYP3A4 Inhib (dose dependent) **CI:** w/ Pimozide, terfenadine, astemizole, or cisapride **Disp:** Inj 115 mg **SE:** N/D, weakness, hiccups, dizziness, HA, dehydration, hot flushing, dyspepsia, Abd pain, neutropenia **Interactions:** ↑ Effects OF dexamethasone, methylprednisolone, midazolam, alprazolam, triazolam; ↓ effect OF OCP & warfarin, phenytoin, tolbutamide **Labs:** ↑ LFTs; monitor INR PRN **Disp:** Inj site discomfort; see also Aprepitant (Emend, Oral)

Foscarnet (Foscavir) [Antiviral] **Uses:** *CMV retinitis*; acyclovir-resistant *herpes Infxns* **Action:** ↓ Viral DNA polymerase & RT **Dose:** *CMV retinitis: Induction:* 60 mg/kg IV q8h or 100 mg/kg q12h × 14–21 d *Maint:* 90–120 mg/kg/d IV (Mon–Fri). *Acyclovir-resistant HSV: Induction:* 40 mg/kg IV q8–12h × 14–21 d; use central line; ↓ w/ renal impair **Caution:** [C, –] ↑ Sz potential w/ fluoroquinolones; avoid nephrotoxic Rx (cyclosporine, aminoglycosides, amphotericin B, protease Inhibs) **CI:** CrCl < 0.4 mL/min/kg **Disp:** Inj 24 mg/mL **SE:** Nephrotox, electrolyte abnormalities **Interactions:** ↑ Risks of Sz W/ quinolones; ↑ risks of nephrotox W/ aminoglycosides, amphotericin B, didanosine, pentamidine, vancomycin **Labs:** ↑ LFTs, BUN, SCr; ↓ HMG, Hct, Ca²⁺, Mg²⁺, K⁺, P; monitor ionized Ca²⁺ **NIPE:** ↑ Fluids; perioral tingling, extremity numbness & paresthesia indicates lytes imbalance; Na loading (500 mL 0.9% NaCl) before & after helps minimize nephrotox

Fosfomycin (Monurol) [Antibiotic] Uses: *Uncomp UTI* **Action:** ↓ Cell wall synth *Spectrum:* Gram(+) *Enterococcus*, staphylococci, enterococci; gram(−) (*E coli, Salmonella, Shigella, H influenzae, Neisseria*, indole-negative *Proteus, Providencia*); *B fragilis* & anaerobic gram(−) cocci are resistant **Dose:** 3 g PO in 90–120 mL of H_2O single dose; ↓ in renal impair **Caution:** [B, ?] ↓ Absorption w/ antacids/Ca salts **CI:** Component sensitivity **Disp:** Granule packets 3 g **SE:** HA, GI upset **Interactions:** ↓ Effects W/ antacids, metoclopramide **Labs:** ↑ LFTs; ↓ HMG, Hct **NIPE:** May take w/o regard to food; may take 2–3 d for Sxs to improve

Fosinopril (Monopril) [Antihypertensive/ACEI] Uses: *HTN, CHF*, DN **Action:** ACE Inhib **Dose:** 10 mg/d PO initial; max 40 mg PO; ↓ in elderly; ↓ in renal impair **Caution:** [D, +] ↑ K^+ w/ K^+ supls, ARBs, K^+-sparing diuretics; ↓ renal after effects w/ NSAIDs, diuretics, hypovolemia **CI:** Hereditary/idiopathic angioedema or angioedema w/ ACE Inhib, bilateral RAS **Disp:** Tabs 10, 20, 40 mg **SE:** Cough, dizziness, angioedema **Interactions:** ↑ Effects W/ antihypertensives, diuretics; ↑ effects *OF* Li; ↑ risk of hyperkalemia W/ K^+-sparing diuretics, salt substitutes; ↑ cough W/ capsaicin; ↓ effects W/ antacids, ASA, NSAIDs **Labs:** ↑ LFTs, K^+; ↓ HMG, Hct **NIPE:** ⊘ PRG, breast-feeding

Fosphenytoin (Cerebyx) [Anticonvulsant/Hydantoin] Uses: *Status epilepticus* **Action:** ↓ Sz spread in motor cortex **Dose:** As phenytoin equivalents (PE) *Load:* 15–20 mg PE/kg *Maint:* 4–6 mg PE/kg/d; ↓ dosage, monitor levels in hepatic impair **Caution:** [D, +] May ↑ phenobarbital **CI:** Sinus bradycardia, SA block, 2nd-/3rd-degree AV block, Adams–Stokes synd, rash during Rx **Disp:** Inj 75 mg/mL **SE:** ↓ BP, dizziness, ataxia, pruritus, nystagmus **Interactions:** ↑ Effects W/ amiodarone, chloramphenicol, cimetidine, diazepam, disulfiram, estrogens, INH, omeprazole, phenothiazine, salicylates, sulfonamides, tolbutamide; ↓ effects W/ TCAs, antiTB drugs, carbamazepine, EtOH, nutritional supls, ginkgo; ↓ effects *OF* anticoagulants, corticosteroids, digitoxin, doxycycline, OCPs, folic acid, Ca, vit D, rifampin, quinidine, theophylline **Labs:** ↑ Serum glucose, alk phos; ↓ serum thyroxine, Ca **NIPE:** Breast-feeding, for short-term use; 15 min to convert fosphenytoin to phenytoin; administer < 150 mg PE/min to prevent ↓ BP; administer w/ BP monitoring

Frovatriptan (Frova) [Migraine Suppressant/5-HT Agonist] Uses: *Rx acute migraine* **Action:** Vascular serotonin receptor agonist **Dose:** 2.5 mg PO repeat in 2 h PRN, 7.5 mg/d max PO dose; max 7.5 mg/d **Caution:** [C, ?/−] **CI:** Angina, ischemic heart Dz, coronary artery vasospasm, hemiplegic or basilar migraine, uncontrolled HTN, ergot use, MAOI use w/in 14 d **Disp:** Tabs 2.5 mg **SE:** N, V, dizziness, hot flashes, paresthesias, dyspepsia, dry mouth, hot/cold sensation, CP, skeletal pain, flushing, weakness, numbness, coronary vasospasm, HTN **Interactions:** ↑ Vasoactive Rxn W/ ergot drugs; serotonin 5-HT_1 agonists; ↑ effects W/ hormonal contraceptives, propranolol; ↑ risk of serotonin synd W/ SSRIs **NIPE:** Risk of photosensitivity; reports of severe cardiac events w/ this drug

Fulvestrant (Faslodex) [Antineoplastic/Antiestrogen] Uses: *HR(+) met breast CA in postmenopausal women w/ progression following antiestrogen therapy* Action: Estrogen receptor antagonist Dose: 250 mg IM monthly, as single 5-mL Inj or two concurrent 2.5-mL IM Inj in buttocks Caution: [X, ?/–] ↑ Effects w/ CYP3A4 Inhibs (Table 10); w/ hepatic impair CI: PRG Disp: Prefilled syringes 50 mg/mL (single 5 mL, dual 2.5 mL) SE: N/V/D, constipation, Abd pain, HA, back pain, hot flushes, pharyngitis, Inj site Rxns Interactions: ↑ Risk of bleeding W/ anticoagulants NIPE: ⊘ PRG, breast-feeding; use barrier contraception; only use IM

Furosemide (Lasix) [Antihypertensive/Loop Diuretic] Uses: *CHF, HTN, edema*, ascites Action: Loop diuretic; ↓ Na & Cl reabsorption in ascending loop of Henle & distal tubule Dose: *Adults.* 20–80 mg PO or IV bid *Peds.* 1 mg/kg/dose IV q6–12h; 2 mg/kg/dose PO q12–24h (max 6 mg/kg/dose); ↑ doses w/ renal impair Disp: Tabs 20, 40, 80 mg; soln 10 mg/mL, 40 mg/5 mL; Inj 10 mg/mL SE: ↓ BP, hyperglycemia Interactions: ↑ Nephrotoxic effects W/ cephalosporins; ↑ risk of digoxin tox & ototox W/ aminoglycosides, cisplatin (esp in renal dysfunction); ↑ risk of hypokalemia W/ antihypertensives, carbenoxolone, corticosteroids, digitalis glycosides, terbutaline; ↓ effects W/ barbiturates, cholestyramine, colestipol, NSAIDs, phenytoin, dandelion, ginseng; ↓ effects OF hypoglycemics Labs: ↑ BUN, Cr; cholesterol, glucose, uric acid, ↓ serum K+, Na+, Ca2+, Mg2+, monitor lytes, renal Fxn NIPE: Risk of photosensitivity—use sunblock; high doses IV may cause ototox; monitor ECG for hypokalemia (flattened T waves)

Gabapentin (Neurontin) [Anticonvulsant] Uses: Adjunct in *partial Szs; postherpetic neuralgia (PHN)*; chronic pain synds Action: Anticonvulsant; GABA analogue Dose: *Adults & Peds > 12 y. Anticonvulsant:* 300 mg PO tid, ↑ max 3600 mg/d. *PHN:* 300 mg d 1, 300 mg bid d 2, 300 mg tid d 3, titrate (1800–3600 mg/d) *Peds 3–12 y.* Start 0–15 mg/kg/d ÷ tid, ↑ over 3 d *3–4 y.* 40 mg/kg/d given tid = *5 y.* 25–35 mg/kg/d ÷ tid, 50 mg/kg/d max; ↓ w/ renal impair Caution: [C, ?] Use in peds 3–12 y w/ epilepsy may ↑ CNS-related adverse events CI: Component sensitivity Disp: Caps 100, 300, 400 mg; soln 250 mg/5 mL; scored tab 600, 800 mg SE: Somnolence, dizziness, ataxia, fatigue Interactions: ↑ Effects W/ CNS depressants; ↓ effects W/ antacids, ginkgo Labs: ↓ WBCs; NIPE: Take w/o regard to food; not necessary to monitor levels; taper ↑ or ↓ over 1 wk

Galantamine (Razadyne, Razadyne ER) [Cholinesterase Inhibitor] Uses: *Mild–mod Alzheimer Dz* Action: ? Acetylcholinesterase Inhib Dose: *Razadyne:* 4 mg PO bid, ↑ to 8 mg bid after 4 wk; may ↑ to 16 mg bid in 4 wk; target 16–24 mg/d ÷ bid *Razadyne ER:* Start 8 mg/d, ↑ to 16 mg/d after 4 wk, then to 24 mg/d after 4 more wk; give qAM w/ food Caution: [B, ?] Caution w/ heart block, ↑ risk of death w/ mild impair CI: Severe renal/hepatic impair Disp: *Razadyne* tabs 4, 8, 12 mg; soln 4 mg/mL; *Razadyne ER* caps 8, 16, 24 mg SE: GI disturbances, ↓ wgt, sleep disturbances, dizziness, HA Interactions: ↑ Effects W/ amiodarone, amitriptyline, bethanechol, cimetidine, digoxin, diltiazem, erythromycin, fluoxetine, fluvoxamine, ketoconazole, NSAIDs, paroxetine, quinidine, succinylcholine, verapamil; ↓ effect W/ anticholinergics **Labs:** ↓ HMG, Hct **NIPE:** ↑ Dosage q4wk, if D/C several d then restart at lowest dose; take w/ food & maint adequate fluid intake; caution w/ urinary outflow obst, Parkinson Dz, severe asthma/COPD, severe heart Dz or ↓ BP; monitor ECG for conduction abnormalities

Gallium Nitrate (Ganite) [Hormone] **WARNING:** ↑ Risk of severe renal Insuff w/ concurrent use of nephrotoxic drugs (eg, aminoglycosides, amphotericin B). D/C if use of potentially nephrotoxic drug is indicated; hydrate several d after administration. D/C w/ SCr > 2.5 mg/dL **Uses:** * ↑ Ca^{2+} of malignancy*; bladder CA **Action:** ↓ Bone resorption of Ca^{2+} **Dose:** ↑ Ca^{2+}: 100–200 mg/m²/d × 5 d. *CA:* 350 mg/m² cont Inf × 5 d to 700 mg/m² rapid IV Inf q2wk in antineoplastic settings (per protocols) **Caution:** [C, ?] Do not give w/ live or rotavirus vaccine **CI:** SCr > 2.5 mg/dL **Disp:** Inj 25 mg/mL **SE:** Renal Insuff, ↓ Ca^{2+}, hypophosphatemia, ↓ bicarbonate, < 1% acute optic neuritis **Interactions:** ↑ Risks of nephrotox W/ amphotericin B, aminoglycosides, vancomycin **NIPE:** Monitor SCr, adequate fluids; bladder CA, use in combo w/ vinblastine & ifosfamide; monitor ECG for cardiac abnormalities

Ganciclovir (Cytovene, Vitrasert) [Antiviral/Synthetic Nucleoside] **Uses:** *Rx & prevent CMV retinitis, prevent CMV Dz* in transplant recipients **Action:** ↓ viral DNA synth **Dose:** *Adults & Peds.* IV: 5 mg/kg IV q12h for 14–21 d, then maint 5 mg/kg/d IV × 7 d/wk or 6 mg/kg/d IV × 5 d/wk. *Ocular impair:* One implant q5–8mo *Adults.* PO: Following induction, 1000 mg PO tid. *Prevention:* 1000 mg PO tid; w/ food; ↓ in renal impair **Caution:** [C, −] ↑ Effect w/ immunosuppressives, imipenem/cilastatin, zidovudine, didanosine, other nephrotoxic Rx **CI:** ANC < 500 cells/mm³, plt < 25,000 cells/mm³, intravitreal implant **Disp:** Caps 250, 500 mg; Inj 500 mg, ocular implant 4.5 mg **SE:** Granulocytopenia & ↓ plt, fever, rash, GI upset **Interactions:** ↑ Effects W/ cytotoxic drugs, immunosuppressive drugs, probenecid; ↑ risks of nephrotox W/ amphotericin B, cyclosporine; ↑ effects W/ didanosine **Labs:** ↑ LFTs; ↓ blood glucose **NIPE:** Take w/ food; ⊘ PRG, breast-feeding, EtOH, NSAIDs; photosensitivity—use sunblock; not a cure for CMV; handle Inj w/ cytotoxic cautions; no systemic benefit w/ implant

Ganciclovir, Ophthalmic Gel (Zirgan) [Nucleoside Analogue] **Uses:** * Acute herpetic keratitis (dendritic ulcers)* **Action:** ↓ Viral DNA synth **Dose:** Adult & Peds ≥ 2 y. 1 gtt affected eye/s 5 × daily (q3h while awake) until ulcer heals, then 1 gtt tid × 7d **Caution:** [C, ?/−] **CI:** None **Disp:** Gel, 5 g tube **SE:** Blurred vision, eye irritation, punctate keratitis, conjunctival hyperemia **Labs:** Correct ↓ Ca^{2+} before use; ✓ Ca^{2+} **NIPE:** Remove contact lenses during therapy

Gefitinib (Iressa) [Antineoplastic] **Uses:** *Rx locally advanced or met NSCLC after platinum-based & docetaxel chemotherapy fails* **Action:** Selective TKI of EGFR **Dose:** 250 mg/d PO **Caution:** [D, −] **Disp:** Tabs 250 mg **SE:** D, rash, acne, dry skin, N/V, interstitial lung Dz, ↑ transaminases **Interactions:** ↑

Effects **W/** ketoconazole, itraconazole, & other CYP3A4 Inhibs; ↑ risk of bleeding **W/** warfarin; ↓ effects **W/** cimetidine, ranitidine, & other H$_2$-receptor antagonists, phenytoin, rifampin, & other CYP3A4 inducers **Labs:** ↑ LFTs (monitor) **NIPE:** ⊘ PRG or breast-feeding; take w/o regard to food; ↑ risk of corneal erosion/ulcer; only give to pts who have already received drug—no new pts because it has not been shown to ↑ survival

Gemcitabine (Gemzar) [Antineoplastic/Nucleoside Analogue]
Uses: *Pancreatic CA, brain mets, NSCLC*, gastric CA **Action:** Antimetabolite; ↓ ribonucleotide reductase; produces false nucleotide base-inhibiting DNA synth **Dose:** 1000–1250 mg/m^2 over 30 min–1 h IV Inf/wk × 3–4 wk or 6–8 wk; modify dose based on hematologic Fxn (per protocol) **Caution:** [D, ?/–] **CI:** PRG **Disp:** Inj 200 mg, 1 g **SE:** ↓ BM, N/V/D, drug fever, skin rash **Interactions:** ↑ BM depression **W/** radiation therapy, antineoplastic drugs; ↓ live virus vaccines **Labs:** ↑ LFTs, BUN, SCr (monitor) **NIPE:** ⊘ EtOH, NSAIDs, immunizations, PRG; reconstituted soln 38 mg/mL

Gemfibrozil (Lopid) [Antilipemic/Fibric Acid Derivative] Uses: *Hypertriglyceridemia, CHD* **Action:** Fibric acid **Dose:** 1200 mg/d PO ÷ bid 30 min ac AM & PM **Caution:** [C, ?] ↑ Warfarin effect, sulfonylureas; ↑ risk of myopathy w/ HMG-CoA reductase Inhibs; ↓ effects w/ cyclosporine **CI:** Renal/hepatic impair (SCr > 2.0 mg/dL), gallbladder Dz, primary biliary cirrhosis **Disp:** Tabs 600 mg **SE:** Cholelithiasis, GI upset **Interactions:** ↑ Effects **OF** anticoagulants, sulfonylureas; ↑ risk of rhabdomyolysis **W/** HMG-CoA reductase Inhibs; ↓ effects **W/** rifampin; ↓ effects **W/** cyclosporine **Labs:** ↑ LFTs & serum lipids, (monitor) **NIPE:** Avoid w/ HMG-CoA reductase Inhib

Gemifloxacin (Factive) [Antibiotic/Fluoroquinolone] Uses: *CAP, acute exacerbation of chronic bronchitis* **Action:** ↓ DNA gyrase & topoisomerase IV *Spectrum:* S pneumoniae (including multidrug-resistant strains), H influenzae, H parainfluenzae, M catarrhalis, M pneumoniae, C pneumoniae, K pneumoniae **Dose:** 320 mg PO daily × 5–7 d; CrCl < 40 mL/min: 160 mg PO/d **Caution:** [C, ?/–]; Peds < 18 y; h/o of ↑ QTc interval, lytes disorders, w/ Class Ia/III antiarrhythmics, erythromycin, TCAs, antipsychotics, ↑ INR & bleeding risk w/ warfarin **CI:** Fluoroquinolone allergy **Disp:** Tabs 320 mg **SE:** Rash, N/V/D, C difficile enterocolitis, ↑ risk of Achilles tendon rupture, tendonitis, Abd pain, dizziness, xerostomia, arthralgia, allergy/anaphylactic Rxns, peripheral neuropathy, tendon rupture **Interactions:** ↑ Risk of prolonged QT interval **W/** amiodarone, antipsychotics, erythromycin, procainamide, quinidine, sotalol, TCAs; ↑ effect **OF** warfarin; ↑ effects **W/** probenecid; ↓ effects **W/** antacids, didanosine, Fe, sucralfate **Labs:** ↑ LFTs **NIPE:** ↑ Fluid intake; D/C if c/o tenderness/pain in muscles/tendons; ⊘ excessive sunlight exposure—use sunblock; take 3 h before or 2 h after Al/Mg antacids, Fe^{2+}, Zn^{2+} or other metal cations; ↑ rash risk w/ ↑ duration of therapy; monitor ECG for ↑ QT interval

Gentamicin (Garamycin, G-Myticin, Others) [Antibiotic/Aminoglycoside] Uses: *Septicemia, serious bacterial Infxn of CNS, urinary tract, resp tract, GI tract, including peritonitis, skin, bone, soft tissue, including burns; severe Infxn *P aeruginosa* w/ carbenicillin; group D streptococci endocarditis w/ PCN-type drug; serious staphylococcal Infxns, but not the antibiotic of 1st choice; mixed Infxn w/ staphylococci & gram(−))* **Action:** Aminoglycoside, bactericidal; ↓ protein synth **Spectrum:** Gram(−) (not *Neisseria, Legionella, Acinetobacter*); weaker gram(+) but synergy w/ PCNs **Dose:** *Adults. Standard:* 1–2 mg/kg IV q8–12h or daily dosing 4–7 mg/kg q24h IV. *Gram(+) synergy:* 1 mg/kg q8h **Peds. Infants < 7 d < 1200 g.** 2.5 mg/kg dose q18–24h **Infants > 1200 g.** 2.5 mg/kg/dose q12–18h **Infants > 7 d.** 2.5 mg/kg/dose IV q8–12h **Children.** 2.5 mg/kg/d IV q8h; ↓ w/ renal Insuff; if obese, dose based on IBW **Caution:** [C, +/−] Avoid other nephrotoxics **CI:** Aminoglycoside sensitivity **Disp:** Premixed Infs 40, 60, 70, 80, 90, 100, 120 mg; ADD-Vantage Inj vials 10 mg/mL; Inj 40 mg/mL; IT preservative-free 2 mg/mL **SE:** Nephro-/oto-/neurotox **Notes:** *Levels: Peak:* 30 min after Inf; *Trough:* < 0.5 h before next dose; *Therapeutic: Peak:* 5–8 mcg/mL; *Trough:* < 2 mcg/mL, if > 2 mcg/mL associated w/ renal tox **Interactions:** ↑ Ototox, neurotox, nephrotox *W/* aminoglycosides, amphotericin B, cephalosporins, loop diuretics, PCNs; ↑ effects *W/* NSAIDs; ↓ effects *W/* carbenicillin **Labs:** Monitor CrCl, SCr, & serum conc for dose adjustments; ↑ LFTs, BUN, Cr; ↓ HMG, Hct, plts, WBC **NIPE:** Photosensitivity—use sunblock; use IBW to dose (use adjusted if obese > 30% IBW); OK to use intraperitoneal for peritoneal dialysis-related Infxns

Gentamicin & Prednisolone, Ophthalmic (Pred-G Ophthalmic) [Antibiotic/Anti-Inflammatory]
Uses: *Steroid-responsive ocular & conjunctival Infxns* sensitive to gentamicin **Action:** Bactericidal; ↓ protein synth w/ antiinflammatory. **Spectrum:** *Staphylococcus, E coli, H influenzae, Klebsiella, Neisseria, Pseudomonas, Proteus,* & *Serratia* sp **Dose:** *Oint:* 1/2 in in conjunctival sac daily–tid. *Susp:* 1 gtt bid–qid, up to 1 gtt/h for severe Infxns **CI:** Aminoglycoside sensitivity **Caution:** [C, ?] **Disp:** Oint, ophthal: Prednisolone acetate 0.6% & gentamicin sulfate 0.3% (3.5 g). *Susp, ophthal:* Prednisolone acetate 1% & gentamicin sulfate 0.3% (2, 5, 10 mL) **SE:** Local irritation; **NIPE:** Systemic effects w/ long-term use

Gentamicin, Ophthalmic (Garamycin, Genoptic, Gentacidin, Gentak, Others) [Antibiotic]
Uses: *Conjunctival Infxns* **Action:** Bactericidal; ↓ protein synth **Dose:** *Oint:* Apply 1/2 in bid–tid. *Soln:* 1–2 gtt q2–4h, up to 2 gtt/h for severe Infxn **Caution:** [C, ?] **CI:** Aminoglycoside sensitivity **Disp:** Soln & oint 0.1% & 0.3% **SE:** Local irritation **NIPE:** Do not use other eye drops w/in 5–10 min; do not touch dppr to eye

Gentamicin, Topical (Garamycin, G-myticin) [Antibiotic]
Uses: *Skin Infxns* caused by susceptible organisms **Action:** Bactericidal; ↓ protein synth **Dose:** *Adults & Peds > 1 y.*Apply tid–qid **Caution:** [C, ?] **CI:** Aminoglycoside sensitivity **Disp:** Cream & oint 0.1% **SE:** Irritation **NIPE:** ⊘ Apply to large denuded areas

Glimepiride (Amaryl) [Hypoglycemic/Sulfonylurea]
Uses: *Type 2 DM* **Action:** Sulfonylurea; ↑ pancreatic insulin release; ↑ peripheral insulin

sensitivity; ↓ hepatic glucose output/production **Dose:** 1–4 mg/d, max 8 mg **Caution:** [C, –] **CI:** DKA **Disp:** Tabs 1, 2, 4 mg **SE:** HA, N, hypoglycemia **Interactions:** ↑ Effects W/ ACEIs, adrenergic antagonists, BBs, chloramphenicol, MAOIs, NSAIDs, probenecid, salicylates, sulfonamides, warfarin, ginseng, garlic; ↓ effects W/ corticosteroids, estrogens, INH, OCPs, nicotinic acid, phenytoin, sympathomimetics, thiazide diuretics, thyroid hormones **Labs:** ↑ LFTs, BUN, Cr; ↓ HMG, Hct, plts, WBC, RBC, glucose **NIPE:** Antabuse-like effect w/ EtOH (rare); Give w/ 1st meal of d; BB may mask hypoglycemia

Glimepiride/Pioglitazone (Duetact) [Hypoglycemic/Sulfonylurea/Thiazolidinedione]
Uses: *Adjunct to exercise type 2 DM not controlled by single agent* **Action:** Sulfonylurea (↓ glucose) w/ agent that ↑ insulin sensitivity & ↓ gluconeogenesis **Dose:** initial 30 mg/2 mg PO qAM; 45 mg pioglitazone/8 mg glimepiride/d max; w/ food **Caution:** [C, ?/–] w/ Liver impair, elderly **CI:** Component hypersensitivity, DKA **Disp:** Tabs 30/2, 30 mg/4 mg **SE:** URI, ↑ wgt, edema, HA, N/D, may ↑ CV mortality **Interactions:** ↑ Effects W/ ACEIs, adrenergic antagonists, BBs, chloramphenicol, MAOIs, NSAIDs, probenecid, salicylates, sulfonamides, warfarin, ginseng, garlic; ↓ effects W/ corticosteroids, estrogens, INH, OCPs, nicotinic acid, phenytoin, sympathomimetics, thiazide diuretics, thyroid hormones **Labs:** ↑ LFTs, BUN, Cr; ↓ HMG, Hct, plts, WBC, RBC, glucose; monitor CBC, ALT, Cr **NIPE:** Monitor wgt; BB may mask hypoglycemia

Glipizide (Glucotrol, Glucotrol XL) [Hypoglycemic/Sulfonylurea]
Uses: *Type 2 DM* **Action:** Sulfonylurea; ↑ pancreatic insulin release; ↑ peripheral insulin sensitivity; ↓ hepatic glucose output/production; ↓ intestinal glucose absorption **Dose:** 5 mg initial, ↑ by 2.5–5 mg/d, max 40 mg/d; XL max 20 mg; 30 min ac; hold if NPO **Caution:** [C, ?/–] Severe liver Dz **CI:** DKA, type 1 DM, sulfonamide sensitivity **Disp:** Tabs 5, 10 mg; XL tabs 2.5, 5, 10 mg **SE:** HA, anorexia, N/V/D, constipation, fullness, rash, urticaria, photosensitivity **Interactions:** ↑ Effects W/ azole antifungals, anabolic steroids, BB, chloramphenicol, cimetidine, clofibrate, MAOIs, NSAIDs, probenecid, salicylates, sulfonamides, TCAs, warfarin, celery, coriander, dandelion root, fenugreek, ginseng, garlic, juniper berries; ↓ effects W/ amphetamines, corticosteroids, epinephrine, estrogens, glucocorticoids, OCPs, phenytoin, rifampin, sympathomimetics, thiazide diuretics, thyroid hormones, tobacco **Labs:** ↑ BUN, Cr, AST, lipids; ↓ glucose, HMG, WBC, plts **NIPE:** Antabuse-like effect w/ EtOH (rare); give 30 min ac; hold dose if pt NPO; counsel about DM management; wait several d before adjusting dose; monitor glucose; BB can mask hypoglycemia

Glucagon [Antihypoglycemic/Hormone]
Uses: Severe *hypoglycemic *Rxns in DM w/ sufficient liver glycogen stores; BB/CCB OD **Action:** Accelerates liver gluconeogenesis **Dose:** *Adults.* 0.5–1 mg SQ, IM, or IV; repeat in 20 min PRN *ECC 2010:* β-Blocker or CCB OD: 3–10 mg slow IV over 3–5 min; follow with Inf of 3–5 mg/h Hypoglycemia: 1 mg IV, IM, or SQ *Peds. Neonates.*

0.3 mg/kg/dose SQ, IM, or IV q4h PRN *Children*. 0.025–0.1 mg/kg/dose SQ, IM, or IV; repeat in 20 min PRN **Caution:** [B, M] **CI:** Pheo **Disp:** Inj 1 mg **SE:** N/V, ↓ BP **Interactions:** ↑ Effect W/ epinephrine, phenytoin; ↑ effects *OF* anticoagulants **Labs:** ↓ Serum K+ **NIPE:** Response w/in 20 min after Inj; administration of dextrose IV necessary; ineffective in starvation, adrenal Insuff, or chronic hypoglycemia

Glyburide (DiaBeta, Micronase, Glynase) [Hypoglycemic/Sulfonylurea] Uses: *Type 2 DM* **Action:** Sulfonylurea; ↑ pancreatic insulin release; ↑ peripheral insulin sensitivity; ↓ hepatic glucose output/production; ↓ intestinal glucose absorption **Dose:** 1.25–10 mg daily–bid, max 20 mg/d. *Micronized:* 0.75–6 mg daily–bid, max 12 mg/d **Caution:** [C, ?] Renal impair, sulfonamide allergy **CI:** DKA, type 1 DM **Disp:** Tabs 1.25, 2.5, 5 mg; micronized tabs 1.5, 3, 6 mg **SE:** HA, hypoglycemia, cholestatic jaundice, & hep; may cause liver failure **Interactions:** Many medications can enhance hypoglycemic effects such as: ↑ Effects W/ anticoagulants, anabolic steroids, BBs, chloramphenicol, cimetidine, clofibrate, MAOIs, NSAIDs, probenecid, salicylates, sulfonamides, TCAs, EtOH, celery, coriander, dandelion root, fenugreek, ginseng, garlic, juniper berries; ↓ effects W/ amphetamines, corticosteroids, baclofen, epinephrine, glucocorticoids, OCPs, phenytoin, rifampin, sympathomimetics, thiazide diuretics, thyroid hormones, tobacco **Labs:** ↑ LFTs, BUN; ↓ glucose, HMG, Hct, plts, WBC **NIPE:** Antabuse-like effect w/ EtOH (rare); not OK for CrCl < 50 mL/min; hold dose if NPO, hypoglycemia may be difficult to recognize; many medications can enhance hypoglycemic effects

Glyburide/Metformin (Glucovance) [Hypoglycemic/Sulfonylurea & Biguanide] Uses: *Type 2 DM* **Action:** *Sulfonylurea:* ↑ Pancreatic insulin release. *Metformin:* Peripheral insulin sensitivity; ↓ hepatic glucose output/production; ↓ intestinal glucose absorption **Dose:** 1st-line (naive pts), 1.25/250 mg PO daily–bid; 2nd-line, 2.5/500 mg or 5/500 mg bid (max 20/2000 mg); take w/ meals, slowly ↑ dose; hold before & 48 h after ionic contrast media **Caution:** [C, –] **CI:** SCr > 1.4 mg/dL in females or > 1.5 mg/dL in males; hypoxemic conditions (sepsis, recent MI); alcoholism; metabolic acidosis; liver Dz **Disp:** Tabs 1.25/250, 2.5/500, 5/500 mg **SE:** HA, hypoglycemia, lactic acidosis, anorexia, N/V, rash; see Glyburide **Interactions:** ↑ Effects W/ amiloride, ciprofloxacin cimetidine, digoxin, miconazole, morphine, nifedipine, procainamide, quinidine, quinine, ranitidine, triamterene, TMP, vancomycin; ↓ effects W/ CCBs, INH, phenothiazines **Labs:** Monitor folate levels (megaloblastic anemia) **NIPE:** Avoid EtOH; hold dose if NPO, see Glyburide

Glycerin Suppository [Laxative] Uses: *Constipation* **Action:** Hyperosmolar laxative **Dose:** *Adults.* 1 adult supp PR PRN *Peds.* 1 infant supp PR daily–bid PRN **Caution:** [C, ?] **Disp:** Supp (adult, infant); Liq 4 mL/applicator-full **SE:** D **Interactions:** ↑ Effects W/ diuretics **Labs:** ↑ Serum triglycerides, phosphatidylglycerol in amniotic fluid; ↓ serum Ca **NIPE:** Insert & retain for 15 min

Golimumab (Simponi)[Antirheumatics/DMARDs/TNF Blocker]
WARNING: Serious Infxns (bacterial, fungal, TB, opportunistic) possible. D/C w/ severe Infxn/sepsis, test & monitor for TB w/ Tx; lymphoma/other CA possible in children/adolescents **Uses:** *Mod/severe RA w/ methotrexate, psoriatic arthritis w/ or w/o methotrexate, ankylosing spondylitis* **Action:** TNF blocker **Dose:** 50 mg SQ 1 × /mo **Caution:** [B, ?/–] Do use w/ active Infxn; w/ malignancies, CHF, demyelinating Dz; do use w/ abatacept, anakinra, live vaccines **CI:** None **Disp:** Prefilled syringe & SmartJect Auto-injector 50 mg/0.5 mL **SE:** URI, nasopharyngitis,Inj site Rxn, LFTs, Infxn, hep B reactivation, new onset psoriasis **Interactions:** ↑ Risk of serious Infxns **W/** abatacept, anakinra, corticosteroids, methotrexate; immunosuppresants; ↓ effects **W/** live virus vaccines; monitor CYP450 substrates w/ narrow therapeutic index: cyclosporine, theophylline, warfarin **Labs:** ↑ LFTs; monitor CBC; **NIPE:** ⊘ w/ live virus vaccines; monitor for signs serious Infxn (fever, malaise, wgt loss, sweats, cough, dyspnea); monitor for new or > CHF; monitor for exacerbation or new onset psoriasis

Gonadorelin (Factrel) [Gonadotropin-Releasing Hormone] Uses: *Primary hypothalamic amenorrhea* **Action:** ↑ Pituitary release of LH & FSH **Dose:** 5 mcg IV over 1 min q90min × 21 d using pump kit **Caution:** [B, M] ↑ Levels w/ androgens, estrogens, progestins, glucocorticoids, spironolactone, levodopa; ↓ levels w/ OCP, digoxin, DA antagonists **CI:** Condition exacerbated by PRG or reproductive hormones, ovarian cysts, causes of anovulation other than hypothalamic, hormonally dependent tumor **Disp:** Inj 100 mcg **SE:** Multiple PRG risk **Interactions:** ↑ Effects **W/** androgens, estrogens, glucocorticoids, levodopa, progestins, spironolactone; ↓ effects **W/** digoxin, DA antagonists, OCPs, phenothiazines **Labs:** Monitor LH, FSH **NIPE:** Inj site pain

Goserelin (Zoladex) [Antineoplastic/Gonadotropin-Releasing Hormone] Uses: Advanced *CA Prostate* & w/ radiation for localized high-risk Dz, *endometriosis, breast CA* **Action:** LHRH agonist, transient ↑ then ↓ in LH, w/ ↓ testosterone **Dose:** 3.6 mg SQ (implant) q28d or 10.8 mg SQ q3mo; usually upper Abd wall **Caution:** [X, –] PRG, breast-feeding, 10.8-mg implant not for women **Disp:** SQ implant 3.6 (1 mo), 10.8 mg (3 mo) **SE:** Hot flashes, ↓ libido, gynecomastia, & transient exacerbation of CA-related bone pain ("flare Rxn" 7–10 d after 1st dose) **Interactions:** None noted **Labs:** ↑ LFTs, glucose, cholesterol, triglycerides; initial ↑ then ↓ after 1–2 wk FSH, LH, testosterone **NIPE:** Inject SQ into fat in Abd wall; do not aspirate; females must use contraception

Granisetron (Kytril) [Antiemetic/5-HT$_3$ Antagonist] Uses: *Rx & prevention of N/V (chemotherapy/radiation/post-op)* **Action:** Serotonin (5-HT$_3$) receptor antagonist **Dose:** *Adults & Peds. Chemotherapy:* 10 mcg/kg/dose IV 30 min prior to chemotherapy *Adults.* Inj 0.1, 1 mg/mL *Chemotherapy:* 2 mg PO qd 1 h before chemotherapy, then 12 h later. *Post-op N/V:* 1 mg IV over 30 s before end of case **Caution:** [B, +/–] St. John's wort ↓ levels **CI:** Liver Dz, children < 2 y **Disp:** Tabs 1 mg; Inj 0.1, 1 mg/mL; soln 2 mg/10 mL **SE:** HA, asthenia, somnolence,

D, constipation, Abd pain, dizziness, insomnia **Interactions:** ↑ Serotonergic effects W/ horehound; ↑ extrapyramidal Rxns W/ drugs causing these effects **Labs:** ↑ ALT, AST; ↓ HMG, Hct, plts, WBC **NIPE:** May cause anaphylactic Rxn

Guaifenesin (Robitussin, Others) [Expectorant/Propanediol Derivative] Uses: *Relief of dry, nonproductive cough* **Action:** Expectorant **Dose:** *Adults.* 200–400 mg (10–20 mL) PO q4h SR 600–1200 mg PO bid, (max 2.4 g/d) *Peds 2–5 y.* 50–100 mg (2.5–5 mL) PO q4h (max 600 mg/d) *6–11 y.* 100–200 mg (5–10 mL) PO q4h (max 1.2 g/d) **Caution:** [C, ?] **Disp:** Tabs 100, 200 mg; SR tabs 600, 1200 mg; caps 200 mg; SR caps 300 mg; Liq 100 mg/5 mL **SE:** GI upset **Interactions:** ↑ Bleeding W/ heparin **Labs:** ↓ Serum uric acid level, HMG, plts, WBCs **NIPE:** Give w/ large amount of H_2O; some dosage forms contain EtOH

Guaifenesin & Codeine (Robitussin AC, Brontex, Others) [Expectorant/Analgesic/Antitussive] [C-V] Uses: *Relief of dry cough* **Action:** Antitussive w/ expectorant **Dose:** *Adults.* 5–10 mL or 1 tab PO q6–8h (max 60 mL/24 h) *Peds 2–6 y.* 1–1.5 mg/kg codeine/d ÷ dose q4–6h (max 30 mg/24 h) *6–12 y.* 5 mL q4h (max 30 mL/24 h) **Caution:** [C, +] **Disp:** Brontex tab 10 mg codeine/300 mg guaifenesin; Liq 2.5 mg codeine/75 mg guaifenesin/5 mL; others 10 mg codeine/100 mg guaifenesin/5 mL **SE:** Somnolence, constipation **Interactions:** ↑ CNS depression W/ barbiturates, antihistamines, glutethimide, methocarbamol, cimetidine, EtOH; ↓ effects W/ quinidine **Labs:** ↑ Urine morphine; ↓ serum uric acid level, HMG, plts, WBCs **NIPE:** Take w/ food

Guaifenesin & Dextromethorphan (Many OTC Brands) [Expectorant/Antitussive] Uses: *Cough* d/t upper resp tract irritation **Action:** Antitussive w/ expectorant **Dose:** *Adults & Peds > 12 y.* 10 mL PO q6–8h (max 40 mL/24 h) *Peds 2–6 y.* Dextromethorphan 1–2 mg/kg/24 h ÷ 3–4 ×/d (max 10 mL/d) *6–12 y.* 5 mL q6–8h (max 20 mL/d) **Caution:** [C, +] **CI:** Administration w/ MAOI **Disp:** Many OTC formulations **SE:** Somnolence **Interactions:** ↑ Effects W/ quinidine, terbinafine; ↓ effects OF isocarboxazid, MAOIs, phenelzine; ↑ risk of serotonin synd W/ sibutramine **Labs:** ↓ Serum uric acid level, HMG, plts, WBCs **NIPE:** Give w/ plenty of fluids; some forms contain EtOH

Guanfacine (Intuniv, Tenex) [Central Alpha-2A Agonist/Hypertension] Uses: *ADHD (peds > 6 y)*; *HTN (adults)* **Action:** Central α_{2A}-adrenergic agonist; **Dose:** *Adults.* 1–3 mg/d IR PO hs (Tenex), ↑ by 1 mg q3–4 wk PRN 3 mg/d max *Peds.* 1–4 mg/d XR PO (Intuniv), ↑ by 1 mg q1wk PRN 4 mg/d max **Caution:** [B; +/–] **Disp:** Tabs IR 1, 2 mg; tabs XR 1, 2, 3, 4 mg **SE:** Somnolence, dizziness, HA, fatigue, constipation, Abd pain, xerostomia, hypotension, bradycardia, syncope **Interactions:** ↑ Effects W/ CYP3A4/5 Inhibs (eg, ketoconazole), antihypertensives, CNS depressants; ↑effects OF valproic acid; ↓ effects W/ CYP3A4 inducers (eg, rifampin) **NIPE:**Rebound ↑ BP, anxiety, nervousness w/ abrupt D/C

Haemophilus B Conjugate Vaccine (ActHIB, HibTITER, Hiberix, PedvaxHIB, Prohibit, TriHIBit, Others) [Vaccine/Inactivated] Uses: Routine *immunization* of children against *H influenzae* type B Dzs

Action: Active immunization against *Haemophilus* B **Dose: Peds.** 0.5 mL (25 mg) IM in deltoid or vastus lateralis 2 doses 2 & 4 mo; booster at 12–15 mo or 2, 4, & 6 mo booster at 12–15 mo depending on formulation **Caution:** [C, +] **CI:** Component sensitivity, febrile illness, immunosuppressive, allergy to thimerosal **Disp:** Inj 7.5, 10, 15, 25 mcg/0.5 mL **SE:** Fever, restlessness, fussiness, anorexia, observe for anaphylaxis; edema, ↑ risk of *Haemophilus* B Infxn the wk after vaccination **Interactions:** ↓ Effects *W/* immunosuppressives, steroids **NIPE:** Prohibit & TriHIBit cannot be used in children < 12 mo; *Hiberix*-approved ages 15 mo–4 y, single dose; booster beyond 5 y not required; report SAE to Vaccine Adverse Events Reporting System (VAERS: 1-800-822-7967); dosing varies, check w/ each product; pain/redness at Inj site

Haloperidol (Haldol) [Antipsychotic/Butyrophenone] WARNING: ↑ Mortality in elderly w/ dementia-related psychosis, death w/ IV administration at higher doses **Uses:** *Psychotic disorders, agitation, Tourette disorders, hyperactivity in children* **Action:** Butyrophenone; antipsychotic, neuroleptic **Dose: Adults.** *Mod Sxs:* 0.5–2 mg PO bid–tid *Severe Sxs/agitation:* 3–5 mg PO bid–tid or 1–5 mg IM q4h PRN (max 100 mg/d) **Peds 3–6 y.** 0.01–0.03 mg/kg/24 h PO daily **6–12 y.** *Initial:* 0.5–1.5 mg/24 h PO; ↑ by 0.5 mg/24 h to maint of 2–4 mg/24 h (0.05–0.1 mg/kg/24 h) or 1–3 mg/dose IM q4–8h to 0.1 mg/kg/24 h max; Tourette Dz may require up to 15 mg/24 h PO; ↓ in elderly **Caution:** [C, ?] ↑ Effects w/ SSRIs, CNS depressants, TCA, indomethacin, metoclopramide; avoid levodopa (↓ antiparkinsonian effects) **CI:** NAG, severe CNS depression, coma, Parkinson Dz, BM suppression, severe cardiac/hepatic Dz **Disp:** Tabs 0.5, 1, 2, 5, 10, 20 mg; conc Liq 2 mg/mL; Inj 5 mg/mL; decanoate Inj 50, 100 mg/mL **SE:** Extrapyramidal Sxs (EPS), tardive dyskinesia, neuroleptic malignant synd, ↓ BP, anxiety, dystonias, risk for torsades de pointes, & QT prolongation **Interactions:** ↑ Effects *W/* CNS depressants, quinidine, EtOH; ↑ hypotension *W/* antihypertensives, nitrates; ↑ anticholinergic effects *W/* antihistamines, antidepressants, atropine, phenothiazine, quinidine, disopyramide; ↓ effects *W/* antacids, carbamazepine, Li, nutmeg, tobacco; ↓ effects *OF* anticoagulants, levodopa, guanethidine **Labs:** ↑ LFTs, monitor for leukopenia, neutropenia, & agranulocytosis; follow CBC if WBC counts ↓ **NIPE:** ↑ Risk of photosensitivity—use sunblock; do not give decanoate IV; dilute PO conc Liq w/ H₂O/juice; monitor for EPS; ECG monitoring w/ off-label IV use

Hep A Vaccine (Havrix, Vaqta) [Vaccine/Inactivated] **Uses:** *Prevent hep A* in high-risk individuals (eg, travelers, certain professions eg, day care workers if 1 or more children or workers are infected, high-risk behaviors, children at ↑ risk), in chronic liver Dz **Action:** Active immunity **Dose: Adults.** *Havrix* 1-mL IM w/ 1-mL booster 6 oster 6 w/ 1 *Vaqta*: 1 mL IM w/ 1 mL IM booster 6 ELISA units **Peds ≥ 12 mo.** Havrix 0.5-mL IM, w/ 0.5-mL booster 6 A units [EL.U.]), certain PR w/ booster 0.5 mL 66/0.5-mL booster **Caution:** [C, +] **CI:** Component sensitivity **Disp:** *Havrix:* Inj 720 EL.U./0.5 mL, 1440 EL.U./1 mL; *Vaqta* 50 units/mL **SE:** Fever, fatigue, HA, Inj site pain **NIPE:** Give primary at least 2 wk before anticipated exposure; do not give Havrix in gluteal region; report SAE to VAERS (1-800-822-7967)

Hep A (Inactivated) & Hep B (Recombinant) Vaccine (Twinrix) [Vaccine/Inactivated] Uses: *Active immunization against hep A/B in pts >18 y* **Action:** Active immunity **Dose:** 1 mL IM at 0, 1, & 6 mo; accelerated regimen 1 mL IM d0, 7, & 21–20 then booster at 12 mo; 720 EL.U. hep A antigen, 20 mcg/mL hep B surface antigen **Caution:** [C, +/–] **CI:** Component sensitivity **Disp:** Single-dose vials, syringes **SE:** Fever, fatigue, pain/redness at site, HA **Interactions:** ↓ Immune response W/ corticosteroids, immunosuppressants **NIPE:** ↑ Response if Inj in deltoid vs gluteus; booster OK 6–12 mo after vaccination; report SAE to Vaccine Adverse Events Reporting System (VAERS: 1-800-822-7967)

Hep B Immune Globulin (HyperHep, HepaGam B, Nabi-HB, H-BIG) [Hepatitis B Prophylaxis/Immunoglobulin] Uses: *Exposure to HBsAg(+) material (eg, blood, accidental needlestick, mucous membrane contact, PO, or sexual contact), prevent hep B in HBsAg(+) liver Tx pt* **Action:** Passive immunization **Dose:** *Adults & Peds.* 0.06 mL/kg IM 5 mL max; w/in 24 h of exposure; w/in 14 d of sexual contact; repeat 1 mo if nonresponder or refused initial Tx; liver Tx per protocols **Caution:** [C, ?] **CI:** Allergies to γ-globulin or anti-immunoglobulin Ab; allergies to thimerosal; IgA deficiency **Disp:** Inj **SE:** Inj site pain, dizziness, HA, myalgias, arthralgias, anaphylaxis **Interactions:** ↓ Immune response if given W/ live virus vaccines **NIPE:** IM in gluteal or deltoid; W/ continued exposure, give hep B vaccine; not for active hep B; ineffective for chronic hep B

Hep B Vaccine (Engerix-B, Recombivax HB) [Vaccine/Inactivated] Uses: *Prevent hep B* men: men who have sex w/ men, people who inject street drugs; chronic renal/liver Dz, healthcare workers exposed to blood, body fluids; sexually active not in monogamous relationship, people seeking eval for or w/ STDs, household contacts & partners of hep B infected persons, travelers to countries w/ hep B prevalence, clients/staff working w/ people w/ developmental disabilities **Action:** Active immunization; recombinant DNA **Dose:** *Adults.* 3 IM doses 1 mL each; 1st 2 doses 1 mo apart; the 3rd 6 mo after the 1st *Peds.* 0.5 IM adult schedule **Caution:** [C, +] ↓ Effect w/ immunosuppressives **CI:** Yeast allergy, component sensitivity **Disp:** *Engerix-B:* Inj 20 mcg/mL; peds Inj 10 mcg/0.5 mL. *Recombivax HB:* Inj 10 & 40 mcg/mL; peds Inj 5 mcg/0.5 mL **SE:** Fever, HA, Inj site pain **Interactions:** ↓ Immune response W/ corticosteroids, immunosuppressants **NIPE:** ↑ Response Inj in deltoid vs gluteus; deltoid IM Inj adults/older peds; younger peds, use anterolateral thigh

Heparin (Generic) [Anticoagulant/Antithrombotic] Uses: *Rx & prevention of DVT & PE*, unstable angina, AF w/ emboli, & acute arterial occlusion **Action:** Acts w/ antithrombin III to inactivate thrombin & ↓ thromboplastin formation **Dose:** *Adults. Prophylaxis:* 3000–5000 units SQ q8–12h. *DVT/PE Rx:* Load 50–80 units/kg IV (max 10,000 units), then 10–20 units/kg IV qh (adjust based on PTT) *ECC 2010:* STEMI: Bolus 60 units/kg (max 4000 units); then 12 units/kg/h (max 1000 units/h) round to nearest 50 units; keep aPTT 1.5–2 × control 48 h or until angiography *Peds. Infants.* Load 50 units/kg IV bolus, then 20 units/kg/h IV by cont Inf *Children.* Load 50 units/kg IV, then 15–25 units/kg cont Inf or 100 units/kg/dose q4h IV intermittent bolus (adjust based on PTT) **Caution:** [B, +] ↑ Risk of hemorrhage w/ anticoagulants, ASA, antiplts, cephalosporins w/ MTT side chain **CI:** Uncontrolled bleeding, severe ↓ plt, suspected ICH **Disp:** Unfractionated Inj 10, 100, 1000, 2000, 2500, 5000, 7500, 10,000, 20,000, 40,000 units/mL **SE:** Bruising, bleeding, ↓ plt **Interactions:** ↑ Effects *W/* anticoagulants, antihistamines, ASA, clopidogrel, cardiac glycosides, cephalosporins, pyridamole, NSAIDs, quinine, tetracycline, ticlopidine, feverfew, ginkgo, ginger, valerian; ↓ effects *W/* nitroglycerine, ginseng, goldenseal, ↓ effects *OF* insulin **Labs:** ↑ LFTs; follow PTT, thrombin time, or ACT; little PT effect; therapeutic PTT 1.5–2 × control for most conditions; monitor for HIT w/ plt counts **NIPE:** Monitor for signs bleeding: Bleeding gums, nosebleed, unusual bruising, black tarry stools, hematuria, < Hct, guaiac + stool; new itor for signs blepharin is ~ 10% less effective than older formulations

Hetastarch (Hespan) [Plasma Volume Expander] Uses: *Plasma vol expansion* adjunct in shock & leukapheresis **Action:** Synthetic colloid; acts similar to albumin **Dose:** *Vol expansion:* 500–1000 mL (1500 mL/d max) IV (20 mL/kg/h max rate). *Leukapheresis:* 250–700 mL; ↓ in renal failure **Caution:** [C, +] **CI:** Severe bleeding disorders, CHF, oliguric/anuric renal failure **Disp:** Inj 6 g/100 mL **SE:** Bleeding **Labs:** ↑ PT, PTT, bleed time; monitor CBC, PT, PTT **NIPE:** Observe for anaphylactic Rxns; not blood or plasma substitute

Human Papillomavirus Recombinant Vaccine (Cervarix [Types 16, 18], Gardasil (Types 6, 11, 16, 18) Uses: *Prevent cervical CA, precancerous genital lesions (Cervarix & Gardasil), genital warts, anal CA & oral CA (Gardasil) d/t HPV types 16, 18 (Cervarix) & types 6, 11, 16, 18 (Gardasil) in females 9–26 y*; prevent genital warts, anal CA & anal intraepithelial neoplasia in males 9–26 y (Gardasil) **Action:** Recombinant vaccine, passive immunity **Dose:** 0.5 mL IM initial, then 1 & 6 mo (Cervarix), or 2 & 6 mo (Gardasil) (upper thigh or deltoid) **Caution:** [B, ?/–] **Disp:** SDV & prefilled syringe: 0.5 mL **SE:** Erythema, pain at Inj site, fever, syncope, venous thromboembolism **Interactions:** May be ↓ response *W/* immunosuppressants, may get ↓ response **NIPE:** 1st CA prevention vaccine; 90% effective in preventing CIN 2 or more severe dx in HPV naive populations; report adverse events to Vaccine Adverse Events Reporting System (VAERS: 1-800-822-7967); IM in upper thigh or deltoid; continue cervical CA screening; h/o genital warts, abnormal Pap smear, or (+) HPV DNA test is not CI to vaccination

Hydralazine (Apresoline, Others) [Antihypertensive/Vasodilator] Uses: *Mod–severe HTN; CHF* (w/ Isordil) **Action:** Peripheral vasodilator **Dose:** *Adults.* Initial 10 mg PO 3–4 × /d, ↑ to 25 mg 3–4 × /d, 300 mg/d max *Peds.* 0.75–3 mg/kg/24 h PO ÷ q6–12h; ↓ in renal impair; (CBC & ANA before) **Caution:** [C, +]

↓ Hepatic Fxn & CAD; ↑ tox w/ MAOI, indomethacin, BBs **CI:** Dissecting aortic aneurysm, mitral valve/rheumatic heart Dz **Disp:** Tabs 10, 25, 50, 100 mg; Inj 20 mg/mL **SE:** SLE-like synd w/ chronic high doses; SVT following IM route, peripheral neuropathy **Interactions:** ↑ Effects *W/* antihypertensives, diazoxide, diuretics, MAOIs, nitrates, EtOH; ↓ pressor response *W/* epinephrine; ↓ effects *W/* NSAIDs **NIPE:** Take w/ food; compensatory sinus tachycardia eliminated w/ BBs

Hydrochlorothiazide (HydroDIURIL, Esidrix, Others) [Antihypertensive/Thiazide Diuretic] **Uses:** *Edema, HTN* prevent stones in hypercalciuria **Action:** Thiazide diuretic; ↓ distal tubule Na⁺ reabsorption **Dose:** *Adults.* 25–100 mg/d PO single or ÷ doses; 200 mg/d max *Peds < 6 mo.* 2–3 mg/kg/d in 2 ÷ doses > *6 mo.* 2 mg/kg/d in 2 ÷ doses **Caution:** [D, +] **CI:** Anuria, sulfonamide allergy, renal Insuff **Disp:** Tabs 25, 50, mg; caps 12.5 mg; PO soln 50 mg/5 mL **SE:** ↓ K⁺, hyperglycemia, hyperuricemia, ↓ Na⁺ **Interactions:** ↑ Hypotension *W/* ACEIs, antihypertensives, carbenoxolone, ↑ hypokalemia *W/* carbenoxolone, corticosteroids; ↑ hyperglycemia *W/* BBs, diazoxide, hypoglycemic drugs; ↑ effects *OF* Li; ↓ effects *W/* amphetamines, cholestyramine, colestipol, NSAIDs, quinidine, dandelion **Labs:** ↑ Glucose, cholesterol, Ca, uric acid levels; ↓ K⁺, Na⁺, HMG, Hct, plts, WBCs; follow K⁺, may need supplementation **NIPE:** Take w/ food; ↑ risk of photosensitivity—use sunblock; monitor ECG for hypokalemia (flattened T waves)

Hydrochlorothiazide & Amiloride (Moduretic) [Antihypertensive/Thiazide & K⁺-Sparing Diuretic] **Uses:** *HTN* **Action:** Combined thiazide & K⁺-sparing diuretic **Dose:** 1–2 tabs/d PO **Caution:** [D, ?] **CI:** Renal failure, sulfonamide allergy **Disp:** Tabs (amiloride/HCTZ) 5 mg/50 mg **SE:** ↓ BP, photosensitivity, hyperglycemia, hyperlipidemia, hyperuricemia **Interactions:** ↑ Hypotension *W/* ACEIs, antihypertensives, carbenoxolone, ↑ hypokalemia *W/* amphotericin B, carbenoxolone, corticosteroids, licorice; ↑ risk of hyperkalemia *W/* ACE-I, K⁺-sparing diuretics, NSAIDs, & K⁺ salt substitutes; ↑ hyperglycemia *W/* BBs, diazoxide, hypoglycemic drugs; ↑ effects *OF* amantadine, antihypertensives, digoxin, Li, MTX; ↑ effects *W/* CNS depressants; ↑ effects *W/* amphetamines, cholestyramine, colestipol, NSAIDs, quinidine, dandelion **Labs:** ↑ Glucose, cholesterol, Ca, uric acid levels; ↓ Na⁺, HMG, Hct, plts, WBCs; ↑ K⁺/↓ K⁺; interferes w/ GTT; monitor lytes, LFTs, uric acid **NIPE:** Take w/ food, I&O, daily wgt, ⊘ salt substitutes, bananas, & oranges ↑ risk of photosensitivity—use sunblock; monitor ECG for hypo-/hyperkalemia (flattened or peaked T waves)

Hydrochlorothiazide & Spironolactone (Aldactazide) [Antihypertensive/Thiazide & K⁺-Sparing Diuretic] **Uses:** *Edema, HTN* **Action:** Thiazide & K⁺-sparing diuretic **Dose:** 25–200 mg each component/d, ÷ doses **Caution:** [D, +] **CI:** Sulfonamide allergy **Disp:** Tabs (HCTZ mg/spironolactone mg) 25/25, 50/50 **SE:** Photosensitivity, ↓ BP, hyperglycemia, hyperlipidemia, hyperuricemia **Interactions** ↑ Risk of hyperkalemia *W/* ACEIs, K⁺-sparing diuretics, K⁺ supls, salt substitutes; ↓ effects *OF* digoxin **Labs:** ↑ or ↓ K⁺, ↓ Na⁺ **NIPE:** DC drug 3 d before GTT; monitor ECG for hypo-/hyperkalemia (flattened or peaked T waves)

Hydrochlorothiazide & Triamterene (Dyazide, Maxzide) [Anti-hypertensive/Thiazide & K+-Sparing Diuretic] Uses: *Edema & HTN* Action: Combo thiazide & K+-sparing diuretic Dose: *Dyazide:* 1–2 caps PO daily–bid. *Maxzide:* 1 tab/d PO Caution: [D, +/–] CI: Sulfonamide allergy Disp: (Triamterene/HCTZ mg) 37.5/25, 75/50 SE: Photosensitivity, ↓ BP, hyperglycemia, hyperlipidemia, hyperuricemia Interactions: ↑ Risk of hyperkalemia W/ ACEIs, K+-sparing diuretics, K+ supls, salt substitutes; ↑ effects W/ cimetidine, licorice root, ↓ effects *OF* digoxin Labs: ↑ or ↓ K+, ↓ Na+, ↑ serum glucose, BUN, Cr, Mg^{2+}, uric acid, urinary Ca^{2+}; interference w/ assay of quinidine & lactic dehydrogenase NIPE: Urine may turn blue; HCTZ component in Maxzide more bio-available than in Dyazide; monitor ECG for hypo-/hyperkalemia (flattened or peaked T waves)

Hydrocodone & Acetaminophen (Lorcet, Vicodin, Hycet, Others) [C-III] [Narcotic Analgesic/Antitussive] Uses: *Mod–severe pain* Action: Narcotic analgesic w/ nonnarcotic analgesic Dose: *Adults.* 1–2 caps or tabs PO q4–6h PRN; soln 15 mL q4–6h *Peds.* Soln (Hycet) 0.27 mL/kg q4–6h Caution: [C, M] CI: CNS depression, severe resp depression Disp: Many formulations; specify hydrocodone mg/APAP mg dose; caps 5/500; tabs 2.5/500, 5/325, 5/400, 5/500, 7.5/325, 7.5/400, 7.5/500, 7.5/650, 7.5/750, 10/325, 10/400, 10/500, 10/650, 10/660, 10/750; soln *Hycet* (fruit punch) (7.5 mg hydrocodone/325 mg APAP/15 mL) SE: GI upset, sedation, fatigue Interactions: ↑ Effects W/ antihistamines, cimetidine, CNS depressants, dextroamphetamines, glutethimide, MAOIs, protease Inhibs, TCAs, EtOH, St. John's wort; ↑ effects *OF* warfarin ↓ effects W/ phenothiazine Labs: False ↑ amylase, lipase NIPE: Take w/ food, ↑ fluid intake; do not exceed > 4 g APAP/d

Hydrocodone & Aspirin (Lortab ASA, Others) [C-III] [Narcotic Analgesic] Uses: *Mod–severe pain* Action: Narcotic analgesic w/ NSAID Dose: 1–2 PO q4–6h PRN, w/ food/milk Caution: [C, M] ↓ Renal Fxn, gastritis/PUD CI: Component sensitivity; children w/ chickenpox (Reye synd) Disp: 5 mg hydrocodone/500 mg ASA/tabs SE: GI upset, sedation, fatigue NIPE: Monitor for GI bleed

Hydrocodone & Guaifenesin (Hycotuss Expectorant, Others) [C-III] [Narcotic/Expectorant] Uses: *Nonproductive cough*associated w/ resp Infxn Action: Expectorant w/ cough suppressant Dose: *Adults & Peds > 12 y.* 5 mL q4h pc & hs *Peds < 2 y.* 0.3 mg/kg/d ÷ qid *2–12 y.* 2.5 mL q4h pc & hs Caution: [C, M] CI: Component sensitivity Disp: Hydrocodone 5 mg/guaifenesin 100 mg/5 mL SE: GI upset, sedation, fatigue Interactions: ↑ Risk of bleeding W/ heparin

Hydrocodone & Homatropine (Hycodan, Hydromet, Others) [C-III] [Narcotic Analgesic/Antitussive] Uses: *Relief of cough* Action: Combo antitussive Dose: (Based on hydrocodone) *Adults.* 5–10 mg q4–6h *Peds.* 0.6 mg/kg/d ÷ tid–qid Caution: [C, M] CI: NAG, ↑ ICP, depressed ventilation Disp: Syrup 5 mg hydrocodone/5 mL; tabs 5 mg hydrocodone **SE:** Sedation, fatigue, GI upset **Labs:** ↑ ALT, AST **NIPE:** Do not give < q4h; see individual drugs

Hydrocodone & Ibuprofen (Vicoprofen) [C-III] [Narcotic Analgesic/ NSAID] Uses: *Mod–severe pain (< 10 d)* **Action:** Narcotic w/ NSAID **Dose:** 1–2 tabs q4–6h PRN **Caution:** [C, M] Renal Insuff; **CI:** Component sensitivity **Disp:** Tabs 7.5 mg hydrocodone/200 mg ibuprofen **SE:** Sedation, fatigue, GI upset **Interactions:** ↑ Effect W/ CNS depressants, EtOH, MAOI, ASA, TCA, anticoagulants; ↓ effects OF ACEIs, diuretics; ↓ effect W/ ACE Inhibs & diuretics; ↑ risk of bleeding W/ heparin

Hydrocodone & Pseudoephedrine (Detussin, Histussin-D, Others) [C-III] [Antitussive/Decongestant] Uses: *Cough & nasal congestion* **Action:** Narcotic cough suppressant w/ decongestant **Dose:** 5 mL qid, PRN **Caution:** [C, M] **CI:** MAOIs **Disp:** Hydrocodone/pseudoephedrine 5 mg/60 mg, 3 mg/15 mg; tabs 5 mg/60 mg **SE:** ↑ BP, GI upset, sedation, fatigue **Interactions:** ↑ Effects W/ sympathomimetics **NIPE:** ↑ Bleeding w/ heparin

Hydrocodone, Chlorpheniramine, Phenylephrine, Acetaminophen, & Caffeine (Hycomine Compound) [C-III] [Narcotic Analgesic/Antitussive/Antihistamine] Uses: *Cough & Sxs of URI* **Action:** Narcotic cough suppressant w/ decongestants & analgesic **Dose:** 1 tab PO q4h PRN **Caution:** [C, M] **CI:** NAG **Disp:** Hydrocodone 5 mg/chlorpheniramine 2 mg/ phenylephrine 10 mg/APAP 250 mg/caffeine 30 mg/tab **SE:** ↑ BP, GI upset, sedation, fatigue; see individual agents

Hydrocortisone, Rectal (Anusol-HC Suppository, Cortifoam Rectal, Proctocort, Others) [Corticosteroid] Uses: *Painful anorectal conditions*, radiation proctitis, UC **Action:** Anti-inflammatory steroid **Dose:** *Adults. UC:* 10–100 mg PR daily–bid for 2–3 wk **Caution:** [B, ?/–] **CI:** Component sensitivity **Disp:** *Hydrocortisone acetate:* Rectal aerosol 90 mg/applicator; supp 25 mg *Hydrocortisone base:* Rectal 0.5%, 1%, 2.5%; rectal susp 100 mg/60 mL **SE:** Minimal systemic effect **NIPE:** Administer after BM, insert supp blunt end 1st, administer enema w/ pt lying on side & retain for 1 h

Hydrocortisone, Topical & Systemic (Cortef, Solu-Cortef) [Corticosteroid] See Steroids Tables 2 & 3 **Peds. ECC 2010:** Adrenal insufficiency: 2 mg/kg IV/IO bolus; max dose 100 mg **Caution:** [B, –] **CI:** Viral, fungal, or tubercular skin lesions; serious Infxns (except septic shock or TB meningitis) **SE:** *Systemic:* ↑ Appetite, insomnia, hyperglycemia, bruising **Notes:** May cause hypothalamic-pituitary-adrenal axis suppression **Interactions:** ↑ Effects W/ cyclosporine, estrogens; ↑ effects OF cardiac glycosides, cyclosporine; ↑ risk of GI bleed W/ NSAIDs; ↓ effects W/ aminoglutethimide, antacids, barbiturates, cholestyramine, colestipol, ephedrine, phenobarbital, phenytoin, rifampin; ↓ effects OF anticoagulants, hypoglycemics, insulin, INH, salicylates **Labs:** ↑ Glucose, cholesterol; ↓ K$^+$, Ca$^+$ **NIPE:** ⊘ EtOH, live virus vaccines, abrupt D/C of drug; take w/ food; may mask S/Sxs Infxn

Hydromorphone (Dilaudid) [C–II] [Narcotic Analgesic]   WARNING:
A potent Schedule II opioid agonist; highest potential for abuse & risk of resp depression. HP formula is highly concentrated; do not confuse w/ standard formulations, OD & death could result. Alcohol, other opioids, CNS depressants ↑ resp depressant effects **Uses:** *Mod/severe pain* **Action:** Narcotic analgesic **Dose:** 1–4 mg PO, IM, IV, or PR q4–6h PRN; 3 mg PR q6–8h PRN; ↓ w/ hepatic failure **Caution:** [B (D if prolonged use or high doses near term), ?] ↑ Resp depression & CNS effects CNS depressants, phenothiazines, TCA **CI:** HP lesion w/ ↑ ICP, COPD, cor pulmonale, emphysema, kyphoscoliosis, status asthmaticus; HP-Inj form in OB analgesia **Disp:** Tabs 2, 4 mg, 8 mg scored; Liq 5 mg/5 mL or 1 mg/mL; Inj 1, 2, 4, HP is 10 mg/mL; supp 3 mg **SE:** Sedation, dizziness, GI upset **Interactions:** ↑ Effects W/ CNS depressants, phenothiazines, TCAs, EtOH, St. John's wort; ↓ effects W/ nalbuphine, pentazocine **Labs:** ↑ Serum amylase, lipase **NIPE:** Take w/ food; ↑ fluids & fiber to prevent constipation; morphine 10 mg IM = hydromorphone 1.5 mg IM

Hydromorphone, Extended Release (Exalgo) [C–II] [Opioid Analgesic]   WARNING: Use in opioid tolerant only; high potential for abuse, criminal diversion & resp depression. Not for post-op pain or PRN use. OD & death esp in children. Do not break/crush/chew tabs, may result in OD **Uses:** *Mod/severe chronic pain requiring around the clock opioid analgesic* **Action:** Narcotic analgesic **Dose:** 8–64 mg PO/d titrate to effect; ↓ w/ hepatic/renal impair & elderly **Caution:** [C, –] Abuse potential; ↑ resp depression & CNS effects, w/ CNS depressants, pts susceptible to intracranial effects of CO_2 retention **CI:** Opioid intolerant patients, ↓ pulm Fxn, ileus, GI tract narrowing/obst, component hypersensitivity; w/in 14 d of MAOI **Disp:** Tabs 8,12,16 mg **SE:** Constipation, N/V, somnolence, HA, dizziness **Interactions:** Anticholinergics may ↑ SE; ↑ effects W/ CNS depressants, TCA, phenothiazines, EtOH **NIPE:** See label for opioid conversion; do not use w/in 14 d of MAOI. Not for opioid naïve; swallow whole; withdraw gradually

Hydroxocobalamin (Cyanokit) [Antidote]   Uses: *Cyanide poisoning* **Action:** Binds cyanide to form nontoxic cyanocobalamin excreted in urine **Dose:** 5 mg IV over 15 min, repeat PRN 5 g IV over 15 min–2 h, total dose 10 g **Caution:** [C, ?] **CI:** None known **Disp:** Kit 2-, 2.5-g vials w/ Inf set **SE:** ↑ BP (can be severe) anaphylaxis, chest tightness, edema, urticaria, rash, chromaturia, N, HA **NIPE:** Inj site Rxns

Hydroxyurea (Hydrea, Droxia) [Antineoplastic/Antimetabolite]
Uses: *CML, head & neck, ovarian & colon CA, melanoma, ALL, sickle cell anemia, polycythemia vera, HIV* **Action:** ↓ Ribonucleotide reductase **Dose:** (Per protocol) 50–75 mg/kg for WBC > 100,000 cells/mL; 20–30 mg/kg in refractory CML *HIV:* 1000–1500 mg/d in single or ÷ doses; ↓ in renal Insuff **Caution:** [D, –] **CI:** Severe anemia, BM suppression, WBC < 2500 cells/mL or plt < 100,000 cells/mm^3, PRG **Disp:** Caps 200, 300, 400, 500 mg, tabs 1000 mg **SE:** ↓ BM (mostly leukopenia), N/V, rashes, facial erythema, radiation recall Rxns, renal impair

Interactions: ↑ Effects *W/* zidovudine, zalcitabine, didanosine, stavudine, 5-FU, ↑ risk of pancreatitis *W/* didanosine, indinavir, stavudine; ↑ BM suppression *W/* antineoplastic drugs or radiation therapy **Labs:** ↑ Serum uric acid, BUN, Cr **NIPE:** ↑ Fluids 10–12 glasses/d, use barrier contraception, ↑ risk of infertility; empty caps into H_2O

Hydroxyzine (Atarax, Vistaril) [Antipsychotic, Sedative/Hypnotic/Antihistamine]
Uses: *Anxiety, sedation, itching* **Action:** Antihistamine, antianxiety **Dose:** *Adults. Anxiety/sedation:* 50–100 mg PO or IM qid or PRN (max 600 mg/d) *Itching:* 25–50 mg PO or IM tid–qid **Peds.** 0.5–1.0 mg/kg/24 h PO or IM q6h; ↓ w/ hepatic impair **Caution:** [C, +/–] ↑ Effects w/ CNS depressants, anticholinergics, EtOH **CI:** Component sensitivity **Disp:** Tabs 10, 25, 50 mg; caps 25, 50 mg; syrup 10 mg/5 mL; susp 25 mg/5 mL; Inj 25, 50 mg/mL **SE:** Drowsiness, anticholinergic effects **Interactions:** ↑ Effects *W/* antihistamines, anticholinergics, CNS depressants, EtOH **Labs:** False(–) skin allergy tests; false ↑ in urinary 17-hydroxycorticosteroid levels **NIPE:** Used to potentiate narcotic effects; not for IV/SQ (thrombosis & digital gangrene possible)

Hyoscyamine (Anaspaz, Cystospaz, Levsin, Others) [Antispasmodic/Anticholinergic]
Uses: *Spasm w/ GI & bladder disorders* **Action:** Anticholinergic **Dose:** *Adults.* 0.125–0.25 mg (1–2 tabs) SL/PO tid–qid, ac & hs; 1 SR caps q12h **Caution:** [C, +] ↑ Effects w/ amantadine, antihistamines, antimuscarinics, haloperidol, phenothiazines, TCA, MAOI **CI:** BOO, GI obst, NAG, MyG, paralytic ileus, UC, MI **Disp:** (Cystospaz-M, Levsinex) time-release caps 0.375 mg; elixir (EtOH); soln 0.125 mg/5 mL; Inj 0.5 mg/mL; tab 0.125 mg; tab (Cystospaz) 0.15 mg; XR tab (Levbid) 0.375 mg; SL (Levsin SL) 0.125 mg **SE:** Dry skin, xerostomia, constipation, anticholinergic effects, heat prostration w/ hot weather **Interactions:** ↑ Effects *W/* amantadine, antimuscarinics, haloperidol, phenothiazine, quinidine, TCAs, MAOIs; ↓ effects *W/* antacids, antidiarrheals; ↓ effects *OF* levodopa **NIPE:** ↑ Risk of heat intolerance; photophobia; administer tabs ac/food

Hyoscyamine, Atropine, Scopolamine, & Phenobarbital (Donnatal, Others) [Antispasmodic Anticholinergic]
Uses: *Irritable bowel, spastic colitis, peptic ulcer, spastic bladder* **Action:** Anticholinergic, antispasmodic **Dose:** 0.125–0.25 mg (1–2 tabs) tid–qid, 1 caps q12h (SR), 5–10 mL elixir tid–qid or q8h **Caution:** [D, M] **CI:** NAG **Disp:** Many combos/manufacturers *Caps (Donnatal, others):* Hyoscyamine 0.1037 mg/atropine 0.0194 mg/scopolamine 0.0065 mg/phenobarbital 16.2 mg *Tabs (Donnatal, others):* Hyoscyamine 0.1037 mg/atropine 0.0194 mg/scopolamine 0.0065 mg/phenobarbital 16.2 mg. *LA (Donnatal):* Hyoscyamine 0.311 mg/atropine 0.0582 mg/scopolamine 0.0195 mg/phenobarbital 48.6 mg. *Elixirs (Donnatal, others):* Hyoscyamine 0.1037 mg/atropine 0.0194 mg/scopolamine 0.0065 mg/phenobarbital 16.2 mg/5 mL **SE:** Sedation, xerostomia, constipation **Interactions:** ↑ Anticholinergic effects *W/* amantadine, antihistamines, disopyramide; merperidine, procainamide, quinidine, TCA; ↑ effects *OF* atenolol; ↓ effects *W/* antacids **NIPE:** Take drug w/o food

Ibandronate (Boniva) [Bone Resorption Inhibitor/Bisphosphonate]
Uses: *Rx & prevent osteoporosis in postmenopausal women* **Action:** Bisphosphonate, ↓ osteoclast-mediated bone-resorption **Dose:** 2.5 mg PO daily or 150 mg once/mo on same d (do not lie down for 60 min after); 3 mg IV over 15–30 s q3mo **Caution:** [C, ?/–] Avoid w/ CrCl < 30 mL/min **CI:** Uncorrected ↓ Ca²⁺; inability to stand/sit upright for 60 min (PO) **Disp:** Tabs 2.5, 150 mg, Inj IV 3 mg/3 mL **SE:** Jaw osteonecrosis (avoid extensive dental procedures) N/D, HA, dizziness, asthenia, HTN, Infxn, dysphagia, esophagitis, esophageal/gastric ulcer, musculoskeletal pain **Interactions:** ↑ GI upset **W/** ASA, NSAIDs; ↓ absorption **W/** antacids, vits, supl or other drugs containing Ca⁺, Mg⁺, Fe; EtOH, food, milk **Labs:** ↑ Cholesterol; ↓ alk phos **NIPE:** ↑ Risk of photophobia, constipation, urinary hesitancy; take 1st thing in AM W/ H₂O (6–8 oz) > 60 min before 1st food/beverage & any meds w/ multivalent cations; give adequate Ca²⁺& vit D supls; possible association between bisphosphonates & severe musculo/bone/Jt pain; may ↑ atypical subtrochanteric femur fxs

Ibuprofen, Oral (Motrin, Motrin IB, Rufen, Advil, Others) [OTC] [Anti-Inflammatory, Antipyretic, Analgesic/NSAID] WARNING: May ↑ risk of CV events & GI bleeding **Uses:** *Arthritis, pain, fever* **Action:** NSAID **Dose:** *Adults.* 200–800 mg PO bid–qid (max 2.4 g/d) *Peds.* 30–40 mg/kg/d in 3–4 ÷ doses (max 40 mg/kg/d); w/ food **Caution:** [B, +] May interfere w/ ASA's antiplt effect if given 8 h before ASA **CI:** 3rd tri PRG, severe hepatic impair, allergy, use w/ other NSAIDs, upper GI bleeding, ulcers **Disp:** Tabs 100, 200, 400, 600, 800 mg; chew tabs 50, 100 mg; caps 200 mg; susp 50 mg/1.25 mL, 100 mg/2.5 mL, 100 mg/5 mL, 40 mg/mL (Motrin IB & Advil OTC 200 mg are the OTC forms) **SE:** Dizziness, peptic ulcer, plt inhibition, worsening of renal Insuff **Interactions:** ↑ Effects **W/** ASA, corticosteroids, probenecid, EtOH; ↑ effects **OF** aminoglycosides, anticoagulants, digoxin, hypoglycemics, Li, MTX; ↑ risks of bleeding **W/** abciximab, cefotetan, valproic acid, thrombolytic drugs, warfarin, ticlopidine, garlic, ginger, ginkgo; ↓ effects **W/** feverfew; ↓ effects **OF** antihypertensives **Labs:** ↑ BUN, Cr, LFTs; ↓ HMG, Hct, BS, plts, WBCs **NIPE:** Take w/ food

Ibuprofen, Parenteral (Caldolor) [NSAID/Propionic Acid Derivative] WARNING: May risk of CV events & GI bleeding **Uses:** *Mild/mod pain, as adjunct to opioids, ↓ fever* **Action:** NSAID **Dose:** *Pain:* 400–800 mg IV over 30 min q6h PRN *Fever:* 400 mg IV over 30 min, then 400 mg q4–6h or 100–200 mg q4h PRN **Caution:** [C < 30 wk, D after 30 wk, ?/–] may ↑ ACE effects; avoid w/ ASA, & < 17 y **CI:** Hypersensitivity NSAIDs; asthma, urticaria, or allergic Rxns w/ NSAIDs, perioperative CABG **Disp:** Vials 400 mg/4 mL, 800 mg/8 mL **SE:** N/V, HA, flatulence, hemorrhage, dizziness **Interactions:** ↑ risk of GI bleed **W/** anticoagulants; oral corticosteroids; EtOH, tobacco; ↑ Li, methotrexate; ↓ effects **OF** ACEI, diuretics **Labs:** Monitor LFTs, BUN/SCr **NIPE:** Make sure pt well hydrated; use lowest dose & shortest duration possible

Ibutilide (Corvert) [Antiarrhythmic/Ibutilide Derivative] Uses: *Rapid conversion of AF/A flutter* **Action:** Class III antiarrhythmic **Dose:** *Adults.*

> 60 kg 1 mg IV over 10 min; may repeat × 1; < 60 kg use 0.01 mg/kg *ECC 2010:* **SVT (AF & aflutter):** Adults ≥ 60 kg, 1 mg (10 mL) over 10 min; 2nd dose may be used; < 60 kg, 0.01 mg/kg over 10 min.Consider DC cardioversion **Caution:** [C, –] **CI:** w/ Class I/III antiarrhythmics (Table 9); QTc > 440 ms **Disp:** Inj 0.1 mg/mL **SE:** Arrhythmias, HA **Interactions:** ↑ effects *W/* amiodarone, disopyramide, procainamide, quinidine, sotalol; ↑ QT interval *W/* antihistamines, antidepressants, erythromycin, phenothiazine, TCAs **Labs:** Monitor K+, Mg2+ **NIPE:** Give w/ ECG monitoring

Idarubicin (Idamycin) [Antineoplastic/Anthracycline] WARNING: Administer only under supervision of an MD experienced in leukemia & in an institution w/ resources to maint a pt compromised by drug tox **Uses:** *Acute leukemias* (AML, ALL), *CML in blast crisis, breast CA* **Action:** DNA intercalating agent; ↓ DNA topoisomerases I & II **Dose:** (Per protocol) 10–12 mg/m²/d for 3–4 d; ↓ in renal/hepatic impair **Caution:** [D, –] PRT: Bilirubin > 5 mg/dL, PRG **Disp:** Inj 1 mg/mL (5-, 10-, 20-mg vials) **SE:** ↓ BM, cardiotox, N/V, mucositis, alopecia, & IV site Rxns, rarely ↓ renal/hepatic Fxn **Interactions:** ↑ Myelosuppression *W/* antineoplastic drugs & radiation therapy; ↓ effects *OF* live virus vaccines **Labs:** ↑ BUN, Cr, uric acid, LFTs; ↓ HMG, Hct, plts, RBCs, WBCs **NIPE:** ↑ Fluids to 2–3 L/d; avoid extrav, potent vesicant; IV only

Ifosfamide (Ifex, Holoxan) [Antineoplastic/Alkylating Agent] WARNING: Administer only under supervision of an MD experienced in chemotherapy; hemorrhagic cystitis, myelosuppression; confusion, coma possible **Uses:** *Testis*, lung, breast, pancreatic & gastric CA, Hodgkin lymphoma/NHL, soft-tissue sarcoma **Action:** Alkylating agent **Dose:** (Per protocol) 1.2 g/m²/d for 5 d bolus or cont Inf; 2.4 g/m²/d for 3 d; w/ mesna uroprotection; ↓ in renal/hepatic impair **Caution:** [D, M] **CI:** ↓ BM Fxn, PRG **Disp:** Inj 1, 3 g **SE:** Hemorrhagic cystitis, nephrotox, N/V, mild–mod leukopenia, lethargy & confusion, alopecia, ↑ LFTs **Interactions:** ↑ Risk of bleeding *W/* anticoagulants, ASA, NSAIDs; ↑ effects *W/* barbiturates, carbamazepine, chloral hydrate, phenobarbital, phenytoin; ↑ myelosuppression *W/* antineoplastic drugs & radiation therapy; ↓ effects *OF* live virus vaccines; ↓ effects *W/* corticosteroids, St. John's wort **Labs:** ↑ LFTs, uric acid; ↓ plts, WBCs **NIPE:** ↑ Fluids to 2–3 L/d; administer w/ MESNA to prevent hemorrhagic cystitis; WBC nadir 10–14 d; recovery 21–28 d

Iloperidone (Fanapt) [Antipsychotics/Piperidinyl-Benzisoxazole Atypical] WARNING: Risk for torsades de pointes & ↑ QT. Elderly pts at risk of death, CVA **Uses:** *Acute schizophrenia* **Action:** Atypical antipsychotic **Dose:** *Initial:* 1 mg IV, daily to goal 12–24 mg/d ÷ bid **Caution:** [?, ?] **Contra:** Component hypersensitivity **Disp:** Tabs:1, 2, 4, 6, 8, 10, 12 mg **SE:** Orthostatic↓ BP, dizziness, dry mouth, ↑ wgt; **Interactions:** ↑ Risk of prolonged QTc *W/* amiodarone, antiarrhythmics, antipsychotics, chlorpromazine, gatifloxacin, levomethadyl, methadone, moxifloxacin, pentamidine, procainamide, quinidine, thioridazine; ↑ effects *OF* CYP2D6 & CYP3A4 Inhibs, clarithromycin, fluoxetine, ketoconazole, paroxetine; ↑ risks of orthostatic hypotension *W*/ antihypertensives; ↑ risks of impaired thermoregulation *W*/ anticholinergics **Labs:** Monitor CBC, K⁺, Mg **NIPE:** Titrate to ↓ BP risk; monitor ECG for prolonged QT interval

Iloprost (Ventavis) [Prostaglandin Analog] **WARNING:** Associated w/ syncope; may require dosage adjustment **Uses:** *NYHA Class III/IV pulm arterial HTN* **Action:** Prostaglandin analogue **Dose:** Initial 2.5 mcg; if tolerated, ↑ to 5 mcg Inh 6–9 × /d at least 2 h apart while awake **Caution:** [C, ?/–] Antiplt effects, ↑ bleeding risk w/ anticoagulants; additive hypotensive effects **CI:** SBP < 85 mm Hg **Disp:** Inh soln 10 mcg/mL **SE:** Syncope, ↓ BP, vasodilation, cough, HA, trismus, D, dysgeusia, rash, oral irritation **Interactions:** ↑ Effects *OF* anticoagulants, antihypertensives, antiplts **Labs:** ↑ Alk phos **NIPE:** Instruct pt of syncope risk; monitor BP; requires *Pro-Dose AAD* or *I-neb ADD* system nebulizer; counsel on syncope risk; do not mix w/ other drugs; monitor vital signs during initial Rx

Imatinib (Gleevec) [Antineoplastic/Tyrosine Kinase Inhibitor] **Uses:** *Rx CML Ph(+), CML blast crisis, ALL Ph(+), myelodysplastic/myeloproliferative Dz, aggressive systemic mastocytosis, chronic eosinophilic leukemia, GIST, dermatofibrosarcoma protuberans* **Action:** BCL-ABL; TKI **Dose:** *Adults. Typical:* 400–600 mg PO daily; w/ meal *Peds. CML Ph(+) newly diagnosed:* 340 mg/m²/d, 600 mg/d max *Recurrent:* 260 mg/m²/d PO ÷ daily–bid, to 340 mg/m²/d max **Caution:** [D, ?/–] w/ CYP3A4 meds (Table 10), warfarin **CI:** Component sensitivity **Disp:** Tab 100, 400 mg **SE:** GI upset, fluid retention, muscle cramps, musculoskeletal pain, arthralgia, rash, HA, neutropenia, ↓ plt **Interactions:** ↑ Effects *OF* cyclosporine, CCB, HMG-CoA reductase Inhibs, triazolobenzodiazepines, erythromycin, itraconazole, ketoconazole; ↑ risk of liver tox *W*/ APAP; ↓ effects *W*/ carbamazepine, dexamethasone, phenobarbital, phenytoin, rifampin, St. John's wort **Labs:** ↑ LFTs; ↓ HMG, Hct, neutrophils, plts; follow CBCs & LFTs baseline & monthly **NIPE:** Take w/ large glass of H₂O & food to ↓ GI irritation; use barrier contraception

Imipenem–Cilastatin (Primaxin) [Antibiotic/Carbapenems] **Uses:** *Serious Infxns* d/t susceptible bacteria **Action:** Bactericidal; ↓ cell wall synth. *Spectrum:* Gram(+) (*S aureus*, group A & B streptococci), gram(–) (not *Legionella*), anaerobes **Dose:** *Adults.* 250–1000 mg (imipenem) IV q6–8h, 500–750 mg IM *Peds.* 60–100 mg/kg/24 h IV ÷ q6h; ↓ if CrCl is < 70 mL/min **Caution:** [C, +/–] Probenecid ↑ tox **CI:** Ped pts w/ CNS Infxn (↑ Sz risk) & < 30 kg w/ renal impair **Disp:** Inj (imipenem/cilastatin mg) 250/250, 500/500 **SE:** Szs if drug accumulates, GI upset, ↓ plt **Interactions:** ↑ Risks of Szs *W*/ cyclosporine, ganciclovir; ↑ effects *W*/ probenecid **Labs:** ↑ LFTs, BUN, Cr; ↓ HMG, Hct, plts, WBCs **NIPE:** Eval for super Infxn; ↑ risk of Sz

Imipramine (Tofranil) [Antidepressant/TCA] **WARNING:** Close observation for suicidal thinking or unusual changes in behavior **Uses:** *Depression, enuresis*, panic attack, chronic pain **Action:** TCA; ↑ CNS synaptic serotonin or norepinephrine **Dose:** *Adults. Hospitalized:* Initial 100 mg/24 h PO in ÷ doses; ↑ over several wk 300 mg/d max *Outpatient:* Maint 50–150 mg PO hs, 300 mg/24 h max *Peds. Antidepressant:* 1.5–5 mg/kg/24 h ÷ daily–qid. *Enuresis:* **> 6 y:** 10–25 mg PO qhs; ↑ by 10–25 mg at 1–2-wk intervals (max 50 mg for 6–12 y, 75 mg for > 12 y); Rx for 2–3 mo, then taper **Caution:** [D, ?/–] **CI:** Use w/ MAOIs, NAG, acute recovery from MI, PRG, CHF, angina, CV Dz, arrhythmias **Disp:** Tabs 10, 25, 50 mg; caps 75, 100, 125, 150 mg **SE:** CV Sxs, dizziness, xerostomia, discolored urine **Interactions:** ↑ Effects **W/** amiodarone, anticholinergics, BBs, cimetidine, diltiazem, Li, OCPs, quinidine, phenothiazine, ritonavir, verapamil, EtOH, evening primrose oil; ↑ effects **OF** CNS depressants, hypoglycemics, warfarin; ↑ risk of serotonin synd **W/** MAOIs; ↓ effects **W/** tobacco; ↓ effects **OF** clonidine **Labs:** ↑ Serum glucose, LFTs **NIPE:** D/C 48 h before surgery; D/C MAOIs 2 wk before administration of this drug; 4–6 wk for full effects; take w/ food; less sedation than amitriptyline

Imiquimod Cream, 5% (Aldara) [Topical Immunomodulator]
Uses: *Anogenital warts, HPV, condylomata acuminata* **Action:** Unknown; ? cytokine induction **Dose:** Apply 3 × /wk, leave on 6–10 h & wash off w/ soap & H₂O, continue 16 wk max **Caution:** [B, ?] **CI:** Component sensitivity **Disp:** Single-dose packets 5% (250 mg cream) **SE:** Local skin Rxns **NIPE:** Not a cure; may weaken condoms/Vag diaphragms, wash hands before & after use

Immune Globulin, IV (Gamimune N, Gammaplex, Gammar IV, Sandoglobulin, Others) [Immune Serum/Immunologic Agent]
Uses: *IgG deficiency Dz states, B-cell CLL, CIDP, HIV, hep A prophylaxis, ITP*, Kawasaki dx, travel to ↑ prevalence area & hep A vaccination w/in 2 wk of travel **Action:** IgG supl **Dose:** *Adults & Peds. Immunodeficiency:* 200–(300 *Gammaplex*)–800 mg/kg/mo IV at 0.012 wk of (*Gammaplex*) mL/kg/min; initial dose 0.01 mL/kg/min *B-cell CLL:* 400 mg/kg/dose IV q3wk, *CIDP:* 2000 over 2 initial dose 0.01 mL/kg/min in 2 wk of *ITP:* 400 mg/kg/dose IV daily × 5 d *BMT:* 500 mg/kg/wk; ↓ in renal Insuff **Caution:** [C, ?] Separate live vaccines by 3 mo **CI:** IgA deficiency w/ Abs to IgA, severe ↓ IgA, coagulation disorders **Disp:** Inj **SE:** Associated mostly w/ Inf rate; GI upset, thrombotic events, hemolysis, renal failure/ dysfunction, TRALI **Interactions:** ↓ Effects **OF** live virus vaccines **Labs:** ↑ BUN, Cr **NIPE:** Monitor vitals during Inf; do not give if vol depleted; hep A prophylaxis w/ Ig is no better than w/ vaccination; advantages to using vaccination, cost similar

Immune Globulin, Subcutaneous (Vivaglobin) [Immune Serum]
Uses: *Primary immunodeficiency* **Action:** IgG supl **Dose:** 100–200 mg/kg body wgt SQ weekly **Caution:** [C, ?] **CI:** h/o Anaphylaxis to immune globulin; IgA deficiency if known IgA Abs **Disp:** 3-,10-, 20-mL vials w/ 160 mg/mL **SE:** Inj site Rxns, HA, arthralgia, GI complaint, fever, N, D, rash, sore throat **NIPE:** May instruct in home administration; keep refrigerated; discard unused drug; dose > 15 mL divided between sites

Inamrinone [Amrinone] (Inocor) [Inotropic/Vasodilator] **Uses:** *Acute CHF, ischemic cardiomyopathy* **Action:** Inotrope w/ vasodilator **Dose:** *Adults.* IV bolus 0.75 mg/kg over 2–3 min; maint 5–10 mcg/kg/min, 10 mg/kg/d max; ↓ if CrCl < 10 mL/min *Peds. ECC 2010:* CHF in post-op CV surgery pts, shock w/ ↑ SVR: 0.75–1 mg/kg IV/IO load over 5 min; repeat × 2 PRN; max 3 mg/kg;

cont Inf 5–10 mcg/kg/min **Caution:** [C, ?] **CI:** Bisulfite allergy **Disp:** Inj 5 mg/mL **SE:** Monitor fluid, lytes, & renal changes **Interactions:** Diuretics cause sig hypovolemia; ↑ effects *OF* cardiac glycosides **Labs:** Monitor LFTs **NIPE:** Monitor I&O, daily wgt, BP, pulse; incompatible w/ dextrose solns; observe for arrhythmias

Indapamide (Lozol) [Antihypertensive/Thiazide Diuretic] **Uses:** *HTN, edema, CHF* **Action:** Thiazide diuretic; ↑ Na, Cl, & H_2O excretion in distal tubule **Dose:** 1.25–5 mg/d PO **Caution:** [D, ?] ↑ Effect w/ loop diuretics, ACE Inhibs, cyclosporine, digoxin, Li **CI:** Anuria, thiazide/sulfonamide allergy, renal Insuff, PRG **Disp:** Tabs 1.25, 2.5 mg **SE:** ↓ BP, dizziness, photosensitivity **Interactions:** ↑ Effects *W/* antihypertensives, diazoxide, nitrates, EtOH; ↑ effects *OF* ACEIs, Li; ↑ risk of hypokalemia *W/* amphotericin B, corticosteroids, mezlocillin, piperacillin, ticarcillin; ↓ effects *W/* cholestyramine, colestipol, NSAIDs **Labs:** ↑ Serum glucose, cholesterol, uric acid, ↓ K^+, Na, Cl **NIPE:** ↑ Risk photosensitivity—use sunblock; take w/ food or milk; no additional effects w/ doses > 5 mg; take early to avoid nocturia

Indinavir (Crixivan) [Antiretroviral/Protease Inhibitor] **Uses:** *HIV Infxn* **Action:** Protease Inhib; ↓ maturation of noninfectious virions to mature infectious virus **Dose:** Typical 800 mg PO q8h in combo w/ other antiretrovirals (dose varies); on empty stomach; ↓ w/ hepatic impair **Caution:** [C, ?] Numerous drug interactions, esp CYP3A4 Inhib (Table 10) *W/* triazolam, midazolam, pimozide, ergot alkaloids, simvastatin, lovastatin, sildenafil, St. John's wort, amiodarone **Disp:** Caps 100, 200, 333, 400 mg **SE:** Nephrolithiasis, dyslipidemia, lipodystrophy, N/V **Interactions:** ↑ Effects *W/* azole antifungals, clarithromycin, delavirdine, ILs, quinidine, zidovudine; ↑ effects *OF* amiodarone, cisapride, clarithromycin, ergot alkaloids, fentanyl, HMG-CoA reductase Inhibs, INH, OCPs, phenytoin, rifabutin, ritonavir, sildenafil, stavudine, zidovudine; ↓ effects *W/* efavirenz, fluconazole, phenytoin, rifampin, St. John's wort, high-fat/-protein foods, grapefruit juice; ↓ effects *OF* midazolam, triazolam **Labs:** ↑ Bilirubin, Serum glucose, LFTs, ↓ HMG, plts, neutrophils **NIPE:** ↑ Fluids—drink six 8-oz glasses of H_2O/d; caps moisture sensitive—keep desiccant in container

Indomethacin (Indocin) [Analgesic, Anti-Inflammatory, Antipyretic/ NSAID] **WARNING:** May ↑ risk of CV events & GI bleeding **Uses:** *Arthritis; close ductus arteriosus; ankylosing spondylitis* **Action:** ↓ Prostaglandins **Dose:** *Adults.* 25–50 mg PO bid–tid, max 200 mg/d **Peds.** *Infants.* 0.2–0.25 mg/kg/dose IV; may repeat in 12–24 h up to 3 doses; w/ food **Caution:** [B, +] **CI:** ASA/NSAID sensitivity, peptic ulcer/active GI bleed, precipitation of asthma/urticaria/rhinitis by NSAIDs/ASA, premature neonates w/ NEC ↓ renal Fxn, active bleeding, ↓ plt, 3rd tri PRG **Disp:** Inj 1 mg/vial; caps 25, 50 mg; SR caps 75 mg; susp 25 mg/5 mL **SE:** GI bleeding or upset, dizziness, edema **Interactions:** ↑ Effects *W/* APAP, anti-inflammatories, gold compounds, diflunisal, probenecid; ↑ effects *OF* aminoglycosides, anticoagulants, digoxin, hypoglycemics, Li, MTX, nifedipine, phenytoin, penicillamine, verapamil; ↓ effects *W/* ASA; ↓ effects *OF* antihypertensives **Labs:** ↑

LFTs, serum K+, BUN, Cr, ↓ HMG, Hct, leukocytes, plts; monitor renal Fxn **NIPE:** Take w/ food, monitor ECG for hyperkalemia (peaked T waves)

Infliximab (Remicade) [Anti-Inflammatory/Monoclonal Antibody] **WARNING:** TB, invasive fungal Infxns, & other opportunistic Infxns reported, some fatal; perform TB skin testing prior to use; possible association w/ rare lymphoma Uses: *Mod–severe Crohn Dz; fistulizing Crohn Dz; UC; RA (w/ MTX) psoriasis, ankylosing spondylitis* **Action:** IgG1K neutralizes TNF-α **Dose:** *Adults. Crohn Dz:* Induction: 5 mg/kg IV Inf, w/ doses 2 & 6 wk after *Maint:* 5 mg/kg IV Inf q8wk *RA:* 3 mg/kg IV Inf at 0, 2, 6 wk, then q8wk *Peds > 6 y.* 5 mg/ kg IV q8wk **Caution:** [B, ?/–] Active Infxn, hepatic impair, h/o or risk of TB, hep B **CI:** Murine allergy, mod–severe CHF, w/ live vaccines (eg, smallpox) **Disp:** 100 mg Inj **SE:** Allergic Rxns; HA, fatigue, GI upset, Inf Rxns; hepatotox; reactivation hep B, pneumonia, BM suppression, systemic vasculitis, pericardial effusion, new psoriasis **Interactions:** May ↓ effects *OF* live virus vaccines **Labs:** Monitor LFTs; PPD at baseline; monitor hep B carrier **NIPE:** ↑ Susceptibility to Infxn; skin exam for malignancy w/ psoriasis; can premedicate w/ antihistamines, APAP, and/or steroids to ↑ Inf Rxns

Influenza Monovalent Vaccine (H1N1), Inactivated (CSL, ID Biomedical, Novartis, Sanofi Pasteur) The 2010, Sanofi Pasteur (HUS/Canada) will be the trivalent influenza vaccine that includes pandemic H1N1 influenza A. The monovalent vaccine against H1N1 influenza A will no longer be administered

Influenza Vaccine, Inactivated (Afluria, Agriflu, Fluarix, FluLaval, Fluvirin, Fluzone) [Antiviral/Vaccine] Uses: *Prevent influenza (not H1N1 swine flu)* in adults > 50 y, children 6–59 mo, PRG women (2nd/3rd tri during flu season), nursing home residents, chronic Dzs (asthma, CAD, DM, chronic liver or renal Dz, hematologic Dzs, immunosuppression), healthcare workers, household contacts, & caregivers of high-risk pts, children < 5 y & adults > 50 y **Action:** Active immunization **Dose:** *Adults & Peds > 9 y.* 0.5 mL/dose IM annually *Peds 6 mo–3 y.* 0.25 mL IM annually; 0.25 mL IM × 2 doses > 4 wk apart 1st vaccination; give 2 doses in 2nd vaccination y if only 1 dose given in 1st y *3–8 y.* 0.5 mL IM annually, start 0.5 mL IM × 2 doses > 4 wk apart in 1st vaccination y **Caution:** [C, +] **CI:** Egg hypersensitivity; neomycin, polymyxin (Afluria); kanamycin, neomycin (Agriflu); gentamicin (Fluarix); polymyxin, neomycin (Fluvirin)/ thimerosal allergy (FluLaval, Fluvirin, & multidose Fluzone); Infxn at site, acute resp or febrile illness, h/o Guillain-Barré, immunocompromised **Disp:** Based on manufacturer, 0.25- & 0.5-mL prefilled syringes **SE:** Inj site soreness, fever, chills, insomnia, myalgia, malaise, rash, urticaria, anaphylactoid Rxns, Guillain-Barré synd **Interactions:** ↑ Effects *OF* theophylline, warfarin; ↓ effects *W/* corticosteroids, immunosuppressants; ↓ effects *OF* aminopyrine, phenytoin **NIPE:** Not for swine flu H1N1; can be administered at the same time. Fluarix & Agriflu not labeled for peds; optimal in United States Oct–Nov, protection begins 1–2 wk after, lasts up to 6 mo; each y, vaccines based on predictions of flu active in flu season

(Nov–Apr in United States though sporadic cases all y); whole or split virus for adults; peds < 13 y split virus or purified surface antigen to ↓ febrile Rxns; see www.cdc.gov/flu for more info; 2010 labeled for peds; optimal in United States Oct–Nov, protection begins 1–2 wk after, lasts up to 6 mo

Influenza Virus Vaccine Live, Intranasal [LAIV] (FluMist) [Antiviral/ Vaccine] Uses: *Prevent influenza* Action: Live attenuated vaccine Dose: *Adults 18–49 y.* 0.1 mL each nostril × 1 annually *Peds 2–8 y.* 0.1 mL each nostril × 1 annually; initial 0.1 mL each nostril × 2 doses > 6 wk apart in 1st vaccination y > 9 y. See Adults dose Caution: [C, ?/–] CI: Age < 2 y, egg, gentamicin, gelatin, or arginine allergy, peds 2–17 y on ASA, PRG, h/o Guillain-Barré, known/ suspected immune deficiency, asthma or reactive airway Dz, acute febrile illness Disp: Prefilled, single-use, intranasal sprayer; shipped frozen, store 35–46°F SE: Runny nose, nasal congestion, HA, cough NIPE: Do not give w/ other vaccines; avoid contact w/ immunocompromised individuals for 21 d; live influenza vaccine more effective in children than inactivated influenza vaccine; 2010 nl US trivalent vaccine will protect against 3 different flu viruses: H3N2, influenza B, H1N1

Insulin, Injectable [Hypoglycemic/Hormone] (See Table 4) Uses: *Type 1 or 2 DM refractory to diet or PO hypoglycemic agents; acute life-threatening ↑ K+* Action: Insulin supl Dose: Based on serum glucose; usually SQ (upper arms, Abd wall [most rapid absorption site], upper legs, buttocks; can give IV (only regular)/IM; type 1 DM typical start dose 0.5–1 units/kg/d; type 2 DM 0.3–0.4 units/kg/d; renal failure ↓ insulin needs Caution: [B, +] CI: Hypoglycemia Disp: Table 4 ; can dispensed w/ preloaded insulin cartridge pens w/ 29-, 30-, or 31-gauge needles & dosing adjustments SE: Hypoglycemia. Highly purified insulins ↑ free insulin; monitor for several wk when changing doses/agents Interactions: ↑ Hypoglycemic effects W/ α-blockers, anabolic steroids, BBs, clofibrate, fenfluramine, guanethidine, MAOIs, NSAIDs, pentamidine, phenylbutazone, salicylates, sulfinpyrazone, tetracyclines, EtOH, celery, coriander, dandelion root, fenugreek, ginseng, garlic, juniper berries; ↓ hypoglycemic effects W/ corticosteroids, dextrothyroxine, diltiazem, dobutamine, epinephrine, niacin, OCPs, protease Inhib antiretrovirals, rifampin, thiazide diuretics, thyroid preps, marijuana, tobacco NIPE: If mixing insulins, draw up shortacting preps 1st in syringe; specific agent/regimen based on pt/healthcare provider choices for glycemic control. Typical type 1 DM regimens use basal daily insulin w/ premeal Injs of rapidly acting insulins. Insulin pumps may achieve basal insulin levels. ↑ Malignancy risk w/ glargine controversial

Interferon Alfa (Roferon-A, Intron-A) [Antineoplastic/Immuno-modulator] WARNING: Can cause or aggravate fatal or life-threatening neuropsychological, autoimmune, ischemic, & infectious disorders. Monitor closely Uses: *HCL, Kaposi sarcoma, melanoma, CML, chronic hep B & C, follicular NHL, condylomata acuminata* Action: Antiproliferative; modulates host immune response; ↓ viral replication in infected cells Dose: Per protocols. Adults. Per protocols HCL: α_{2a} (Roferon-A): 3 MU/d for 16–24 wk SQ/IM, then 3 MU

$3 \times$ /wk $\times$ 6–24 mo; α_{2b} *(Intron-A):* 2 MU/m² IM/SQ $3 \times$ /wk for 2–6 mo. *Chronic hep B:* α_{2b} *(Intron-A):* 3 MU/m² SQ $3 \times$ /wk $\times$ 1 wk, then 6 MU/m² $3 \times$ /wk (max 10 MU $3 \times$ /wk, total duration 16–24 wk). *Follicular NHL* (Intron-A): 5 MU $3 \times$ /wk for 18 mo *Melanoma* (Intron-A): 20 MU/m² IV $\times$ 5 d/wk $\times$ 4 wk, then 10 MU/m² SQ $3 \times$ / wk $\times$ 48 wk *Kaposi sarcoma (Intron-A):* 30 MU/m² IM/SQ $3 \times$ /wk $\times$ 10–12 wk, then 36 MU IM/SQ $3 \times$ /wk. *Chronic hep C (Intron-A):* 3 MU $3 \times$ /wk $\times$ 16 wk (continue 18–24 mo if response) *Roferon A:* 3 MU $3 \times$ /wk for 12 mo SQ/IM. *Condyloma (Intron-A):* 1 MU/lesion (max 5 lesions) $3 \times$ /wk for 3 wk. **Peds.** *CML:* α_{2a} *(Roferon-A):* 2.5–5 MU /m² IM daily **CI:** Benzyl alcohol sensitivity, decompensated liver Dz, autoimmune Dz, immunosuppressed, neonates, infants **Disp:** Inj forms (see also Polyethylene Glycol [PEG]-Interferon) **SE:** Flu-like Sxs, fatigue, anorexia, neurotox at high doses; up to 40% neutralizing Ab w/ Rx **Interactions:** ↑ Effects *OF* antineoplastics, CNS depressants, doxorubicin, theophylline; ↓ effects *OF* live virus vaccine **Labs:** ↑ LFTs, BUN, SCr, glucose, P, ↓ HMG, Hct, Ca **NIPE:** ASA & EtOH use may cause GI bleed, ↑ fluids to 2–3 L/d

Interferon Alfa-2b & Ribavirin Combo (Rebetron) [Antineoplastic/ Immunomodulator] **WARNING:** Can cause or aggravate fatal or life-threatening neuropsychological, autoimmune, ischemic, & infectious disorders. Monitor pts closely. CI in PRG females & their male partners **Uses:** *Chronic hep C w/ compensated liver Dz who relapse after α-interferon therapy* **Action:** Combo antiviral agents (see individual agents) **Dose:** 3 MU Intron-A SQ $3 \times$ /wk w/ 1000– 1200 mg of Rebetron PO ÷ bid dose for 24 wk *Pts < 75 kg:* 1000 mg of Rebetron/d **Caution:** [X, ?] **CI:** PRG, males w/ PRG female partner, autoimmune hep, CrCl < 50 mL/min **Disp:** *Pts < 75 kg:* Combo packs: 6 vials Intron-A (3 mill units/ 0.5 mL) w/ 6 syringes & EtOH swabs, 70 Rebetol caps; one 18-MU multidose vial of Intron-A Inj (22.8 mill units/3.8 mL; 3 MU/0.5 mL) & 6 syringes & swabs, 70 Rebetol caps; one 18-mill units Intron-A Inj multidose pen (22.5 MU/1.5 mL; 3 mill units/0.2 mL) w/ 6 needles & swabs, 70 Rebetol caps *Pts > 75 kg:* Identical except 84 Rebetol caps/pack **SE:** See Warning, flu-like synd, HA, anemia **NIPE:** Monthly PRG test; instruct in self-administration of SQ Intron-A

Interferon Alfacon-1 (Infergen) [Immunomodulator] **WARNING:** Can cause or aggravate fatal or life-threatening neuropsychological, autoimmune, ischemic, & infectious disorders. Monitor closely **Uses:** *Chronic hep C* **Action:** Biologic response modifier **Dose:** 9 mcg SQ $3 \times$ /wk $\times$ 24 wk **Caution:** [C, M] **CI:** *E coli* product allergy **Disp:** Inj 9, 15 mcg **SE:** Flu-like synd, depression, blood dyscrasias, colitis, pancreatitis, hepatic decompensation, ↑ SCr, eye disorders **Interactions:** ↑ Effects *OF* theophylline **Labs:** ↑ Triglycerides, TSH; ↑ SCr ; ↓ HMG, Hct;↓ thyroid enzymes; monitor CBC, plt, SCr, TFT **NIPE:** Refrigerate; ⊘ shake; use barrier contraception; allow > 48 h between Inj

Interferon Beta-1a (Rebif) [Immunomodulator] **WARNING:** Can cause or aggravate fatal or life-threatening neuropsychological, autoimmune, ischemic, & infectious disorders. Monitor closely **Uses:** *MS, relapsing* **Action:** Biologic response modifier **Dose:** 44 mcg SQ 3 × /wk; start 8.8 mcg SQ 3 × /wk × 2 wk, then 22 mcg SQ 3 × /wk × 2 wk **Caution:** [C, ?] w/ hepatic impair, depression, Sz disorder, thyroid Dz **CI:** Human albumin allergy **Disp:** 0.5-mL prefilled syringes w/ 29-gauge needle Titrate Pak 8.8 & 22 mcg; 22 or 44 mcg **SE:** Inj site Rxn, HA, flu-like Sxs, malaise, fatigue, rigors, myalgia, depression w/ suicidal ideation, hepatotox, ↓ BM **Interactions:** Caution w/ other hepatotoxic drugs **Labs:** Monitor CBC 1, 3, 6 mo; ✓ TFTs q6mo w/ h/o thyroid Dz **NIPE:** Dose > 48 h apart; D/C if jaundice occurs; may have abortifacient effects

Interferon Beta-1b (Betaseron, Extavia) [Immunomodulator]

Uses: *MS, relapsing/remitting/secondary progressive* **Action:** Biologic response modifier **Dose:** 0.0625 mg (2 MU) (0.25 mL) qod SQ, ↑ by 0.0625 mg q2wk to target dose 0.25 mg (1 mL) qod **Caution:** [C, ?] **CI:** Human albumin sensitivity **Disp:** Powder for Inj 0.3 mg (32 MU interferon [IFN]) **SE:** Flu-like synd, depression, blood dyscrasias, Inj site necrosis, anaphylaxis **Interactions:** ↑ Effects *OF* theophylline, zidovudine **Labs:** ↑ AST/ALT/GGT, BUN, urine protein; monitor LFTs, CBC 1, 3, 6 mo, TFT q6mo **NIPE:** ↑ Risk *OF* photosensitivity—use sunscreen, abortion; ↑ fluid intake, use barrier contraception; pt self Inj, rotate sites; consider stopping w/ depression

Interferon Gamma-1b (Actimmune) [Immunomodulator]

Uses: *↓ Incidence of serious Infxns in chronic granulomatous Dz (CGD), osteoporosis* **Action:** Biologic response modifier **Dose:** *Adults. CGD:* 50 mcg/m² SQ (1.5 MU/m²) BSA > 0.5 m²; if BSA < 0.5 m², give 1.5 mcg/kg/dose; given 3 × /wk **Caution:** [C, ?] **CI:** Allergy to *E coli*–derived products **Disp:** Inj 100 mcg (2 MU) **SE:** Flu-like synd, depression, blood dyscrasias, dizziness, altered mental status, gait disturbance, hepatic tox **Interactions:** ↑ Myelosuppression *W/* myelosuppressive drugs **Labs:** ↑ LFTs; ↓ neutrophils, plts **NIPE:** Small frequent meals will ↓ GI upset; rotate Inj sites; may ↑ deaths in interstitial pulm fibrosis

Ipecac Syrup [OTC] [Antidote]

Uses: *Drug OD, certain cases of poisoning* (Note: Usage is falling out of favor & is no longer recommended by some groups) **Action:** Irritation of the GI mucosa; stimulation of the chemoreceptor trigger zone **Dose:** *Adults.* 15–30 mL PO, followed by 200–300 mL of H₂O; if no emesis in 20 min, repeat once *Peds 6–12 y.* 5–10 mL PO, followed by 10–20 mL/kg of H₂O; if no emesis in 20 min, repeat once *1–12 y.* 15 mL PO followed by 10–20 mL of H₂O; if no emesis in 20 min, repeat once **Caution:** [C, ?] **CI:** Ingestion of petroleum distillates, strong acid, base, or other caustic agents; comatose/unconscious **Disp:** Syrup 15, 30 mL (OTC) **SE:** Lethargy, D, cardiotox, protracted V **Interactions:** ↑ Effects *OF* myelosuppressives, theophylline, zidovudine **NIPE:** ↑ Fluids to 2–3 L/d; ⊘ EtOH, CNS depressants; caution in CNS depressant OD; activated charcoal considered more effective (www.clintox.org/PosStatements/Ipecac.htm)

Ipilimumab (Yervoy) [Cytotoxic T-Lymphocyte Antigen 4 (CTLA-4)-Blocking Antibody]

WARNING: Severe fatal immune Rxns possible; D/C & Tx w/ high-dose steroids w/ severe Rxn; assess for enterocolitis, dermatitis, neuropathy, endocrinopathy before each dose **Uses:** *Unresectable/met melanoma* **Action:** Human CTLA-4-blocking Ab; ↑ T-cell proliferation/activation **Dose:** 3 mg/kg IV q3wk× 4 doses; Inf over 90 min **Caution:** [X,–] Can cause immune mediated adverse Rxns; endocrinopathies may require Rx; hep **CI:** None **Disp:** IV 50 mg/10 mL, 200 mg/40 mL **SE:** Fatigue, D, pruritus, rash, colitis **Labs:** ✓ LFTs, TFT, chemistries baseline/pre Inf

Ipratropium (Atrovent HFA, Atrovent nasal) [Bronchodilator/ Anticholinergic] **Uses:** *Bronchospasm w/ COPD, rhinitis, rhinorrhea* **Action:** Synthetic anticholinergic similar to atropine; antagonizes ACH receptors, inhibits mucous gland secretions **Dose:** *Adults & Peds > 12 y.* 2–4 puffs qid, max 12 Inh/d *Nasal:* 2 sprays/nostril bid–tid *Nebulization:* 500 mcg 3–4 × /d *ECC 2010:* Asthma: 250–500 mcg by nebulizer/MDI q20min × 3 **Caution:** [B, +/–] w/ inhaled insulin **CI:** Allergy to soya lecithin–related foods **Disp:** *HFA:* Metered-dose inhaler 18 mcg/dose; Inh soln 0.02%; nasal spray 0.03%, 0.06% **SE:** Nervousness, dizziness, HA, cough, bitter taste, nasal dryness, URI, epistaxis **Interactions:** ↑ Effects *W/* albuterol; ↑ effects *OF* anticholinergics, antimuscarinics; ↓ effects *W/* jaborandi tree, pill-bearing spurge **NIPE:** Adequate fluids; separate Inh of other drugs by 5 min; not for acute bronchospasm

Irbesartan (Avapro) [Antihypertensive/ARB] **WARNING:** D/C stat if PRG detected **Uses:** *HTN, DN*, CHF **Action:** Angiotensin II receptor antagonist **Dose:** 150 mg/d PO, may ↑ to 300 mg/d **Caution:** [C (1st tri; D 2nd/3rd tri), ?/–] **Disp:** Tabs 75, 150, 300 mg **SE:** Fatigue, ↓ BP **Interactions:** ↑ Risk of hyperkalemia *W/* K+-sparing diuretics, TMP, K+ supls; ↑ effects *OF* Li **Labs:** ↑ K+ (monitor) **NIPE:** ⊘ PRG, breast-feeding; monitor ECG for hyperkalemia (peaked T waves)

Irinotecan (Camptosar) [Antineoplastic] **WARNING:** D & myelosuppression **Uses:** *Colorectal* & lung CA **Action:** Topoisomerase I Inhib; ↓ DNA synth **Dose:** Per protocol; 125–350 mg/m² qwk–q3wk (↓ hepatic dysfunction, as tolerated per tox) **Caution:** [D, –] **CI:** Allergy to component **Disp:** Inj 20 mg/mL **SE:** ↓ BM, N/V/D, Abd cramping, alopecia; D is dose limiting; Rx acute D w/ atropine; Rx subacute D w/ loperamide **Interactions:** ↑ Effects *OF* antineoplastics; ↑ risk of akathisia *W/* prochlorperazine **Labs:** ↑ LFTs **NIPE:** Use barrier contraception; N exposure to Infxn; D correlated to levels of metabolite SN-38

Iron Dextran (Dexferrum, INFeD) [Iron Supplement] **WARNING:** Anaphylactic Rxn w/ death reported; proper personnel & equipment should be available. Use test dose on only if PO Fe not possible **Uses:** *Fe deficiency anemia where PO administration not possible* **Dose:** See also tables/formula to calculate dose. Estimate Fe deficiency; total dose (mL) = [0.0442 × (desired Hgb−observed Hgb) × lean body wgt] + (0.26 × lean body wgt); Fe replacement, blood loss: Total dose (mg) = blood loss (mL) × Hct (as decimal fraction) max 100 mg/d **IV use:** *Test Dose:* 0.5 mL IV over 30 s, if OK, 2 mL or less daily IV over 1 mL/ min to calculated total dose **IM use:** *Test Dose:* 0.5 mL deep IM in buttock. Administer calculated total dose not to exceed daily doses as follows: Infants < 5 kg: 1 mL

Children < 10 kg. All others 2 mL (100 mg of Fe). **Caution:** [C, M] w/ Hx allergy/asthma. Keep epi available (1:1000) for acute Rxn **CI:** Component hypersensitivity, non–Fe-deficiency anemia **Disp:** Inj 50 mg Fe/mL in 2 mL vials (*InFeD*) & 1 & 2-mL vials (*Dexferrrum*) **Interactions:** ↓ Effects *W/* chloramphenicol, ↓ absorption *OF* oral Fe **Labs:** False ↓ serum Ca; false(+) guaiac test; ✓ Hgb/Hct. Also Fe, TIBC, & % saturation transferrin may be used to monitor **NIPE:** Not recorded in infants < 4 mo. Reticulocyte count best early indicator of response (several d). IM use "Z-track" technique; give test dose > 1 h before; ⊘ take oral Fe

Iron Sucrose (Venofer) [Iron Supplement] Uses: *Fe-deficiency anemia in CKD, w/ or w/o dialysis, w/ or w/o erythropoietin* **Action:** Fe supl **Dose:** 100 mg on dialysis; 200 mg slow IV over 25 min × 5 doses over 14-d period. Total cum dose 1000 mg **W/P:** [B, ?] Hypersensitivity. ↓ BP, Fe overload, may interfere w/ MRI **CI:** non–Fe-deficiency anemia; Fe overload; component sensitivity **Disp:** Inj 20 mg Fe/mL, 2.5, 5, 10 mL vials **SE:** Muscle cramps, N/V, strange taste in the mouth, D, constipation, HA, cough, back/Jt pain, Jt pain, dizziness, swelling of the arms/legs **Interactions:** ↓ Absorption *OF* oral Fe supls **Labs:** Monitor ferritin, HMG, Hct, transferrin saturation; Fe levels 48 h > IV dose; ↑ LFTs **NIPE:** Safety in peds not established; ⊘ use oral & IV supls together; most pts require cumulative doses of 1000 mg; give slowly

Isoniazid (INH) [Antitubercular] Uses: *Rx & prophylaxis of TB* **Action:** Bactericidal; interferes w/ mycolic acid synth, disrupts cell wall **Dose:** *Adults. Active TB:* 5 mg/kg/24 h PO or IM (usually 300 mg/d) or DOT: 15 mg/kg (max 900 mg) 3 × /wk *Prophylaxis:* 300 mg/d PO for 6–12 mo or 900 mg 2 × /wk *Peds. Active TB:* 10–15 mg/kg/d PO or IM 300 mg/d max *Prophylaxis:* 10 mg/kg/24 h PO; ↓ in hepatic/renal dysfunction **Caution:** [C, +] Liver Dz, dialysis; avoid EtOH **CI:** Acute liver Dz, h/o INH hep **Disp:** Tabs 100, 300 mg; syrup 50 mg/5 mL; Inj 100 mg/mL **SE:** Hep, peripheral neuropathy, GI upset, anorexia, dizziness, skin Rxn **Interactions:** ↑ Effects *OF* APAP, anticoagulants, carbamazepine, cycloserine, diazepam, meperidine, hydantoins, theophylline, valproic acid, EtOH; ↑ effects *W/* rifampin; ↓ effects *W/* Al salts; ↓ effects *OF* anticoagulants, ketoconazole **Labs:** ↑ LFTs, glucose; ↓ HMG, plts, WBCs **NIPE:** Only take w/ food if GI upset; use w/ 2–3 other drugs for active TB, based on INH resistance patterns when TB acquired & sensitivity results; prophylaxis w/ INH alone. IM rarely used. ↓ Peripheral neuropathy w/ pyridoxine 50–100 mg/d. See CDC guidelines (*MMWR*) for current recommendations

Isoproterenol (Isuprel) [Bronchodilator/Sympathomimetic] Uses: *Shock, cardiac arrest, AV nodal block* **Action:** β_1- & β_2-receptor stimulant **Dose:** *Adults.* 2–10 mcg/min IV Inf; titrate; 2–10 mcg/min titrate (*ECC 2005*) *Peds.* 0.2–2 mcg/kg/min IV Inf; titrate **Caution:** [C, ?] **CI:** Angina, tachyarrhythmias (digitalis-induced or others) **Disp:** 0.02 mg/mL, 0.2 mg/mL **SE:** Insomnia, arrhythmias, HA, trembling, dizziness **Interactions:** ↑ Effects *W/* albuterol, guanethidine, oxytocic drugs, sympathomimetics, TCAs; ↑ risk of arrhythmias *W/* amitriptyline, bretylium, cardiac glycosides, K⁺-depleting drugs, theophylline; ↓ effects *W/* BBs **Labs:** False ↑ serum AST, bilirubin, glucose **NIPE:** Saliva may turn pink in color, ↑ fluids to 2–3 L/d; more specific β₂-agonists preferred d/t excessive β₁ cardiac stimulation of drug; drug induces ischemia & dysrhythmias; pulse > 130 BPM may induce arrhythmias

Isosorbide Dinitrate (Isordil, Sorbitrate, Dilatrate-SR) [Antianginal/Nitrate] **Uses:** *Rx & prevent angina*, CHF (w/ hydralazine) **Action:** Relaxes vascular smooth muscle **Dose:** *Acute angina:* 5–10 mg PO (chew tabs) q2–3h or 2.5–10 mg SL PRN q5–10 min; do not give > 3 doses in a 15–30-min period *Angina prophylaxis:* 5–40 mg PO q6h; do not give nitrates on a chronic q6h or qid basis > 7–10 d; tolerance may develop; provide 10–12-h drug-free intervals; *CHF:* Initial 20 mg 3–4x/d, target 120–160 mg/d **Caution:** [C, ?] Severe anemia, NAG, postural ↓ BP, cerebral hemorrhage,**Disp:** Tabs 5, 10, 20, 30 mg; SR tabs 40 mg; SL tabs 2.5, 5 mg; SR caps 40 mg **SE:** HA, ↓ BP, flushing, tachycardia, dizziness **Interactions:** ↑ Hypotension *W/* antihypertensives, ASA, CCBs, phenothiazides, sildenafil, EtOH; head trauma (can ↑ ICP), w/ sildenafil, tadalafil, vardenafil **Labs:** False ↓ serum cholesterol **NIPE:** ⊘ Nitrates for an 8–12-h period/d to avoid tolerance; begin PO dose needed for same results as SL forms

Isosorbide Dinitrate & Hydralazine HCL (BiDil) [Antianginal, Antihypertensive/Vasodilator, Nitrate] **Uses:** HF in AA pts; improve survival & functional status, prolong time between hospitalizations for HF **Action:** Relaxes vascular smooth muscle; peripheral vasodilator **Dose:** *Initially:* 1 tab tid PO (if not tolerated reduce to 1/2 tab tid), titrate > 3–5 d as tolerated *Max:* 2 tabs tid **Caution:** [C, ?/–] recent MI, syncope, hypovolemia, hypotension, hep impair **CI:** ⊘ For children, concomitant use w/ PDE5 Inhibs (sildenafil) **Disp:** Isosorbide dinitrate 20 mg/hydralazine HCL 37.5 mg tabs **SE:** HA, dizziness, orthostatic hypotension, sinusitis, GI distress, tachycardia, paresthesia, amblyopia **Interactions:** ↑ Risk of severe hypotension *W/* antihypertensives, ASA, CCBs, MAOIs, phenothiazides, sildenafil, tadalafil, vardenafil, ETOH; ↓ pressor response *W/* epinephrine; ↓ effects *W/* NSAIDs **Labs:** False ↑ serum cholesterol **NIPE:** ⊘ Nitrates for an 8–12-h period/d to avoid tolerance; take w/ food

Isosorbide Mononitrate (Ismo, Imdur) [Antianginal/Nitrate] **Uses:** *Prevention/Rx of angina pectoris* **Action:** Relaxes vascular smooth muscle **Dose:** 5–10 mg PO bid, w/ the 2 doses 7 h apart or XR (Imdur) 30–60 mg/d PO, max 240 mg **Caution:** [C, ?] **CI:** Head trauma/cerebral hemorrhage (can ↑ ICP), w/ sildenafil, tadalafil, vardenafil **Disp:** Tabs 10, 20 mg; XR 30, 60, 120 mg **SE:** HA, dizziness, ↓ BP **Interactions:** ↑ Hypotension *W/* ASA, CCB, nitrates, sildenafil, EtOH **Labs:** False ↓ serum cholesterol **NIPE:** Metabolite of isosorbide dinitrate

Isotretinoin [13-cis Retinoic Acid] (Accutane, Amnesteem, Claravis, Sotret) [Antiacne Agent] **WARNING:** Must not be used by PRG females; can induce severe birth defects; pt must be capable of complying w/ mandatory contraceptive measures; prescribed according to product-specific risk-management system. Because of teratogenicity, is approved for marketing only under a special restricted distribution FDA program called iPLEDGE **Uses:** *Refractory severe acne* **Action:** Retinoic acid derivative **Dose:** 0.5–2 mg/kg/d PO ÷ bid; ↓ in hepatic Dz, take w/ food **Caution:** [X, –] Avoid tetracyclines **CI:** Retinoid sensitivity, PRG **Disp:** Caps 10, 20, 30, 40 mg **SE:** *Rare:* Depression, psychosis, suicidal thoughts; derm sensitivity, xerostomia, photosensitivity, LFTs, triglycerides **Interactions:** ↑ Effects w/ corticosteroids, phenytoin, vit A; ↑ risk of pseudotumor cerebri w/ tetracyclines; ↑ triglyceride levels w/ EtOH; ↓ effects OF carbamazepine **Labs:** ↑ LFTs, triglycerides; monitor LFTs & lipids **NIPE:** ↑ Risk of photosensitivity—use sunblock, take w/ food, ⊘ PRG; low-dose progesterone-only hormonal contraceptives may not be adequate birth control alone; risk-management program requires 2 (–) PRG tests before Rx & use of 2 forms of contraception 1 mo before, during, & after therapy; to prescribe isotretinoin, the prescriber must access the iPLEDGE system via the Internet (www.ipledgeprogram.com)

Isradipine (DynaCirc) [Antihypertensive/CCB] **Uses:** *HTN* **Action:** CCB **Dose: Adults.** 2.5–5 mg PO bid **Caution:** [C, ?] **CI:** Severe heart block, sinus bradycardia, CHF, dosing w/in several h of IV BBs **Disp:** Caps 2.5, 5 mg; tabs CR 5, 10 mg **SE:** HA, edema, flushing, fatigue, dizziness, palpitations **Interactions:** ↑ Effects w/ antihypertensives, azole antifungals, BBs, cimetidine; fentanyl, nitrates, quinidine, EtOH, grapefruit juice; ↑ effects OF carbamazepine, cyclosporine, digitalis glycosides, prazosin, quinidine; ↑ risk of bradycardia/conduction defects/CHF w/ BB, digoxin, disopyramide, phenytoin; ↓ effects w/ Ca, NSAIDs, rifampin; ↓ effects OF lovastatin **Labs:** ↑ LFTs **NIPE:** ⊘ D/C abruptly

Itraconazole (Sporanox) [Antifungal] **WARNING:** CI w/ cisapride, pimozide, quinidine, dofetilide, or levacetylmethadol. Serious CV events (eg, ↑ QT, torsades de pointes, VT, cardiac arrest, and/or sudden death) reported w/ these meds & other CYP3A4 Inhibs. Do not use for onychomycosis w/ ventricular dysfunction **Uses:** *Fungal Infxns* (aspergillosis, blastomycosis, histoplasmosis, candidiasis)* **Action:** Azole antifungal, ↓ ergosterol synth **Dose:** 200 mg PO daily–bid (caps w/ meals or cola/grapefruit juice); PO soln on empty stomach; avoid antacids **Caution:** [C, ?] Numerous interactions **CI:** See Warning; PRG or considering PRG; ventricular dysfunction **Disp:** Caps 100 mg; soln 10 mg/mL **SE:** N/V, rash, hepatotoxic, CHF, ↑ BP, neuropathy **Interactions:** ↑ Effects w/ clarithromycin, erythromycin; ↑ effects OF alprazolam, anticoagulants, atevirdine, atorvastatin, buspirone, cerivastatin, chlordiazepoxide, cyclosporine, diazepam, digoxin, felodipine, fluvastatin, indinavir, lovastatin, methadone, methylprednisolone, midazolam, nelfinavir, pravastatin, ritonavir, saquinavir, simvastatin, tacrolimus, tolbutamide, triazolam, warfarin; ↑ QT prolongation w/ astemizole, cisapride, pimozide, quinidine, terfenadine; ↓ effects w/ antacids, Ca, cimetidine, didanosine, famotidine, lansoprazole, Mg, nizatidine, omeprazole, phenytoin, rifampin, sucralfate, grapefruit juice **Labs:** ↑ LFTs, BUN, SCr; ↓ K+; monitor LFTs **NIPE:** Take caps w/ food & soln w/o food; ⊘ PRG or breast-feeding; ↑ risk of disulfiram-like response w/ EtOH; PO soln & caps not interchangeable; useful in pts who cannot take amphotericin B, can cause ↑ QTc in combo w/ other drugs—monitor ECG

Ixabepilone Kit (Ixempra) [Epothilone Microtubule Inhibitor]
WARNING: CI in combo w/ capecitabine w/ AST/ALT > 2.5× ULN or bilirubin > 1× ULN d/t ↑ tox & neutropenia-related death Uses: *Met /locally advanced breast CA after failure of an anthracycline, a taxane, & capecitabine* **Action:** Microtubule Inhib Dose: 40 mg/m² IV over 3 h q3wk Caution: [D, ?/–] CI: Hypersensitivity to Cremophor EL; baseline ANC < 1500 cells/mm³ or plt < 100,000 cells/mm³; AST/ALT > 2.5× UNL , bilirubin > 1× ULN Disp: Inj 15, 45 mg SE: Neutropenia, leukopenia, anemia, ↓ plt, peripheral sensory neuropathy, fatigue/asthenia, myalgia/arthralgia, alopecia, N/V/D, stomatitis/ mucositis Interactions: ↑ Effects W/ strong CYP3A4 Inhibs (azole antifungals, protease Inhibs, certain macrolides, nefazodone, grapefruit juice); ↓ effects W/ CYP3A4 inducers (phenytoin, carbamazepine, rifampin, phenobarbital) Labs: Monitor LFTs, neutropenia NIPE: Monitor for neuropathy; D/C if cardiac ischemia or cardiac dysfunction occurs

Japanese Encephalitis Vaccine, Inactivated, Adsorbed [Vaccine]
(Ixiaro, Je-Vax) Uses: *Prevent Japanese encephalitis* **Action:** Inactivated vaccine Dose: *Adults.* 0.5 mL IM, repeat 28 d later *Peds.* Use Je-Vax *1–3 y:* Three 0.5 mL SQ doses on d 0, 7, 30 *> 3 y:* Three 1 mL SQ doses on d 0, 7, 30 Caution: [B (Ixiaro)/C (Je-Vax), ?] SE: HA, fatigue, Inj site pain, flu-like synd, hypersensitivity Rxns Interactions: ↓ Response W/ other vaccines, immunosuppressants (eg. radiation, chemotherapy, high-dose steroids) NIPE: Abbreviate administration schedules of 3 doses on d 0, 7, & 14; booster dose recommended after 2 y. Avoid EtOH 48 h after dose

Kaolin-Pectin (Kaodene, Kao-Spen, Kapectolin) [Antidiarrheal/ Absorbent] [OTC] Uses: *D* **Action:** Absorbent demulcent Dose: *Adults.* 60–120 mL PO after each loose stool or q3–4h PRN *Peds.* *3–6 y.* 15–30 mL/dose PO PRN *6–12 y.* 30–60 mL/dose PO PRN Caution: [C, +] CI: D d/t pseudomembranous colitis Disp: Multiple OTC forms; also available w/ opium (Parepectolin [CII]) SE: Constipation, dehydration Interaction: ↓ Effects OF ciprofloxacin, clindamycin, digoxin, lincomycin, lovastatin, penicillamine, quinidine, tetracycline NIPE: Take other meds 2–3 h before or after this drug

Ketamine (Ketalar) [CIII] Uses: *Induction/maint of anesthesia* (in combo w/ sedatives), sedation, analgesia Action: Dissociative anesthesia; IV onset 30 s, duration 5–10 min Dose: *Adults.* 1–4.5 mg/kg IV, typical 2 mg/kg; 3–8 mg/kg IM *Peds.* 0.5–2 mg/kg IV; 0.5–1 mg/kg for minor procedure sedation (also IM/PO regimens) Caution: [C, ?/–] w/ CAD, ↓ BP, tachycardia, EtOH use/abuse CI: When ↑ BP hazardous Disp: Soln 10, 50, 100 mg/mL SE: Arrhythmia, bradycardia, ↓/↓ BP, ↓ HR, N/V, resp depression, emergence Rxns, ↑ CSF pressure Interactions: CYP2B6 Inhibs ↓ metabolism (see Table 10) NIPE: Used in RSI protocols; street drug of abuse

Ketoconazole (Nizoral) [Antifungal/Imidazole] **WARNING:** (Oral use) Risk of fatal hepatotox. Concomitant terfenadine, astemizole, & cisapride are CI d/t serious CV adverse events Uses: *Systemic fungal Infxns (Candida, blastomycosis, histoplasmosis, etc); refractory topical dermatophyte Infxn*; PCa when rapid ↓ testosterone needed or hormone refractory Action: Azole, ↓ fungal cell wall synth;

high dose blocks P450 to ↓ testosterone production **Dose:** *PO:* 200 mg PO daily; ↑ to 400 mg PO daily for serious Infxn *PCa:* 400 mg PO tid w/ hydrocortisone 20–40 mg ÷ bid; best on empty stomach **Caution:** [C, +/−] w/ Agent that ↑ gastric pH (↓ absorption); may enhance anticoagulants; w/ EtOH (disulfiram-like Rxn); numerous interactions including statins, niacin **CI:** CNS fungal Infxns, w/ astemizole, triazolam **Disp:** Tabs 200 mg **SE:** N, rashes, hair loss, HA, ↑ wgt gain, dizziness, disorientation, fatigue, impotence, hepatox, adrenal suppression, acquired cutaneous adherence ("sticky skin synd") **Interactions:** ↑ Effects *OF* alprazolam, anticoagulants, atevirdine, atorvastatin, buspirone, chlordiazepoxide, cyclosporine, diazepam, felodipine, fluvastatin, indinavir, lovastatin, methadone, methylprednisolone, midazolam, nelfinavir, pravastatin, ritonavir, saquinavir, simvastatin, tacrolimus, tolbutamide, triazolam, warfarin; ↑ QT prolongation *W/* astemizole, cisapride, quinidine, terfenadine; ↓ effects *W/* antacids, Ca, cimetidine, didanosine, famotidine, lansoprazole, Mg, nizatidine, omeprazole, phenytoin, rifampin, sucralfate **Labs:** ↑ LFTs; monitor LFTs w/ systemic use; can rapidly ↓ testosterone levels **NIPE:** Take tabs w/ citrus juice, take w/ food; shampoo wet hair 1 min, rinse, repeat for 3 min; ⊘ PRG or breast-feeding

Ketoconazole, Topical (Extina, Kuric, Nizoral A-D Shampoo, Xolegel) [Antifungal/Imidazole] [Shampoo–OTC] Uses: *Topical for seborrheic dermatitis, shampoo for dandruff* local fungal Infxns d/t dermatophytes & yeast **Action:** Azole, ↓ fungal cell wall synth **Dose:** *Topical:* Apply qd-bid **Caution:** [C, +/−] **CI:** Broken/inflamed skin **Disp:** Tabs 200 mg; topical cream 2%; (*Xolegel*) gel 2%, (*Extina*) foam 2%, shampoo 1% & 2% **SE:** Irritation, pruritus, stinging **NIPE:** Do not dispense foam into hands

Ketoprofen (Orudis, Oruvail) [Analgesic/NSAID]   WARNING: May ↑ risk of CV events & GI bleeding; CI for perioperative pain in CABG surgery **Uses:** *Arthritis (RA/OA), pain* **Action:** NSAID; ↓ prostaglandins **Dose:** 25–75 mg PO tid–qid, 300 mg/d/max; SR 200 mg/d; w/ food; ↓ w/ hepatic/renal impair, elderly **Caution:** [C (D 3rd tri). −] w/ ACE, diuretics **CI:** NSAID/ASA sensitivity **Disp:** Caps 50, 75 mg; caps, SR 200 mg **SE:** GI upset, peptic ulcers, dizziness, edema, rash, ↑ BP, renal dysfunction **Interactions:** Effects *W/* ASA, corticosteroids, NSAIDs, probenecid, EtOH; ↑ effects *OF* antineoplastics, hypoglycemics, insulin, Li, MTX, warfarin; ↑ risk of nephrotox *W/* aminoglycosides, cyclosporines; ↑ risk of bleeding *W/* anticoagulants, defamandole, cefotetan, cefoperazone, clopidogrel, eptifibatide, plicamycin, thrombolytics, tirofiban, valproic acid, dong quai, feverfew, garlic, ginkgo, ginger, horse chestnut, red clover; ↓ effects *OF* antihypertensives, diuretics **Labs:** ↑ LFTs, BUN, Cr, PT; ↓ plts, WBCs **NIPE:** ↑ Risk of photosensitivity—use sunblock, take w/ food

Ketorolac (Toradol) [Analgesic/NSAID]   WARNING: For short-term (= 5 d) Rx of mod–severe acute pain; CI w/ PUD, GI bleed, postcoronary artery bypass graft, anticipated major surgery, severe renal Insuff, bleeding diathesis, L&D, nursing, & w/ ASA/NSAIDs. NSAIDs may cause an ↑ risk of CV thrombotic events (MI, stroke). PO CI in peds < 16 y **Uses:** *Pain* **Action:** NSAID; ↓ prostaglandins

Dose: *Adults.* 15–30 mg IV/IM q6h; 10 mg PO qid only after IM/IV; max IV/IM 120 mg/d, max PO 40 mg/d *Peds 2–16 y.* 1 mg/kg IM × 1 30 mg max *IV:* 0.5 mg/kg, 15 mg max; do not use for > 5 d; ↓ if > 65 y, elderly, w/ renal impair,< 50 kg **Caution:** [C (D 3rd tri), −] w/ ACE Inhi, diuretics, BP meds, warfarin **CI:** See Warning **Disp:** Tabs 10 mg; Inj 15 mg/mL, 30 mg/mL **SE:** Bleeding, PUD, ↑ BP, edema, dizziness, allergy **Interactions:** ↑ Effects *W/* ASA, corticosteroids, NSAIDs, probenecid, EtOH; ↑ effects *OF* antineoplastics, hypoglycemics, insulin, Li, MTX; ↑ risk of nephrotox *W/* aminoglycosides, cyclosporines; ↑ risk of bleeding *W/* anticoagulants, defamandole, cefotetan, cefoperazone, clopidogrel, eptifibatide, plicamycin, thrombolytics, tirofiban, valproic acid, dong quai, feverfew, garlic, ginkgo, ginger, horse chestnut, red clover; ↓ effects of antihypertensives, diuretics **Labs:** ↑ LFTs, Cr, PT; ↓ HMG, Hct **NIPE:** 30-mg dose equals comparative analgesia of meperidine 100 mg or morphine 12 mg; PO only as continuation of IM/IV therapy

Ketorolac Nasal (Sprix) [NSAID] WARNING: For short-term (< 5 d) use; CI w/ PUD, GI bleed, suspected bleeding risk, post-op CABG, advanced renal Dz or risk of renal failure w/ vol depletion; ↑ risk CV thrombotic events (MI, stroke) **Uses:** *Short-term (< 5 d) Rx pain requiring opioid level analgesia* **Action:** NSAID; ↑ prostaglandins **Dose:** *< 65 y:* 31.5 mg (one 15.75 mg spray each nostril) q6–8h; max 126 mg/d = 65 y / *renal impair or < 50 kg:* 15.75 mg (one 15.75 mg spray in only 1 nostril) q6–8 h; max 63 mg/d **Caution:** [C (D 3rd tri), −] do not use w/ other NSAIDs; can cause severe allergic Rxns; do not use w/ critical bleeding risk; w/ CHF **CI:** See Warning; prophylactic to major surgery L&D; w/ Hx allergy to other NSAIDs **Disp:** Nasal spray 15.75 mg ketorolac/100 uL spray (8 sprays/bottle) **SE:** Nasal discomfort/rhinitis, ↑ lacrimation, throat irritation, oliguria, rash, ↓ HR, ↓ urine output, ↑ BP **Interactions:** ↑ Effects *W/* ASA, corticosteroids, NSAIDs; ↑ risk of hallucinations *W/* fluoxetine, thiothixene, alprazolam; ↓ effects *OF* furosemide, thiazides, ACE Inhibs, angiotensin II receptor antagonists **LABS:** ↑ ALT/ AST **NIPE:** Not for peds; discard open bottle after 24 h

Ketorolac Ophthalmic (Acular, Acular LS, Acular PF) [Analgesic, Anti-Inflammatory/NSAID] Uses: *Ocular itching w/ seasonal allergies; inflammation w/ cataract extraction*; pain/photophobia w/ incisional refractive surgery (Acular PF); pain w/ corneal refractive surgery (*Acular LS*) **Action:** NSAID **Dose:** 1 gtt qid **Caution:** [C, +] possible cross-sensitivity to NSAIDs, ASA **CI:** Hypersensitivity **Disp:** *Acular LS:* 0.4% 5 mL; *Acular:* 0.5% 3, 5, 10 mL; *Acular PF:* Soln 0.5% **SE:** Local irritation, ↑ bleeding ocular tissues, hyphemas, slow healing, keratitis **NIPE:** Do not use w/ contacts; teach use of eye drops

Ketotifen (Alaway, Zaditor) [Ophthalmic Antihistamine/Histamine Antagonist & Mast Cell Stabilizer] [OTC] Uses: *Allergic conjunctivitis* **Action:** Antihistamine H_1-receptor antagonist, mast cell stabilizer **Dose:** *Adults & Peds > 3 y.* 1 gtt in eye(s) q8–12h **Caution:** [C, ?/−] **Disp:** Soln 0.025%/5 & 10 mL **SE:** Local irritation, HA, rhinitis, keratitis, mydriasis **Notes:** Wait 10 min before inserting contacts; ⊘ wear contact lenses if eyes red

Kunecatechins [Sinecatechins] (Veregen) [Botanical] Uses: *External genital/perianal warts* Action: Unknown; green tea extract Dose: Apply 0.5-cm ribbon to each wart 3 × /d until all warts clear; not > 16 wk Caution: [C, ?] Disp: Oint 15% SE: Erythema, pruritus, burning, pain, erosion/ulceration, edema, induration, rash, phimosis NIPE: Wash hands before/after use; not necessary to wipe off prior to next use; avoid on open wounds

Labetalol (Trandate) [Antihypertensive/Alpha Blocker & BB] Uses: *HTN* & hypertensive emergencies (IV) Action: α- & β-adrenergic blocker Dose: Adults. HTN: Initial, 100 mg PO bid, then 200–400 mg PO bid. Hypertensive emergency: 20–80 mg IV bolus, then 2 mg/min IV Inf, titrate up to 300 mg ECC 2010: 10 mg IV over 1–2 min; repeat or double dose q10min (150 mg max); or initial bolus, then 2–8 mg/min Peds. PO: 1–3 mg/kg/d in ÷ doses, 1200 mg/d max Hypertensive emergency: 0.4–1.5 mg/kg/h IV cont Inf Caution: [C (D in 2nd or 3rd tri), +] CI: Asthma/COPD, cardiogenic shock, uncompensated CHF, heart block, sinus bradycardia Disp: Tabs 100, 200, 300 mg; Inj 5 mg/mL SE: Dizziness, N, ↓ BP, fatigue, CV effects Interactions: ↑ Effects W/ cimetidine, diltiazem, nitroglycerine, quinidine, paroxetine, verapamil; ↑ tremors W/ TCAs; ↓ effects W/ glutethimide, NSAIDs, salicylates; ↓ effects OF antihypertensives, β-adrenergic bronchodilators, sulfonylureas Labs: False(+) amphetamines in urine drug screen; ↑ LFTS NIPE: May have transient tingling of scalp

Lacosamide (Vimpat) [Antiepileptic] WARNING: Antiepileptics associated w/ ↑ risk of suicide ideation Uses: *Adjunct in partial-onset Szs* Action: Anticonvulsant Dose: Initial: 50 mg IV or PO bid, ↑ weekly Maint: 200–400 mg/d; 300 mg/d max if CrCl < 30 mL/min or mild/mod hepatic Dz Caution: [C, ?] Contra: None Disp: IV: 200 mg/mL; tabs: 50, 100, 150, 200 mg; oral soln 10 mg/mL SE: Dizziness, N/V, ataxia, HA, diplopia NIPE: ⊘ Abrupt cessation—withdraw over 1 wk; ↓ ECG before dosing & periodically—may ↑ PR interval

Lactic Acid & Ammonium Hydroxide [Ammonium Lactate] (LacHydrin) [Emollient] Uses: *Severe xerosis & ichthyosis* Action: Emollient moisturizer, humectant Dose: Apply bid Caution: [B, ?] Disp: Cream, lotion, lactic acid 12% w/ ammonium hydroxide SE: Local irritation, photosensitivity NIPE: ⊘ Children < 2 y; ↓ sun exposure—use sunblock; risk of hyperpigmentation; shake well before use

Lactobacillus (Lactinex Granules) [Antidiarrheal] [OTC] Uses: *Control of D*, esp after antibiotic Rx Action: Replaces nl intestinal flora, lactase production; L acidophilus &L helveticus Dose: Adults & Peds > 3 y. 1 packet, 1–2 caps, or 4 tabs qd–qid Caution: [A, +] Some products may contain whey CI: Milk/lactose allergy Disp: Tabs, caps; granules in packets (all OTC) SE: Flatulence NIPE: May take granules on food

Lactulose (Constulose, Generlac, Enulose, Others) [Laxative/Osmotic] Uses: *Hepatic encephalopathy; constipation* Action: Acidifies the colon, allows ammonia to diffuse into colon; osmotic effect to ↑ peristalsis Dose:

Acute hepatic encephalopathy: 30–45 mL PO q1h until soft stools, then tid–qid, adjust 2–3 stools/d. *Constipation:* 15–30 mL/d, ↑ to 60 mL/d 1–2 ÷ doses, adjust to 2–3 stools. *Rectally:* 200 g in 700 mL of H_2O PR, retain 30–60 min q4–6h **Peds. Infants.** 2.5–10 mL/24 h ÷ tid–qid *Other Peds.* 40–90 mL/24 h ÷ tid–qid *Peds constipation:* 5 g (7.5 mL) PO after breakfast **Caution:** [B, ?] **CI:** Galactosemia **Disp:** Syrup 10 g/15 mL, soln 10 g/15 mL, 10, 20 g/packet **SE:** Severe D, N/V, cramping, flatulence; life-threatening lytes disturbances **Interactions:** ↓ Effects *W/* antacids, antibiotics, neomycin **Labs:** ↓ Serum ammonia **NIPE:** May take 24–48 h for results

Lamivudine (Epivir, Epivir-HBV, 3TC [Many Combo Regimens]) [Antiretroviral/NRTI] **WARNING:** Lactic acidosis & severe hepatomegaly w/ steatosis reported w/ nucleoside analogues **Uses:** *HIV Infxn, chronic hep B* **Action:** NRTI, ↓ HIV RT & hep B viral polymerase, causes viral DNA chain termination **Dose:** *HIV:* **Adults & Peds > 16 y.** 150 mg PO bid or 300 mg PO daily **Peds able to swallow pills.** *14–21 kg.* 75 mg bid *22–29 kg.* 75 mg qAM, 150 mg qPM *> 30 kg.* 150 mg bid **Neonates < 30 d.** 2 mg/kg bid *Epivir-HBV.* **Adults.** 100 mg PO **Peds 2–17 y.** 3 mg/kg/d PO, 100 mg max; ↓ w/ CrCl < 50 mL/min **Caution:** [C, –] w/ Interferon-α & ribavirin may cause liver failure; do not use w/ zalcitabine or w/ ganciclovir/valganciclovir **Disp:** Tabs 100 mg (*Epivir-HBV*) 150, 300 mg; soln 5 mg/mL (*Epivir-HBV*), 10 mg/mL **SE:** Malaise, fatigue, N/V/D, HA, pancreatitis, lactic acidosis, peripheral neuropathy, fat redistribution, rhabdomyolysis hyperglycemia, nasal Sxs **Interactions:** ↑ Effects *W/* cotrimoxazole, TMP/SMX; ↑ risk of lactic acidosis *W/* antiretrovirals, RT Inhibs **Labs:** ↑ LFTs; ↓ HMG, Hct, plts **NIPE:** Take w/ food to < GI upset; differences in formulations; do not use Epivir-HBV for hep in pt w/ unrecognized HIV d/t rapid emergence of HIV resistance

Lamotrigine (Lamictal) [Anticonvulsant/Phenyltriazine] **WARNING:** Serious rashes requiring hospitalization & D/C of Rx reported; rash less frequent in adults; ↑ suicidality risk for antiepileptic drug; highest for those w/ epilepsy vs those using drug for psychological indications **Uses:** *Partial Szs, tonic–clonic Szs, bipolar disorder, Lennox–Gastaut synd* **Action:** Phenyltriazine antiepileptic, ↓ glutamate, stabilize neuronal membrane **Dose:** *Adults.* **Szs:** Initial 50 mg/d PO, then 50 mg PO bid for × 1–2 wk, maint 300–500 mg/d in 2 ÷ doses **Bipolar.** Initial 25 mg/d PO × 1–2 wk, 50 mg PO daily for 2 wk, 100 mg PO daily for 1 wk, maint 200 mg/d **Peds.** 0.6 mg/kg in 2 ÷ doses for wk 1 & 2, then 1.2 mg/kg for wk 3 & 4, q1–2wk to maint 5–15 mg/kg/d (max 400 mg/d) 1–2 ÷ doses; ↓ in hepatic Dz or if w/ enzyme inducers or valproic acid **Caution:** [C, –] Interactions w/ other antiepileptics, estrogen, rifampin **Disp:** Tabs 25, 100, 150, 200 mg; chew tabs 2, 5, 25 mg (color coded for those on interacting meds) **SE:** Photosensitivity, HA, GI upset, dizziness, diplopia, blurred vision, blood dyscrasias, ataxia, rash (may be much more life-threatening to peds than to adults) **Interactions:** ↑ Effects *OF* valproic acid; ↑ effects *OF* carbamazepine; ↓ effects *W/* APAP, OCPs, phenobarbital, phenytoin, primidone **NIPE:** ↑ Risk of photosensitivity—use sunblock; value of therapeutic monitoring uncertain, taper w/ D/C

Lamotrigine Extended Release (Lamictal XR) [Anticonvulsant/ Phenyltriazine] WARNING: Life-threatening serious rashes, including SJS & toxic epidermal necrolysis, and/or rash-related death reported; D/C at first sign of rash **Uses:** *Adjunct primary generalized tonic–clonic Sz, conversion to monotherapy in pt > 13 y w/ partial Szs* **Action:** Phenyltriazine antiepileptic, ↓ glutamate, stabilize neuronal membrane **Dose:** Adjunct target 200–60 mg/d; monotherapy conversion target dose 25–300 mg/d **Adults:** *w/ Valproate*: wk 1–2: 25 mg qod; wk 3–4: 25 mg qd; wk 5: 50 mg qd; wk 6: 100 mg qd; wk 7: 150 mg qd; then maint 200–250 mg qd.w/o *carbamazepine, penytoin, phenobarbital, primidone or valproate:* Wk 1–2 25 mg qd; wk 3–4: 50 mg qd; wk 5: 100 mg qd; wk 6: 150 mg qd; wk 7: 200 mg qd then maint: 300–400 mg qd *Convert IR to ER tabs:* Initial dose = total daily dose of IR. *Convert adjunctive to monotherapy:* Maint: 250–300mg qd. Refer to PI for specifics. W/ *Estrogen-containing OCP*: See package insert **Peds > 13 y.** See Adults **Caution:** [C, –] Withdrawal Szs **CI:** Component hypersensitivity (See Warning) **Disp:** Tabs 25, 100, 150, 200 mg **SE:** Dizziness, tremor/intention tremor, V, & diplopia. Rash (may be much more life-threatening to peds than to adults), aseptic meningitis, blood dyscrasias **Interactions:** w/ Other antiepileptics, estrogen (OCP), rifampin; valproic acid ↑ levels at least 2X; ↑ suicidal ideation **Labs:** Monitor CBC **NIPE:** Taper over 2 wk w/ D/C; can have withdrawal Szs

Lansoprazole (Prevacid, Prevacid IV, Prevacid 24HR [OTC]) [Antisecretory/Proton Pump Inhibitor] **Uses:** *Duodenal ulcers, prevent & Rx NSAID gastric ulcers, active gastric ulcers, *H pylori* Infxn, erosive esophagitis, & hypersecretory conditions, GERD. Pediatric erosive esophagitis, pediatric GERD.* **Action:** PPI **Dose:** 15–30 mg/d PO *NSAID ulcer prevention:* 15 mg/d PO = 12 wk *NSAID ulcers:* 30 mg/d PO × 8 wk *Hypersecretory condition:* 60 mg/d before food; *H Pylori* eradication-triple therapy 30 mg bid for 10–14 d, dual therapy is 30 mg tid for 14 d; erosive esophagitis short term 30 mg qd for 8 wks; Ped GERD and erosive esophagitis 15 mg qd for 12 wks for < 30 kg; 30 mg qd > 30 kg for 12 wks; ↓ w/ severe hepatic impair **Caution:** [B, ?/–] w/ clopidogrel **Disp:** ***Prevacid:*** DR caps 15, 30 mg; Prevacid 24HR (OTC) 15 mg; Prevacid SoluTab (ODT) 15 mg, 30 mg (contains phenylalanine); granules for susp 15, 30 mg, once–daily tabs 15, 30 mg **SE:** N/V Abd pain HA, fatigue **Interactions:** ↓ Effects ***W/*** sucralfate; ↓ effects ***OF*** ampicillin, digoxin, Fe, ketoconazole, atazanavir **Labs:** Monitor theophylline & warfarin levels if taking these drugs **NIPE:** Take ac; do not crush/chew; granules can be given w/ applesauce or apple juice (NG tube) only; ? ↑ risk of fxs w/ all PPI; caution w/ ODT in feeding tubes; risk of hypomagnesemia w/ long-term use, monitor; may give antacids concomitantly

Lansoprazole 30 mg, Amoxicillin 500 mg, Clarithromycin 500 mg (Prevpac) [Proton Pump Inhibitor + Antibiotics (Penicillin + Macrolide)] Uses: Eradication *H pylori* to reduce risk of duodenal ulcer recurrence **Action:** PPI + antibiotics **Dose:** Lansoprazole 30 mg + amoxicillin 1000 mg + clarithromycin 500 mg all bid for 10–14 d **Caution:** [C,–] w/ Clopidogrel; w/ severe renal impairment **Disp:** Lansoprazole 30 mg (2 caps containing e–c granules), amoxicillin 500 mg (4 caps), clarithromycin 500 mg (2 tabs); per pack. **SE:** N/V Abd pain HA, fatigue, abnormal taste, diarrhea, blood dyscrasias **Interactions:** ↑ Effects *W/* probenecid; ↑ effects *OF/* theophylline, carbamazepine, omeprazole, phenytoin, digoxin, warfarin, ergot alkaloids, triazolam, cyclosporine, hexobarbital, tacrolimus, alfentanil, disopyramide, bromocriptine, valproate, rifabutin, statins; ↓ effects *W/* sucralfate; ↓ effects *OF* ampicillin, digoxin, Fe, ketoconazole, atazanavir **Labs:** ↑ BUN, monitor theophylline & warfarin levels if taking these drugs; may cause false(+) glucose test with Clinitest, Benedict's or Fehling's soln; **NIPE:** Take ac; ↑ risk of fx w/ all PPI; risk of hypomagnesemia w/ long-term use, monitor

Lanthanum Carbonate (Fosrenol) [Renal & GU Agent/Phosphate Binder] Uses: *Hyperphosphatemia in renal Dz* **Action:** Phosphate binder **Dose:** 750–1500 mg PO daily ÷ doses, w/ or stat after meal; titrate q2–3wk based on PO_4^{2-} levels **Caution:** [C, ?/–] No data in GI Dz; not for peds **Disp:** Chew tabs 250, 500, 750, 1000 mg **SE:** N/V, graft occlusion, HA, ↓ BP **Labs:** ↑ Serum Ca level; monitor serum phosphate levels **NIPE:** Use cautiously w/ GI Dz; monitor for bone pain or deformity; chew tabs before swallowing; separate from meds that interact w/ antacids by 2 h

Lapatinib (Tykerb) [Tyrosine Kinase Inhibitor] Uses: *Advanced breast CA w/ capecitabine w/ tumors that overexpress HER2 & failed w/ anthracycline, taxane, & trastuzumab* **Action:** TKI **Dose:** Per protocol, 1250 mg PO d 1–21 w/ capecitabine 2000 mg/m²/d ÷ 2 doses/d d 1–14; ↓ w/ severe cardiac or hepatic impair **Caution:** [D, ?] Avoid CYP3A4 Inhibs/inducers **CI:** w/ Phenothiazines **Disp:** Tabs 250 mg **SE:** N/V/D, anemia, ↑ QT interval, hand–foot synd, rash, ↓ LVEF, interstitial lung Dz & pneumonitis **Interactions:** ↑ Effects *W/* potent CYP3A4 Inhibs (eg, ketoconazole), grapefruit; ↓ effects *W/* potent CYP3A4 inducers (eg, carbamazepine) **Labs:** ↑ LFTs; ↓ plt, neutropenia **NIPE:** Consider baseline LVEF & periodic ECG; take 1 h before or 1 h after a meal

Latanoprost (Xalatan) [Glaucoma Agent/Prostaglandin] Uses: *Open-angle glaucoma, ocular HTN* **Action:** Prostaglandin, ↑ outflow of aqueous humor **Dose:** 1 gtt eye(s) hs **Caution:** [C, ?] **Disp:** 0.005% soln **SE:** May darken light irides; blurred vision, ocular stinging, & itching, ↑ number & length of eyelashes **Interactions:** ↑ Risk *OF* precipitation if mixed w/ eye drops w/ thimerosal **NIPE:** Wait 15 min before using contacts; separate from other eye products by 5 min

Leflunomide (Arava) [Antirheumatic DMARDs/Immunomodulator] WARNING: PRG must be excluded prior to start of Rx Uses: *Active RA, orphan drug for organ rejection* **Action:** DMARD, ↓ pyrimidine synth **Dose:** Initial 100 mg/d PO for 3 d, then 10–20 mg/d **Caution:** [X, –] w/ Bile acid sequestrants, warfarin, rifampin, MTX **CI:** PRG **Disp:** Tabs 10, 20, 100 mg **SE:** D, Infxn, HTN, alopecia, rash, N, Jt pain, hep, interstitial lung Dz, immunosuppression **Interactions:** ↑ Effects *W/* rifampin; ↑ risk of hepatotox *W/* hepatotoxic drugs, MTX; ↑ effects *OF* NSAIDs; ↓ effects *W/* activated charcoal, cholestyramine

Labs: ↑ LFTs; monitor LFTs, CBC, PO_4 during initial therapy **NIPE:** ⊘ PRG, breast-feeding, live virus vaccines; vaccine should be up-to-date

Lenalidomide (Revlimid) [Immunomodulator] WARNING: Sig teratogen; pt must be enrolled in RevAssist risk-reduction program; hematologic tox, DVT & PE risk **Uses:** *MDS, combo w/ dexamethasone in multiple myeloma in pt failing 1 prior therapy **Action:** Thalidomide analogue, immune modulator **Dose:** *Adults.* 10 mg PO daily; swallow whole w/ H_2O; multiple myeloma 25 mg/d d 1–21 of 28-d cycle w/ protocol dose of dexamethasone **Caution:** [X, –] w/ Renal impair **Disp:** Caps 5, 10, 15, 25 mg **SE:** D, pruritus, rash, fatigue, night sweats, edema, nasopharyngitis, thromboembolism **Interactions:** Monitor digoxin **Labs:** ↓ BM (plt, WBC)—monitor CBC, ↑ K^+, ↑ LFTs; routine PRG tests required **NIPE:** Monitor for myelosuppression, thromboembolism, hepatotox; Rx only in 1-mo increments; limited distribution network; males must use condom & not donate sperm; use at least 2 forms of contraception > 4 wk beyond D/C

Lepirudin (Refludan) [Anticoagulant/Thrombin Inhibitor] Uses: *HIT* **Action:** Direct thrombin Inhib **Dose:** *Bolus:* 0.4 mg/kg IV, then 0.15 mg/kg/h Inf; if > 110 kg 44 mg of Inf 16.5 mg/kg/h max; ↓ dose & Inf rate w/ CrCl < 60 mL/min or if used w/ thrombolytics **Caution:** [B, ?/–] Hemorrhage event or severe HTN **CI:** Active bleeding **Disp:** Inj 50 mg **SE:** Bleeding, anemia, hematoma, anaphylaxis **Interactions:** ↑ Risk of bleeding *W/* antiplt drugs, cephalosporins, NSAIDs, thrombolytics, salicylates, feverfew, ginkgo, ginger, valerian **Labs:** Adjust based on aPTT ratio, maint aPTT 1.5–2 × control **NIPE:** Monitor for bleeding: Bleeding gums, nosebleed, unusual bruising, tarry stools, hematuria, guaiac + stool

Letrozole (Femara) [Antineoplastic/Aromatase Inhibitor] Uses: *Breast Ca:* Adjuvant w/ postmenopausal hormone receptor positive early Dz; adjuvant in postmenopausal women w/ early breast CA w/ prior adjuvant tamoxifen therapy; 1st/2nd line in postmenopausal women w/ hormone receptor positive or unknown Dz* **Action:** Nonsteroidal aromatase Inhib **Dose:** 2.5 mg/d PO; qod w/ severe liver Dz or cirrhosis **Caution:** [D, ?] **CI:** PRG, premenopausal **Disp:** Tabs 2.5 mg **SE:** Anemia, N, hot flashes, arthralgia **Interactions:** ↑ Risk of interference *W/* action of drug *W/* estrogens & OCPs **Labs:** ↑ LFTs, cholesterol; monitor CBC, thyroid Fxn, lytes, LFT, & SCr

Leucovorin (Wellcovorin) [Folic Acid Derivative/Vitamin] Uses: *OD of folic acid antagonist; megaloblastic anemia, augment 5-FU impaired MTX elimination; w/ 5-FU in colon CA* **Action:** Reduced folate source; circumvents action of folate reductase Inhibs (eg, MTX) **Dose:** *Leucovorin rescue:* 10 mg/m² PO/IM/IV q6h; start w/in 24 h after dose or 15 mg PO/IM/IV q6h, 25 mg max PO *Folate antagonist OD (eg, Pemetrexed):* 100 mg/m² IM/IV × 1, then 50 mg/m² IM/IV q6h × 8 d 100 mg/m² × 1 *5-FU adjuvant Tx, colon CA per protocol Low dose* 20 mg/m²/d IV × 5 d w/ 5-FU 425 mg/m²/d IV × 5 d, repeat q4–5wk × 6 *High dose:* 500 mg/m² IV qwk × 6, w/ 5-FU 500 mg/m² IV qwk × 6 wk, repeat after 2 wk off × 4 *Megaloblastic anemia:* 1 mg IM/IV daily **Caution:** [C, ?/–] **CI:** Pernicious anemia **Disp:** Tabs 5, 10, 15, 25 mg; Inj 50, 100, 200, 350, 500 mg **SE:** Allergic Rxn, N/V/D, fatigue, wheezing **Interactions:** ↑ Effects *OF* 5-FU; ↓ effects *OF* MTX, phenobarbital, phenytoin, primidone, TMP/SMX **Labs:** ↑ Plt; monitor Cr, methotrexate levels q24h w/ leucovorin rescue; w/ 5-FU monitor CBC w/ different plt, LFTs, lytes **NIPE:** ↑ Fluids to 3 L/d; do not use intravenously/intraventricularly

Leuprolide (Lupron, Lupron DEPOT, Lupron DEPOT-Ped, Viadur, Eligard) [Antineoplastic/GnRH Analogue] Uses: *Advanced PCa (all except Depot-Ped), endometriosis (Lupron), uterine fibroids (Lupron), & precocious puberty (Lupron-Ped)* **Action:** LHRH agonist; paradoxically ↓ release of GnRH w/ ↓ LH from anterior pituitary; in men ↓ testosterone **Dose:** *Adults. PCa: Lupron DEPOT:* 7.5 mg IM q28d or 22.5 mg IM q3mo or 30 mg IM q4mo *Eligard:* 7.5 mg SQ q28d or 22.5 mg SQ q3mo or 30 mg SQ q4mo or 45 mg SQ 6 mo *Endometriosis (Lupron DEPOT):* 3.75 mg IM qmo × 6 or 11.25 IM q3mo × 2 *Fibroids:* 3.75 mg IM qmo × 3 or 11.25 mg IM × 1 *Peds. CPP (Lupron DEPOT-Ped):* 50 mcg/kg/d SQ Inj; ↑ by 10 mcg/kg/d until downregulation achieved *Lupron DEPOT: < 25 kg.* 7.5 mg IM q4wk *> 25–37.5 kg.* 11.25 mg IM q4wk *> 37.5 kg.* 15 mg IM q4wk, ↑ by 3.75 mg q4wk until response **Caution:** [X, –] w/ Impending cord compression in PCa **CI:** AUB, implant in women/peds; PRG **Disp:** Inj 5 mg/mL; *Lupron DEPOT* 3.75 (1 mo for fibroids, endometriosis) *Lupron DEPOT for PCa:* 7.5 mg (1 mo), 11.25 mg (3 mo), 22.5 mg (3 mo), 30 mg (4 mo) *Eligard depot for PCa:* 7.5 mg (1 mo); 22.5 mg (3 mo), 30 mg (4 mo), 45 mg (6 mo) *Viadur:* 65 mg 12-mo SQ implant (unavailable to new Rx after April 2008) *Lupron DEPOT-Ped:* 7.5, 11.25, 15 mg **SE:** Hot flashes, gynecomastia, N/V, alopecia, anorexia, dizziness, HA, insomnia, paresthesias, depression exacerbation, peripheral edema, & bone pain (transient "flare Rxn" at 7–14 d after the 1st dose [LH/testosterone surge before suppression]); ↓ BMD w/ > 6 mo use, bone loss possible **Interactions:** ↓ Effects *W/* androgens, estrogens **Labs:** ↑ LFTs, BUN, Cr, uric acid, lipids, MBG; ↓ PT, PTT, plts **NIPE:** Non-steroidal antiandrogen (eg, bicalutamide) may block flare in men w/ PCa

Levalbuterol (Xopenex, Xopenex HFA) [Bronchodilator/Beta-2 Agonist] Uses: *Asthma (Rx & prevention of bronchospasm)* **Action:** Sympathomimetic bronchodilator; *R*-isomer of albuterol **Dose:** Based on NIH Guidelines 2007 *Adults.* Acute-severe exacerbation Xopenex HFA 4–8 puffs q20min up to 4 h, then q1–4h PRN or nebulizer 1/25–2.5 mg q20min × 3, then 1.25–5 mg q1–4h PRN *Peds < 4 y.* Quick relief 0.31–1.25 mg q4–6h PRN, severe 1.25 mg q20min × 3, then 0.075–0.15 mg/kg q1–4h PRN, 5 mg max *5–11 y.* Acute-severe exacerbation 1.25 mg q20min × 3, then 0.075–0.15 mg/kg q1–4h PRN, 5 mg max *> 11 y.* 0.63–1.25 mg nebulizer q6–8h **Caution:** [C, ?] w/ non–K⁺-sparing diuretics, CAD, HTN, arrhythmias **CI:** w/ Phenothiazines & TCAs, MAOI w/in 14 d **Disp:** MDI (Xopenex HFA) 45 mcg/puff (15 g); soln nebulizer Inh 0.31, 0.63, 1.25 mg/3 mL; concentrate 1.25 mg/0.5 mL **SE:** Parabox bronchospasm, anaphylaxis, angioedema, tachycardia, nervousness, V **Interactions:** ↑ Effects *W/* MAOIs, TCAs; ↑ risk of hypokalemia *W/* loop & thiazide diuretics; ↓ effects *W/* BBs; ↓ effects *OF* digoxin **Labs:** ↑ Serum glucose, ↓ serum K⁺ **NIPE:** May ↓ CV SE compared w/ albuterol; do not mix w/ other nebulizers or dilute; use other inhalants 5 min after this drug; monitor ECG for hypokalemia (flattened T waves)

Levetiracetam (Keppra) [Anticonvulsant/ Pyrrolidine Agent]
Uses: *Adjunctive PO Rx in partial onset Sz (adults & peds ≥ 4 y), myoclonic Szs (adults & peds ≥ 12 y) w/ JME, primary generalized tonic–clonic (PGTC) Szs (adults & peds ≥ 6 y) w/ idiopathic generalized epilepsy. Adjunctive Inj Rx partial-onset Szs in adults w/ epilepsy & myoclonic Szs in adults w/ JME. Inj alternative for adults (≥ 16 y) when PO not possible* **Action:** Unknown **Dose:** *Adults & Peds > 16 y.* 500 mg PO bid, titrate q2wk, may ↑ 3000 mg/d max *Peds 4–15 y.* 10–20 mg/kg/d ÷ in 2 doses, 60 mg/kg/d max (↓ in renal Insuff) **Caution:** [C, ?/–] Elderly, renal impair, psychological disorders; ↑ suicidality risk for antiepileptic drugs, higher for those w/ epilepsy vs those using drug for psychological indications; Inj not for < 16 y **CI:** Component allergy **Disp:** Tabs 250, 500, 750, 1000 mg, soln 100 mg/mL; Inj 100 mg/mL **SE:** Dizziness, somnolence, HA, N/V hostility, aggression, hallucinations, myelosuppression, impaired coordination **Interactions:** ↑ Effects W/ antihistamines, TCAs, benzodiazepines, narcotics, phenytoin; EtOH **NIPE:** May take w/ food; do not D/C abruptly—may cause Szs; post-market hepatic failure & pancytopenia reported

Levobunolol (A-K Beta, Betagan) [Glaucoma Agent/Beta-Adrenergic Blocker] **Uses:** *Open-angle glaucoma, ocular HTN* **Action:** β-Adrenergic blocker **Dose:** 1 gtt daily–bid **Caution:** [C, ?] w/ Verapamil or systemic BBs **CI:** Asthma, COPD sinus bradycardia, heart block (2nd-, 3rd-degree) CHF **Disp:** Soln 0.25%, 0.5% **SE:** Ocular stinging/burning, bradycardia, ↓ BP **Interactions:** ↑ Effects W/ BBs; ↑ risk of hypotension & bradycardia W/ quinidine, verapamil; ↓ IOP W/ carbonic anhydrase Inhibs, epinephrine, pilocarpine **NIPE:** Night vision & acuity may be ↓; possible systemic effects if absorbed

Levocetirizine (Xyzal) [Antihistamine] **Uses:** *Perennial/seasonal allergic rhinitis, chronic urticaria* **Action:** ↓ Antihistamine **Dose:** *Adults.* 5 mg qd *Peds 6–11 y.* 2.5 mg qd **Caution:** [B, ?] ↓ Adult dose w/ renal impair, CrCl 50–80 mL/ min 2.5 mg daily, 30–50 mL/min 2.5 mg qod 10–30 mL/min 2.5 mg 2 × /wk **CI:** Peds 6–11 y w/ renal impair, adults w/ ESRD **Disp:** Tab 5 mg, soln 0.5 mL/mL (150 mL) **SE:** CNS depression, drowsiness, fatigue, xerostomia **Interactions:** ↑ Effects W/ theophylline, ritonavir **NIPE:** Take in evening; avoid EtOH, CNS depressants

Levofloxacin (Levaquin) [Antibiotic/Fluoroquinolone] **WARNING:** ↑ Risk Achilles tendon rupture & tendonitis **Uses:** *Skin/skin structure Infxn (SSSI), UTI, chronic bacterial prostatitis, acute pyelo, acute bacterial sinusitis, acute bacterial exacerbation of chronic bronchitis, CAP, including multidrug-resistant S pneumoniae, nosocomial pneumonia; Rx inhalational anthrax in adults & peds ≥ 6 mo* **Action:** Quinolone, ↓ DNA gyrase *Spectrum:* Excellent gram(+) except MRSA & E faecium; excellent gram(–) except S maltophilia & Acinetobacter sp; poor anaerobic **Dose:** *Adults = 18 y.* IV/PO: Bronchitis: 500 mg qd × 7 d CAP: 500

mg qd × 7–14 d or 750 mg qd × 5 d *Sinusitis:* 500 mg qd × 10–14 d or 750 mg qd × 5 d. *Prostatitis:* 500 mg qd × 28 d *Uncomp SSSI:* 500 mg qd × 7–10 d *Comp SSSI/ nosocomial pneumonia:* 750 mg qd × 7–14 d *Anthrax:* 500 mg qd × 60 d *Uncomp UTI:* 250 mg qd × 3 d *Comp UTI/acute pyelo:* 250 mg qd × 10 d or 750 mg qd × 5 d, CrCl 10–19 mL/min; 250 mg, then 250 mg q48h or 750 mg, then 500 mg q48h *HD:* 750 mg, then 500 mg q48h *Peds ≥ 6 mo. Anthrax only: > 50 kg:* 500 mg q24h × 60 d *< 50 kg:* 8 mg/kg (250 mg/dose max) q12h for 60 d ↓ w/ renal impair avoid antacids w/ PO; oral soln 1 h before, 2 h after meals **Caution:** [C, –] w/ Cation-containing products (eg, antacids), w/ drugs that ↑ QT interval **CI:** Quinolone sensitivity **Disp:** Tabs 250, 500, 750 mg; premixed IV 250, 500, 750 mg, Inj 25 mg/ mL; Leva-Pak 750 mg × 5 d **SE:** N/D, dizziness, rash, GI upset, photosensitivity, CNS stimulant w/ IV use, *C difficile* enterocolitis; rare fatal hepatox **Interactions:** ↑ Effects *OF* cyclosporine, digoxin, theophylline, warfarin, caffeine; ↑ risk of Szs *W/* foscarnet, NSAIDs; ↑ risk of hyper-/hypoglycemia *W/* hypoglycemic drugs; ↓ effects *W/* antacids, antineoplastics, Ca, cimetidine, didanosine, famotidine, Fe, lansoprazole, Mg, nizatidine, omeprazole, phenytoin, ranitidine, NaHCO₃, sucralfate, zinc **NIPE:** Risk of tendon rupture & tendonitis—D/C if pain or inflammation; use w/ steroids ↑ tendon risk; ↑ fluids, use sunscreen, antacids 2 h before or after this drug; only for anthrax in peds

Levofloxacin Ophthalmic (Quixin, Iquix) [Antibiotic/Fluoroquinolone]

Uses: *Bacterial conjunctivitis* **Action:** See Levofloxacin **Dose:** *Ophthal:* 1–2 gtt in eye(s) q2h while awake × 2 d, then q4h while awake × 5 d **Caution:** [C, –] **CI:** Quinolone sensitivity **Disp:** 25 mg/mL ophthal soln 0.5% (Quixin), 1.5% (Iquix) **SE:** Ocular burning/pain, ↓ vision, fever, foreign body sensation, HA, pharyngitis, photophobia

Levonorgestrel (Next Choice, Plan B One Step) [Progestin/Hormone]

Uses: *Emergency contraceptive ("morning-after pill")*; prevents PRG if taken < 72 h after unprotected sex/contraceptive failure **Action:** Progestin, alters tubal transport & endometrium to implantation **Dose:** *Adults & Peds (postmenarche females).* w/in 72 h of unprotected intercourse: *Next Choice* 0.75 mg q12h × 2; *Plan B One Step* 1.5 mg × 1 **Caution:** [X, +] w/ AUB; may ↑ ectopic PRG risk **CI:** Known/suspected PRG **Disp:** *Next Choice:* Tab 0.75 mg, 2 blister pack *Plan B One Step:* Tab 1.5 mg, 1 blister pack **SE:** N/V/D, Abd pain, fatigue, HA, menstrual changes, dizziness, breast changes **Interactions:** ↓ Effects *W/* barbiturates, carbamazepine, modafinil, phenobarbital, phenytoin, pioglitazone, rifabutin, rifampin, ritonavir, topiramate, St. John's wort **NIPE:** Will not induce abortion; ↑ risk of ectopic PRG; OTC ("behind the counter") if > 17 y, RX if < 17 y but varies by state; if V occurs w/in 2 h of ingesting drug—may consider repeating dose

Levonorgestrel IUD (Mirena) [Progestin/Hormone]

Uses: *Contraception, long term* **Action:** Progestin, alters endometrium, thicken cervical mucus, inhibits ovulation & implantation **Dose:** Up to 5 y, insert w/in 7 d menses onset or stat after 1st tri abortion; wait 6 wk if postpartum; replace any time during menstrual cycle **Caution:** [C, ?] **CI:** PRG, w/ active hepatic Dz or tumor, uterine anomaly, breast CA, acute/h/o of PID, postpartum endometriosis, infected abortion last 3 mo, gynecological neoplasia, abnormal Pap, AUB, untreated cervicitis/vaginitis, multiple sex partners, ↑ susceptibility to Infxn **Disp:** 52 mg IUD **SE:** Failed insertion, ectopic PRG, sepsis, PID, infertility, PRG comps w/ IUD left in place, abortion, embedment, ovarian cysts, perforation uterus/cervix, intestinal obst/perforation, peritonitis, N, Abd pain, ↑ BP, acne, HA **NIPE:** Inform pt does not protect against STD/HIV; see package insert for insertion instructions; reexamine placement after 1st menses; 80% PRG w/in 12 mo of removal

Levorphanol (Levo-Dromoran) [C-II] [Narcotic Analgesic]   Uses: *Mod–severe pain; chronic pain* **Action:** Narcotic analgesic, morphine derivative **Dose:** 2–4 mg PO PRN q6–8h; ↓ in hepatic impair **Caution:** [B/D (prolonged use/ high doses at term), ?/–] w/ ↑ ICP, head trauma, adrenal Insuff **CI:** Component allergy **Disp:** Tabs 2 mg **SE:** Tachycardia, ↓ BP, drowsiness, GI upset, constipation, resp depression, pruritus **Interactions:** ↑ CNS effects **W/** antihistamines, cimetidine, CNS depressants, glutethimide, methocarbamol, EtOH, St. John's wort **Labs:** ↑ Amylase, lipase **NIPE:** ↓ Fluids & fiber, take w/ food

Levothyroxine (Synthroid, Levoxyl, Others) [Thyroid Hormone]: **WARNING:** Not for obesity or wgt loss; tox w/ high doses, esp when combined w/ sympathomimetic amines **Uses:** *Hypothyroidism, pituitary TSH suppression, myxedema coma* **Action:** T₄ supl L-thyroxine **Dose:** *Adults. Hypothyroid:* Titrate until euthyroid > 50 y w/ heart Dz or < 50 y w/ heart Dz 25–50 mcg/d, ↑ q6–8wk; > 50 y w/ heart Dz 12.5–25 mcg/d, ↑ q6–8wk; usual 100–200 mcg/d *Myxedema:* 200–500 mcg IV, then 100–300 mcg/d **Peds.** *Hypothyroid: 0–3 mo.* 10–15 mcg/kg/24 h PO *3–6 mo.* 8–10 mcg/kg/d PO. *6–12 mo.* 6–8 mcg/kg/d PO *1–5 y.* 5–6 mcg/kg/d PO *6–12 y.* 4–5 mcg/kg/d PO *>12 y.* 2–3 mcg/kg/d PO; if growth & puberty complete ↑ 1.7 mcg/kg/d; ↓ dose by 50% if IV; titrate based on response & thyroid tests; dose can ↑ rapid in young/ middle-aged; best on empty stomach **Caution:** [A, +] **CI:** Recent MI, uncorrected adrenal Insuff; many drug interactions; in elderly w/ CV Dz **Disp:** Tabs 25, 50, 75, 88, 100, 112, 125, 137, 150, 175, 200, 300 mcg; Inj 200, 500 mcg **SE:** Insomnia, wgt loss, N/V/D, irregular periods, ↓ BMD, alopecia, arrhythmia **Interactions:** ↑ Effects *OF* anticoagulants, sympathomimetics, TCAs, warfarin; ↓ effects *W/* antacids, BBs, carbamazepine, cholestyramine, estrogens, Fe salts, phenytoin, phenobarbital, rifampin, simethicone, sucralfate, ↓ effects *OF* digoxin, hypoglycemics, theophylline **Labs:** ↑ LFTs—Monitor; ↓ thyroid Fxn tests; drug alters thyroid uptake of radioactive I—D/C drug 4 wk before studies **NIPE:** ⊘ Switch brands d/t different bioavailabilities; take w/ full glass of H₂O (prevents choking); PRG may ↑ need for higher doses; takes 6 wk to see effect on TSH; wait 6 wk before checking TSH after dose change

Lidocaine, Systemic (Xylocaine, Others) [Antiarrhythmic]   Uses: *Rx cardiac arrhythmias* **Action:** Class Ib antiarrhythmic **Dose:** *Adults. Antiarrhythmic, ET:* 5 mg/kg; follow w/ 0.5 mg/kg in 10 min if effective *IV load:* 1 mg/ kg/dose bolus over 2–3 min; repeat in 5–10 min; 200–300 mg/h max; cont Inf

20–50 mcg/kg/min or 1–4 mg/min *ECC 2010:* **Cardiac arrest from VF/VT refractory VF:** *Initial:* 1–1.5 mg/kg IV/IO, additional 0.5–0.75 mg/kg IV push, repeat in 5–10 min, max total 3 mg/kg *ET:* 2–4 mg/kg as last resort **Reperfusing stable VT, wide complex tachycardia or ectopy:** Doses of 0.5–0.75 mg/kg to 1–1.5 mg/kg may be used initially; repeat 0.5–0.75 mg/kg q5–10min; max dose 3 mg/kg *Peds.* *ECC 2010:* **VF/pulseless VT, wide-complex tachycardia (w/ pulses):** 1 mg/kg IV/ IO, then maint 20–50 mcg/kg/min (repeat bolus if Inf started > 15 min after initial dose) **RSI:** 1–2 mg/kg IV/IO bolus **Caution:** [B, +] Corn allergy **CI:** Adams–Stokes synd; heart block **Disp:** Inj IV: 1% (10 mg/mL), 2% (20 mg/mL); admixture 4%, 10%, 20% *IV Inf:* 0.2%, 0.4% **SE:** Dizziness, paresthesias, & convulsions associated w/ tox **Interactions:** ↑ Effects *W/* amprenavir, BBs, cimetidine; ↑ neuromuscular blockade *W/* aminoglycosides, tubocurarine; ↑ cardiac depression *W/* procainamide, phenytoin, propranolol, quinidine, tocainide; ↑ effects *OF* succinylcholine **Labs:** ↑ SCr, ↑ CPK for 48 h after Inj **NIPE:** 2nd line to amiodarone in ECC; dilute ET dose 1–2 mL w/ NS; for IV forms, ↓ w/ liver Dz or CHF *Systemic levels:* Steady state 6–12 h *Therapeutic:* 1.2–5 mcg/mL *Toxic:* > 6 mcg/mL *1/2-life:* 1.5 h

Lidocaine; Lidocaine with Epinephrine (Anestacon Topical, Xylocaine, Xylocaine Viscous, Xylocaine MPF, Others) [Anesthetic]

Uses: *Local anesthetic, epidural/caudal anesthesia, regional nerve blocks, topical on mucous membranes (mouth/pharynx/urethra)* **Action:** Anesthetic; stabilizes neuronal membranes; inhibits ionic fluxes required for initiation & conduction **Dose:** *Adults. Local Inj anesthetic:* 4.5 mg/kg max total dose or 300 mg; w/ epi 7 mg/kg or total 500 mg max dose *Oral:* 15 mL viscous swish & spit or *pharyngeal gargle & swallow, do not use < 3-h intervals or > 8 × in 24 h Urethra* 10–15 mL (200–300 mg) jelly in men, 5 mL female urethra; 600 mg/24 h max *Peds. Topical:* Apply max 3 mg/kg/dose *Local Inj anesthetic:* Max 4.5 mg/kg (Table 1) **Caution:** [B, +] Corn allergy; epi-containing solns may interact w/ TCA or MAOI & cause severe ↑ BP **CI:** Do not use lidocaine w/ epi on digits, ears, or nose (vasoconstriction & necrosis) **Disp:** Inj local: 0.5%, 1%, 1.5%, 2%, 4%, 10%, 20%; Inj w/ epi 0.5%/1:200,000,0 1%/1:100,000, 2%/1:100,000; (MPF) 1%/1:200,000, 1.5%/1:200,000, 2%/1:200,000; (Dental formulations) 2%/1:50,000, 2%/1:100,000; cream 2%; gel 2, 2.5%; oint 2.5%, 5%; Liq 2.5%; soln 2%, 4%; viscous 2% **SE:** Dizziness, paresthesias, & convulsions associated w/ tox **Notes:** See Table 1 **NIPE:** Oral spray/soln may impair swallowing; epi may be added for local anesthesia to ↑ effect & ↓ bleeding

Lidocaine Powder Intradermal Injection System (Zingo) [Topical Anesthetic]

Uses: *Local anesthesia before venipuncture or IV in peds 3–18 y* **Action:** Local amide anesthetic **Dose:** Apply 3 min before procedure **Caution:** [N/A, N/A] Only on intact skin **CI:** Lidocaine allergy **Disp:** 6.5-in device to administer under pressure 0.5 mg lidocaine powder in 2-cm area, single use **SE:** Skin Rxn, edema, petechiae

Lidocaine/Prilocaine (EMLA, LMX) [Topical Anesthetic]

Uses: *Topical anesthetic for intact skin or genital mucous membranes*; adjunct to phlebotomy or dermal procedures **Action:** Amide local anesthetics **Dose:** *Adults.* *EMLA cream, anesthetic disc (1 g/10 cm²):* Thick layer 2–2.5 g to intact skin, cover w/ occlusive dressing (eg, Tegaderm) for at least 1 h *Anesthetic disc:* 1 g/10 cm² for at least 1 h *Peds. Max Dose:* < *3 mo or* < *5 kg.* 1 g/10 cm² for 1 h *3–12 mo & > 5 kg.* 2 g/20 cm² for 4 h *1–6 y & > 10 kg.* 10 g/100 cm² for 4 h *7–12 y & > 20 kg.* 20 g/200 cm² for 4 h **Caution:** [B, +] Methemoglobinemia **CI:** Use on mucous membranes, broken skin, eyes; allergy to amide-type anesthetics **Disp:** Cream 2.5% lidocaine/2.5% prilocaine; anesthetic disc (1 g); periodontal gel 2.5/2.5% **SE:** Burning, stinging, methemoglobinemia **NIPE:** Longer contact time ↑ effect; low risk of systemic adverse effects

Lidocaine/Tetracaine Transdermal (Synera) [Topical Anesthetic]
Uses: Topical anesthetic; adjunct to phlebotomy or dermal procedures **Action:** Topical anesthetic **Dose:** *Adults & Children > 3 y. Phlebotomy:* Apply to intact skin 20–30 min prior to venipuncture *Dermal procedures:* Apply to intact skin 30 min prior to procedure **Caution:** [B, ±] **CI:** Pts w/ allergy to lidocaine/tetracaine/ amide & ester-type anesthetics; use on mucous membranes, broken skin; pts w/ PABA hypersensitivity **Disp:** TD patch lidocaine 70 mg/tetracaine 70 mg **SE:** Erythema, blanching, edema, rash, burning, dizziness, HA, paresthesias **Interactions:** ↑ Systemic effects *OF* Class I antiarrhythmic drugs (tocainide, mexiletine); ↑ systemic effects *W/* other local anesthetics **NIPE:** ⊗ Cut patch/remove top cover—may cause thermal injury; low risk of systemic adverse effects; ⊗ use multiple patches simultaneously or sequentially

Linagliptin (Tradjenta) [Dipeptidyl Peptidase-4 Inhibitor] **Uses:** *Type-2 DM alone or combo (w/ metformin or glimepiride)* **Action:** ↑ Insulin release; blocks enzyme dipeptidyl peptidase-4 **Dose:** 5 mg/d w/ or w/o food **Caution:** [B,?] **CI:** N **Disp:** Tabs 5 mg **SE:** URI, stuffy nose, sore throat, muscle pain, HA **Interactions:** ↓ Effects *W/* CYP3A4 inducers such as rifampin; ↑ risk of hypoglycemia *W/* sulfonylureas—↓ secretagogue dose **NIPE:** Not for Type 1 DM or DKA; use as adjunct to diet & exercise; use as monotherapy or combo therapy

Lindane (Kwell, Others) [Scabicide/Pediculicide] **WARNING:** Only for pts intolerant/failed 1st-line therapy w/ safer agents. Szs & deaths reported w/ repeat/prolonged use. Caution d/t ↑ risk of neurotox in infants, children, elderly, w/ other skin conditions, & if < 50 kg. Instruct pts on proper use & inform that itching occurs after successful killing of scabies or lice **Uses:** *Head lice, pubic "crab" lice, body lice, scabies* **Action:** Ectoparasiticide & ovicide **Dose:** *Adults& Peds.* *Cream or lotion:* Thin layer to dry skin after bathing, leave for 8–12 h, pour on laundry *Shampoo:* Apply 30 mL to dry hair, develop a lather w/ warm H₂O for 4 min, comb out nits **Caution:** [C, +/−] **CI:** Premature infants, uncontrolled Sz disorders open wounds **Disp:** Lotion 1%; shampoo 1% **SE:** Arrhythmias, Szs, local irritation, GI upset, ataxia, alopecia, N/V, aplastic anemia **Interactions:** Oil-based hair creams ↑ drug absorption **NIPE:** Apply to dry hair/dry, cool skin; caution w/ overuse (may be absorbed); may repeat Rx in 7 d; try OTC 1st w/ pyrethrins (Pronto, Rid, others)

Linezolid (Zyvox) [Antibiotic/Oxazolidinones] Uses: *Infxns caused by gram(+) bacteria (including VRE), pneumonia, skin Infxns* **Action:** Unique, binds ribosomal bacterial RNA; bacteriocidal for streptococci, bacteriostatic for enterococci & staphylococci *Spectrum:* Excellent gram(+) including VRE & MRSA **Dose:** *Adults.* 400–600 mg IV or PO q12h *Peds.* 10 mg/kg IV or PO q8h (q12h in preterm neonates) **Caution:** [C, ?/–] w/ MAOI, w/ ↓ BM **Disp:** Inj 200, 600 mg; tabs 600 mg; susp 100 mg/5 mL **SE:** Lactic acidosis, peripheral/optic neuropathy, HTN, N/D, HA, insomnia, GI upset, ↓ BM, tongue discoloration **Interactions:** ↑ Risk of serotonin synd **W/** SSRIs, sibutramine, trazodone, venlafaxine; ↑ HTN **W/** amphetamines, dextromethorphan, DA, epinephrine, levodopa, MAOIs, meperidine, metaraminol, phenylephrine, phenylpropanolamine, pseudoephedrine, tyramine, ginseng, ephedra, ma huang, tyramine-containing foods; ↑ risk of bleeding **W/** antiplts **Labs:** Follow weekly CBC **NIPE:** Take w/o regard to food; avoid foods w/ tyramine & cough/cold products w/ pseudoephedrine; not for gram(−) Infxn, ↑ deaths in catheter-related Infxns

Liothyronine (Cytomel, Triostat, T$_3$) [Thyroid Hormone] **WARNING:** Not for obesity or wgt loss Uses: *Hypothyroidism, nontoxic goiter, myxedema coma, thyroid suppression therapy* **Action:** T$_3$ replacement **Dose:** *Adults.* Initial 25 mcg/24 h, titrate q1–2wk to response & TFT; maint of 25–100 mcg/d PO *Myxedema coma:* 25–50 mcg IV *Myxedema:* 5 mcg/d, PO ↑ 5–10 mcg/d q1–2wk; maint 50–100 mcg/d *Nontoxic goiter:* 5 mcg/d PO, ↑ 5–10 mcg/d q1–2wk, usual dose 75 mcg/d *T$_3$ suppression test:* 75–100 mcg/d × 7d *Peds.* Initial 5 mcg/24 h, titrate by 5-mcg/24-h increments at q3–4d intervals; maint peds 1–3 y: 50 mcg/d *Infants–12 mo.* 20 mcg/d *> 3 y.* Adult dose; ↓ in elderly & CV **Dz Caution:** [A, +] **CI:** Recent MI, uncorrected adrenal Insuff, uncontrolled HTN, thyrotoxicosis, artificial rewarming **Disp:** Tabs 5, 25, 50 mcg; Inj 10 mcg/mL **SE:** Alopecia, arrhythmias, CP, HA, sweating, twitching, ↑ HR, ↑ BP, MI, CHF, fever **Interactions:** ↑ Effects *OF* anticoagulants; ↓ effects **W/** bile acid sequestrants, carbamazepine, estrogens, phenytoin, rifampin; ↓ effects *OF* hypoglycemics, theophylline **Labs:** Monitor TFT; monitor glucose w/ DM meds **NIPE:** Monitor cardiac status, take in AM; separate antacids by 4 h; when switching from IV to PO, taper IV slowly

Liraglutide Recombinant (Victoza) [Glucagon-Like Peptide-1 (GLP-1) Receptor Agonist] **WARNING:** CI w/ personal or family Hx of medullary thyroid Ca (MCT) or w/ multiple endocrine neoplasia synd type 2 (MEN 2) Uses: *Type 2 DM* **Action:** Glucagon-like peptide-1 receptor agonist **Dose:** 1.8 mg/d; begin 0.6 mg/d any time of d SQ (Abd/thigh/upper arm), ↑ to 1.2 mg after 1 wk, may ↑ to 1.8 mg/d after **Caution:** [C; ?/–] **CI:** See Warning **Disp:** Multidose pens, 0.6, 1.2, 1.8 mg/dose, 6 mg/mL **SE:** Pancreatitis, MCT, HA, N/D **Interactions:** ↓ Glucose w/ sulfonylurea **NIPE:** Delays gastric emptying

Lisdexamfetamine Dimesylate (Vyvanse) [Stimulant] [C-II] **WARNING:** Amphetamines have high potential for abuse; prolonged administration may lead to dependence; misuse may cause sudden death & serious CV events

Uses: *ADHD* Action: CNS stimulant Dose: *Adults & Peds 6–12 y.* 30 mg daily, ↑ qwk 10–20 mg/d, 70 mg/d max Caution: [C, ?/–] w/ Potential for drug dependency in pt w/ psychological or Sz disorder, Tourette synd, HTN CI: Severe arteriosclerotic CV Dz, mod–severe ↑ BP, ↑ thyroid, sensitivity to sympathomimetic amines, NAG, agitated states, h/o drug abuse, w/ or w/in 14 d of MAOI Disp: Caps 30, 50, 70 mg SE: HA, insomnia, ↓ appetite Interactions: Risk of HTN crisis W/ MAOIs, furazolidone; ↑ effects W/ TCA, propoxyphene; ↑ effects OF meperidine, norepinephrine, phenobarbital, TCA; ↓ effects W/ haloperidol, chlorpromazine, Li; ↓ effects OF adrenergic blockers, antihistamines, antihypertensives Labs: Monitor phenytoin levels; may interfere w/ urinary steroid tests NIPE: OK to open & dissolve in H_2O; AHA statement April 2008: All children diagnosed w/ ADHD who are candidates for stimulant meds should undergo CV assessment prior to use

Lisinopril (Prinivil, Zestril) [Antihypertensive/ACEI] WARNING: ACE Inhibs can cause fetal injury/death in 2nd/3rd tri; D/C w/ PRG Uses: *HTN, CHF, prevent DN & AMI* Action: ACE Inhib Dose: 5–40 mg/24 h PO daily–bid, CHF target 40 mg/d *AMI:* 5 mg w/in 24 h of MI, then 5 mg after 24 h, 10 mg after 48 h, then 10 mg/d; ↓ in renal Insuff; use low dose, ↑ slowly in elderly Caution: [D, –] CI: Bilateral RAS, PRG ACE Inhib sensitivity (angioedema) Disp: Tabs 2.5, 5, 10, 20, 30, 40 mg SE: Dizziness, HA, cough, ↓ BP, angioedema Interactions: ↑ Effects W/ α-blockers, diuretics ↑ risk of hyperkalemia W/ K⁺-sparing diuretics, TMP, salt substitutes; ↑ risk of cough W/ capsaicin; ↑ effects OF insulin, Li; ↓ effects W/ ASA, indomethacin, NSAIDs Labs: ↑ LFTs, serum K⁺, Cr, BUN, monitor levels; rare ↓ BM-monitor WBC NIPE: Max effect may take several wk; to prevent DN, start when urinary microalbuminuria begins; monitor ECG for hyperkalemia (peaked T waves)

Lisinopril & Hydrochlorothiazide (Prinzide, Zestoretic, Generic) [Antihypertensive/ACEI/HCTZ] WARNING: ACE Inhib can cause fetal injury/death in 2nd/3rd tri; D/C w/ PRG Uses:*HTN* Action: ACE Inhib w/ diuretic (HCTZ) Dose: Initial 10 mg lisinopril/12.5 mg HCTZ, titrate upward to effect; > 80 mg/d lisinopril or > 50 mg/d HCTZ are not recommended; ↓ in renal Insuff; use low dose, ↑ slowly in elderly Caution: [C (1st tri; D after), –] w/ AS/ cardiomyopathy CI: Bilateral RAS, PRG, ACE Inhib sensitivity (angioedema) Disp: Tabs (mg lisinopril/mg HCTZ) 10/12.5, 20/12.5; Zestoretic also available as 20/25 SE: Anaphylactoid Rxn (rare), dizziness, HA, cough, fatigue, ↓ BP, angioedema,rare ↓ BM/cholestatic jaundice Interactions: ↑ Effects W/ α-blockers, diuretics ↑ risk of hyperkalemia W/ K⁺-sparing diuretics, TMP, salt substitutes; ↑ risk of cough W/ capsaicin; ↑ effects OF insulin, Li; ↓ effects W/ ASA, indomethacin, NSAIDs Labs: ↑/↓ K⁺, ↑ Cr; ✓ K⁺, BUN, Cr, K⁺, WBC NIPE: Use only when monotherapy fails; monitor ECG for hyperkalemia (peaked T waves)

Lithium Carbonate (Eskalith, Lithobid, Others) [Antipsychotic] WARNING: Li tox related to serum levels & can be seen at close to therapeutic levels Uses: *Manic episodes of bipolar Dz*, augment antidepressants, aggression, posttraumatic stress disorder **Action:** Effects shift toward intraneuronal metabolism of catecholamines **Dose: *Adults. Bipolar, acute mania:*** 1800 mg/d PO in 2–3 ÷ doses (target serum 1–1.5 mEq/L (check 2 × /wk until stable) *Bipolar maint:* 900–1200 /d PO in 2–3 ÷ doses (target serum 0.6–1.2 mEq/L) ***Peds = 12 y.*** See Adults; ↓ in renal Insuff, elderly **Caution:** [D, –] Many drug interactions; avoid ACE Inhib or diuretics; thyroid Dz **CI:** Severe renal impair or CV Dz, lactation **Disp:** Caps 150, 300, 600 mg; tabs 300 mg; SR tabs 300 mg, CR tabs 450 mg; syrup & soln 300 mg/5 mL **SE:** Polyuria, polydipsia, nephrogenic DI, long term may affect renal conc ability & cause fibrosis; tremor; Na retention or diuretic use may ↑ tox; arrhythmias, dizziness, alopecia, goiter ↓ thyroid, N/V/D, ataxia, nystagmus, ↓ BP **Notes:** Levels: *Trough:* Just before next dose *Therapeutic:* 0.8–1.2 mEq/mL *Toxic:* > 1.5 mEq/mL *1/2-life:* 18–20h. Follow levels q1–2mo on maint **Interactions:** ↑ Effects *OF* TCA; ↑ effects *W/* ACEIs, bumetanide, carbamazepine, ethacrynic acid, fluoxetine, furosemide, methyldopa, NSAIDs, phenytoin, phenothiazine, probenecid, tetracyclines, thiazide diuretics, dandelion, juniper; ↓ effects *W/* acetazolamide, antacids, mannitol, theophylline, urea, verapamil, caffeine **Labs:** ↑ Serum glucose, I-131 uptake, WBC; ↓ uric acid, T_3, T_4 **NIPE:** Several wk before full effects of med, ↑ fluid intake to 2–3 L/d

Lodoxamide (Alomide) [Antihistamine] Uses: *Vernal conjunctivitis/keratitis* **Action:** Stabilizes mast cells **Dose: *Adults & Peds > 2 y.*** 1–2 gtt in eye(s) qid = 3 mo **Caution:** [B, ?] **Disp:** Soln 0.1% **SE:** Ocular burning, stinging, HA **NIPE:** Do not use soft contacts during use

Loperamide (Diamode, Imodium) [Antidiarrheal] [OTC] Uses: *D* **Action:** Slows intestinal motility **Dose: *Adults.*** Initial 4 mg PO, then 2 mg after each loose stool, up to 16 mg/d ***Peds. 2–5 y, 13–20 kg.*** 1 mg PO tid *6–8 y, 20–30 kg.* 2 mg PO bid *8–12 y, > 30 kg.* 2 mg PO tid **Caution:** [C, +] Not for acute D caused by *Salmonella, Shigella,* or *C difficile;* w/ HIV may cause toxic megacolon **CI:** Pseudomembranous colitis, bloody D, Abd pain w/o D, < 2 y **Disp:** Caps 2 mg; tabs 2 mg; Liq 1 mg/5 mL, 1 mg/7.5 mL (OTC) **SE:** Constipation, sedation, dizziness, Abd cramp, N **Interactions:** ↑ Effects *W/* antihistamines, CNS depressants, phenothiazines, TCAs, EtOH

Lopinavir/Ritonavir (Kaletra) [Antiretroviral/Protease Inhibitor] Uses: *HIV Infxn* **Action:** Protease Inhib **Dose: *Adults. Tx naive:*** 800/200 mg PO daily or 400/100 mg PO bid *Tx experienced pt:* 400/100 mg PO bid (↑ dose if w/ amprenavir, efavirenz, fosamprenavir, nelfinavir, nevirapine); do not use qd dosing w/ concomitant Rx ***Peds. 7–15 kg.*** 12/3 mg/kg PO bid *15–40 kg.* 10/2.5 mg/kg PO bid *> 40 kg.* Adult dose; w/ food **Caution:** [C, ?/–] Numerous interactions, w/ hepatic impair **CI:** w/ Drugs dependent on CYP3A/CYP2D6 (Table10), statins, St. John's wort, fluconazole, w/α₁-adrenoreceptor antagonist (alfuzosin)/w/ PDE5 Inhib sildenafil **Disp:** (lopinavir mg/ritonavir mg) Tab 100/25, 200/50, soln 400/100/5 mL **SE:** Avoid disulfiram (soln has EtOH), metronidazole, GI upset, asthenia, pancreatitis; protease metabolic synd **Interactions:** ↑ Effects *W/* clarithromycin, erythromycin; ↑ effects *OF* amiodarone, amprenavir, azole antifungals, bepridil, cisapride, cyclosporine, CCBs, ergot alkaloids, flecainide, flurazepam, HMG-CoA reductase Inhibs, indinavir, lidocaine, meperidine, midazolam, pimozide, propafenone, propoxyphene, quinidine, rifabutin, saquinavir, sildenafil, tacrolimus, terfenadine, triazolam, zolpidem; ↓ effects *W/* barbiturates, carbamazepine, dexamethasone, didanosine, efavirenz, nevirapine, phenytoin, rifabutin, rifampin, St. John's wort; ↓ effects *OF* OCPs, warfarin **Labs:** ↑ LFTs, cholesterol, triglycerides **NIPE:** Take w/ food, use barrier contraception

Loratadine (Claritin, Alavert) [Antihistamine] Uses: *Allergic rhinitis, chronic idiopathic urticaria* **Action:** Nonsedating antihistamine **Dose: *Adults.*** 10 mg/d PO *Peds 2–5 y.* 5 mg PO daily > 6 *y.* Adult dose; on empty stomach; ↓ in hepatic Insuff; qod dose w/ CrCl < 30 mL/min **Caution:** [B, +/–] **CI:** Component allergy **Disp:** Tabs 10 mg (OTC); rapidly disintegrating RediTabs 10 mg; chew tabs 5 mg; syrup 1 mg/mL **SE:** HA, somnolence, xerostomia, hyperkinesis in peds **Interactions:** ↑ Effects *W/* CNS depressants, erythromycin, ketoconazole, MAOIs, protease Inhibs, procarbazine, ETOH **NIPE:** Take w/o food; licorice consumption may prolong QT interval

Lorazepam (Ativan, Others) [C-IV] [Anxiolytic, Sedative/Hypnotic/ Benzodiazepine] Uses: *Anxiety & anxiety w/ depression; sedation; control status epilepticus; EtOH withdrawal; antiemetic* **Action:** Benzodiazepine; antianxiety agent; works via postsynaptic GABA receptors **Dose: *Adults.*** *Anxiety:* 1–10 mg/d PO in 2–3 ÷ doses *Pre-op:* 0.05 mg/kg to 4 mg max IM 2 h before or 0.044 mg/ kg–2 mg dose max IV 15–20 min before surgery *Insomnia:* 2–4 mg PO hs *Status epilepticus:* 4 mg/dose slow over 2–5 min IV PRN q10–15min; usual total dose 8 mg *Antiemetic:* 0.5–2 mg IV or PO q4–6h PRN *EtOH withdrawal:* 2–5 mg IV or 1–2 mg PO initial depending on severity; titrate *Peds. Status epilepticus:* 0.05–0.1 mg/kg/ dose IV over 2–5 min, repeat at 1–20-min intervals × 2 PRN *Antiemetic, 2–15 y:* 0.05 mg/kg (to 2 mg/dose) prechemotherapy; ↓ in elderly; do not administer IV > 2 mg/ min or 0.05 mg/kg/min **Caution:** [D, ?/–] w/ Hepatic impair, other CNS depression, COPD; ↓ dose by 50% w/ valproic acid & probenecid **CI:** Severe pain, severe ↓ BP, sleep apnea, NAG, allergy to propylene glycol or benzyl alcohol **Disp:** Tabs 0.5, 1, 2 mg; soln, PO conc 2 mg/mL; Inj 2, 4 mg/mL **SE:** Sedation, memory impair, EPS, dizziness, ataxia, tachycardia, ↓ BP constipation, resp depression **Interactions:** ↑ Effects *W/* cimetidine, disulfiram, probenecid, calendula, catnip, hops, lady's slipper, passion-flower, kava kava, valerian; ↑ effects *OF* phenytoin; ↑ CNS depression *W/* anticonvulsants, antihistamines, CNS depressants, MAOIs, scopolamine, EtOH; ↓ effects *W/* caffeine, tobacco; ↓ effects *OF* levodopa **Labs:** ↑ LFTs **NIPE:** ⊘ D/C abruptly; ~ 10 min for effect if IV; IV Inf requires in-line filter

Losartan (Cozaar) [Antihypertensive/ARB] **WARNING:** Can cause fatal injury & death if used in 2nd & 3rd tri. D/C Rx if PRG detected Uses: *HTN, DN, prevent CVA in HTN & LVH* **Action:** Angiotensin II receptor antagonist **Dose: *Adults.*** 25–50 mg PO daily–bid, max 100 mg; ↓ in elderly/hepatic impair *Peds ≥ 6 y.*

HTN: Initial 0.7 mg/kg qd, ↑ to 50 mg/d PRN; 1.4 mg/kg/d or 100 mg/d max **Caution:** [C (1st tri, D 2nd & 3rd tri), ?/–) w/ NSAIDs, supls may cause ↑ K⁺; w/ RAS, hepatic impair **CI:** PRG, component sensitivity **Disp:** Tabs 25, 50, 100 mg **SE:** ↓ BP in pts on diuretics; GI upset, facial/angioedema, dizziness, cough, weakness, ↓ renal Fxn **Interactions:** ↑ Risk of hyperkalemia **W/** K⁺-sparing diuretics, K⁺ supls, TMP; ↑ effects *OF* Li; ↓ effects **W/** diltiazem, fluconazole, phenobarbital, rifampin **Labs:** ↑ K⁺ **NIPE:** ⊘ PRG, breast-feeding

Lovastatin (Mevacor, Altoprev) [Antilipemic/HMG-CoA Reductase Inhibitor] Uses: *Hypercholesterolemia to ↓ risk of MI, angina* **Action:** HMG-CoA reductase Inhib **Dose:** *Adults.* 20 mg/d PO w/ PM meal; may ↑ at 4-wk intervals to 80 mg/d max or 60 mg ER tab; take w/ meals *Peds 10–17 y (at least 1-y postmenarchal). Familial ↑ cholesterol:* 10 mg PO qd, ↑ q4wk PRN to 40 mg/d max (IR w/ PM meal) **Caution:** [X, –] Avoid w/ gemfibrozil; dose escalation w/ renal impair **CI:** Active liver Dz, PRG, lactation **Disp:** Tabs generic 10, 20, 40 mg; Mevacor 20, 40 mg; Altoprev ER tabs 20, 40, 60 mg **SE:** HA & GI intolerance common; promptly report any unexplained muscle pain, tenderness, or weakness (myopathy) **Interactions:** ↑ Effects **W/** [grapefruit juice]; ↑ risk of severe myopathy **W/** azole antifungals, cyclosporine, erythromycin, gemfibrozil, HMG-CoA Inhibs, niacin; ↑ effects *OF* warfarin; ↓ effects **W/** isradipine, pectin **Labs:** ↑ LFTs; monitor LFT q12wk × 1 y, then q6mo; may alter TFT **NIPE:** ⊘ PRG; take drug PM; periodic eye exams; maint cholesterol-lowering diet

Lubiprostone (Amitiza) [Laxative] Uses: *Chronic idiopathic constipation in adults, IBS w/ constipation in females ≥ 18 y* **Action:** Selective Cl⁻ channel activator; ↑ intestinal motility **Dose:** *Adults. Constipation:* 24 mcg PO bid w/ food; w/ food & water (reduce w/ mod to severe hepatic impairment) *IBS:* 8 mcg bid; w/ food & water (reduce w/severe hepatic impairment) **CI:** Mechanical GI obst **Caution:** [C, ?/–] Severe D, severe renal or mod–severe hepatic impair **Disp:** Gelcaps 8, 24 mcg **SE:** N/D, HA, GI distention, Abd pain **Labs:** Monitor LFTs & BUN/Cr; requires (–) PRG test before Tx **NIPE:** Utilize contraception; periodically reassess drug need; not for chronic use; suspend drug if D; ⊘ breast-feeding; not approved in males; may experience severe dyspnea w/in 1 h of dose, usually resolves w/in 3 h

Lurasidone (Latuda) [Atypical Antipsychotic/Serotonin Receptor Antagonist] WARNING: Elderly w/ dementia-related psychosis at ↑ death risk. Not approved for dementia-related psychosis Uses: *Schizophrenia* **Action:** Atypical antipsychotic: Central DA type 2 (D2) & serotonin type 2 (5HT2A) receptor antagonist **Dose:** 40–80 mg/d PO ;40 mg max w/ CrCl 10–49 mL/min or mod–severe hepatic impair **Caution:** [B; –] **CI:** w/ Strong CYP3A4 Inhib/inducer **Disp:** Tabs 40, 80 mg **SE:** Somnolence, agitation, tardive dyskinesia, akathisia, parkinsonism, stroke, TIAs, Sz, orthostatic hypotension, syncope, dysphagia, neuroleptic malignant synd, body temperature dysregulation, N, ↑ wgt, type 2 DM, hyperprolactinemia **Interactions:** Do not use w/ concomitant strong CYP3A4 Inhibs (eg, ketoconazole) & inducers (eg, rifampin); ↑ CNS effects **W/** Etoh & other CNS depressants **Labs:** ↓ WBC; ↑ lipids; monitor CBC, during first few mo of therapy; monitor FBS **NIPE:** w/ DM risk ✓ glucose; take w/ food

Lutropin Alfa (Luveris) [Hormone] **Uses:** *Infertility w/ profound LH deficiency* **Action:** Recombinant LH **Dose:** 75 units SQ w/ 75–150 units FSH, 2 separate Inj max 14 d **Caution:** [X, ?/M] potential for arterial thromboembolism **CI:** Primary ovarian failure, uncontrolled thyroid/adrenal dysfunction, intracranial lesion, AUB, hormone-dependent GU tumor, ovarian cyst, PRG **Disp:** Inj 75 units **SE:** HA, N, ovarian hyperstimulation synd, ovarian torsion, Abd pain d/t ovarian enlargement, breast pain, ovarian cysts; ↑ risk of multiple births **NIPE:** Rotate Inj sites; do not exceed 14 d duration unless signs of imminent follicular development; monitor ovarian ultrasound & serum estradiol; specific pt info packets given

Lymphocyte Immune Globulin [Antithymocyte Globulin, ATG] (Atgam) [Immunosuppressant] **WARNING:** Should only be used by healthcare provider experienced in immunosuppressive Tx or management of solid-organ and/or BM transplant pts Adequate lab & supportive resources must be readily available **Uses:** *Allograft rejection in renal transplant pts; aplastic anemia if not candidates for BMT*, prevent rejection of other solid-organ transplants, GVHD after BMT **Action:** ↓ Circulating antigen-reactive T lymphocytes; human & equine product **Dose:** *Adults. Prevent rejection:* 15 mg/kg/d IV × 14 d, then qod × 14 d; initial dose w/in 24 h before/after transplant *Rx rejection:* Same except use 10–15 mg/kg/d; max 21 doses in 28 d, qd 1st 14 d *Aplastic anemia:* 10–20 mg/kg/d × 8–14 d, then qod × 7 doses for total 21 doses in 28 d *Peds. Prevent renal allograft rejection:* 5–25 mg/kg/d IV; aplastic anemia 10–20 mg/kg/d IV **Caution:** [C, –] **CI:** h/o Previous Rxn or Rxn to other equine γ-globulin prep **Disp:** Inj 50 mg/mL **SE:** D/C w/ severe ↓ plt & WBC; rash, fever, chills, ↓ BP, HA, CP, edema, N/V/D, lightheadedness **Notes:** *Test* Dose: 0.1 mL 1:1000 in NS **Interactions:** ↑ Immunosuppression *W/* azathioprine, corticosteroids, immunosuppressants **Labs:** ↑ LFTs, ↑ K⁺, ↓ plt & WBC; monitor WBC, plt; plt counts usually return to nl w/o D/C Rx therapy **NIPE:** A systemic Rxn precludes use; give via central line; consider preTx w/ antipyretic, antihistamine, and/or steroids

Magaldrate (Riopan-Plus) [Antacid/Aluminum & Magnesium Salt] [OTC] **Uses:** *Hyperacidity associated w/ peptic ulcer, gastritis, & hiatal hernia* **Action:** Low-Na antacid **Dose:** 5–10 mL PO between meals & hs, on empty stomach **Caution:** [C, ?/+] **CI:** UC, diverticulitis, appendicitis, ileostomy/colostomy, renal Insuff (Mg²⁺ content) **Disp:** Susp (magaldrate mg/simethicone mg) 540/20 & 1080/40/5 mL (OTC) **SE:** White flecked feces, constipation, N/V/D **Notes:** < 0.3 mg Na⁺/tab or tsp **Interactions:** ↑ Effects *OF* levodopa, quinidine; ↓ effects *OF* allopurinol, anticoagulants, cefpodoxime, ciprofloxacin, clindamycin, digoxin, indomethacin, INH, ketoconazole, lincomycin, phenothiazine, quinolones, tetracyclines **Labs:** ↑ Mg²⁺, ↓ PO₄ **NIPE:** ⊘ Other meds w/in 1–2 h

Magnesium Citrate (Citroma, Others) [Laxative/Magnesium Salt] [OTC] **Uses:** *Vigorous bowel prep*; constipation **Action:** Cathartic laxative

Dose: *Adults.* 120–300 mL PO PRN *Peds.* 0.5 mL/kg/dose, q4–6h to 200 mL PO max; w/ a beverage **Caution:** [B, +] w/ neuromuscular Dz **CI:** Severe renal Dz, heart block, N/V, rectal bleeding intestinal obst/perforation/impaction, colostomy, ileostomy, UC, diverticulitis **Disp:** Soln 290 mg/5 mL (300 mL); 100 mg tabs **SE:** Abd cramps, gas, ↓ BP, resp depression **Interactions:** ↓ Effects *OF* anticoagulants, digoxin, fluoroquinolones, ketoconazole, nitrofurantoin, phenothiazine, tetracyclines **Labs:** ↑ Mg^{2+}, ↓ protein, Ca^{2+}, K^+ **NIPE:** ⊘ Other meds w/in 1–2 h; only for occasional use w/ constipation

Magnesium Hydroxide (Milk of Magnesia) [OTC] [Laxative/Magnesium Salt]
Uses: *Constipation*, hyperacidity, Mg^{2+} replacement **Action:** NS laxative **Dose:** *Adults. Antacid:* 5–15 mL (400 mg/5 mL) or 2–4 mL (311 mg) tabs PO PRN qid *Mg^{2+} replacement:* 2–4 (500 mg) tabs PO qhs or ÷ doses *Laxative:* 30–60 mL (400 mg/5 mL) or 15–30 mL (800 mg/5 mL) or 8 mL (311 mg) tabs PO qhs or ÷ doses *Peds. Antacid & Mg^{2+} replacement:* < 12 y not recommended *Laxative:* < 2 y not recommended *2–5 y.* 5–15 mL (400 mg/5 mL) PO qhs or ÷ doses *6–11 y.* 15–30 mL (400 mg/5 mL) or 7.5–15 mL (800 mg/5 mL) PO qhs or ÷ doses *3–5 y.* 2 mL (311-mg) tabs PO qhs or ÷ doses *6–11 y.* 4 mL (311-mg) tabs PO qhs or ÷ doses **Caution:** [B, +] w/ Neuromuscular Dz or renal impair **CI:** Renal Insuff, intestinal obst, ileostomy/colostomy **Disp:** Chew tabs 311, 500 mg; Liq 400, 800 mg/5 mL (OTC) **SE:** D, Abd cramps **Interactions:** ↓ Effects *OF* chlordiazepoxide, dicumarol, digoxin, indomethacin, INH, quinolones, tetracyclines **Labs:** ↑ Mg^{2+}, ↓ protein, Ca^{2+}, K^+ **NIPE:** ⊘ Other meds w/in 1–2 h; for occasional use in constipation

Magnesium Oxide (Mag-Ox 400, Others) [OTC] [Antacid, Magnesium Supplement/Magnesium Salt]
Uses: *Replace low Mg^{2+} levels* **Action:** Mg^{2+} supl **Dose:** 400–800 mg/d or ÷ w/ food in full glass of H_2O; ↓ w/ renal impair **Caution:** [B, +] w/ neuromuscular Dz & renal impair, w/ bisphosphonates, calcitriol, CCBs, neuromuscular blockers, tetracyclines, quinolones **CI:** UC, diverticulitis, ileostomy/colostomy, heart block **Disp:** Caps 140, 250, 500, 600 mg; tabs 400 mg (OTC) **SE:** D, N **Interactions:** ↓ Effects *OF* chlordiazepoxide, dicumarol, digoxin, indomethacin, INH, quinolones, tetracyclines **Labs:** ↑ Mg^{2+}, ↓ protein, Ca^{2+}, K^+ **NIPE:** ⊘ Other meds w/in 1–2 h

Magnesium Sulfate (Various) [Magnesium Supplement/Magnesium Salt]
Uses: *Replace low Mg^{2+}; preeclampsia, eclampsia, & premature labor, cardiac arrest, AMI arrhythmias, cerebral edema, barium poisoning, Szs, pediatric acute nephritis*; refractory ↓ K^+ & ↓ Ca^{2+} **Action:** Mg^{2+} supl, bowel evacuation, ↓ ACH in nerve terminals, ↓ rate of sinoatrial node firing **Dose:** *Adults.* 3 g PO q6h × 4 PRN *Supl:* 1–2 g IM or IV; repeat PRN *Preeclampsia/premature labor:* 4-g load, then 1–4 g/h IV Inf *ECC 2010:* **VF/pulseless VT arrest w/ torsades de pointes:** 1–2 g IV push (2–4 mL 50% soln) in 10 mL D_5W. If pulse present then 1–2 g in 50–100 mL D_5W over 5–60 min *Peds.* 25–50 mg/kg/dose IM, IV, IO q4–6h for 3–4 doses; repeat PRN; q8–12h in neonates; max 2-g single dose

ECC 2010: **Pulseless VT w/ torsades:** 25–50 mg/kg IV/IO bolus; max dose 2g **Pulseless VT w/ torsades or hypomagnesemia:** 25–50 mg/kg IV/IO over 10–20 min; max dose 2 g **Status asthmaticus:** 25–50 mg/kg IV/IO over 15–30 min **Caution:** [A/C (manufacturer specific), +] w/ neuromuscular Dz interactions; see Magnesium Oxide & Aminoglycosides **CI:** Heart block, renal failure; ↓ dose w/ low urinary output or renal Insuff **Disp:** Premix Inj: 10, 20, 40, 80 mg/mL; Inj 125, 500 mg/mL; oral/topical powder 227, 454, 480, 1810, 1920, 2721 g **SE:** CNS depression, D, flushing, heart block, ↓ BP, vasodilation **Interactions:** ↑ CNS depression *W/* antidepressants, antipsychotics, anxiolytics, barbiturates, hypnotics, narcotics; EtOH; ↑ neuromuscular blockade *W/* aminoglycosides, atracurium, gallamine, pancuronium, tubocurarine, vecuronium **Labs:** ↑ Mg²⁺; ↓ Ca²⁺, K⁺ **NIPE:** Check for absent patellar reflexes; different formulation may contain Al²⁺

Mannitol (Various) [Osmotic Diuretic]   **Uses:** *Cerebral edema, ↑ IOP, renal impair, poisonings, GU irrigation* **Action:** Osmotic diuretic **Dose:** Test **Dose:** 0.2 g/kg/dose IV over 3–5 min; if no diuresis w/in 2 h, D/C *Oliguria:* 50–100 g IV over 90 min; ↑ IOP: 0.5–2 g/kg IV over 30 min *Cerebral edema:* 0.25–1.5 g/kg/dose IV > 30 min **Caution:** [C, ?/M] w/ renal overload, w/ nephrotoxic drugs & Li **CI:** Anuria, dehydration, HF, PE **Disp:** Inj 5%, 10%, 15%, 20%, 25%; GU soln 5% **SE:** May exacerbate CHF, N/V/D, ↓/↑ BP, ↑ HR **Interactions:** ↑ Effects *OF* cardiac glycosides; ↓ effects *OF* barbiturates, imipramine, Li, salicylates **Labs:** ↑/↓ Lytes **NIPE:** Monitor for vol depletion

Maraviroc (Selzentry) [CCR5 Coreceptor Antagonist]   **WARNING:** Possible drug-induced hepatotox **Uses:** *Tx of CCR5-tropic HIV Infxn* **Action:** Antiretroviral, CCR5 coreceptor antagonist **Dose:** 300 mg bid **Caution:** [B, −] w/ concomitant CYP3A inducers/Inhibs **CI:** None **Disp:** Tab 150, 300 mg **SE:** Fever, URI, cough, rash **Interactions:** ↑ effects *W/* CYP3A Inhibits (most protease Inhibs, delavirdine, ketoconazole, itraconazole, clarithromycin, nefazodone, telithromycin) & ↓ effects *W/* CYP3A inducers (efavirenz, rifampin, carbamazepine, phenobarbital, phenytoin); substantial ↓ effect *W/* St. John's wort **Labs:** ↑ LFTs **NIPE:** Swallow whole; monitor for immune reconstitution synd, Infxns, malignancies; ⊘ breastfeeding; ⊘ for < 16 y; take w/ or w/o food; must be given w/ another antiretroviral

Measles, Mumps, & Rubella Vaccine Live [MMR] (M-M-R II)[Live Attenuated Vaccine]   **Uses:** *Vaccination against measles, mumps, & rubella 12 mo & older* **Action:** Active immunization, live attenuated viruses **Dose:** 1 (0.5-mL) SQ Inj, 1st dose 12 mo, 2nd dose 4–6 y, at least 3 mo between doses (28 d if > 12 y), adults born after 1957 unless CI, h/o measles & mumps or documented immunity & childbearing age women w/ rubella immunity documented **Caution:** [C, ?/M] h/o cerebral injury, Szs, family h/o Szs (febrile Rxn), ↓ plt **CI:** Component & gelatin sensitivity, h/o anaphylaxis to neomycin, blood dyscrasia, lymphoma, leukemia, malignant neoplasias affecting BM, immunosupprression, fever, PRG, h/o active untreated TB **Disp:** Inj, single dose **SE:** Fever, febrile Szs (5–12 d after vaccination), Inj site Rxn, rash **Interactions:** ↑ Immunosuppression w/ other immunosuppresents **Labs:** ↓ plt; may interfere w/ tuberculin test **NIPE:** Per FDA, CDC of febrile Sz (2 ×) w/ MMRV vs MMR & varicella separately; preferable to use 2 separate vaccines; allow 1 mo between Inj & any other measles vaccine or 3 mo between any other varicella vaccine; limited availability of MMRV; avoid those who have not been exposed to varicella for 6 wk post-Inj; may contain albumin or trace egg antigen; avoid salicylates for 6 wk postvaccination; avoid PRG for 3 mo following vaccination; do not give w/in 3 mo of transfusion or immune globulin

Measles, Mumps, Rubella, & Varicella Virus Vaccine Live [MMRV] (ProQuad) [Vaccine/Live Attenuated] **Uses:** *Vaccination against measles, mumps, rubella, & varicella **Action:** Active immunization, live attenuated viruses **Dose:** 1 (0.5-mL) vial SQ Inj 12 mo–12 y or for 2nd dose of measles, mumps, & rubella (MMR)*, at least 3 mo between doses (28 d if > 12 y) **Caution:** [C, ?/M] h/o cerebral injury or Szs (febrile Rxn), w/ ↓ plt **CI:** Component & gelatin sensitivity, h/o anaphylaxis to neomycin, blood dyscrasia, lymphoma, leukemia, malignant neoplasias affecting BM, w/ immunosuppression, febrile illness, untreated TB, PRG **Disp:** Inj **SE:** Fever, febrile Szs, (5–12 d after vaccination, Inj site Rxn, rash **LABs:** ↓ plt **NIPE:** Per FDA, CDC ↑ of febrile Sz (2 ×) w/ combo vaccine (MMRV) vs MMR & varicella separately; preferable to use 2 separate vaccines; allow 1 mo between Inj & any other measles vaccine or 3 mo between any other varicella vaccine; limited availability of MMRV; substitute MMR II or Varivax; avoid those who have not been exposed to varicella for 6 wk post-Inj; may contain albumin or trace egg antigen; avoid salicylates

Mecasermin (Increlex, Iplex) [Human IGF-1] **Uses:** *Growth failure in severe primary IGF-1 deficiency or human growth hormone (HGH) antibodies* **Action:** Human IGF-1 (recombinant DNA origin) **Dose:** *Peds.* 0.04–0.08 mg/kg SQ bid; may ↑ by 0.04 mg/kg per dose to 0.12 mg/kg bid; take w/in 20 min of meal d/t insulin-like hypoglycemic effect **Caution:** [C, ?/M] Contains benzyl alcohol **CI:** Closed epiphysis, neoplasia, not for IV **Disp:** Vial 40 mg **SE:** Tonsillar hypertrophy, ↑ AST, ↑ LDH, HA, Inj site Rxn, V, hypoglycemia **Labs:** Rapid dose ↑ may cause hypoglycemia; consider monitoring glucose until dose stable **NIPE:** Initial funduscopic exam & during Tx; limited distribution; rotate Inj site

Mechlorethamine (Mustargen) [Antineoplastic/Alkylating Agent] WARNING: Highly toxic, handle w/ care, limit use to experienced physicians; avoid exposure during PRG; vesicant **Uses:** *Hodgkin Dz (stages III, IV), cutaneous T-cell lymphoma (mycosis fungoides), lung CA, CML, malignant PEs, CLL, polycythemia vera*, psoriasis **Action:** Alkylating agent, nitrogen analogue of sulfur mustard **Dose:** Per protocol: 0.4 mg/kg single dose or 0.1 mg/kg/d for 4 d, repeat at 4–6-wk intervals; 6 mg/m² IV on d 1 & 8 of 28-d cycle *Intracavitary* 0.2–0.4 mg/kg × 1, may repeat PRN *Topical:* 0.01–0.02% soln, lotion, oint **Caution:** [D, ?/–] **CI:** PRG, known infect Dz, severe myelosuppression **Disp:** Inj 10 mg; topical soln, lotion, oint **SE:** ↓ BM, thrombosis, thrombophlebitis at site; tissue damage w/ extrav (Na thiosulfate used topically to Rx); N/V/D, skin rash/allergic dermatitis w/ contact, amenorrhea, sterility (esp in men), secondary leukemia if treated for Hodgkin Dz, chromosomal alterations, hepatotox, peripheral neuropathy **Interactions:** ↑ Risk of blood dyscrasias *W/* amphotericin B; ↑ risk of bleeding *W/* anticoagulants, NSAIDs, plt Inhibs, salicylates; ↑ myelosuppression *W/* antineoplastic drugs, radiation therapy; ↓ effects *OF* live virus vaccines **Labs:** ↑ Serum uric acid **NIPE:** Highly volatile & emetogenic; give w/in 30–60 min of prep; ↑ fluids to 2–3 L/d; ⊘ PRG, breast-feeding, vaccines, exposure to Infxn; ↑ risk of tinnitus

Meclizine (Antivert) (Bonine, Dramamine [OTC]) [Antiemetic/ Antivertigo/Anticholinergic] Uses: *Motion sickness, vertigo* **Action:** Antiemetic, anticholinergic, & antihistaminic properties **Dose:** *Adults & Peds > 12 y. Motion sickness:* 12.5–25 mg PO 1 h before travel, repeat PRN q12–24h *Vertigo:* 25–100 mg/d ÷ doses **Caution:** [B, ?/–] NAG, BPH, BOO, elderly, asthma **Disp:** Tabs 12.5, 25, 50 mg; chew tabs 25 mg; caps 25, 30 mg (OTC) **SE:** Drowsiness, xerostomia, blurred vision, thickens bronchial secretions **Interactions:** ↑ Sedation *W/* antihistamines, CNS depressants, neuroleptics, EtOH; ↑ anticholinergic effects *W/* anticholinergics, atropine, disopyramide, haloperidol, phenothiazine, quinidine **NIPE:** Use prophylactically; ↑ risk of heat exhaustion

Medroxyprogesterone (Provera, Depo Provera, Depo-Sub Q Provera) [Antineoplastic/Progestin] WARNING: Do not use in the prevention of CV Dz or dementia; ↑ risk MI, stroke, breast CA, PE, & DVT in postmenopausal women (50–79 y). ↑ Dementia risk in postmenopausal women (≥ 65 y). Risk of sig bone loss Uses: *Contraception; secondary amenorrhea; endometrial CA ↓ endometrial hyperplasia* AUB caused by hormonal imbalance **Action:** Progestin supl **Dose:** *Contraception:* 150 mg IM q3mo depo or 104 mg SQ q3mo (depo SQ) *Secondary amenorrhea:* 5–10 mg/d PO for 5–10 d *AUB:* 5–10 mg/d PO for 5–10 d beginning on the 16th or 21st d of menstrual cycle *Endometrial CA:* 400–1000 mg/wk IM *Endometrial hyperplasia:* 5–10 mg/d × 12–14 d on d 1 or 16 of cycle; ↓ in hepatic Insuff **Caution:** *Provera* [X, –] *Depo Provera* [X, +] **CI:** Thrombophlebitis/embolic disorders, cerebral apoplexy, CA breast/genital organs, undiagnosed Vag bleeding, missed abortion, PRG, as a diagnostic test for PRG **Disp:** *Provera* tabs 2.5, 5, 10 mg; depot Inj 150, 400 mg/mL; depo SQ Inj 104 mg/ 10.65 mL **SE:** Breakthrough bleeding, spotting, altered menstrual flow, breast tenderness, galactorrhea, depression, insomnia, jaundice, N, wgt gain, acne, hirsutism, vision changes **Interactions:** ↓ Effects *W/* aminoglutethimide, phenytoin, carbamazepine, phenobarbital, rifampin, rifabutin **Labs:** ↑ LFTs **NIPE:** Sunlight exposure may cause melasma; if GI upset take w/ food; perform breast exam & Pap smear before contraceptive therapy; obtain PRG test if last Inj > 3 mo

Megestrol Acetate (Megace, Megace-ES) [Antineoplastic/Progestin] Uses: *Breast/endometrial CAs; appetite stimulant in cachexia (CA & HIV)* **Action:** Hormone; antileuteinizing; progesterone analogue **Dose:** *CA:* 40–320 mg/d PO in ÷ doses *Appetite* 800 mg/d PO ÷ dose or *Megace ES* 625 mg/d **Caution:**

[X, −] Thromboembolism; handle w/ care **CI:** PRG **Disp:** Tabs 20, 40 mg; susp 40 mg/mL, *Megace ES* 125 mg/mL **SE:** DVT, edema, menstrual bleeding, photosensitivity, N/V/D, HA, mastodynia, insomnia, rash, ↑ BP, CP, palpitations **Interactions:** ↑ Effects *OF* warfarin **Labs:** ↑ CA, glucose; ↓ BM **NIPE:** ↑ Risk of photosensitivity—use sunblock; do not D/C abruptly; Megace ES not equivalent to others mg/mg; Megace ES approved only for anorexia

Meloxicam (Mobic) [Analgesic/Anti-Inflammatory/NSAIDs]
WARNING: May ↑ risk of CV events & GI bleeding; CI in post-op CABG **Uses:** *OA, RA, JRA* **Action:** NSAID w/ ↑ COX-2 activity **Dose:** *Adults.* 7.5–15 mg/d PO *Peds > 2 y.* 0.125 mg/kg/d, max 7.5 mg; ↓ in renal Insuff; take w/ food **Caution:** [C, D (3rd tri) ?/−] w/ Severe renal Insuff, CHF, ACE Inhib, diuretics, Li²⁺, MTX, warfarin **CI:** Peptic ulcer, NSAID, or ASA sensitivity, PRG, post-op CABG **Disp:** Tabs 7.5, 15 mg; susp. 7.5 mg/5 mL **SE:** HA, dizziness, GI upset, GI bleeding, edema, ↑ BP, renal impair, rash (SJS) **Interactions:** ↑ Effects *OF* ASA, anticoagulants, corticosteroids, Li, NSAIDs, EtOH, tobacco; ↓ effects *W/* cholestyramine; ↓ effects *OF* antihypertensives **Labs:** ↑ LFTs, BUN, Cr; ↓ HMG, WBCs, plt **NIPE:** Take w/ food, may take several d for full effect; ↑ risk of GI bleed w/ concurrent use of EtOH & tobacco

Melphalan [L-PAM] (Alkeran) [Antineoplastic/Alkylating Agent]
WARNING: Administer under the supervision of a qualified physician experienced in the use of chemotherapy; severe BM depression, leukemogenic, & mutagenic **Uses:** *Multiple myeloma, ovarian CAs*, breast & testicular CA, melanoma; allogenic & ABMT (high dose), neuroblastoma, rhabdomyosarcoma **Action:** Alkylating agent, nitrogen mustard **Dose:** *Adults. Multiple myeloma:* 16 mg/m² IV q2wk × 4 doses then at 4-wk intervals after tox resolves; w/ renal impair ↓ IV dose 50% or 6 mg PO qd × 2–3 wk, then D/C up to 4 wk, follow counts then 2 mg qd *Ovarian CA:* 0.2 mg/kg qd × 5 d, repeat q4–5wk based on counts **Peds.** *Off-label rhabdomyosarcoma:* 10–35 mg/m²/dose IV q21–28d. *w/ BMT for neuroblastoma:* 100–220 mg/m²/dose IV × 1 or ÷ 2–5 daily doses, Inf over 60 min; ↓ in renal Insuff **Caution:** [D, ?/−] w/ cisplatin, digitalis, live vaccines **CI:** Allergy or resistance **Disp:** Tabs 2 mg; Inj 50 mg **SE:** N/V, secondary malignancy, AF, ↓ LVEF, ↓ BM, secondary leukemia, alopecia, dermatitis, stomatitis, pulm fibrosis; rare allergic Rxns **Interactions:** ↑ Risk of nephrotox *W/* cisplatin, cyclosporine; ↓ effects *W/* cimetidine, interferon-α **Labs:** ↓ HMG, RBCs, WBCs, plt; false(+) direct Coombs test **NIPE:** ◊ Fluids, ⊘ PRG, breast-feeding; take PO on empty stomach

Memantine (Namenda, Namenda XR) [N-Methyl-ᴅ-Aspartate (NMDA) Receptor Antagonist]
Uses: *Mod/severe Alzheimer Dz*, mild–mod vascular dementia, mild cognitive impair **Actions:** NMDA receptor antagonist **Dose:** *Namenda* Target 20 mg/d, start 5 mg/d, ↑ to 20 mg/d, wait > 1 wk before ↑ dose; use ÷ doses if > 5 mg/d *Vascular dementia:* 10 mg PO bid *Namenda XR (Alzheimer)* 7 mg inital 1 × qd, ↑ each wk to maint 28 mg/d × 1; ↓ to 14 mg w/ severe renal impair **Caution:** [B, ?/−] Hepatic/mod renal impair; Sx disorders

Disp: *Namenda* Tabs 5, 10 mg, combo pack: 5 mg × 28 + 10 mg × 21; soln 2 mg/mL. *Namenda XR 7,14,21,28 mg* **CI:** Component hypersensitivity **SE:** Dizziness, HA, D **Interactions:** ↑ Effects *W/* amantadine, carbonic anhydrase Inhibits, dextromethorphan, ketamine, NaHCO₃ ; ↑ effects *W/* any drug, herb, food that alkalinizes urine **Labs:** Monitor BUN, SCr NIPE: Take w/o regard to food; EtOH ↑ adverse effects & ↓ effectiveness; renal clearance ↓ by alkaline urine (↓ 80% at pH 8)

Meningococcal Conjugate Vaccine [Quadrivalent, MCV4] (Menactra, Menveo) [Vaccine/Live] **Uses:** *Immunize against *N meningitidis* (meningococcus) high risk 2–10 & 19–55 y & everyone 11–18* high risk (college freshman, military recruits, travel to endemic areas, terminal complement deficiencies, asplenia); if given age 11–12, give booster at 16, should have booster w/in 5 y of college freshman **Action:** Active immunization; *N meningitidis* A, C, Y, W-135 polysaccharide conjugated to diphtheria toxoid (*Menactra*) or lyophilized conjugate component (*Menveo*) **Dose:** *Adults.* *18–55 y* *Peds* > 2 y. 0.5 mL IM x 1 **Caution:** [C, ?/–] w/ Immunosuppression (↓ response) & bleeding disorders **CI:** Allergy to class/diphtheria toxoid/compound/latex; Hx Guillain-Barré **Disp:** Inj **SE:** Inj site Rxns, HA, N/V/D, anorexia, fatigue, irritability, arthralgia, Guillain-Barré **Interactions:** ↓ Effects *W/* Ig if administer w/in 1 mo NIPE: IM only, reported accidental SQ ; keep epi available for Rxns; use polysaccharide *Menomune* (MPSV4) if > 55 y; do not confuse w/ *Menactra,Menveo*; ACIP rec: MCV4 for 2–55 y, ↑ local Rxn compared to *Menomune* (MPSV4) but ↑ Ab titers; peds 2–10, Ab levels ↓ 3 y w/ MPSV4, revaccinate in 2–3 y, use MCV4 for revaccination

Meningococcal Polysaccharide Vaccine [MPSV4] (Menomune A/C/Y/W-135) [Immunization] **Uses:** *Immunize against *N meningitidis* (meningococcus)* in high risk (college freshman, military recruits, travel to endemic areas, terminal complement deficiencies, asplenia) **Action:** Active immunization **Dose:** *Adults & Peds* > 2 y. 0.5 mL SQ only; may repeat 3–5 y if high risk; repeat in 2–3 y if 1st dose given 2–4 y **Caution:** [C, ?/–] If immunocompromised (↓ response) **CI:** Thimerosal/latex sensitivity; w/ pertussis or typhoid vaccine, < 2 y **Disp:** Inj **SE:** *Peds 2–10 y:* Inj site Rxns, drowsiness, irritability *11–55 y:* Inj site Rxns, HA, fatigue, malaise, fever, D NIPE: Keep epi (1:1000) available for Rxns. Recommended > 55 y, but also alternative to MCV4 in 2–55 y if no MCV4 available (MCV4 is preferred). Active against serotypes A, C, Y, & W-135 but not group B; Ab levels ↓ 3 y, high-risk revaccination q3–5 y (use MCV4)

Meperidine (Demerol, Meperitab) [C–II] [Opioid Analgesic] **Uses:** *Mod–severe pain*, post-op shivering, rigors form amphotericin B **Action:** Narcotic analgesic **Dose:** *Adults.* 50–150 mg PO or IV/IM/SQ q3–4h PRN *Peds.*1–1.5 mg/kg/dose PO or IM/SQ q3–4h PRN, up to 100 mg/dose; ↓ in elderly/hepatic impair, avoid in renal impair **Caution:** [C/D (prolonged use or high dose at term), +] ↓ Sz threshold, adrenal Insuff, head injury, ↑ ICP, hepatic impair, not recommended in sickle cell Dz **CI:** w/ MAOIs, renal failure, PRG **Disp:** Tabs 50, 100 mg; syrup/ soln 50 mg/5 mL; Inj 10, 25, 50, 75, 100 mg/mL **SE:** Resp/CNS depression, Szs, sedation, constipation, ↓ BP, rash N/V, biliary & urethral spasms, dyspnea **Interactions:** ↑ Effects W/ antihistamines, barbiturates, cimetidine, MAOIs, neuroleptics, selegiline, TCAs, St. John's wort, EtOH; ↑ effects OF INH; ↓ effects W/ phenytoin **Labs:** ↑ Serum amylase, lipase **NIPE:** Analgesic effects potentiated w/ hydroxyzine; 75 mg IM = 10 mg morphine IM; not best in elderly; do not use oral for acute pain; not recommended for repetitive use in ICU setting

Meprobamate (Various) [C-IV] [Antianxiety]
Uses: *Short-term relief of anxiety* muscle spasm, TMJ relief Action: Mild tranquilizer; antianxiety Dose: Adults. 400 mg PO tid–qid, max 2400 mg/d Peds 6–12 y. 100–200 mg PO bid–tid; ↓ in renal/liver impair Caution: [D, +/–] Elderly, Sz Dz CI: NAG, porphyria, PRG Disp: Tabs 200, 400 mg SE: Drowsiness, syncope, tachycardia, edema, rash (SJS), N/V/D, agranulocytosis Interactions: ↑ Effects W/ antihistamines, barbiturates, CNS depressants, narcotics, EtOH; Labs: ↓ WBC—monitor NIPE: Do not abruptly D/C

Mercaptopurine [6-MP] (Purinethol) [Antineoplastic/Antimetabolite]
Uses: *ALL* 2nd-line Rx for CML & NHL, maint ALL in children, immunosuppressant w/ autoimmune Dzs (Crohn Dz, UC) Action: Antimetabolite, mimics hypoxanthine Dose: Adults. ALL induction: 1.5–2.5 mg/kg/d Maint: 80–100 mg/m²/d or 2.5–5 mg/kg/d; w/ allopurinol use 67–75% ↓ dose of 6-MP (interference w/ xanthine oxidase metabolism) Peds. ALL induction: 2.5–5 mg/kg/d PO or 70–100 mg/m²/d Maint: 1.5–2.5 mg/kg/d PO or 50–75 mg/m²/d qd; ↓ w/ renal/hepatic Insuff; take on empty stomach Caution: [D, ?] w/ allopurinol, immunosuppression, TMP–SMX, warfarin, salicylates CI: Prior resistance, severe hepatic Dz, BM suppression, PRG Disp: Tabs 50 mg SE: Mild hematotox, mucositis, stomatitis, D, rash, fever, eosinophilia, jaundice, hep, hyperuricemia, hyperpigmentation, alopecia Interactions: ↑ Effects W/ allopurinol; ↑ risk of BM suppression W/ TMP–SMX; ↓ effects OF warfarin Labs: False ↑ serum glucose, uric acid; ↑ LFTs; ↓ HMG, RBCs, WBC, plt NIPE: ↑ Fluid intake to 2–3 L/d, may take 4+ wk for improvement; handle properly; limit use to experienced healthcare providers; for ALL, evening dosing may ↓ risk of relapse; low emetogenicity

Meropenem (Merrem) [Antibiotic/Carbapenem]
Uses: *Intra-Abd Infxns, bacterial meningitis, skin Infxn* Action: Carbapenem; ↓ cell wall synth Spectrum: Excellent gram(+) (except MRSA, MRSE, & E faecium) excellent gram(−) including extended-spectrum β-lactamase producers; good anaerobic Dose: Adults. Abd Infxn: 1–2 g IV q8h Skin Infxn: 50 mg IV q8h Meningitis: 2 g IV q8h. Peds = 3 mo, < 50 kg. Abd Infxn: 20 mg/kg IV q8h Skin Infxn: 20 mg/kg IV q8h Meningitis: 40 mg/kg IV q8h Peds > 50 kg. Use adult dose; max 2 g IV q8h; ↓ in renal Insuff (see package insert) Caution: [B, ?] w/ Probenecid, VPA CI: β-Lactam sensitivity Disp: Inj 1 g, 500 mg SE: Less Sz potential than imipenem; C difficile enterocolitis, D, ↓ plt Interactions: ↑ Effects W/ probenecid Labs: ↑ LFTs, BUN, Cr, eosinophils ↓ HMG, Hct, WBCs, plt NIPE: Monitor for super Infxn; overuse ↑ bacterial resistance

Mesalamine (Asacol, Canasa, Lialda, Pentasa, Rowasa) [Anti-Inflammatory/Salicylate] Uses: *Rectal: Mild–mod distal UC, proctosigmoiditis, proctitis; oral: Tx/maint of mild–mod UC* **Action:** 5-ASA derivative, may inhibit prostaglandins, may ↓ leukotrienes & TNF-α **Dose:** *Rectal:* 60 mL qhs, retain 8 h (enema), 500 mg bid–tid or 1000 mg qhs (supp) *PO:* Caps: 1 g PO qid Tabs: 1.6–2.4 g/d ÷ doses (tid–qid); DR 2.4–4.8 g PO daily 8 wk max, do not cut/crush/chew w/ food; ↓ initial dose in elderly **Caution:** [B, M] w/ digitalis, PUD, pyloric stenosis, renal Insuff, elderly **CI:** Salicylate sensitivity **Disp:** Tabs ER (*Asacol*) 400, 800 mg; ER caps (*Pentasa*) 250, 500 mg; DR tab (*Lialda*) 1.2 g; supp 500, (*Canasa*) 1000 mg; (*Rowasa*) rectal susp 4 g/60 mL **SE:** Yellow-brown urine, HA, malaise, Abd pain, flatulence, rash, pancreatitis, pericarditis, dizziness, rectal pain, hair loss, intolerance synd (bloody D) **Interactions:** ↓ Effect *OF* digoxin **Labs:** ✓ CBC, Cr, BUN **NIPE:** May discolor urine yellow-brown; retain rectally 1–3 h; Sx may ↑ when starting

Mesna (Mesnex) [Uroprotectant/Antidote] Uses: *Prevent hemorrhagic cystitis d/t ifosfamide or cyclophosphamide* **Action:** Antidote, reacts w/ acrolein & other metabolites to form stable compounds **Dose:** Per protocol; dose as % of ifosfamide or cyclophosphamide dose *IV bolus:* 20% (eg, 10–12 mg/kg) IV at 0, 4, & 8 h, then 40% at 0, 1, 4, & 7 h *IV Inf:* 20% prechemotherapy, 50–100% w/ chemotherapy, then 25–50% for 12 h following chemotherapy *Oral:* 100% ifosfamide dose given as 20% IV at 0 h, then 40% PO at 4 & 8 h; if PO dose vomited repeat or give dose IV; mix PO w/ juice **Caution:** [B, ?/–] **CI:** Thiol sensitivity **Disp:** Inj 100 mg/mL; tabs 400 mg **SE:** ↓ BP, ↑ HR, ↑ RR allergic Rxns, HA, GI upset, taste perversion **Labs:** ↑ LFTs, ↓ plt **NIPE:** Hydration helps ↓ hemorrhagic cystitis; higher dose for BMT; IV contains benzyl alcohol

Metaproterenol (Alupent, Metaprel) [Bronchodilator/Beta-Adrenergic Agonist] Uses: *Asthma & reversible bronchospasm, COPD* **Action:** Sympathomimetic bronchodilator **Dose:** *Adults. Nebulized:* 5% 2.5 mL q4–6h or PRN *MDI:* 1–3 Inh q3–4h, 12 Inh max/24 h; wait 2 min between Inh *PO:* 20 mg q6–8h *Peds = 12 y. MDI:* 2–3 Inh q3–4h, 12 Inh/d max *Nebulizer:* 2.5 mL (soln 0.4, 0.6%) tid–qid, up to q4h *> 9 y or > 27 kg.* 20 mg PO tid–qid *6–9 y or < 27 kg.* 10 mg PO tid–qid; ↓ in elderly **Caution:** [C, ?/–] w/ MAOI, TCA, sympathomimetics; avoid w/ BBs **CI:** Tachycardia, other arrhythmias **Disp:** Aerosol 0.65 mg/Inh; soln for Inh 0.4%, 0.6%; tabs 10, 20 mg; syrup 10 mg/5 mL **SE:** Nervousness, tremor, tachycardia, HTN, ↑ IOP **Interactions:** ↑ Effects *W/* sympathomimetic drugs, xanthines; ↑ risk of arrhythmias *W/* cardiac glycosides, halothane, levodopa, theophylline, thyroid hormones; ↑ HTN *W/* MAOIs; ↓ effects *W/* BBs **Labs:** ↓ Glucose, ↓ K+ **NIPE:** Separate additional aerosol use by 5 min; fewer β_1 effects than isoproterenol & longer acting, but not a 1st-line β-agonist. Use w/ face mask < 4 y; oral ↑ ADR; contains ozone-depleting CFCs; will be gradually removed from US market

Metaxalone (Skelaxin) [Skeletal Muscle Relaxant] Uses: *Painful musculoskeletal conditions* **Action:** Centrally acting skeletal muscle relaxant

Dose: 800 mg PO tid–qid **Caution:** [C, ?/–] w/ Elderly, EtOH & CNS depression, anemia **CI:** Severe hepatic/renal impair; drug-induced, hemolytic, or other anemias **Disp:** Tabs 800 mg **SE:** N/V, HA, drowsiness, hep **Interactions:** ↑ Sedating effects *W/* CNS depressants, antihistamines, opioid analgesics, sedative/hypnotics, chamomile, kava kava, valerian, EtOH **Labs:** False(+) urine glucose using Benedict test **NIPE:** Monitor elderly for sedation & weakness

Metformin (Glucophage, Glucophage XR) [Hypoglycemic/Biguanide] **WARNING:** Associated w/ lactic acidosis, risk ↑ w/ sepsis, dehydration, renal/hepatic impair, ↑ alcohol, acute CHF; Sxs include myalgias, malaise, resp distress, Abd pain, somnolence; Labs: ↓ pH, ↑ anion gap, ↑ blood lactate; D/C stat & hospitalize if suspected **Uses:** *Type 2 DM*, polycystic ovary synd (PCOS) HIV lipodystrophy **Action:** Biguanide; ↓ hepatic glucose production & intestinal absorption of glucose; ↑ insulin sensitivity **Dose:** *Adults. Initial:* 500 mg PO bid; or 850 mg daily, titrate 1–2-wk intervals, may ↑ to 2550 mg/d max; take w/ AM & PM meals; can convert total daily dose to daily dose of XR *Peds 10–16 y.* 500 mg PO bid, ↑ 500 mg/wk to 2000 mg/d max in ÷ doses; do not use XR formulation in peds **Caution:** [B, +/–] Avoid EtOH; hold dose before & 48 h after ionic contrast; hepatic impair, renal impair **CI:** SCr > 1.4 mg/dL in females or > 1.5 mg/dL in males; hypoxemic conditions (eg, acute CHF/sepsis); metabolic acidosis **Disp:** Tabs 500, 850, 1000 mg; XR tabs 500, 750, 1000 mg; soln 100 mg/mL **SE:** Anorexia, N/V/D, flatulence, weakness, myalgia, rash **Interactions:** ↑ Effects *W/* amiloride, cimetidine, digoxin, furosemide, MAOIs, morphine, procainamide, quinidine, quinine, ranitidine, triamterene, TMP, vancomycin; ↓ effects *W/* corticosteroids, CCBs, diuretics, estrogens, INH, OCPs, phenothiazine, phenytoin, sympathomimetics, thyroid drugs, tobacco **Labs:** Monitor LFTs, BUN/Cr, serum vit B_{12} **NIPE:** Take w/ food; avoid dehydration, EtOH, before surgery

Methadone (Dolophine, Methadose) [C-II] [Opioid Analgesic] **WARNING:** Deaths reported during initiation & conversion of pain pts to methadone Rx from Rx w/ other opioids. Resp depression & QT prolongation, arrhythmias observed. Only dispensed by certified opioid Tx programs for addiction. Analgesic use must outweigh risks **Uses:** *Severe pain not responsive to nonnarcotics; detox w/ maint of narcotic addiction* **Action:** Narcotic analgesic **Dose:** *Adults.* 2.5–10 mg IM/IV/SQ q8–12h or 5–15 mg PO q8h; titrate as needed; see package insert for conversion from other opioids *Peds.* (Not FDA approved) 0.1 mg/kg q4–12h IV; ↑ slowly to avoid resp depression; ↓ in renal impair **Caution:** [C, +] Avoid w/ severe liver Dz **CI:** Resp depression, acute asthma, ileus **Disp:** Tabs 5, 10 mg; tabs dispersible 40 mg; PO soln 5, 10 mg/5 mL; PO conc 10 mg/mL; Inj 10 mg/mL **SE:** Resp depression, sedation, constipation, urinary retention, ↑ QT interval, arrhythmias, ↓ HR, syncope **Interactions:** ↑ Effects *W/* cimetidine, CNS depressants, protease Inhibits, EtOH; ↑ effects *OF* anticoagulants, EtOH, antihistamines, barbiturates, glutethimide, methocarbamol; ↓ effects *W/* carbamazepine, nelfinavir, phenobarbital, phenytoin, primidone, rifampin, ritonavir **Labs:** ↓ K+,

↓ Mg^{2+} **NIPE:** *Parenteral:* Oral 1:2; equianalgesic w/ parenteral morphine; longer 1/2-life; resp depression occurs later & lasts longer than analgesic effect; use w/ caution to avoid iatrogenic OD

Methenamine Hippurate (Hiprex) Methenamine Mandelate (UROQUID-Acid No. 2) [Urinary Anti-Infective] Uses: *Suppress recurrent UTI long term. Use only after Infxn cleared by antibiotics* **Action:** Converted to formaldehyde & ammonia in acidic urine; nonspecific bactericidal action **Dose:** *Adults. Hippurate:* 1 g PO bid *Mandelate:* Initial 1 g qid PO pc & hs, maint 1–2 g/d *Peds 6–12 y. Hippurate:* 0.5–1 g PO bid PO ÷ bid *> 2 y. Mandelate:* 50–75 mg/kg/d PO ÷ qid; take w/ food, ascorbic acid w/ hydration **Caution:** [C, +] **CI:** Renal Insuff, severe hepatic Dz, & severe dehydration **Disp:** *Methenamine hippurate* (Hiprex, Urex): Tabs 1 g *Methenamine mandelate:* 500 mg, 1 g EC tabs **SE:** Rash, GI upset, dysuria, super Infxn w/ prolonged use, *C difficile*–associated D **Interactions:** ↓ Effects *W/* acetazolamide, antacids **Labs:** ↑ LFTs **NIPE:** ↑ Fluids to 2–3 L/d; take w/ food; use w/ sulfonamides may precipitate in urine; hippurate not indicated in peds < 6 y; not for pts w/ indwelling catheters as dwell time in bladder required for action

Methimazole (Tapazole) [Antithyroid Agent] Uses: *Hyperthyroidism, thyrotoxicosis*, prep for thyroid surgery or radiation **Action:** Blocks T_3 & T_4 formation, but does not inactivate circulating T_3, T_4 **Dose:** *Adults. Initial based on severity:* 15–60 mg/d PO q8h *Maint:* 5–15 mg PO daily *Peds.* Initial: 0.4–0.7 mg/kg/24 h PO q8h *Maint:* 1/3–2/3 of initial dose PO daily; take w/ food **Caution:** [D, –] w/ other meds **CI:** Breast-feeding **Disp:** Tabs 5, 10, 20 mg **SE:** GI upset, dizziness, blood dyscrasias, dermatitis, fever, hepatic Rxns, lupus-like synd **Interactions:** ↑ Effects *OF* digitalis glycosides, metoprolol, propranolol; ↓ effects *OF* anticoagulants, theophylline; ↓ effects *W/* amiodarone **Labs:** ↑ LFTs, PT; follow clinically & w/ TFT, CBC w/ diff **NIPE:** Take w/ food

Methocarbamol (Robaxin) [Skeletal Muscle Relaxant/Centrally Acting] Uses: *Relief of discomfort associated w/ painful musculoskeletal conditions* **Action:** Centrally acting skeletal muscle relaxant **Dose:** *Adults & Peds > 16 y.* 1.5 g PO qid for 2–3 d, then 1 g PO qid maint *Tetanus:* 1–2 g IV q6h × 3 d, then use PO *< 16 y.* 15 mg/kg/dose or 500 mg/m² IV, may repeat PRN (tetanus only), max 1.8 g/m²/d × 3 d **Caution:** Sz disorders [C, +] **CI:** MyG, renal impair w/ IV **Disp:** Tabs 500, 750 mg; Inj 100 mg/mL **SE:** Can discolor urine, lightheadedness, drowsiness, GI upset, ↓ HR, ↓ BP **Interactions:** ↑ Effects *W/* CNS depressant, EtOH **Labs:** ↑ Urine 5-HIAA **NIPE:** Monitor for blurred vision, orthostatic hypotension; tabs can be crushed & added to NG; do not operate heavy machinery

Methotrexate (Rheumatrex Dose Pack, Trexall) [Antineoplastic, Antirheumatic (DMARDs), Immunosuppressant/Antimetabolite] **WARNING:** Administration only by experienced healthcare provider; do not use in women of childbearing age unless absolutely necessary (teratogenic); impaired elimination w/ impaired renal Fxn, ascites, PE; severe ↓ BM w/ NSAIDs; hepatotox, occasionally fatal; can induce life-threatening pneumonitis; D & ulcerative stomatitis require D/C; lymphoma risk; may cause tumor lysis synd; can cause severe skin Rxn, opportunistic Infxns; w/ RT can ↑ tissue necrosis risk. Preservatives make this agent unsuitable for IT or higher dose use **Uses:** *ALL, AML, leukemic meningitis, trophoblastic tumors (choriocarcinoma, hydatidiform mole), breast, lung, head, & neck CAs, Burkitt lymphoma, mycosis fungoides, osteosarcoma, Hodgkin Dz & NHL, psoriasis; RA, JRA, SLE*, chronic Dz **Action:** ↓ Dihydrofolate reductase-mediated product of tetrahydrofolate, causes ↓ DNA synth **Dose:** *Adults. CA:* Per protocol *RA:* 7.5 mg/wk PO 1/wk 1 or 2.5 mg q12h PO for 3 doses/wk *Psoriasis:* 2.5–5 mg PO q12h × 3 d/wk or 10–25 mg PO/IM qwk *Chronic:* 15–25 mg IM/SQ qwk, then 15 mg/wk **Peds.** 10 mg/m² PO/IM qwk, then 5–14 mg/m² × 1 or as 3 ÷ doses 12 h apart; ↓ elderly, w/ renal/hepatic impair **Caution:** [D, –] w/ other nephro-/hepatotox meds, multiple interactions; w/ Sz, profound ↓ BM other than CA related **CI:** Severe renal/hepatic impair, PRG/lactation **Disp:** Dose pack 2.5 mg in 8, 12, 16, 20, or 24 doses; tabs 2.5, 5, 7.5, 10, 15 mg; Inj 25 mg/mL; Inj powder 20 mg, 1 g **SE:** ↓ BM, N/V/D, anorexia, mucositis, hepatotox (transient & reversible; may progress to atrophy, necrosis, fibrosis, cirrhosis), rashes, dizziness, malaise, blurred vision, alopecia, photosensitivity, renal failure, pneumonitis; rare pulm fibrosis; chemical arachnoiditis & HA w/ IT delivery **Notes:** *Systemic levels: Therapeutic:* > 0.01 mcmol *Toxic:* > 10 mcmol over 24 h **Interactions:** ↑ Effects *W/* chloramphenicol, cyclosporine, etretinate, NSAIDs, phenylbutazone, phenytoin, PCN, probenecid, salicylates, sulfonamides, sulfonylureas, EtOH; ↑ effects *OF* cyclosporine, tetracycline, theophylline; ↑ effects *W/* antimalarials, aminoglycosides, binding resins, cholestyramine, folic acid; ↓ effects *OF* digoxin **Labs:** Monitor CBC, LFTs, Cr, MTX levels & CXR **NIPE:** "High dose" > 500 mg/m² requires leucovorin rescue to ↓ tox; w/ IT, use preservative-free/alcohol-free soln; ↑ risk of photosensitivity—use sunscreen, ↑ fluids 2–3 L/d

Methyldopa (Aldomet) [Antihypertensive/Centrally Acting Antiadrenergic]

Uses: *HTN* **Action:** Centrally acting antihypertensive, ↓ sympathetic outflow **Dose:** *Adults.* 250–500 mg PO bid–tid (max 2–3 g/d) or 250 mg–1 g IV q6–8h *Peds neonates.* 2.5–5 mg/kg PO/IV q8h *Other peds.* 10 mg/kg/24 h PO in 2–3 ÷ doses or 5–10 mg/kg/dose IV q6–8h to max 65 mg/kg/24 h; ↓ in renal Insuff/elderly **Caution:** [B(PO), C(IV), +] **CI:** Liver Dz, w/ MAOIs, bisulfate allergy **Disp:** Tabs 250, 500 mg; Inj 50 mg/mL **SE:** Discolors urine; initial transient sedation/drowsiness, edema, hemolytic anemia, hepatic disorders, fevers, nightmares **Interactions:** ↑ Effects *W/* anesthetics, diuretics, levodopa, Li, methotrimeprazine, thioxanthenes, vasodilators, verapamil; ↑ effects *OF* haloperidol, Li, tolbutamide; ↓ effects *W/* amphetamines, Fe, phenothiazine, TCAs; ↓ effects *OF* ephedrine **Labs:** ↑ BUN, Cr; ↓ LFTs, HMG, RBC, WBC, plt; false(+) Coombs test **NIPE:** Tolerance may occur

Methylergonovine (Methergine) [Oxytocic/Ergot Alkaloid]

Uses: *Postpartum bleeding (atony, hemorrhage)* **Action:** Ergotamine derivative, rapid

& sustained uterotonic effect **Dose:** 0.2 mg IM after anterior shoulder delivery or puerperium, may repeat in 2–4-h intervals or 0.2–0.4 mg PO q6–12h for 2–7 d **Caution:** [C, ?] w/ sepsis, obliterative vascular Dz, hepatic/renal impair, w/ CYP3A4 Inhibs (Table 10) **CI:** HTN, PRG, toxemia **Dose:** 0.2 mg/mL; tabs 0.2 mg **SE:** HTN, N/V, CP, ↓ BP, Sz **Interactions:** ↑ Vasoconstriction *W/* ergot alkaloids, sympathomimetics, tobacco **NIPE:** ⊘ Smoking; give IV only if absolutely necessary over > 1 min w/ BP monitoring

Methylnaltrexone Bromide (Relistor) [Opioid Antagonist] Uses: *Opioid-induced constipation in pt w/ advanced illness such as CA* **Action:** Peripheral opioid antagonist **Dose: Adults.** *Wgt based < 38 kg/> 114 kg:* 0.15 mg/kg SQ *38–61 kg:* 8 mg SQ *62–114 kg:* 12 mg SQ, dose qod PRN, max 1 dose q24hr **Caution:** [B, NR] w/ CrCl < 30 mL/min ↓ dose 50% **Disp:** Inj 12 mg/0.6 mL **SE:** N/D, Abd pain, dizziness **NIPE:** Does not change opioid analgesic effects or induce withdrawal; not recommended for children

Methylphenidate, Oral (Concerta, Metadate CD, Methylin Ritalin, Ritalin LA, Ritalin SR, Others) [CII] [CNS Stimulant/Piperidine Derivative] **WARNING:** w/ Hx of drug or alcohol dependence, avoid abrupt D/C; chronic use can lead to dependence or psychotic behavior; observe closely during withdrawal of drug **Uses:** *ADHD, narcolepsy*, depression **Action:** CNS stimulant, blocks reuptake of norepinephrine & DA **Dose: Adults.** *Narcolepsy:* 10 mg PO 2–3 × /d, 60 mg/d max *Depression:* 2.5 mg qAM; ↑ slowly, 20 mg/d max, ÷ bid 7 AM & 12 PM; use regular-release only **Adults & Peds > 6 y.** *ADHD:* IR: 5 mg PO bid, ↑ 5–10 mg/d to 60 mg/d, max 2 mg/kg/d *ER/SR:* Use total IR dose qd *CD/LA:* 20 mg PO qd, ↑ 10–20 mg qwk to 60 mg/d max *Concerta:* 18 mg PO qAM Rx naïve or already on 20 mg/d, 36 mg PO qAM if on 40 mg/d or 54 mg PO qAM if on 60 mg/d **Caution:** [C, +/–] w/ h/o EtOH/drug abuse, CV Dz, HTN, bipolar Dz, Sz; separate from MAOIs by 14 d **Disp:** Chew tabs 2.5, 5, 10 mg; tabs scored IR (*Ritalin*) 5, 10, 20 mg; caps ER (*Ritalin LA*) 10, 20, 30, 40 mg; caps ER (*Metadate CD*) 10, 20, 30, 40, 50, 60 mg (*Methylin ER*) 10, 20 mg; tabs SR (*Ritalin SR*) 20 mg; ER tabs (*Concerta*) 18, 27, 36, 54 mg; oral soln 5, 10 mg/5 mL **SE:** CV/CNS stimulation, growth retard, GI upset, pancytopenia **CI:** Marked anxiety, tension, agitation, NAG, motor tics, family h/o or diagnosis of Tourette synd, severe HTN, angina, arrhythmias, CHF, recent MI, ↑ thyroid; w/ or w/in 14 d of MAOI **Interactions:** ↑ Risk of hypertensive crisis *W/* MAOIs; ↑ effects *OF* anticonvulsants, anticoagulants, TCA, SSRIs; ↓ effects *OF* guanethidine, antihypertensives **Labs:** ↑ LFTs; monitor CBC, plts, LFTs **NIPE:** See also transdermal form; titrate dose; take 30–45 min ac; do not chew or crush; Concerta "ghost tab" may appear in stool—avoid w/ GI narrowing; abuse & diversion concerns; D/C if Sz or agitation occurs; Metadate contains sucrose, avoid w/ lactose/galactose problems; do not use these meds w/ halogenated anesthetics; AHA rec all ADHD peds need CV assessment & consideration for ECG before Rx

Methylphenidate, Transdermal (Daytrana) [CNS Stimulant] [CII] **WARNING:** w/ h/o of drug or alcohol dependence; chronic use can lead to dependence or psychotic behavior; observe closely during withdrawal of drug **Uses:** *ADHD in children 6–17 y* **Action:** CNS stimulant, blocks reuptake of norepinephrine & DA **Dose:** *Adults & Peds ≥ 6 y.* Apply to hip in AM (2 h before desired effect), remove 9 h later; titrate 1st wk 10 mg/9 h, 2nd wk 15 mg/9 h, 3rd wk 20 mg/9 h, 4th wk 30 mg/9 h **Caution:** [C, +/–] See Methylphenidate, oral sensitization may preclude subsequent use of oral forms; abuse & diversion concerns **CI:** Sig anxiety, agitation; component allergy; glaucoma; w/ or w/in 14 d of MAOI; tics, or family Hx Tourette synd **Disp:** Patches 10, 15, 20, 30 mg **SE:** Local Rxns, N/V, nasopharyngitis, ↓ wgt, ↓ appetite, lability, insomnia, tic **Interactions:** ↑ Effects *OF* oral anticoagulants, phenobarbital, phenytoin, primidone, SSRIs, TCAs; ↑ risk *OF* hypertensive crisis *W/* MAOIs; caution *W/* pressor drugs **NIPE:** Titrate dose weekly; effects last h after removal; eval BP, HR at baseline & periodically; avoid heat exposure to patch, may cause OD, AHA rec all ADHD peds need CV assessment & consideration for ECG before Rx

Methylprednisolone (Solu-Medrol) [See Steroids Table 2]

Metoclopramide (Metozolv, Reglan, Generic) [Antiemetic/Dopamine Antagonist]

WARNING: Chronic use may cause tardive dyskinesia; D/C if Sxs develop; avoid prolonged use (> 12 wk) **Uses:** *Diabetic gastroparesis, symptomatic GERD; chemotherapy & post-op N/V, facilitate small-bowel intubation & upper GI radiologic eval,* *GERD, diabetic gastroparesis (Metozolv)* **Action:** ↑ Upper GI motility; blocks DA in chemoreceptor trigger zone, sensitized tissues to ACH **Dose:** *Adults. Gastroparesis:* (Reglan) 10 mg PO 30 min ac & hs for 2–8 wk PRN, or same dose IM/IV for 10 d, then PO *Reflux:* 10–15 mg PO 30 min ac & hs *Chemotherapy antiemetic:* 1–3 mg/kg/dose IV 30 min before chemotherapy, then q2h × 2 doses, then q3h × 3 doses *Post-op:* 10–20 mg IV/IM q4–6h PRN *Adults & Peds > 14 y. Intestinal intubation:* 10 mg IV × 1 over 1–2 min *Peds. Reflux:* 0.1 mg/kg/dose PO 30 min ac & hs, max 0.3–0.75 mg/kg/d × 2 wk–6 mo *Chemotherapy antiemetic:* 1–2 mg/kg/dose IV as adults *Post-op:* 0.25 mg/kg IV q6–8h PRN *Peds intestinal intubation: 6–14 y.* 2.5–5 mg IV × 1 over 1–2 min; *< 6 y.* Use 0.1 mg/kg IV × 1 **Caution:** [B, –] Drugs w/ extrapyramidal ADRs, MAOIs, TCAs, sympathomimetics **CI:** w/ EPS meds, GI bleeding, Pheo, Sz disorders, GI obst **Disp:** Tabs 5, 10 mg; syrup 5 mg/5 mL; Inj 5 mg/mL; ODT (Metozolv) 5,10 g **SE:** Dystonic Rxns common w/ high doses (Rx w/ IV diphenhydramine), fluid retention, restlessness, D, drowsiness **Interactions:** ↑ Risk of serotonin synd *W/* sertraline, venlafaxine; ↑ effects *OF* APAP, ASA, CNS depressants, cyclosporine, levodopa, Li, succinylcholine, tetracyclines, EtOH; ↓ effects *W/* anticholinergics, narcotics; ↓ effects *OF* cimetidine, digoxin **Labs:** ↑ Serum ALT, AST, amylase; ✓ baseline Cr **NIPE:** Monitor for extrapyramidal effects; ↓ w/ renal impair/elderly

Metolazone (Zaroxolyn) [Antihypertensive/Thiazide Diuretic]

Uses: *Mild–mod essential HTN & edema of renal Dz or cardiac failure* **Action:** Thiazide-like diuretic; ↓ distal tubule Na reabsorption **Dose:** *HTN:* 2.5–5 mg PO maint 5–20 mg PO qd *Edema:* 2.5–20 mg/d PO **Caution:** [D, +] Avoid w/ Li, gout, digitalis, SLE, many interactions **CI:** Anuria, hepatic coma or precoma **Disp:** Tabs 2.5, 5, 10 mg **SE:** Monitor fluid/lytes; dizziness; ↓ BP, ↑ HR, CP **Interactions:** ↑ Effects *W/* antihypertensives, barbiturates, narcotics, nitrates, EtOH, food; ↑ effects *OF* digoxin, Li; ↑ hyperglycemia *W/* BBs, diazoxide; ↑ hypokalemia *W/* amphotericin B, corticosteroids, mezlocillin, piperacillin, ticarcillin; ↓ effects *W/* cholestyramine, colestipol, hypoglycemics, insulin, NSAIDs, salicylates; ↑ effects *OF* methenamine **Labs:** ↑ Uric acid; ↓ K⁺, NA⁺, Mg⁺, monitor lytes **NIPE:** ↑ Risk of photosensitivity—use sunblock; ↑ risk of gout; monitor ECG for hypokalemia (flattened T waves)

Metoprolol Tartrate (Lopressor) Metoprolol Succinate (Toprol XL) [Antihypertensive/BB]   **WARNING:** Do not acutely D/C Rx as marked worsening of angina can result; taper over 1–2 wk **Uses:** *HTN, angina, CHF (XL form)* **Action:** β₁-Adrenergic receptor blocker **Dose:** *Adults. Angina:* 50–200 mg PO bid max 400 mg/d; ER form dose qd *HTN:* 50–200 mg PO bid max 450 mg/d, ER form dose qd *AMI:* 5 mg IV q2min × 3 doses, then 50 mg PO q6h × 48 h, then 100 mg PO bid (*XL form preferred*): 12.5–25 mg/d PO × 2 wk, ↑ at 1- to 2-wk intervals, 200 mg/max, use low dose w/ greatest severity *ECC 2010:* AMI: 5 mg slow IV q5min, total 15 mg; then 50 mg PO, titrate to effect **Peds. 1–17 y.** HTN IR form 1–2 mg/kg/d PO, max 6 mg/kg/d (200 mg/d) *> 6 y.* HTN ER form 1 mg/kg/d PO, initial max 50 mg/d, ↑ PRN to 2 mg/kg/d max; ↓ w/ hepatic failure; take w/ meals **Caution:** [C, +] Uncompensated CHF, bradycardia, heart block, hepatic impair, MyG, PVD, Raynaud, thyrotoxicosis **CI:** For HTN/angina SSS (unless paced), severe PVD, Pheo. For MI sinus bradycardia < 45 BPM, 1st-degree block (PR > 0.24 s), 2nd-, 3rd-degree block, SBP < 100 mm Hg, severe CHF, cardiogenic shock **Disp:** Tabs 25, 50, 100 mg; ER tabs 25, 50, 100, 200 mg; Inj 1 mg/mL **SE:** Drowsiness, insomnia, ED, bradycardia, bronchospasm **Interactions:** ↑ Effects *W/* cimetidine, dihydropyridine, diltiazem, fluoxetine, hydralazine, methimazole, OCPs, propylthiouracil, quinidine, quinolones; ↑ effects *OF* hydralazine; ↑ bradycardia *W/* digoxin, dipyridamole, verapamil; ↓ effects *W/* barbiturates, NSAIDs, rifampin; ↓ effects *OF* isoproterenol, theophylline **Labs:** ↑ BUN, SCr, LFTs, uric acid **NIPE:** *IR:*ER 1:1 daily dose but ER/XL is qd. OK to split XL tabs but do not crush/chew; take w/ food, ⊘ D/C abruptly—withdraw over 2 wk

Metronidazole (Flagyl, MetroGel) [Antibacterial, Antiprotozoals] **WARNING:** Carcinogenic in rats **Uses:** *Bone/Jt, endocarditis, intra-Abd, meningitis, & skin Infxns; amebiasis & amebic liver abscess; trichomoniasis in pt & partner; bacterial vaginosis; PID; giardiasis; antibiotic associated pseudomembranous colitis (*C difficile*), eradicate *H pylori* w/ combo therapy, rosacea, prophylactic in post-op colorectal surgery* **Action:** Interferes w/ DNA synth **Spectrum:** Excellent anaerobic, *C difficile* **Dose:** *Adults. Anaerobic Infxns:* 500 mg IV q6–8h *Amebic dysentery: 500*–750 mg/d PO q8h × 5–10 d *Trichomonas:* 250 mg PO tid for 7 d or 2 g PO × 1 (Rx partner) *C difficile:* 500 mg PO or IV q8h for 7–10 d (PO preferred;

IV only if pt NPO), if no response, change to PO vancomycin *Vaginosis:* 1 applicator intraVag qd or bid × 5 d, or 500 mg PO bid × 7 d or 750 mg PO qd × 7 d *Acne rosacea/skin:* Apply bid *Giardia:* 500 mg PO bid × 5–7 d *H pylori:* 250–500 mg PO w/ meals & hs × 14 d, combine w/ other antibiotic & a PPI or H₂ antagonist **Peds.** 30 mg/kg PO/IV/d ÷ q6h, 4 g/d max ÷ *Amebic dysentery:* 35–50 mg/kg/24 h PO in 3 ÷ doses for 5–10 d; Rx 7–10 d for *C difficile Trichomonas:* 15–30 mg/kg/d PO ÷ q8h × 7 d *C difficile:* 20 mg/kg/d PO ÷ q6h × 10 d, max 2 g/d; ↓ w/ severe hepatic/renal impair **Caution:** [B, +/–] Avoid EtOH, w/ warfarin, CYP3A4 substrates (Table 10), ↑ Li levels **CI:** 1st tri of PRG **Disp:** Tabs 250, 500 mg; XR tabs 750 mg; caps 375 mg; IV 500 mg/100 mL; lotion 0.75%; gel 0.75%, 1%; intravag gel 0.75% (5 g/applicator 37.5 mg in 70-g tube), cream 0.75%,1% **SE:** Disulfiram-like Rxn; dizziness, HA, GI upset, anorexia, urine discoloration, flushing, metallic taste **Interactions:** ↑ Effects *W/* cimetidine; ↑ effects *OF* carbamazepine, 5-FU, Li, warfarin; ↓ effects *W/* barbiturates, cholestyramine, colestipol, phenytoin **Labs:** May cause ↓/0 values for LFTs, triglycerides, glucose **NIPE:** Take w/ food; for trichomoniasis-Rx pt's partner; no aerobic bacteria activity; use in combo w/ serious mixed Infxns; wait 24 h after 1st dose to breast-feed or 48 h if extended therapy, take ER on empty stomach

Mexiletine (Mexitil) [Antiarrhythmic/Lidocaine Analogue]

WARNING: Mortality risks noted for flecainide and/or encainide (Class I antiarrhythmics). Reserve for use in pts w/ life-threatening ventricular arrhythmias **Uses:** *Suppress symptomatic vent arrhythmias* **DN Action:** Class Ib antiarrhythmic (Table 9) **Dose: Adults.** 200–300 mg PO q8h. Initial 200 mg q8h, can load w/ 400 mg if needed, ↑ q2–3d, 1200 mg/d max **Caution:** [C, +] CHF, may worsen severe arrhythmias; interacts w/ hepatic inducers & suppressors **CI:** Cardiogenic shock or 2nd-/3rd-degree AV block w/o pacemaker **Disp:** Caps 150, 200, 250 mg **SE:** Lightheadedness, dizziness, anxiety, incoordination, GI upset, ataxia, hepatic damage, blood dyscrasias, PVCs, N/V, tremor **Interactions:** ↑ Effects *W/* fluvoxamine, quinidine, caffeine; ↑ effects *OF* theophylline; ↓ effects *W/* atropine, hydantoins, phenytoin, phenobarbital, rifampin, tobacco **Labs:** ↑ LFTs; ↓ plts; monitor LFTs & CBC; false(+) ANA **NIPE:** Take w/ food < GI upset

Miconazole (Monistat 1 Combo, Monistat 3, Monistat 7) [OTC] (Monistat-Derm) [Antifungal]

Uses: *Candidal Infxns, dermatomycoses (tinea pedis/tinea cruris/tinea corporis/tinea versicolor/candidiasis)* **Action:** Azole antifungal, alters fungal membrane permeability **Dose:** *Intravag:* 100 mg supp or 2% cream intravag qhs × 7 d or 200 mg supp or 4% cream intravag qhs × 3 d *Derm:* Apply bid, AM/PM *Tinea versicolor:* Apply qd. Treat tinea pedis for 1 mo & other Infxns for 2 wk **Peds ≥ 12 y.** 100 mg supp or 2% cream intravag qhs × 7 d or 200 mg supp or 4% cream intravag qhs × 3 d **Caution:** [C, ?] Azole sensitivity **Disp:** *Monistat-Derm:* (Rx) cream 2% *Monistat 1 Combo:* 2% cream w/ 1200 mg supp *Monistat 3:* Vag cream 4%, supp 200 mg *Monistat 7:* Cream 2%, supp 100 mg; lotion 2%; powder 2%; effervescent tabs 2%, oint 2%, spray 2%; Vag supp 100,

200, 1200 mg; Vag cream 2%, 4%; [OTC] **SE:** Vag burning; on skin contact dermatitis, irritation, burning **Interactions:** ↑ Effects *OF* anticoagulants, cisapride, loratadine, phenytoin, quinidine; ↓ effects *W/* amphotericin B; ↓ effects *OF* amphotericin B **Labs:** ↑ Protein **NIPE:** Antagonistic to amphotericin B in vivo; may interfere w/ condom & diaphragm, do not use w/ tampons

Miconazole, Buccal (Oravig) [Antifungal]   Uses: *Oropharyngeal candidiasis* Action: Azole antifungal, alters fungal membrane permeability Dose:
Adults. Apply one 50 mg buccal tab to gum once daily × 14 d; do not crush/chew/swallow tab **Caution:** [C, ?/–] allergic Rxns may occur **CI:** Hypersensitivity to milk protein or components **Disp:** Tabs buccal 50 mg **SE:** HA, N/V/D, upper Abd pain, dysgeusia **Interactions:** ↑ Effects *OF* anticoagulants (eg, warfarin), cisapride, loratadine, phenytoin, quinidine; ↓ effects *W/* amphotericin B; ↓ effects *OF* amphotericin B **Labs:** Monitor INR

Miconazole/Zinc Oxide/Petrolatum (Vusion) [Antifungal]   Uses:
Candidal diaper rash Action: Combo antifungal Dose: Peds > 4 wk. Apply at each diaper change × 7 d **Caution:** [C, ?] **CI:** None **Disp:** Miconazole/zinc oxide/petrolatum oint 0.25%/15%/81.35%; 50-, 90-g tube **SE:** None **NIPE:** Keep diaper dry, not for prevention

Midazolam (Various) [C-IV] [Sedative/Benzodiazepine]   WARN-ING: Associated w/ resp depression & resp arrest esp when used for sedation in noncritical care settings. Reports of airway obst, desaturation, hypoxia, & apnea w/ other CNS depressants. Cont monitoring required Uses: *Pre-op sedation, conscious sedation for short procedures & mechanically ventilated pts, induction of general anesthesia* Action: Short-acting benzodiazepine Dose: Adults. 1–5 mg IV or IM or 0.02–0.35 mg/kg based on indication; titrate to effect Peds. Pre-op: > 6 mo. 0.25–1 mg/kg PO, 20 mg max Conscious sedation: 0.08 mg/kg × 1 > 6 mo. 0.1–0.15 mg/kg IM × 1 max 10 mg General anesthesia: 0.025–0.1 mg/kg IV q2min for 1–3 doses PRN to induce anesthesia (↓ in elderly, w/ narcotics or CNS depressants) **Caution:** [D, +/–] w/ CYP3A4 substrate (Table 10), multiple drug interactions **CI:** NAG; w/ amprenavir, atazanavir, nelfinavir, ritonavir **Disp:** Inj 1, 5 mg/mL; syrup 2 mg/mL **SE:** Resp depression; ↓ BP w/ conscious sedation, N **Interactions:** ↑ Effects *W/* azole antifungals, antihistamines, cimetidine, CCBs, CNS depressants, erythromycin, INH, phenytoin, protease Inhibs, grapefruit juice, EtOH; ↓ effects *W/* rifampin, tobacco; ↓ effects *OF* levodopa **NIPE:** Monitor for resp depression; reversal w/ flumazenil; not for epidural/IT use

Midodrine (Proamatine) [Antihypotensive/Vasopressor/Alpha-1 Agonist.]   Uses: *Tx orthostatic hypotension* Action: Vasopressor/antihypotensive; α_1-agonist Dose: 10 mg PO tid when pt plans to be upright **Caution:** [C, ?] **CI:** Pheo, renal Dz, thyrotoxicosis, severe heart dz, urinary retention **Disp:** Tabs 2.5,5,10 mg **SE:** Supine HTN, paresthesia, urinary retention **Interactions:** ↑ Risk of bradycardia/AV Block/arrhythmias *W/* cardiac glycosides, BB, CNS drugs; ↑ effects *W/*

pseudoephedrine, ergots, other α-agonists, & fludrocortisone; ↓ effects **W/** prazosin & other α-antagonists **NIPE:** SBP ≥ 200 mm Hg in ~13% pts given 10 mg

Mifepristone [RU 486] (Mifeprex) [Abortifacient/Synthetic Steroid]
WARNING: Pt counseling & info required; associated w/ fatal Infxns & bleeding **Uses:** *Terminate intrauterine PRGs of < 49 d* **Action:** Antiprogestin; ↑ prostaglandins, results in uterine contraction **Dose:** Administered w/ 3 office visits: d 1: 600 mg PO × 1; d 3, unless abortion confirmed, 400 mcg PO of misoprostol (*Cytotec*); about d 14, verify termination of PRG. Surgical termination if Rx fails **Caution:** [X, –] w/ Infxn, sepsis **CI:** Ectopic PRG, undiagnosed adnexal mass, w/ IUD, adrenal failure, w/ long-term steroid therapy, hemorrhagic Dz, w/ anticoagulants, prostaglandin hypersensitivity. Pts who do not have access to medical facilities or unable to understand Tx or comply **Disp:** Tabs 200 mg **SE:** Abd pain & 1–2 wk of uterine bleeding, N/V/D, HA **Interactions:** ↑ Effects **W/** azole antifungals, erythromycin, grapefruit juice; ↓ effects w/ carbamazepine, dexamethasone, phenytoin, phenobarbital, rifampin, St. John's wort **NIPE:** Give under supervision of healthcare provider only 9–16 d Vag bleed on average after using

Miglitol (Glyset) [Hypoglycemic/Alpha-Glucosidase Inhibitor]
Uses: *Type 2 DM* **Action:** α-Glucosidase Inhib; delays carbohydrate digestion of **Dose:** Initial 25 mg PO tid; maint 50–100 mg tid (w/ 1st bite of each meal), titrate over 4–8 wk **Caution:** [B, –] w/ digitalis & digestive enzymes **CI:** DKA, obstructive/inflammatory GI disorders; SCr > 2 mg/dL **Disp:** Tabs 25, 50, 100 mg **SE:** Flatulence, D, Abd pain **Interactions:** ↑ Effects **W/** celery, coriander, juniper berries, ginseng, garlic; ↓ effects w/ INH, niacin, intestinal absorbents, amylase, pancreatin; ↓ effects **OF** digoxin, propranolol, ranitidine **Labs:** ⊘ Use w/ SCr > 2 mg/dL **NIPE:** Use alone or w/ sulfonylureas

Milnacipran HCl (Savella) [Antidepressant/Serotonin & Norepinephrine Reuptake Inhibitor]
WARNING: Antidepressants associated w/ ↑ risk of suicide ideation in children & young adults **Uses:** *Fibromyalgia* **Action:** Antidepressant, SNRI **Dose:** 50 mg PO bid, max 200 mg/d; ↑ to 25 mg bid w/ CrCl < 30 mL/min **Caution:** [C, /?] **CI :** NAG, w/ recent MAOI **Disp:** Tabs: 12.5, 25, 50, 100 mg **SE:** HA, N/V, constipation, dizziness, ↑ HR, ↑ BP **Interactions:** ↓ Effects **OF** anticoagulants ↑ risk of serotonin synd **W/** Li, tramadol, triptans; ↓ effects **OF** clonidine **Labs:** ↑ LFTs **NIPE:** Monitor HR & BP; withdraw gradually; wait 14 d > D/C MAOI to start this drug. Wait 5 d > D/C this drug to start MAOI

Milrinone (Primacor) [Vasodilator/Bipyridine Phosphodiesterase Inhibitor]
Uses: *CHF acutely decompensated* , Ca antagonist intoxication **Action:** Phosphodiesterase Inhib + inotrope & vasodilator; little chronotropic activity **Dose:** 50 mcg/kg, IV over 10 min, then 0.375–0.75 mcg/kg/min IV Inf; ↓ w/ renal impair **Caution:** [C, ?] **CI:** Allergy to drug; w/ inamrinone **Disp:** Inj 200 mcg/mL **SE:** Arrhythmias, ↓ BP, HA **Interactions:** ↑ Hypotension **W/** nesiritide **Labs:** Lytes, CBC, Mg^{2+} **NIPE:** Monitor fluids, BP, HR; not for long-term use

Mineral Oil [OTC] [Emollient Laxative] Uses: *Constipation, bowel irritation, fecal impaction* Action: Lubricant laxative Dose: *Adults. Constipation:* 15–45 mL PO/d PRN *Fecal impaction or after barium:* 118 mL rectally × 1 *Peds. > 6 y. Constipation:* 5–25 mL PO qd *2–12 y. Fecal impaction:* 118 mL rectally × 1 Caution: [C, ?] w/ N/V, difficulty swallowing, bedridden pts; may ↓ absorption of vit A, D, E, & K, warfarin CI: Colostomy/ileostomy, appendicitis, diverticulitis, UC Disp: All [OTC] Liq PO 13.5 mL/15 mL, PO microemulsion 2.5 mL/5 mL, rectal enema 118 mL SE: Lipid pneumonia (aspiration of PO), N/V, temporary anal incontinence Interactions: ↑ Effects *W/* stool softeners; ↓ effects *OF* cardiac glycosides, OCPs, sulfonamides, vits, warfarin NIPE: Rectal incontinence; take PO upright; do not use in peds < 6 y

Mineral Oil-Pramoxine HCl-Zinc Oxide (Tucks Ointment, [OTC]) [Topical Anesthetic] Uses: *Temporary relief of anorectal disorders (itching, etc)* Action: Topical anesthetic Dose: *Adults & Peds ≥ 12 y.* Cleanse, rinse, & dry, apply externally or into anal canal w/ tip 5 × /d × 7 d max Caution: [?/?] Do not place into rectum CI: None Disp: Oint 30-g tube SE: Local irritation NIPE: D/C w/ or if rectal bleeding occurs or if condition worsens or does not improve w/in 7 d

Minocycline (Dynacin, Minocin, Solodyn) [Antibiotic/Tetracycline] Uses: *Mod–severe nonnodular acne (Solodyn),* anthrax, rickettsiae, gonococcus, skin Infxn, URI, UTI, nongonococcal urethritis, amebic dysentery, asymptomatic meningococcal carrier, *M marinum* Action: Tetracycline, bacteriostatic, ↓ protein synth Dose: *Adults & Peds > 12 y. Usual:* 200 mg, then 100 mg q12h or 100–200 mg, then 50 mg qid; *Gonococcal urethritis, men:* 100 mg q12h × 5 d *Syphilis:* Usual dose × 10–15 d *Meningococcal carrier:* 100 mg q12h × 5 d *M marinum:* 100 mg q12h × 6–8 wk *Uncomp urethral, endocervical, or rectal Infxn:* 100 mg q12h × 7 d minimum *Adults & Peds > 12 y. Acne: (Solodyn)* 1 mg/kg PO qd × 12 wk *> 8 y.* 4 mg/kg initially, then 2 mg/kg q12h w/ food to ↓ irritation, hydrate well, ↓ dose or extend interval w/ renal impair Caution: [D, –] Associated w/ pseudomembranous colitis, w/ renal impair, may ↓ OCP, or w/ warfarin may ↑ INR CI: Allergy, women of childbearing potential Disp: Tabs 50, 75, 100 mg; ER *(Solodyn)* 45, 90, 135 mg; caps *(Minocin)* 50, 100 mg, susp 50 mg/mL SE: D, HA, fever, rash, Jt pain, fatigue, dizziness, photosensitivity, hyperpigmentation, SLE synd, pseudotumor cerebri Interactions: ↑ Effects *OF* digoxin, oral anticoagulants; ↑ risk of nephrotox *W/* methoxyflurane; ↓ effects *W/* antacids, cholestyramine, colestipol, laxatives, cimetidine, Fe products; ↓ effects *OF* hormonal contraceptives Labs: ↑ LFTs, BUN; ↓ HMG, plts, WBCs NIPE: Do not cut/crush/chew; keep away from children; risk of photosensitivity—use sunblock; may take *W/* food to < GI upset; tooth discoloration in < 8 y or w/ use last half of PRG

Minoxidil, Oral [Antihypertensive/Vasodilator] WARNING: May cause pericardial effusion, occasional tamponade, & angina pectoris may be exacerbated. For nonresponders to max doses of 2 other antihypertensives & a diuretic. Administer under supervision w/ a BB & diuretic. Monitor for ↓ BP in those receiving guanethidine w/ malignant HTN **Uses:** *Severe HTN* **Action:** Peripheral vasodilator **Dose:** *Adults & Peds > 12 y.* 5 mg PO ÷ daily, titrate q3d, 10 mg/d max *Peds.* 0.2–1 mg/kg/24 h ÷ PO q12–24h, titrate q3d, max 50 mg/d; ↓ w/ elderly, renal Insuff **Caution:** [C, +] **CI:** Pheo, component allergy, CHF, renal impair **Disp:** Tabs 2.5, 10 mg **SE:** Pericardial effusion & vol overload w/ PO use; hypertrichosis w/ chronic use, edema, ECG changes, wgt gain **Interactions:** ↑ Hypotension *W/* guanethidine **Labs:** ↑ Alk phos, BUN, Cr; ↓ HMG, Hct **NIPE:** Take PO drug w/ food to < GI upset; avoid for 1 mo after MI

Minoxidil, Topical (Theroxidil, Rogaine) [OTC] [Topical Hair Growth] **Uses:** *Male & female pattern baldness* **Action:** Stimulates vertex hair growth **Dose:** Apply 1 mL bid to area, D/C if no growth in 4 mo **Caution:** [?, ?] **CI:** Component allergy **Disp:** Soln & aerosol foam 5% **SE:** Changes in hair color/texture **NIPE:** Hypertrichosis w/ chronic use; requires chronic use to maintain hair

Mirtazapine (Remeron, Remeron SolTab) [Tetracyclic Antidepressant] **WARNING:** ↑ Risk of suicidal thinking & behavior in children, adolescents, & young adults w/ major depression & other psychological disorders. Not for peds use **Uses:** *Depression* **Action:** α_2-Antagonist antidepressant, ↑ norepinephrine & 5-HT **Dose:** 15 mg PO hs, up to 45 mg/d hs **Caution:** [C, ?] Has anticholinesterol effects, w/ Sz, clonidine, CNS depressant use, CYP1A2, CYP3A4 inducers/ Inhibs **CI:** MAOIs w/in 14 d **Disp:** Tabs 15, 30, 45 mg; rapid dispersion tabs (SolTab) 15, 30, 45 mg **SE:** Somnolence, constipation, xerostomia, wgt gain, agranulocytosis, ↓ BP, edema, musculoskeletal pain **Interactions:** ↑ Effects *W/* CNS depressants, fluvoxamine; ↑ risk of HTN crisis *W/* MAOIs **Labs:** ↑ ALT, cholesterol, triglycerides **NIPE:** Handle rapid tabs w/ dry hands, do not cut or chew; do not ↑ dose at intervals < q1–2wk

Misoprostol (Cytotec) [Mucosal Protective Agent/Prostaglandin] **WARNING:** Use in PRG can cause abortion, premature birth, or birth defects; do not use to ↓ ulcer risk in women of childbearing age; must comply w/ birth control measures **Uses:** *Prevent NSAID-induced gastric ulcers; medical termination of PRG < 49 d w/ mifepristone; induce labor (cervical ripening); incomplete & therapeutic abortion* **Action:** Prostaglandin (PGE-1), antisecretory & mucosal protection; induces uterine contractions **Dose:** *Ulcer prevention:* 200 mcg PO qid w/ meals; in females, start 2nd/3rd d of next nl period *Induction of labor (term):* 25–50 mcg intravag *PRG termination:* 400 mcg PO on d 3 of mifepristone; take w/ food **Caution:** [X, −] **CI:** PRG, component allergy **Disp:** Tabs 100, 200 mcg **SE:** Miscarriage w/ severe bleeding; HA, D, Abd pain, constipation **Interactions:** ↑ HA & GI Sxs *W/* phenylbutazone **NIPE:** Not used for induction of labor w/ previous C-section or major uterine surgery

Mitomycin (Mutamycin) [Antineoplastic/Alkylating Agent] **WARNING:** Administration only by physician experienced in chemotherapy; myelosuppressive; can induce hemolytic uremic synd w/ irreversible renal failure **Uses:** *Stomach, pancreas*, breast, colon CA; squamous cell carcinoma of the anus; NSCLC, head & neck, cervical; bladder CA (intravesically) **Action:** Alkylating agent; generates oxygen-free radicals w/ DNA strand breaks **Dose:** (Per protocol) 20 mg/m^2 q6–8wk IV or 10 mg/m^2 combo w/ other myelosuppressive drugs q6–8wk *Bladder CA:* 20–40 mg in 40 mL NS via a urethral catheter once/wk × 8 wk, followed by monthly × 12 mo for 1 y; ↓ in renal/hepatic impair **Caution:** [D, –] **CI:** coagulation disorders, Cr > 1.7 mg/dL, ↑ cardiac tox w/ vinca alkaloids/ doxorubicin **Disp:** Inj 5, 20, 40 mg **SE:** ↓ BM (persists for 3–8 wk, may be cumulative; minimize w/ lifetime dose < 50–60 mg/m^2), N/V, anorexia, stomatitis, renal tox, microangiopathic hemolytic anemia w/ renal failure (hemolytic–uremic synd), venoocclusive liver Dz, interstitial pneumonia, alopecia, extrav Rxns, contact dermatitis; CHF **Interactions:** ↑ Bronchospasm *W/* vinca alkaloids; ↑ BM suppression *W/* antineoplastics **Labs:** ↓ Plt, ↓ WBC, Monitor plts, WBCs, differential, Hgb repeatedly during & for at least 8 wk after therapy **NIPE:** Monitor fluid balance & avoid overhydration; ⊘ PRG or breast-feeding

Mitoxantrone (Novantrone) [Antineoplastic/Antibiotic] WARNING: Administration only by physician experienced in chemotherapy; except for acute leukemia, do not use w/ ANC of < 1500 cells/mm^3; severe neutropenia can result in Infxn, follow CBC; cardiotox (CHF), secondary AML reported **Uses:** *AML (w/ cytarabine), ALL, CML, PCA, MS, Lung CA* breast CA, & NHL **Action:** DNA-intercalating agent; ↓ DNA synth by interacting w/ topoisomerase II **Dose:** Per protocol; ↓ w/ hepatic impair, leukopenia, ↓ plt **Caution:** [D, –] Reports of secondary AML, w/ MS ↑ CV risk, do not treat MS pt w/ low LVEF **CI:** PRG, sig ↓ in LVEF **Disp:** Inj 2 mg/mL **SE:** ↓ BM, N/V, stomatitis, alopecia (infrequent), cardiotox, urine discoloration, secretions & scleras may be blue-green **Interactions:** ↑ BM suppression *W/* antineoplastics; ↓ effects *OF* live virus vaccines **Labs:** ↑ AST, ALT, uric acid **NIPE:** ↓ Fluids to 2–3 L/d, maint hydration, ⊘ vaccines, Infxn; baseline CV eval w/ ECG & LVEF; cardiac monitoring prior to each dose; not for IT use

Modafinil (Provigil) [C-IV] [Analeptic/CNS Stimulant] Uses: *Improve wakefulness in pts w/ excess daytime sleepiness (narcolepsy, sleep apnea, SWSD)* **Action:** Alters DA & norepinephrine release, ↓ GABA-mediated neurotransmission **Dose:** 200 mg PO qAM; ↓ dose 50% w/ elderly/hepatic impair **Caution:** [C, ?/–] *CV* Dz; **CI:** Component allergy **Disp:** Tabs 100, 200 mg **SE:** Serious rash incuding SJS, HA, N, D, paresthesias, rhinitis, agitation, psychological Sx **Interactions:** ↑ Effects *OF* CNS stimulants, diazepam, phenytoin, propranolol, TCAs, warfarin; ↓ effect *OF* cyclosporine, OCPs, theophylline **Labs:** ↑ Glucose, AST, GTT **NIPE:** Take w/o regard to food; monitor BP; use barrier contraception; CV assessment before using

Moexipril (Univasc) [Antihypertensive/ACEI] WARNING: ACE Inhibs can cause fatal injury/death in 2nd/3rd tri; D/C w/ PRG **Uses:** *HTN, post-MI*, DN **Action:** ACE Inhib **Dose:** 7.5–30 mg in 1–2 ÷ doses 1 h ac ↓ in renal impair **Caution:** [C (1st tri), D 2nd & 3rd tri), ?] **CI:** ACE Inhib sensitivity

Disp: Tabs 7.5, 15 mg **SE:** ↓ BP, edema, angioedema, HA, dizziness, cough **Interactions:** ↑ Effects *W/* diuretics, antihypertensives, EtOH, probenecid, garlic; ↑ effects *OF* insulin, Li; ↑ risk of hyperkalemia *W/* K⁺ supl, K⁺-sparing diuretics; ↓ effects *W/* antacids, ASA, NSAIDs, ephedra, yohimbe, ginseng **Labs:** ↑ BUN, Cr, K⁺; ↓ Na⁺ **NIPE:** May alter sense of taste, may cause cough, ⊘ salt substitutes, ⊘ PRG, use barrier contraception

Molindone (Moban) [Antipsychotic] Uses: *Schizophrenia* **Action:** Piperazine phenothiazine **Dose:** *Adults.* 50–75 mg/d PO, ↑ to max 225 mg/d q3–4d PRN *Peds. 3–5 y.* 1–2.5 mg/d PO in 4 ÷ doses *5–12 y.* 0.5–1.0 mg/kg/d in 4 ÷ doses **Caution:** [C, ?] NAG **CI:** Drug/EtOH CNS depression, coma **Disp:** Tabs 5, 10, 25, 50 mg scored **SE:** Drowsiness, depression, ↓ BP, tachycardia, arrhythmias, EPS, neuroleptic malignant synd, Szs, constipation, xerostomia, blurred vision **Interactions:** ↑ Effects *W/* antihypertensives; ↑ hyperkalemia *W/* K⁺-sparing diuretics, K⁺ supls, salt substitutes, TMP; ↑ effects *OF* insulin, Li; ↓ effects *W/* ASA, NSAIDs **Labs:** ✓ Lipid profile, fasting glucose, HgA₁c; may ↑ prolactin; ↑ serum K⁺, BUN, Cr **NIPE:** Take w/o food; monitor for persistent cough

Mometasone, Inhaled (Asmanex Twisthaler) [Corticosteroid] Uses: *Maint Rx for asthma* **Action:** Corticosteroid **Dose:** *Adults & Peds > 11 y. On bronchodilators alone or inhaled steroids:* 220 mcg × 1 qPM (max 440 mcg/d) *On oral steroids:* 440 mcg bid (max 880 mcg/d)w/ slow oral taper *Peds 4–11 y.* 110 mcg × 1 qPM (max 110 mcg/d) **Caution:** [C, M] Candida Infxn of mouth/throat; hypersensitivity Rxns possible; may worsen certain Infxn (TB, fungal, etc); Sxs; ↓ bone density; ↓ growth in peds; monitor for NAG or cataracts **CI:** Acute asthma attack; component hypersensitivity/milk proteins **Disp:** MDI inhalmometasone 110 mcg Twisthaler delivers 100 mcg/actuation; 220 mcg Twisthaler delivers 200 mcg/actuation **SE:** HA, allergic rhinitis, pharyngitis, URI, sinusitis, oral candidiasis, dysmenorrhea, musculoskeletal/back pain, dyspepsia **Labs:** Monitor for ↑/↓ cortisol; may ↑ glucose **NIPE:** Rinse mouth after use; treat paradoxical bronchospasm w/ inhaled bronchodilator

Mometasone, Nasal (Nasonex) [Corticosteroid] Uses: *Nasal Sx allergic/seasonal rhinitis; prophylaxis of seasonal allergic rhinitis; nasal polyps in adults* **Action:** Corticosteroid **Dose:** *Adults & Peds > 12 y. Rhinitis:* 2 sprays/each nostril qd *Adults. Nasal polyps:* 2 sprays/each nostril bid *Peds 2–11 y.* 1 spray/each nostril qd **Caution:** [C, M] Monitor for adverse effects on nasal mucosa (bleeding candidal Infxn, ulceration, perfusion); may worsen existing Infxns; monitor for NAG, cataracts; ↓ growth in peds **CI:** Component hypersensitivity **Disp:** 50 mg mometasone/spray **SE:** Viral Infxn, pharyngitis, epistaxis, HA **Labs:** Monitor for ↑/↓ cortisol Sxs

Mometasone & Formoterol (Dulera) [Corticosteroid & Beta-2 Agonist] **WARNING:** ↑ Risk of worseningwheezing or asthma-related death w/ LA β₂-adrenergic agonists; use only if asthma not controlled on agent such as inhaled steroid Uses: *Maint Rx for asthma* **Action:** Corticosteroid (mometasone) w/ LA bronchodilator β₂-agonist (formoterol) **Dose:** *Adults & Peds > 12 y.* 2 Inh q12h **Caution:** [C, M] Candida Infxn of mouth/throat, immunosuppression, adrenal suppression, ↓ bone density,w/ glaucoma/cataracts, other LABA should not be used **CI:** Acute asthma attack; component hypersensitivity **Disp:** MDI 120 Inh/canister (mcg mometasone/mcg formoterol) 100/5, 200/5 **SE:** Nasopharyngitis, sinusitis, HA, palpitations, CP, rapid HR, tremor or nervousness **Interactions:** Not recommended withother LA β₂-agonists (eg, formoterol, arformoterol, salmeterol); ↑ cardiac effects *W/* meds that ↑ QT interval; ↑ effects *W/* potent CYP3A4 Inhibs (eg, ketoconazole, ritonavir)↑ risk of hypokalemia *W/* xanthines, steroids, K⁺ depleting diuretics; ↓ effects *W/* BBs **Labs:** May ↑ glucose, ↓ K⁺ **NIPE:** For pts not controlled on other meds (eg, low–medium dose Inh steroids) or whose Dz severitywarrants 2 maint therapies

Montelukast (Singulair) [Bronchodilator/Leukotriene Receptor Antagonist] **Uses:** *Prevent/chronic Rx asthma ≥ 12 mo; seasonal allergic rhinitis ≥ 2 y; perennial allergic rhinitis ≥ 6 mo; prevent exercise bronchoconstriction (EIB) ≥ 15 y; prophylaxis & Rx of chronic asthma, seasonal allergic rhinitis* **Action:** Leukotriene receptor antagonist **Dose:** *Asthma: Adults & Peds > 15 y.* 10 mg/d PO in PM *6–23 mo.* 4-mg pack granules qd *2–5 y.* 4 mg/d PO qPM *6–14 y.* 5 mg/d PO qPM **Caution:** [B, M] **CI:** Component allergy **Disp:** Tabs 10 mg; chew tabs 4, 5 mg; granules 4 mg/pack **SE:** HA, dizziness, fatigue, rash, GI upset, Churg-Strauss synd, flu, cough, neuropsychological events (agitation, restlessness, suicidal ideation) **Interactions:** ↑/↓ Effects *W/* phenobarbital, rifampin **Labs:** ↑ AST, ALT **NIPE:** Not for acute asthma; do not dose w/in 24 h of previous; recent concern over ↑ suicidal behavior

Morphine (Avinza XR, Astramorph/PF, Duramorph, Infumorph, MS Contin, Kadian SR, Oramorph SR, Roxanol) [C-II] [Analgesic/Opioid Agonist] **WARNING:** Do not crush/chew SR/CR forms **Uses:** *Rx severe pain*AMI, acute pulm edema **Action:** Narcotic analgesic; SR/CR forms for chronic use **Dose:** *Adults. Short-term use PO:* 5–30 mg q4h PRN *IV/IM:* 2.5–15 mg q2–6h *Supp:* 10–30 mg q4h *SR formulations:* 15–60 mg q8–12h (do not chew/crush). *IT/epidural* (Duramorph, Infumorph, Astramorph/PF): Per protocol in Inf device *ECC 2010:* STEMI: 2–4 mg IV (over 1–5 min), then give 2–8 mg IV q5–15min PRN NSTEMI: 1–5 mg slow IV if Sxs unrelieved by nitrates or recur; use w/ caution; can be reversed w/ 0.4–2 mg IV naloxone *Peds > 6 mo.* 0.1–0.2 mg/kg/dose IM/IV q2–4h PRN to 15 mg/dose max; 0.2–0.5 mg/kg PO q4–6h PRN; 0.3–0.6 mg/kg SR tabs PO q12h; 2–4 mg IV (over 1–5 min) q5–30 min *(ECC 2005)* **Caution:** [C, +/–] Severe resp depression possible, w/ head injury *CI:* Severe asthma, resp depression, GI obst **Disp:** IR tabs 15, 30 mg; soln 10, 20, 100 mg/5 mL; supp 5, 10, 20, 30 mg; Inj 2, 4, 5, 8, 10, 15, 25, 50 mg/mL; *MS Contin CR* tabs 15, 30, 60, 100, 200 mg; *Oramorph SR* tabs 15, 30, 60, 100 mg; *Kadian SR* caps 10, 20, 30, 50, 60, 80, 100 mg; *Avinza XR* caps 30, 60, 90, 120 mg; *Duramorph/Astramorph PF* Inj 0.5, 1 mg/mL; *Infumorph* 10, 25 mg/mL **SE:** Narcotic SE (resp depression, sedation, constipation, N/V, pruritus, diaphoresis, urinary retention, biliary colic); granulomas w/ IT **Interactions:** ↑ Effects *W/* cimetidine, CNS depressants, dextroamphetamine, TCAs, EtOH, kava kava, valerian, St. John's wort; ↑ effects *OF* warfarin; ↑ riskof HTN crisis *W/* MAOIs; ↓ effects *W/* opioids, phenothiazines **Labs:** ↑ Serum amylase, lipase **NIPE:** May require scheduled dosing to relieve severe chronic pain; do not crush/chew SR/CR forms

Morphine Liposomal (DepoDur) [Analgesic/Opioid Agonist]
Uses: *Long-lasting epidural analgesia* **Action:** ER morphine analgesia **Dose:** 10–20 mg lumbar epidural Inj (C-section 10 mg after cord clamped) **Caution:** [C, +/−] Elderly, biliary Dz (sphincter of Oddi spasm) **CI:** Ileus, resp depression, asthma, obstructed airway, suspected/known head injury ↑ ICP, allergy to morphine **Disp:** Inj 10 mg/mL **SE:** Hypoxia, resp depression, ↓ BP, retention, N/V, constipation, flatulence, pruritus, pyrexia, anemia, HA, dizziness, tachycardia, insomnia, ileus **NIPE:** Effect = 48 h; not for IT/IV/IM

Morphine & Naltrexone (Embeda) [C-II] [Opioid Receptor Agonist/Antagonist]
WARNING: For mod–severe chronic pain; do not use as PRN analgesic; swallow whole or sprinkle contents of cap on applesauce; do not crush/dissolve, chew caps—rapid release & absorption of morphine may be fatal & of naltrexone may lead to withdrawal in opioid-tolerant pts; do not consume EtOH or EtOH-containing products; 100/4 mg caps for opioid-tolerant pts only **Uses:** *Chronic mod–severe pain* **Action:** mu-Opioid receptor agonist & antagonist **Dose: Adult.** Individualize PO q12–24h; if opioid intolerant start 20/0.8 mg q24h; titrate q48h; ↓ start dose in elderly, w/ hepatic/renal Insuff; taper to D/C **Caution:** [C, ?/−] w/ EtOH, CNS depression, muscle relaxants **CI:** Resp depression, acute/ severe asthma/hypercarbia, ileus, hypersensitivity **Disp:** Caps ER (morphine mg/ naltrexone mg) 20/0.8, 30/1.2, 50/2, 60/2.4, 80/3.2, 100/4 **SE:** N/V/D, constipation, somnolence, dizziness, HA, ↓ BP, pruritus, insomnia, anxiety, resp depression, Szs, MI, apnea, anaphylaxis, biliary spasm **Interactions:** ↑ Morphine absorption *W/* Etoh; ↑ CNS depression *W/* antiemetics, phenothiazines, sedatives, hypnotics, muscle relaxants; ↓ effects *OF* diurtics **NIPE:** Withdrawal w/ abrupt D/C, do not give via NG tube; do not use during or w/in 14 d of MAOIs

Moxifloxacin (Avelox) [Antibiotic/Fluoroquinolone]
WARNING: ↑ Risk of tendon rupture & tendonitis ; ↑ risk w/ age > 60, transplant pts; may ↑ Sx of MG **Uses:** *Acute sinusitis & bronchitis, skin/soft-tissue/intra-Abd Infxns, conjunctivitis, CAP, TB, anthrax, endocarditis* **Action:** 4th-gen quinolone; ↓ DNA gyrase *Spectrum:* Excellent gram(+) except MRSA & *E faecium*; good gram(−) except *P aeruginosa, S maltophilia,* & *Acinetobacter* sp; good anaerobic **Dose:** 400 mg/d PO/IV daily; avoid cation products, antacids tid **Caution:** [C, ?/−] Quinolone sensitivity; interactions w/ Mg^{2+}, Ca^{2+}, Al^{2+}, Fe^{2+}-containing products, & Class Ia & III antiarrhythmic agents (Table 9) **CI:** Quinolone/component sensitivity **Disp:** Tabs 400 mg, *ABC Pak* 5 tabs, Inj **SE:** Dizziness, N, QT prolongation, Szs, photosensitivity **Interactions:** ↑ Effects *W/* probenecid; ↑ effects *OF* diazepam, theophylline, caffeine, metoprolol, propranolol, phenytoin, warfarin; ↓ effects *W/*

antacids, didanosine, Fe salts, Mg, sucralfate, NaHCO₃, Zinc **Labs:** ↑ LFTs, BUN, SCr, amylase, PT, triglycerides, cholesterol; ↓ HMG, Hct **NIPE:** ⊘ Give to children < 18 y; ↑ fluids to 2–3 L/d

Moxifloxacin Ophthalmic (Moxeza, Vigamox) [Antibiotic/Fluoroquinolone] Uses: *Bacterial conjunctivitis* **Action:** See Moxifloxacin **Dose:** Instill into affected eye/eyes: *Moxeza*: 1 gtt bid × 7 d; *Vigamo* × 1 gtt tid × 7 d **Caution:** [C, ?/–] Not well studied in Peds < 12 mo **CI:** Quinolone/component sensitivity **Disp:** Ophthal soln 0.5% **SE:** ↓ Visual acuity, ocular pain, itching, tearing, conjunctivitis **NIPE:** Prolonged use may result in fungal overgrowth, do not wear contacts w/ conjunctivitis

Multivitamins, Oral [OTC] (Table 12)

Mupirocin (Bactroban, Bactroban Nasal) [Topical Anti-Infective] Uses: *Impetigo (oint); skin lesion infect w/ S aureus or S pyogenes; eradicate MRSA in nasal carriers* **Action:** ↓ Bacterial protein synth **Dose:** *Topical:* Apply small amount 3 ×/d × 5–14 d *Nasal:* Apply 1/2 single-use tube bid in nostrils × 5 d **Caution:** [B, ?] **CI:** Do not use w/ other nasal products **Disp:** Oint 2%; cream 2%; nasal oint 2% 1-g single-use tubes **SE:** Local irritation, rash **Interactions:** ↓ Bacterial action **W/** chloramphenicol **NIPE:** Pt to contact healthcare provider if no improvement in 3–5 d

Muromonab-CD3 (Orthoclone OKT3) [Immunosuppressant/ Monoclonal Antibody] **WARNING:** Can cause anaphylaxis; monitor fluid status; cytokine release synd Uses: *Acute rejection following organ transplantation* **Action:** Murine Ab, blocks T-cell Fxn **Dose:** Per protocol *Adults.* 5 mg/d IV for 10–14 d *Ped.< 30 kg.* 2.5 mg/d × 30 kg. 5 mg/d IV for 10–14 d **Caution:** [C, ?/–] w/ h/o of Szs, PRG, uncontrolled HTN **CI:** Murine sensitivity, fluid overload **Disp:** Inj 5 mg/5 mL **SE:** Anaphylaxis, pulm edema, fever/chills w/ 1st dose (premedicate w/ steroid/APAP/antihistamine); cytokine release synd (↓ BP, fever, rigors) **Interactions:** ↑ Effects **W/** immunosuppressives; ↑ effects **OF** live virus vaccines; ↑ risk of CNS effects & encephalopathy **W/** indomethacin **Labs:** ↑ BUN, Cr **NIPE:** ⊘ Immunizations, exposure to Infxn; monitor during Inf; use 0.22-mcm filter

Mycophenolic Acid (Myfortic) [Immunosuppressant/Mycophenolic Acid Derivative] **WARNING:** ↑ Risk of Infxns, lymphoma, other CAs, PML; risk of PRG loss & malformation, female of childbearing potential must use contraception Uses: *Prevent rejection after renal transplant* **Action:** Cytostatic to lymphocytes **Dose:** *Adults.* 720 mg PO bid *Peds. BSA 1.19–1.58 m²:* 540 mg bid. *BSA > 1.8 m²:* Adult dose; used w/ steroids & cyclosporine ↓ w/ renal Insuff/neutropenia; take on empty stomach **Caution:** [D, ?/–] **CI:** Component allergy **Disp:** DR tabs 180, 360 mg **SE:** N/V/D, GI bleed, pain, fever, HA, Infxn, HTN, anemia, leukopenia, pure red cell aplasia, edema **Interactions:** ↓ **OF** phenytoin, theophylline; ↓ **W/** antacids, cholestyramine, Fe **Labs:** ↑ Cholesterol; monitor CBC **NIPE:** If GI distress—take w/ food; avoid crowds & people w/ Infxns

Mycophenolate Mofetil (CellCept) [Immunosuppressant/Mycophenolic Acid Derivative] WARNING: ↑ Risk of Infxns, lymphoma, other CAs, PML; risk of PRG loss & malformation; female of childbearing potential must use contraception Uses: *Prevent organ rejection after transplant* Action: Cytostatic to lymphocytes Dose: *Adults.* 1 g PO bid *Peds. BSA 1.2–1.5 m²:* 750 mg PO bid. *BSA > 1.5 m²:* 1 g PO bid; may taper up to 600 mg/m² PO bid; used w/ steroids & cyclosporine; ↓ in renal Insuff or neutropenia *IV:* Infuse over > 2 h *PO:* Take on empty stomach, do not open caps Caution: [D, ?/–] CI: Component allergy; IV use in polysorbate 80 allergy Disp: Caps 250, 500 mg; susp 200 mg/ mL, Inj 500 mg SE: N/V/D, pain, fever, HA, Infxn, HTN, anemia, leukopenia, edema Interactions: ↑ Effects W/ acyclovir, ganciclovir, probenecid; ↑ effects OF acyclovir, ganciclovir; ↓ effects W/ antacids, cholestyramine, cyclosporine, Fe, food; ↓ effects OF OCPs, phenytoin, theophylline Labs: ↑ Cholesterol; monitor CBC NIPE: Use barrier contraception during & 6 wk after drug therapy; ⊘ exposure to Infxn; take w/o food

Nabilone (Cesamet) [CII] [Synthetic Cannabinoid] WARNING: Psychotomimetic Rxns, may persist for 72 h following D/C; caregivers should be present during initial use or dosage modification; pts should not operate heavy machinery; avoid alcohol, sedatives, hypnotics, other psychoactive substances Uses: *Refractory chemotherapy-induced emesis* Action: Synthetic cannabinoid Dose: *Adults.* 1–2 mg PO bid 1–3 h before chemotherapy, 6 mg/d max; may continue for 48 h beyond final chemotherapy dose Caution: [C, ?/–] Elderly, HTN, HF, w/ psychological illness, substance abuse; high protein binding w/ 1st-pass metabolism may lead to drug interactions Disp: Caps 1 mg SE: Drowsiness, vertigo, xerostomia, euphoria, ataxia, HA, difficulty concentrating, tachycardia, ↓ BP Interactions: ↑ CNS depression W/ benzodiazepines, barbiturates, CNS depressants, EtOH; ↑ effects W/ opioids; ↑ effects OF opioids; cross-tolerance W/ opioids NIPE: May require initial dose evening before chemotherapy; Rx only quantity for single Tx cycle

Nabumetone (Relafen) [Analgesic, Anti-Inflammatory, Antipyretic/NSAID] WARNING: May ↑ risk of CV events & GI bleeding, perforation; CI w/ post-op CABG Uses: *OA & RA*, pain Action: NSAID; ↓ prostaglandins Dose: 1000–2000 mg/d ÷ daily–bid w/ food Caution: [C, –] Severe hepatic Dz CI: w/ Peptic ulcer, NSAID sensitivity, after CABG surgery Disp: Tabs 500, 750 mg SE: Dizziness, rash, GI upset, edema, peptic ulcer, ↑ BP Interactions: ↑ Effects W/ aminoglycosides; ↑ effects OF anticoagulants, hypoglycemics, Li, MTX, thrombolytics; ↑ GI effects W/ ASA, corticosteroids, K⁺ supls, EtOH; ↓ effects OF antihypertensives, diuretics NIPE: Photosensitivity—use sunblock; ↑ risk of GI bleed w/ concurrent use of EtOH & tobacco

Nadolol (Corgard) [Antihypertensive, Antianginal/Beta-Blocker] Uses: *HTN & angina* migraine prophylaxis Action: Competitively blocks β-adrenergic receptors (β₁, β₂) Dose: 40–80 mg/d; ↑ to 240 mg/d (angina) or 320 mg/d

(HTN) at 3–7-d intervals; ↓ in renal Insuff & elderly **Caution:** [C (1st tri, D if 2nd or 3rd tri), +] **CI:** Uncompensated CHF, shock, heart block, asthma **Disp:** Tabs 20, 40, 80, 120, 160 mg **SE:** Nightmares, paresthesias, ↓ BP, bradycardia, fatigue **Interactions:** ↑ Effects *W/* antihypertensives, diuretics, nitrates, EtOH; ↑ effects *OF* aminophylline, lidocaine; ↑ risk of HTN *W/* clonidine, ephedrine, epinephrine, MAOIs, phenylephrine, pseudoephedrine; ↑ bradycardia *W/* digitalis glycosides, ephedrine, epi, phenylephrine, pseudoephedrine; ↓ effects *W/* ampicillin, antacids, clonidine, NSAIDs, thyroid meds; ↓ effects *OF* glucagon, theophylline **NIPE:** May ↑ cold sensitivity; ⊘ D/C abruptly

Nafcillin (Nallpen, Unipen) [Antibiotic/Penicillinase-Resistant Penicillin] Uses: *Infxns d/t susceptible strains of *Staphylococcus* & *Streptococcus** **Action:** Bactericidal; β-lactamase–resistant PCN; ↓ cell wall synth *Spectrum:* Good gram(+) except MRSA & enterococcus, no gram(−), poor anaerobe **Dose:** *Adults.* 1–2 g IV q4–6h *Peds.* 50–200 mg/kg/d ÷ q4–6h **Caution:** [B, ?] PCN allergy **CI:** PCN allergy **Disp:** Inj powder 1, 2 g **SE:** Interstitial nephritis, N/D, fever, rash, allergic Rxn **Interactions:** ↑ Effects *OF* MTX; ↓ effects *W/* chloramphenicol, macrolides, tetracyclines; ↓ effects *OF* cyclosporine, OCPs, tacrolimus, warfarin **Labs:** ↑ Serum protein; no adjustments for renal Fxn **NIPE:** Aminoglycosides not compatible, risk of drug inactivation w/ fruit juice/carbonated drinks; monitor for super Infxn; no adjustment for renal Fxn

Naftifine (Naftin) [Antifungal/Antibiotic] Uses: *Tinea pedis, cruris, & corporis* **Action:** Allylamine antifungal, ↓ cell membrane ergosterol synth **Dose:** Apply daily (cream) or bid (gel) **Caution:** [B, ?] **CI:** Component sensitivity **Disp:** 1% cream; gel **SE:** Local irritation **NIPE:** D/C if irritation occurs. Confirm diagnosis w/ KOH smear and/or culture. Avoid occlusive dressings, mucous membranes

Nalbuphine (Nubain) [Analgesic/Narcotic Agonist-Antagonist] Uses: *Mod–severe pain; pre-op & obstetric analgesia* **Action:** Narcotic agonist–antagonist; ↓ ascending pain pathways **Dose:** *Adults. Pain:* 10 mg/70 kg IV/IM/SQ q3–6h; adjust PRN; 20 mg/dose or 160 mg/d max *Anesthesia: Induction:* 0.3–3 mg/kg IV over 10–15 min *Maint:* 0.25–0.5 mg/kg IV q30min *Peds.* 0.2 mg/kg IV or IM, 20 mg max; ↓ w/ renal/in hepatic impair **Caution:** [B, M] w/ opiate use **CI:** Component sensitivity **Disp:** Inj 10, 20 mg/mL **SE:** CNS depression, drowsiness; caution, ↓ BP **Interactions:** ↑ CNS depression *W/* cimetidine, CNS depressants; EtOH ↑ effects *OF* digitoxin, phenytoin, rifampin **Labs:** ↑ Serum amylase, lipase **NIPE:** Monitor for resp depression

Naloxone (Generic) [Antidote/Opioid Antagonist] Uses: *Opioid addiction (diagnosis) & OD* **Action:** Competitive narcotic antagonist **Dose:** *Adults.* 0.4–2 mg IV, IM, or SQ q2–3min; total dose 10 mg max *Peds.* 0.01–0.1 mg/kg/dose IV, IM, or SQ; repeat IV q3min × 3 doses PRN *ECC 2010:* Total reversal of narcotic effects: 0.1 mg/kg IV q2min PRN; max dose 2 mg; smaller doses (1–5 mcg/kg may be used); cont Inf 2–160 mcg/kg/h **Caution:** [B, ?] May precipitate acute withdrawal in addicts **Disp:** Inj 0.4, 1 mg/mL **SE:** ↓ BP, tachycardia, irritability, GI upset, pulm edema **Interactions:** ↓ Effects *OF* opiates **NIPE:** If no response after 10 mg, suspect nonnarcotic cause

Naltrexone (Depade, ReVia, Vivitrol) [Opioid Antagonist]
WARNING: Can cause hepatic injury, CI w/ active liver Dz **Uses:** *EtOH & narcotic addiction* **Action:** Antagonizes opioid receptors **Dose:** *EtOH/narcotic addiction:* 50 mg/d PO; must be opioid-free for 7–10 d *EtOH dependence:* 380 mg IM q4wk (*Vivitrol*) **Caution:** [C, M] **CI:** Acute hep, liver failure, opioid use **Disp:** Tabs 50 mg; Inj 380 mg (*Vivitrol*) **SE:** Hepatotox; insomnia, GI upset, Jt pain, HA, fatigue **Interactions:** ↑ Lethargy & somnolence *W/* thioridazine; ↓ effects *OF* opioids **Labs:** ↑ LFTs **NIPE:** Give IM in gluteal muscle & rotate

Naphazoline (Albalon, Naphcon, Others), Naphazoline & Pheniramine Acetate (Naphcon A, Visine A) [Ophthalmic Antihistamine] **Uses:** *Relieve ocular redness & itching caused by allergy* **Action:** Sympathomimetic α-adrenergic (vasoconstrictor) & antihistamine (pheniramine) **Dose:** 1–2 gtt up to qid, 3 d max **Caution:** [C, +] **CI:** NAG, in children, w/ contact lenses, component allergy **SE:** CV stimulation, dizziness, local irritation **Disp:** Ophthal 0.012%, 0.025%, 0.1%/15 mL; naphazoline & pheniramine 0.025%/0.3% soln **Interactions:** ↑ Risk of HTN crisis *W/* MAOIs, TCAs

Naproxen (Aleve [OTC], Naprosyn, Anaprox) [Analgesic, Anti-Inflammatory, Antipyretic/NSAID] **WARNING:** May ↑ risk of CV events & GI bleeding **Uses:** *Arthritis & pain* **Action:** NSAID; ↓ prostaglandins **Dose:** *Adults & Peds > 12 y.* 200–500 mg bid–tid to 1500 mg/d max *> 2 y. JRA* 5 mg/kg/dose bid; ↓ in hepatic impair **Caution:** [C, (D 3rd tri), –] **CI:** NSAID or ASA triad sensitivity, peptic ulcer, postcoronary artery bypass graft pain, 3rd tri PRG **Disp:** *Tabs:* 220, 250, 375, 500 mg *DR:* 375, 500 mg *CR:* 375, 550 mg *Susp:* 125 mg/5 mL **SE:** Dizziness, pruritus, GI upset, peptic ulcer, edema **Interactions:** ↑ Effects *W/* aminoglycosides; ↑ effects *OF* anticoagulants, hypoglycemics, Li, MTX, thrombolytics; ↑ GI effects *W/* ASA, corticosteroids, K+ supls, NSAIDs, EtOH; ↓ effects *OF* antihypertensives, diuretics **Labs:** ↑ BUN, Cr, LFTs, PT **NIPE:** Take w/ food to ↓ GI upset

Naproxen & Esomeprazole (Vimovo) [NSAID + Proton Pump Inhibitor] **WARNING:** ↑ Risk MI, stroke, PE; CI, CABG surgery pain; ↑ risk GI bleed, gastric ulcer, gastric/duodenal perforation **Uses:** *Pain and/or swelling, RA, OA, ankylosing spondylitis, ↓ risk NSAID associated w/ gastric ulcers* **Action:** NSAID; ↓ prostaglandins & PPI, ↓ gastric acid **Dose:** 375/20 mg (naproxen/esomeprazole) to 500/20 mg PO bid **Caution:** [C (1st, 2nd tri; D 3rd); –] **CI:** PRG 3rd tri; asthma, urticaria from ASA or NSAID; mod–severe hepatic/ renal **Disp:** Tabs (naproxen/esomeprazole) DR 375/20 mg; 500/20 mg **SE:** N/D, Abd pain, gastritis, ulcer, ↑ BP, CHF, edema, serious skin rxn (eg, SJS, etc), ↓ renal Fxn, papillary necrosis **Interactions:** ↑ Effects *OF* saquinavir, hydantoins, sulfonamides, sulfonyureasl; ↑ Li levels; ↑ risk of GI bleed *W/* oral corticosteroid, SSRIs, smoking, EtOH; ↓ effects *OF* diuretics, BB, ACEI **Labs:** May ↑ Li levels;

may cause MTX tox; may ↑ INR on warfarin; monitor levels Li, MTX, INR **NIPE:** Risk of GI adverse events elderly; atrophic gastritis w/ long-term PPI use; possible ↑ risk of fxs w/ all PPI; may ↓ effect BP meds; may ↓ absorption of drugs requiring acid environment

Naratriptan (Amerge) [Migraine Suppressant/5-HT Agonist]
Uses: *Acute migraine* **Action:** Serotonin 5-HT$_1$ receptor agonist **Dose:** 1–2.5 mg PO once; repeat PRN in 4 h; 5 mg/24 h max; ↓ in mild renal/hepatic Insuff, take w/ fluids **Caution:** [C, M] **CI:** Severe renal/hepatic impair, avoid w/ angina, ischemic heart Dz, uncontrolled HTN, cerebrovascular synds, & ergot use **Disp:** Tabs 1, 2.5 mg **SE:** Dizziness, sedation, GI upset, paresthesias, ECG changes, coronary vasospasm, arrhythmias **Interactions:** ↑ Effects *W/* MAOIs, SSRIs; ↑ effects *OF* ergot drugs; ↓ effects *W/* nicotine **NIPE:** Monitor ECG for ↑ PR or QT interval

Natalizumab (Tysabri) [Immunomodulator/Monoclonal Antibody]
WARNING: PML reported **Uses:** *Relapsing MS to delay disability & ↓ recurrences, Crohn Dz* **Action:** Integrin receptor antagonist **Dose:** *Adults.* 300 mg IV q4wk; 2nd-line Tx only **CI:** PML; immune compromise or w/ immunosuppressant **Caution:** [C, ?/–] Baseline MRI to rule out PML **Disp:** Vial 300 mg **SE:** Infxn, immunosuppression; Inf Rxn precluding subsequent use; HA, fatigue, arthralgia; arthralgia **Interactions:** ↑ Risk of Infxn *W/* corticosteroids, immunosuppressants **Labs:** ↑ LFTs **NIPE:** Give slowly to ↓ Rxns; limited distribution (TOUCH Prescribing Program); D/C stat w/ signs of PML (weakness, paralysis, vision loss, impaired speech, cognitive ↓); eval at 3 & 6 mo, then q6mo thereafter

Nateglinide (Starlix) [Hypoglycemic/Amino Acid Derivative]
Uses: *Type 2 DM* **Action:** ↑ Pancreatic insulin release **Dose:** 120 mg PO tid 1–30 min ac; ↓ to 60 mg tid if near target HbA$_{1c}$ **Caution:** [C, –] w/ CYP2C9 metabolized drug (Table 10) **CI:** DKA, type 1 DM **Disp:** Tabs 60, 120 mg **SE:** Hypoglycemia **Interactions:** ↑ Effects of hypoglycemia *W/* nonselective BBs, MAOIs, NSAIDs, salicylates, ↓ effects *W/* corticosteroids, niacin, sympathomimetics, thiazide diuretics, thyroid meds **Labs:** ↓ Glucose **NIPE:** ⊘ Take med if meal skipped

Nebivolol (Bystolic) [Cardioselective Beta-Blocker]
Uses: *HTN* **Action:** β$_1$-Selective blocker **Dose:** *Adults.* 5 mg PO daily, ↑ q2wk to 40 mg/d max, ↓ w/ CrCl < 30 mL/min **Caution:** [D, +/–] w/ bronchospastic Dz, DM, HF, Pheo, w/ CYP2D6 Inhibs **CI:** Bradycardia, cardiogenic shock, decompensated CHF, severe hepatic impair **Disp:** Tabs 5, 10 mg **SE:** HA, fatigue, dizziness **Interactions:** ↑ Effects *W/* CYP2D6 Inhibs: Quinidine, propafenone, paroxetine, fluoxetine; may block epinephrine; **NIPE:** ⊘ D/C abruptly—taper over 1–2 wk

Nefazodone [Antidepressant/Serotonin Modulator]
WARNING: Fatal hep & liver failure possible, D/C if LFTs > 3 × ULN, do not retreat; closely monitor for worsening depression or suicidality, particularly in ped pts **Uses:** *Depression* **Action:** ↓ Neuronal uptake of serotonin & norepinephrine **Dose:** Initial 100 mg PO bid; usual 300–600 mg/d in 2 ÷ doses **Caution:** [C, M] **CI:** w/ MAOIs, pimozide, carbamazepine, alprazolam; active liver Dz **Disp:** Tabs 50, 100,

150, 200, 250 mg **SE:** Postural ↓ BP & allergic Rxns; HA, drowsiness, xerostomia, constipation, GI upset, liver failure **Interactions:** ↑ Risk of hypotension **W/** antihypertensives, nitrates; ↑ effects **OF** alprazolam, CCB, digoxin, HMG-CoA reductase Inhibs, triazolam; ↑ risk of QT prolongation **W/** astemizole, cisapride, pimozide; ↑ risk of serious and/or fatal Rxn **W/** MAOIs; ↓ effects **OF** propranolol **Labs:** ↑ LFTs, cholesterol; ↓ Hct **NIPE:** Take w/o food; may take 2–4 wk for full therapeutic effects; monitor HR, BP

Nelarabine (Arranon) [Antineoplastic/Antimetabolite] WARNING: Fatal neurotox possible **Uses:** *T-cell ALL or T-cell lymphoblastic lymphoma unresponsive > 2 other regimens* **Action:** Nucleoside (deoxyguanosine) analogue **Dose:** *Adults.* 1500 mg/m² IV over 2 h d 1, 3, 5 of 21-d cycle **Peds.** 650 mg/m² IV over 1 h d 1–5 of 21-d cycle **Caution:** [D, ?/–] **Disp:** Vial 250 mg **SE:** Neuropathy, ataxia, Szs, coma, hematologic tox, GI upset, HA, blurred vision **Labs:** Monitor CBC, ↑ transaminase levels, bilirubin **NIPE:** Prehydration, urinary alkalinization, allopurinol before dose; D/C if = grade 2 neurotox occurs; ⊘ live vaccines

Nelfinavir (Viracept) [Antiretroviral/Protease Inhibitor] **Uses:** *HIV Infxn, other agents* **Action:** Protease Inhib causes immature, noninfectious virion production **Dose:** *Adults.* 750 mg PO tid or 1250 mg PO bid **Peds.** 25–35 mg/kg PO tid or 45–55 mg/kg bid; take w/ food **Caution:** [B, –] Many drug interactions **CI:** PKU, w/ triazolam/midazolam use or drug dependent on CYP3A4 (Table 10) **Disp:** Tabs 250, 625 mg; powder 50 mg/g **SE:** Dyslipidemia, lipodystrophy, D, rash **Interactions:** ↑ Effects **W/** erythromycin, ketoconazole, indinavir, ritonavir; ↑ effects **OF** barbiturates, carbamazepine, cisapride, ergot alkaloids, erythromycin, lovastatin, midazolam, phenytoin, saquinavir, simvastatin, triazolam; ↓ effects **W/** barbiturates, carbamazepine, phenytoin, rifabutin, rifampin, St. John's wort; ↓ effects **OF** OCP **Labs:** ↑ LFTs **NIPE:** Take w/ food ↑ absorption; use barrier contraception; PRG registry; tabs can be dissolved in H₂O

Neomycin, Bacitracin, & Polymyxin B (Neosporin Ointment) (See Bacitracin, Neomycin, & Polymyxin B Topical)

Neomycin, Colistin, & Hydrocortisone (Cortisporin-TC Otic Drops); Neomycin, Colistin, Hydrocortisone, & Thonzonium (Cortisporin-TC Otic Susp) [Antibiotic/Aminoglycoside] **Uses:** *Otitis externa*, Infxns of mastoid/fenestration cavities* **Action:** Antibiotic w/ anti-inflammatory **Dose:** *Adults.* 5 gtt in ear(s) tid–qid **Peds.** 3–4 gtt in ear(s) tid–qid **CI:** Component allergy; HSV, vaccinia, varicella **Caution:** [B, ?] **Disp:** Otic gtt & susp **SE:** Local irritation, rash **NIPE:** Shake well, limit use to 10 d/t minimize hearing loss

Neomycin & Dexamethasone (AK-Neo-Dex Ophthalmic, Neo-Decadron Ophthalmic) [Antibiotic/Corticosteroid] **Uses:** *Steroid-responsive inflammatory conditions of the cornea, conjunctiva, lid, & anterior segment* **Action:** Antibiotic w/ anti-inflammatory corticosteroid **Dose:** 1–2 gtt in eye(s) q3–4h or thin coat tid–qid until response, then ↓ to daily **Caution:** [C, ?] **Disp:** Cream neomycin 0.5%/dexamethasone 0.1%; oint neomycin 0.35%/dexamethasone

0.05%; soln neomycin 0.35%/dexamethasone 0.1% **SE:** Local irritation **NIPE:** Use under ophthalmologist's supervision

Neomycin & Polymyxin B (Neosporin Cream) [OTC] [Antibiotic]
Uses: *Infxn in minor cuts, scrapes, & burns* **Action:** Bactericidal **Dose:** Apply bid–qid **Caution:** [C, ?] **CI:** Component allergy **Disp:** Cream neomycin 3.5 mg/polymyxin B 10,000 units/g **SE:** Local irritation **NIPE:** Different from *Neosporin oint*

Neomycin, Polymyxin B, & Dexamethasone (Maxitrol) [Antibiotic/Corticosteroid] **Uses:** *Steroid-responsive ocular conditions w/ bacterial Infxn* **Action:** Antibiotic w/ anti-inflammatory corticosteroid **Dose:** 1–2 gtt in eye(s) q3–4h; apply oint in eye(s) tid–qid **CI:** Component allergy; viral, fungal, TB eye Dz **Caution:** [C, ?] **Disp:** Oint neomycin sulfate 3.5 mg/polymyxin B sulfate 10,000 units/dexamethasone 0.1%/g; susp identical/5 mL **SE:** Local irritation **NIPE:** Use under supervision of ophthalmologist

Neomycin-Polymyxin Bladder Irrigant [Neosporin GU Irrigant] [Antibiotic] **Uses:** *Cont irrigant prevent bacteriuria & gram(−) bacteremia associated w/ indwelling catheter* **Action:** Bactericidal; not for *Serratia* sp or streptococci **Dose:** 1 mL irrigant in 1 L of 0.9% NaCl; cont bladder irrigation w/ 1 L of soln/24 h 10 d max **Caution:** [D] **CI:** Component allergy **Disp:** Soln neomycin sulfate 40 mg & polymyxin B 200,000 units/mL; amp 1, 20 mL **SE:** Rash, neomycin ototox or nephrotox (rare) **NIPE:** Potential for bacterial/fungal super Infxn; not for Inj; use only 3-way catheter for irrigation

Neomycin, Polymyxin, & Hydrocortisone Ophthalmic (Generic) [Antibiotic/Anti-Inflammatory] **Uses:** *Ocular bacterial Infxns* **Action:** Antibiotic w/ anti-inflammatory **Dose:** Apply a thin layer to the eye(s) or 1 gtt daily–qid **Caution:** [C, ?] **Disp:** Ophthal soln; ophthal oint **SE:** Local irritation

Neomycin, Polymyxin, & Hydrocortisone Otic (Cortisporin Otic Solution, Generic Susp) [Antibiotic/ Anti-Inflammatory] **Uses:** *Otitis externa & infected mastoidectomy & fenestration cavities* **Action:** Antibiotic & anti-inflammatory **Dose:** *Adults.* 3–4 gtt in the ear(s) tid–qid *Peds > 2 y.* 3 gtt in the ear(s) tid–qid **CI:** Viral Infxn, hypersensitivity to components **Caution:** [C, ?] **Disp:** Otic susp (generic); otic soln (Cortisporin) **SE:** Local irritation

Neomycin, Polymyxin B, & Prednisolone (Poly-Pred Ophthalmic) [Antibiotic/Corticosteroid] **Uses:** *Steroid-responsive ocular conditions w/ bacterial Infxn* **Action:** Antibiotic & anti-inflammatory **Dose:** 1–2 gtt in eye(s) q4–6h; apply oint in eye(s) tid–qid **Caution:** [C, ?] **Disp:** Susp neomycin/polymyxin B/prednisolone 0.5%/mL **SE:** Irritation **NIPE:** Use under supervision of ophthalmologist

Neomycin Sulfate (Neo-Fradin, Generic) [Antibiotic] **WARNING:** Systemic absorption of oral route may cause neuro-/oto-/nephrotox; resp paralysis possible w/ any route of administration **Uses:** *Hepatic coma, bowel prep* **Action:** Aminoglycoside, poorly absorbed PO; ↓ GI bacterial flora **Dose:** *Adults.* 3–12 g/24 h PO in 3–4 ÷ doses *Peds.* 50–100 mg/kg/24 h PO in 3–4 ÷ doses **Caution:**

[C, ?/−] Renal failure, neuromuscular disorders, hearing impair **CI:** Intestinal obst **Disp:** Tabs 500 mg; PO soln 125 mg/5 mL **SE:** Hearing loss w/ long-term use; rash, N/V **NIPE:** Do not use parenterally (↑ tox); part of the condon bowel prep; also topical form

Nepafenac (Nevanac) [Analgesic, Anti-Inflammatory, Antipyretic/ NSAID] Uses: *Inflammation postcataract surgery* **Action:** NSAID **Dose:** 1 gtt in eye(s) tid 1 d before, & continue 14 d after surgery **CI:** NSAID/ASA sensitivity **Caution:** [C, ?/−] May ↑ bleeding time, delay healing, cause keratitis **Disp:** Susp 3 mL **SE:** Capsular opacity, visual changes, foreign-body sensation, ↑ IOP **Interactions:** ↑ Effects *OF* oral anticoagulants **NIPE:** Prolonged use ↑ risk of corneal damage; shake well before use; separate from other drops by > 5 min

Nesiritide (Natrecor) [Vasodilator/Human B-Type Natriuretic Peptide] Uses: *Acutely decompensated CHF* **Action:** Human B-type natriuretic peptide **Dose:** 2 mcg/kg IV bolus, then 0.01 mcg/kg/min IV **Caution:** [C, ?/−] When vasodilators are not appropriate **CI:** SBP < 90 mm Hg, cardiogenic shock **Disp:** Vials 1.5 mg **SE:** ↓ BP, HA, GI upset, arrhythmias **Interactions:** ↑ hypotension *W/* ACEIs, nitrates **Labs:** ↑ Cr; **NIPE:** Requires cont BP monitoring; some studies indicate ↑ in mortality

Nevirapine (Viramune) [Antiretroviral/NNRTI] WARNING: Reports of fatal hepatotox even w/ short-term use; severe life-threatening skin Rxns (SJS, toxic epidermal necrolysis, & allergic Rxns); monitor closely during 1st 8 wk of Rx **Uses:** *HIV Infxn* **Action:** NNRI **Dose:** *Adults.* Initial 200 mg/d PO × 14 d, then 200 mg bid *Peds. 2 mo−8 y.* 4 mg/kg/d × 14 d, then 7 mg/kg bid *> 8 y.* 4 mg/ kg/d × 14 d, then 4 mg/kg bid max 200 mg/dose for peds (w/o regard to food) **Caution:** [B, −] OCP **Disp:** Tabs 200 mg; susp 50 mg/5 mL **SE:** Life-threatening rash; HA, fever, D, neutropenia, hep **Interactions:** ↑ Effects *W/* clarithromycin, erythromycin; ↓ effects *W/* rifabutin, rifampin, St. John's wort; ↓ effects *OF* clarithromycin, indinavir, ketoconazole, methadone, OCPs, protease Inhibs, warfarin **NIPE:** Use barrier contraception; HIV resistance when given as monotherapy; always use in combo w/ at least 2 additional antiretroviral agent; ⊘ women if CD4 > 250 mcL or men > 400 mcL unless benefit > risk of hepatotox

Niacin (Nicotinic Acid) (Niaspan, Slo-Niacin, Niacor, Nicolar) [Some OTC Forms] [Antilipemic/Vitamin B Complex] Uses: *Sig hyperlipidemia/hypercholesteremia, nutritional supl* **Action:** Vit B₃; ↓ lipolysis; ↓ esterification of triglycerides; ↑ lipoprotein lipase **Dose:** *Hypercholesterolemia.* Start 500 mg PO qhs, ↑ 500 mg q4wk, maint 1–2 g/d; 2 g/d max; qhs w/ low-fat snack; do not crush/chew; niacin supl 1 ER tab PO qd or 100 mg PO qd *Pellagra.* Up to 500 mg/d **Caution:** [C, +] **CI:** Liver Dz, peptic ulcer, arterial hemorrhage **Disp:** ER tabs *(Niaspan)* 500, 750, 1000 mg & *(Slo-Niacin)* 250, 500, 750 mg; tab 500 mg *(Niacor)*; many OTC: tabs 50, 100, 250, 500 mg, ER caps 125, 250, 400 mg, ER tabs 250, 500 mg, elixir 50 mg/5 mL **SE:** Upper body/facial flushing &

warmth; hepatox, GI upset, flatulence, exacerbate peptic ulcer, HA, paresthesias, liver damage, gout, altered glucose control in DM **Interactions:** ↑ Effects *OF* antihypertensives, anticoagulants; ↓ effects *OF* hypoglycemics, probenecid, sulfinpyrazone **Labs:** ✓ Cholesterol, LFTs, if on statins (eg, Lipitor) ✓ CPK & K+ **NIPE:** EtOH & hot beverages ↑ flushing; flushing ↓ by taking ASA or NSAID 30–60 min prior to dose *RDA adults:* male 16 mg/d, female 14 mg/d

Niacin & Lovastatin (Advicor) [Nicotinic Acid Derivative + HMG-CoA Reductase Inhibitor] **Uses:** *Hypercholesterolemia* **Action:** Combo antilipemic agent, w/ HMG-CoA reductase Inhib **Dose:** *Adults.* Niacin 500 mg/lovastatin 20 mg, titrate q4wk, max niacin 2000 mg/lovastatin 40 mg **Caution:** [X, –] See individual agents, D/C w/ LFTs > 3 × ULN **CI:** PRG **Disp:** Niacin mg/lovastatin mg: 500/20, 750/20, 1000/20, 1000/40 tabs **SE:** Flushing, myopathy/rhabdomyolysis, N, Abd pain **Interactions:** ↑ Effects *OF* gaglionic blockers, vasoactive drugs; separate dosing of bile acid sequestrants by 4–6 h; ↑ risk of myopathy *W/* cyclosporine; ↑ effects *OF* antihypertensives, anticoagulants **Labs:** ↑ LFTs; monitor CK, PT, plts **NIPE:** ↓ Flushing by taking ASA or NSAID 30 min before

Niacin & Simvastatin (Simcor) [HMG-CoA Reductase Inhibitor & a Nicotinic Acid Derivative] **Uses:** *Hypercholesterolemia* **Action:** Combo antilipemic agent w/ HMG-CoA reductase Inhib **Dose:** *Adults.* Niacin 500 mg/simvastatin 20 mg, titrate q4wk not to exceed niacin 2000 mg/simvastatin 40 mg **Caution:** [X, –] See individual agents **CI:** PRG **Disp:** Niacin/simvastatin: 500/20, 750/20, 1000/20 tabs **SE:** Flushing, myopathy/rhabdomyolysis, N, Abd pain **Interactions:** ↑ Effects *W/* amiodarone, verapamil; ↑ risk of postural hypotension *W/* ganglionic blockers, vasoactive drugs **Labs:** ↑ LFTs; monitor blood glucose, PT, plts; D/C therapy if LFTs > 3 × nl **NIPE:** Take hs w/ low-fat snack; swallow whole; separate dosing of bile acid sequestrants by 4–6 h; ↓ flushing by taking ASA or NSAID 30 min before

Nicardipine (Cardene) [Antianginal/Antihypertensive/CCB] **Uses:** *Chronic stable angina & HTN*; prophylaxis of migraine **Action:** CCB **Dose:** *Adults.* PO: 20–40 mg PO tid *SR:* 30–60 mg PO bid *IV:* 5 mg/h IV cont Inf; ↑ by 2.5 mg/h q15min to max 15 mg/h *Peds.* (Not established) *PO:* 20–30 mg PO q8h *IV:* 0.5–5 mcg/kg/min; ↓ in renal/hepatic impair **Caution:** [C, ?/–] Heart block, CAD **CI:** Cardiogenic shock, AS **Disp:** Caps 20, 30 mg; SR caps 30, 45, 60 mg; Inj 2.5 mg/mL **SE:** Flushing, tachycardia, ↓ BP, edema, HA **Notes:** *PO-to-IV conversion:* 20 mg tid = 0.5 mg/h, 30 mg tid = 1.2 mg/h, 40 mg tid = 2.2 mg/h **Interactions:** ↑ Effects *W/* cimetidine, grapefruit juice; ↑ effects *OF* cyclosporine; ↑ hypotension *W/* antihypertensives, fentanyl, nitrates, quinidine, EtOH; ↑ dysrhythmias *W/* digoxin, disopyramide, phenytoin; ↓ effects *W/* NSAIDs, rifampin; high-fat food **Labs:** ↑ LFTs **NIPE:** ↑ Risk of photosensitivity—use sunblock; take w/ food (not high fat)

Nicotine Gum (Nicorette, Others) [OTC] [Smoking Deterrent/ Cholinergic] **Uses:** *Aid to smoking cessation, relieve nicotine withdrawal* **Action:** Systemic delivery of nicotine **Dose:** Wk 1–6 one piece q1–2h PRN; wk

7–9 one piece q2–4h PRN; wk 10–12 one piece q4–8h PRN; max 24 pieces/d **Caution:** [C, ?] **CI:** Life-threatening arrhythmias, unstable angina **Disp:** 2, 4 mg/piece; mint, orange, original flavors **SE:** Tachycardia, HA, GI upset, hiccups **Interactions:** ↑ Effects *W/* cimetidine; ↑ effects *OF* catecholamines, cortisol; ↑ hemodynamic & A-V blocking effects *OF* adenosine; ↓ effects *W/* coffee, cola **NIPE:** Chew 30 min for full dose of nicotine; ↓ absorption *W/* coffee, soda, juices, wine w/in 15 min; must stop smoking & perform behavior modification for max effect; use at least 9 pieces 1st 6 wk; > 25 cigarette/d use 4 mg; < 25 cigarette/d use 2 mg

Nicotine Nasal Spray (Nicotrol NS) [Smoking Deterrent/Cholinergic] Uses: *Aid to smoking cessation, relieve nicotine withdrawal* **Action:** Systemic delivery of nicotine **Dose:** 0.5 mg/activation; 1–2 doses/h, 5 doses/h max; 40 doses/d max **Caution:** [D, M] **CI:** Life-threatening arrhythmias, unstable angina **Disp:** Nasal inhaler 10 mg/mL **SE:** Local irritation, tachycardia, HA, taste perversion **Interactions:** ↑ Effects *W/* cimetidine, blue cohash; ↑ effects *OF* catecholamines, cortisol; ↑ hemodynamic & A-V blocking effects *OF* adenosine **NIPE:** ⊘ In pts w/ chronic nasal disorders or severe reactive airway Dz; ↑ incidence of cough; must stop smoking & perform behavior modification for max effect; 1 dose = 1 spray each nostril = 1 mg

Nicotine Transdermal (Habitrol, Nicoderm CQ [OTC], Others) [Smoking Deterrent/Cholinergic] Uses: *Aid to smoking cessation; relief of nicotine withdrawal* **Action:** Systemic delivery of nicotine **Dose:** Individualized; 1 patch (14–21 mg/d) & taper over 6 wk **Caution:** [D, M] **CI:** Life-threatening arrhythmias, unstable angina **Disp:** *Habitrol & Nicoderm CQ:* 7, 14, 21 mg of nicotine/24 h **SE:** Insomnia, pruritus, erythema, local site Rxn, tachycardia, vivid dreams **Interactions:** ↑ Effects *W/* cimetidine, blue cohash; ↑ effects *OF* catecholamines, cortisol; ↑ hemodynamic & A-V blocking effects *OF* adenosine; ↑ HTN *W/* bupropion **NIPE:** Change application site daily; wear patch 16–24 h; must stop smoking & perform behavior modification for max effect; > 10 cigarette/d start w/ 2-mg patch; < 10 cigarette/d 1-mg patch

Nifedipine (Procardia, Procardia XL, Adalat CC) [Antihypertensive, Antianginal/CCB] Uses: *Vasospastic or chronic stable angina & HTN*; tocolytic **Action:** CCB **Dose:** *Adults.* SR tabs 30–90 mg/d *Tocolysis:* Per local protocol *Peds.* 0.25–0.9 mg/kg/24 h ÷ tid–qid **Caution:** [C, +] Heart block, AS **CI:** IR prep for urgent or emergent HTN; AMI **Disp:** Caps 10, 20 mg; SR tabs 30, 60, 90 mg **SE:** HA common on initial Rx; reflex tachycardia may occur w/ regular-release dosage forms; peripheral edema, ↓ BP, flushing, dizziness **Interactions:** ↑ Effects *W/* antihypertensives, azole antifungals, cimetidine, cisapride, CCBs, diltiazem, famotidine, nitrates, quinidine, ranitidine, EtOH, grapefruit juice; ↑ effects *OF* digitalis glycosides, phenytoin, vincristine; ↓ effects *W/* barbiturates, nafcillin, NSAIDs, phenobarbital, rifampin, St. John's wort, tobacco; ↓ effects *OF* quinidine **Labs:** ↑ LFTs **NIPE:** Adalat CC & Procardia XL not interchangeable; SL administration not OK; ↑ risk of photosensitivity—use sunblock

Nilotinib (Tasigna) [Kinase Inhibitor] WARNING: May ↑ QT interval; sudden deaths reported, use w/ caution in hepatic failure; administration on empty stomach Uses: *Ph(+) CML, refractory or at first diagnosis* Action: TKI Dose: *Adults.* 400 mg bid, on empty stomach 1 h prior or 2 h post meal Caution: [D, ?/–] Avoid w/ CYP3A4 Inhibs/inducers (Table 10), adjust w/ hepatic impair, heme tox, QT ↑, avoid QT-prolonging agents CI: Bilirubin > 3× ULN, AST/ALT > 5× ULN, resume at 400 mg/d once levels return to nl Disp: 200 mg caps SE: Anemia, N/V/D, rash, edema Interactions: ↑ Effects W/ strong Inhibs of CYP3A4 such as ketoconazole, itraconazole, clarithromycin, atazanavir, indinavir, nefazodone, nelfinavir, ritonavir, saquinavir, telithromycin, voriconazole; grapefruit; strong CYP3A4 inducers ↓ effects W/ dexamethasone, phenytoin, carbamazepine, rifampin, phenobarbital; St. John's wort; this drug is an Inhib of CYP3A4, CYP2C8, CYP2C9, CYP2D6, UGT1A1 enzymes & ↑ conc of drugs metabolized by these enzymes Labs: ↓ WBCs, plts; monitor CBCs q2wk for 1st 2 mo, then once monthly; monitor ECG at baseline, after 7 d, then periodically & after dose changes; monitor serum lipase, LFTs NIPE: Use chemotherapy precautions when handling; ⊘ PRG or breast-feeding—use adequate contraception

Nilutamide (Nilandron) [Antineoplastic/Antiandrogen] WARNING: Interstitial pneumonitis possible; most cases in 1st 3 mo; check CXR before & during Rx Uses: *Combo w/ surgical castration for met PCa* Action: Nonsteroidal antiandrogen Dose: 300 mg/d PO in ÷ doses × 30 d, then 150 mg/d Caution: [Not used in females] CI: Severe hepatic impair, resp Insuff Disp: Tabs 150 mg SE: Interstitial pneumonitis, hot flashes, ↓ libido, impotence, N/V/D, gynecomastia, hepatic dysfunction Interactions: ↑ Effects OF phenytoin, theophylline, warfarin Labs: ↑ LFTs (monitor) NIPE: Take w/o regard to food; visual adaptation may be delayed; may cause Rxn when taken w/ EtOH

Nimodipine (Nimotop) [Cerebral Vasodilator/CCB] WARNING: Do not give IV or by other parenteral routes can cause death Uses: *Prevent vasospasm following subarachnoid hemorrhage* Action: CCB Dose: 60 mg PO q4h for 21 d; ↓ in hepatic failure Caution: [C, ?] CI: Component sensitivity Disp: Caps 30 mg SE: ↓BP, HA, constipation Interactions: ↑Effects W/ other CCB; grapefruit juice, EtOH; ↓ effects W/ ephedra, St. John's wort, any food Labs: ↑ LFTs NIPE: Give via NG tube if caps cannot be swallowed whole, PO administration only; ↑ risk of photosensitivity—use sunblock

Nisoldipine (Sular) [Antihypertensive/CCB] Uses: *HTN* Action: CCB Dose: 8.5–34 mg/d PO; take on empty stomach; ↓ start doses w/ elderly or hepatic impair Caution: [C, –] Disp: ER tabs 8.5, 17, 25.5, 34 mg SE: Edema, HA, flushing, ↓ BP Interactions: ↑ Effects W/ antihypertensives, cimetidine, nitrates, EtOH, high-fat foods; ↓ effects W/ phenytoin, St. John's wort NIPE: Do not take w/ grapefruit juice or high-fat meal

Nitazoxanide (Alinia) [Anti-Infective/Antiprotozoal] Uses: *Cryptosporidium or Giardia lamblia-induced D* Action: Antiprotozoal interferes w/

pyruvate ferredoxin oxidoreductase *Spectrum: Cryptosporidium, Giardia* **Dose:** *Adults.* 500 mg PO q12h × 3 d *Peds. 1–3 y.* 100 mg PO q12h × 3 d *4–11 y.* 200 mg PO q12h × 3 d *> 12 y.* 500 mg q12h × 3 d; take w/ food **Caution:** [B, ?] Not effective in HIV or immunocompromised **Dose:** 100 mg/5 mL PO susp, 500 tab **SE:** Abd pain **Interactions:** ↑ Effects W/ warfarin **NIPE:** Susp contains sucrose, interacts w/ highly protein-bound drugs

Nitrofurantoin (Furadantin, Macrodantin, Macrobid) [Urinary Anti-Infective] WARNING: Pulm fibrosis possible **Uses:** *Prophylaxis & Rx UTI* **Action:** Bacteriocidal; interferes w/ carbohydrate metabolism *Spectrum:* Some gram(+) & (−) bacteria; *Pseudomonas, Serratia,* & most *Proteus* resistant **Dose:** *Adults. Prophylaxis:* 50–100 mg/d PO Rx: 50–100 mg PO qid × 7 d *Macrobid:* 100 mg PO bid × 7 d *Peds. Prophylaxis:* 1–2 mg/kg/d ÷ 1–2 doses, max 100 mg/d Rx: 5–7 mg/kg/24 h in 4 ÷ doses (w/ food/milk/antacid) **Caution:** [B, +/not OK if child < 1 mo] Avoid w/ CrCl < 60 mL/min **CI:** Renal failure, infants < 1 mo, PRG at term **Disp:** Caps 25, 50, 100 mg; susp 25 mg/5 mL **SE:** GI effects, dyspnea, various acute/chronic pulm Rxns, peripheral neuropathy, hemolytic anemia w/ G6PD deficiency, rare aplastic anemia **Interactions:** ↑ Effects W/ probenecid, sulfinpyrazone; ↓ effects W/ antacids, quinolones **Labs:** ↑ Serum bilirubin, alk phos **NIPE:** Take W/ food; may turn urine brown; macrocrystals (Macrodantin) cause < N than other forms; not for comp UTI

Nitroglycerin (Nitrostat, Nitrolingual, Nitro-Bid Ointment, Nitro-Bid IV, Nitrodisc, Transderm-Nitro, NitroMist, Others) [Antianginal, Vasodilator/Nitrate] **Uses:** *Angina pectoris, acute & prophylactic therapy, CHF, BP control* **Action:** Relaxes vascular smooth muscle, dilates coronary arteries **Dose:** *Adults. SL:* 1 tab q5min SL PRN for 3 doses *Translingual:* 1–2 metered-doses sprayed onto PO mucosa q3–5min, max 3 doses *PO:* 2.5–9 mg tid *IV:* 5–20 mcg/min, titrated to effect *Topical:* Apply 1/2 in of oint to chest wall tid, wipe off at night *Transdermal:* 0.2–0.4 mg/h/patch daily; *aerosol* 1 spray at 5-min intervals, max 3 doses *ECC 2010: IV bolus:* 12.5–25 mcg (if no spray or SL dose given) *Inf:* Start 10 mcg/min,↑ by 10 mcg/dn q3–5min until desired effect; ceiling dose typically 200 mcg/min *SL:* 0.3–0.4 mg,repeat q5min *Aerosol spray:* Spray 0.5–1 s at 5-min intervals *Peds.* 0.25–0.5 mcg/kg/min IV, titrate *ECC 2010: HF, HTN emergency, Pulm HTN:* Cont Inf 0.25–0.5 mcg/kg/min initial, titrate 1 mcg/kg/min q15–20min (typical dose 1–5 mcg/kg/min) **Caution:** [B, ?] Restrictive cardiomyopathy **CI:** w/ Sildenafil, tadalafil, vardenafil, head trauma, NAG, pericardial tamponade, constrictive pericarditis **Disp:** SL tabs 0.3, 0.4, 0.6 mg; translingual spray 0.4 mg/dose; SR caps 2.5, 6.5, 9 mg; Inj 0.1, 0.2, 0.4 mg/mL (premixed); 5 mg/mL Inj soln; oint 2%; transdermal patches 0.1, 0.2, 0.4, 0.6 mg/h; aerosol (*NitroMist*) 0.4 mg/spray **SE:** HA, ↓ BP, lightheadedness, GI upset **Interactions:** ↑ Hypotensive effects W/ antihypertensives, phenothiazine, sildenafil, tadalafil, vardenafil, EtOH; ↓ effects W/ ergot alkaloids; ↓ effects OF SL tabs & spray W/ antihistamines, phenothiazine, TCAs **Labs:** False ↑ cholesterol, triglycerides **NIPE:**

Nitrate tolerance w/ chronic use after 1–2 wk; minimize by providing 10–12 h nitrate-free period daily, using shorter-acting nitrates tid, & removing LA patches & oint before sleep to ↓ tolerance

Nitroprusside (Nipride, Nitropress) [Antihypertensive/Vasodilator] Uses: *Hypertensive crisis, CHF, controlled ↓ BP perioperation (↓ bleeding)*, aortic dissection, pulm edema **Action:** ↓ Systemic vascular resistance **Dose:** *Adults & Peds.* 0.5–10 mcg/kg/min IV Inf, titrate; usual dose 3 mcg/kg/min *ECC 2010:* 0.1 mcg/kg/min start, titrate dose (max 5–10 mcg/kg/min) *Peds. ECC 2010:* **Cardiogenic shock, severe HTN:** 0.3–1 mcg/kg/min, then titrate to 8 mcg/kg/min PRN **Caution:** [C, ?] ↓ Cerebral perfusion **CI:** High output failure, compensatory HTN **Disp:** Inj 25 mg/mL **SE:** Excessive hypotensive effects, palpitations, HA **Interactions:** ↑ Effects *W/* antihypertensives, anesthetics, sildenafil, tadalafil, vardenafil; ↑ risk of arrhythmias *W/* TCA **Labs:** ↑ Cr **NIPE:** Thiocyanate (metabolite w/ renal excretion) w/ tox at 5–10 mg/dL, more likely if used for > 2–3 d; w/ aortic dissection use w/ BB; discard colored soln other than light brown

Nizatidine (Axid, Axid AR [OTC]) [Gastric Antisecretory/H₂-Receptor Antagonist] Uses: *Duodenal ulcers, GERD, heartburn* **Action:** H₂-Receptor antagonist **Dose:** *Adults. Active ulcer:* 150 mg PO bid or 300 mg PO hs; maint 150 mg PO hs *GERD:* 150 mg PO bid *Heartburn:* 75 mg PO bid *Peds. GERD:* 10 mg/kg PO bid in ÷ doses, 150 mg bid max; ↓ in renal impair **Caution:** [B, ?] **CI:** H₂-Receptor antagonist sensitivity **Disp:** Tabs 75 mg [OTC]; caps 150, 300 mg; soln 15 mg/mL **SE:** Dizziness, HA, constipation, D **Interactions:** ↑ Effects *OF* salicylates, EtOH; ↓ effects *W/* antacids, tomato/mixed veg juice **Labs:** ↑ LFTs, uric acid **NIPE:** Smoking ↑ gastric acid secretion

Norepinephrine (Levophed) [Adrenergic Agonist/Vasopressor/Sympathomimetic] Uses: *Acute ↓ BP, cardiac arrest (adjunct)* **Action:** Peripheral vasoconstrictor of arterial/venous beds **Dose:** *Adults.* 8–30 mcg/min IV, titrate *Peds.* 0.05–0.1 mcg/kg/min IV, titrate **Caution:** [C, ?] **CI:** ↓ BP d/t hypovolemia, vascular thrombosis, do not use w/ cyclopropane/halothane anesthetics **Disp:** Inj 1 mg/mL **SE:** Bradycardia, arrhythmia **Interactions:** ↑ HTN *W/* antihistamines, BBs, ergot alkaloids, guanethidine, MAOIs, methyldopa, oxytocic meds; interaction w/ TCAs leads to severe HTN; ↑ risk of arrhythmias *W/* cyclopropane, halothane **Labs:** ↑ Glucose **NIPE:** Correct vol depletion as much as possible before vasopressors; use large vein to avoid extrav; phentolamine 5–10 mg/10 mL NS injected locally for extrav

Norethindrone Acetate/Ethinyl Estradiol Tablets (Femhrt) (See Estradiol/Norethindrone Acetate)

Norfloxacin (Noroxin, Chibroxin Ophthal) [Antibiotic/Fluoroquinolone] **WARNING:** Use associated w/ tendon rupture & tendonitis Uses: *Comp & uncomp UTI d/t gram(−) bacteria, prostatitis, GC*, infectious D, conjunctivitis **Action:** Quinolone, ↓ DNA gyrase, bactericidal. *Spectrum:* Broad gram(+) & (−) *E faecalis, E coli, K pneumoniae, P mirabilis, P aeruginosa, S epidermidis,* & *S* *saprophyticus* **Dose:** *Uncomp UTI (E coli, K pneumoniae, P mirabilis):* 400 mg PO bid × 3 d; other uncomp UTI Rx × 7–10 d *Comp UTI:* 400 mg q12h for 10–21 d PO bid *GC:* 800 mg × 1 dose *Prostatitis:* 400 mg PO bid × 28 d. *Gastroenteritis, travelers D:* 400 mg PO × 1–3 d; take 1 h ac or 2 h pc *Adults & Peds > 1 y.* *Ophthal:* 1 gtt each eye qid for 7 d; CrCl < 30 mL/min use 400 mg qd **Caution:** [C, −] Quinolone sensitivity w/ some antiarrhythmics **CI:** h/o allergy or tendon problems **Disp:** Tabs 400 mg; ophthal 3 mg/mL **SE:** Photosensitivity, HA, dizziness, asthenia, GI upset, pseudomembranous colitis; ocular burning w/ ophthal **Interactions:** ↑ Effects W/ probenecid; ↑ effects OF diazepam, theophylline, caffeine, metoprolol, propranolol, phenytoin, warfarin; ↓ effects W/ antacids, didanosine, Fe salts, mg, sucralfate, NaHCO₃, Zinc; ↓ effects W/ food **Labs:** ↑ LFTs, BUN, SCr **NIPE:** ⊘ Give to children < 18 y except for opthal sol; ↑ fluids to 2–3 L/d; may cause photosensitivity—use sunblock; good conc in the kidney & urine, poor blood levels; not for urosepsis; CDC suggests do not use for GC; ↑ risk of developing fluoroquinolone-associated tendonitis & tendon rupture is higher in pts > 60 y, in those taking corticosteroids, & in kidney, heart, & lung transplant recipients

Nortriptyline (Pamelor) [Antidepressant/TCA] WARNING: ↑ Suicide risk in pts < 24 y w/ major depressive/other psychological disorders esp during 1st mo of Tx; risk ↓ pts > 65 y; observe all pts for clinical Sxs; not for ped use **Uses:** *Endogenous depression* **Action:** TCA; ↑ synaptic CNS levels of serotonin and/or norepinephrine **Dose:** *Adults.* 25 mg PO tid–qid; > 150 mg/d not OK *Elderly.* 10–25 mg hs *Peds 6–7 y.* 10 mg/d *8–11 y.* 10–20 mg/d *> 11 y.* 25–35 mg/d, ↓ w/ hepatic Insuff **Caution:** [D, −] NAG, CV Dz CI: TCA allergy, use w/ MAOI **Disp:** Caps 10, 25, 50, 75 mg; soln 10 mg/5 mL **SE:** Anticholinergic (blurred vision, retention, xerostomia, sedation) **Interactions:** ↑ Effects W/ antihistamines, CNS depressants, cimetidine, fluoxetine, OCP, phenothiazine, quinidine, EtOH; ↑ effects OF anticoagulants; ↑ risk of HTN W/ clonidine, levodopa, sympathomimetics; ↓ effects W/ barbiturates, carbamazepine, rifampin **Labs:** ↑ Serum bilirubin, alk phos **NIPE:** Concurrent use W/ MAOIs have resulted in HTN, Szs, death; ↑ risk of photosensitivity—use sunscreen; max effect may take > 2–3 wk

Nystatin (Mycostatin) [Anti-Infective/Antifungal] Uses: *Mucocutaneous Candida Infxns (oral, skin, Vag)* **Action:** Alters membrane permeability *Spectrum:* Susceptible Candida sp **Dose:** *Adults & Peds. PO:* 400,000–600,000 units PO "swish & swallow" qid *Vag:* 1 tab vaginally hs × 2 wk *Topical:* Apply bid–tid to area *Peds Infants.* 200,000 units PO q6h **Caution:** [B (C PO), +] **Disp:** PO susp 100,000 units/mL; PO tabs 500,000 units; troches 200,000 units; Vag tabs 100,000 units; topical cream/oint 100,000 units/g, powder 100,000 units/g **SE:** GI upset, SJS **NIPE:** Store susp up to 10 d in refrigerator; not absorbed PO; not for systemic Infxns

Octreotide (Sandostatin, Sandostatin LAR) [Antidiarrheal/ Hormone] Uses: *↓ Severe D associated w/ carcinoid & neuroendocrine GI tumors (eg, vasoactive intestinal peptide-secreting tumor [VIPoma], ZE synd), acromegaly*; bleeding esophageal varices **Action:** LA peptide; mimics natural somatostatin **Dose:** *Adults.* 100–600 mcg/d SQ/IV in 2–4 ÷ doses; start 50 mcg daily–bid *Sandostatin LAR (depot):* 10–30 mg IM q4wk **Peds.** 1–10 mcg/kg/24 h SQ in 2–4 ÷ doses **Caution:** [B, +] Hepatic/renal impair **Disp:** Inj 0.05, 0.1, 0.2, 0.5, 1 mg/mL; 10, 20, 30 mg/5 mL LAR depot **SE:** N/V, Abd discomfort, flushing, edema, fatigue, cholelithiasis, hyper-/hypoglycemia, hep, hypothyroidism **Interactions:** ↓ Effects *OF* cyclosporine, vit B_{12} **Labs:** Small ↑ LFTs, ↓ serum thyroxine, vit B_{12} **NIPE:** May alter effects of hypoglycemics; stabilize for at least 2 wk before changing to LAR form

Ofatumumab (Arzerra) [MoAb] **WARNING:** Administer only by physician experienced in chemotherapy. Do not give IV push d/t severe Inf Rxn **Uses:** *Rx refractory CLL* **Action:** MoAb, binds CD20 molecule on B-lymphocytes w/ cell lysis **Dose:** *Adults.* 300 mg (0.3 mg/mL) IV wk 1, then 2000 mg (2 mg/mL) weekly × 7 doses, then 2000 mg q4wk × 4 doses. Titrate Inf; start 12 mL/h × 30 min, ↑ 25 mL/h for 30 min, ↑ to 50 mL/h × 30 min, ↑ to 100 mL/h × 30 min, then 200 mL/h for duration.**Caution:** [C, ?] **Disp:** Inj 20 mg/mL (5 mL) **SE:** Inf Rxns (bronchospasm, pulm edema, ↑/↓ BP, syncope, cardiac ischemia, angioedema), anemia, fever, fatigue, rash, N/D, pneumonia, Infxns; do not restart if grade 4 Rxn occurs. **Labs:** ↓ WBC, HMG; monitor CBC **NIPE:** Premedicate w/ APAP, antihistamine, & IV steroid; avoid w/ live viral vaccines. Monitor for neurologic changes

Ofloxacin (Floxin) [Antibiotic/Fluoroquinolone] **WARNING:** Use associated w/ tendon rupture & tendonitis **Uses:** *Lower resp tract, skin & skin structure, & UTI, prostatitis, uncomp GC, & Chlamydia Infxns* **Action:** Bactericidal; ↓ DNA gyrase *Broad-spectrum gram(+) & (−): S pneumoniae, S aureus, S pyogenes, H influenzae, P mirabilis, N gonorrhoeae, C trachomatis, & E coli* **Dose:** *Adults & Peds > 1 y* 200–400 mg PO bid or IV q12h *Adults & Peds > 1 y.* Ophthal: 1–2 gtt in eye(s) q2–4h for 2 d, then qid × 5 more d *Adults & Peds > 12 y.* Otic: 10 gtt in ear(s) bid for 10 d *Peds 1–12 y.* Otic: 5 gtt in ear(s) for 10 d; ↓ in renal impair; take on empty stomach **Caution:** [C, −] ↓ Absorption w/ antacids, sucralfate, Al^{2+}-, Ca^{2+}-, Mg^{2+}-, Fe^{2+}-, Zn^{2+}-containing drugs, h/o Szs **CI:** Quinolone allergy **Disp:** Tabs 200, 300, 400 mg; Inj 20, 40 mg/mL; ophthal & otic 0.3% **SE:** N/V/D, photosensitivity, insomnia, HA, local irritation **Interactions:** ↑ Effects *W/* cimetidine, probenecid; ↑ effects *OF* procainamide, theophylline, warfarin; ↑ risk of tendon rupture *W/* corticosteroids; ↓ effects *W/* antacids, antineoplastics, Ca, didanosine, Fe, $NaHCO_3$, sucralfate, Zinc **NIPE:** Take w/o food; use sunscreen; ↑ fluids to 2–3 L/d; ophthal form OK in ears

Ofloxacin Ophthalmic (Ocuflox Ophthalmic) [Antibiotic/Fluoroquinolone] **Uses:** *Bacterial conjunctivitis, corneal ulcer* **Action:** See Ofloxacin **Dose:** *Adults & Peds > 1 y.* 1–2 gtt in eye(s) q2–4h × 2 d, then qid × 5 more d **Caution:** [C, +/−] **CI:** Quinolone allergy **Disp:** Ophthal 0.3% soln **SE:** Burning, hyperemia, bitter taste, chemosis, photophobia **NIPE:** Ophthal form OK in ears

Ofloxacin Otic (Floxin Otic, Floxin Otic Singles) [Antibiotic/Fluoroquinolone] Uses: *Otitis externa; chronic suppurative otitis media w/ perforated drums; otitis media in peds w/ tubes* Action: See Ofloxacin Dose: *Adults & Peds > 13 y. Otitis externa:* 10 gtt in ear(s) × 7–14 d *Peds 1–12 y. Otitis media:* 5 gtt in ear(s) bid × 10 d Caution: [C, –] CI: Quinolone allergy Disp: Otic 0.3% soln 5/10 mL bottles; singles 0.25 mL foil pack SE: Local irritation NIPE: OK w/ tubes/perforated drums; 10 gtt = 0.5 mL

Olanzapine (Zyprexa, Zydis) [Antipsychotic/Thienobenzodiazepine] WARNING: ↑ Mortality in elderly w/ dementia-related psychosis Uses: *Bipolar mania, schizophrenia*, psychotic disorders, acute agitation in schizophrenia Action: DA & serotonin antagonist; atypical antipsychotic Dose: *Bipolar/schizophrenia:* 5–10 mg/d, weekly PRN, 20 mg/d max *Agitation:* 5–10 mg IM q2–4h PRN, 30 mg d/max Caution: [C, –] Disp: Tabs 2.5, 5, 7.5, 10, 15, 20 mg; PO disintegrating tabs (*Zyprexa, Zydis*) 5, 10, 15, 20 mg; Inj 10 mg SE: HA, somnolence, orthostatic ↓ BP, tachycardia, dystonia, xerostomia, constipation, hyperglycemia; ↑ wgt, & sedation may be ↑ in peds Interactions: ↑ Effects W/ fluvoxamine; ↑ sedation W/ CNS depressants, EtOH; ↑ Szs W/ anticholinergics, CNS depressants; ↑ hypotension W/ antihypertensives, diazepam; ↓ effects W/ activated charcoal, carbamazepine, omeprazole, rifampin, St. John's wort, tobacco; ↓ effects OF DA agonists, levodopa Labs: ↑ LFTs, ↑ prolactin levels NIPE: ↑ Risk of tardive dyskinesia, photosensitivity—use sunscreen, body temperature impair; takes wk to titrate dose; smoking ↓ levels; may be confused w/ Zyrtec or Zyprexa Relprevv

Olanzapine, Long-Acting Parenteral (Zyprexa Relprevv): [Antipsychotic/Thienobenzodiazepine] WARNING: ↑ Risk for severe sedation/coma following parenteral Inj, observe closely for 3 h in appropriate facility; restricted distribution; ↑ mortality in elderly w/ dementia-related psychosis; not approved for dementia-related psychosis Uses: *Schizophrenia* Action: See Olanzapine Dose: *IM:* 150 mg/2 wk, 300 mg/4 wk, 210 mg/2 wk, 405 mg/4 wk, or 300 mg/2 wk Caution: [C, –] IM only, do not confuse w/ Zyprexa IM; can cause neuroleptic malignant synd, ↑ glucose/lipids/prolactin, ↓ BP, tardive dyskinesia, cognitive impair, ↓ CBC CI: None Disp: Vials, 210,300,405 mg SE:HA, sedation, ↑ wgt, cough, N/V/D, ↑ appetite,dry mouth, nasopharyngitis, somnolence Interactions: ↑ Risk of hypotension W/ antihypertensives, benzodiazepines, EtOH; ↓ effects W/ rifampin, omeprazole, carbamazepine, others that induce CYP1A2; ↓ effects OF levodopa, DA agonists Labs: ✓ Glucose/lipids/CBC baseline & periodically NIPE: Efficacy shown w/o need for oral supplementation for 2–4 wk depending on dose; smokers may have ↑ metabolism of drug

Olmesartan & Hydrochlorothiazide (Benicar, Benicar HCT) [Antihypertensive/ARB/ARB + HCTZ] WARNING: Use in PRG 2nd/3rd tri can harm fetus; D/C when PRG detected Uses: *Hypertension, alone or in combo* Action: Benicar ARB; Benicar HCT ARB w/ diuretic HCTZ Dose: *Adults. Benicar:* 20–40 mg qd; *Benicar HCT:* 20–40 mg olmesartan w/ 12.5–25 mg HCTZ based on effect *Peds 6–16 y.* Benicar: < 35 Kg, start 10 mg PO, range 10–20 mg qd; ≥ 35 Kg, start 20 mg PO qd, target 20–40 mg qd **Caution:** [C (1st tri, D 2nd, 3rd tri); ?/–] *Benicar HCT* not rec w/ CrCl < 30 mL/min; follow closely if vol depleted with start of med **CI:** Component allergy **Disp:** *Benicar* tabs mg olmesartan 5, 20, 40 *Benicar HCT* mg olmesartan/mg HCTZ 20/12.5, 40/12.5, 40/25 **SE:** Dizziness, ↓ K+ w/ HCTZ product (may require replacement) **Interactions:** ↑ Risk of digitalis, Li tox; ↑ risk of hypokalemia W/ ACTH, amphotericin B, corticosteroids; ↑ risk of hyperkalemia W/K+ supls, K+-sparing diuretics or K+-containing salt substitutes; ↓ effects W/ NSAIDs; ↓ effect OF norepinephrine **Labs:** May interfere w/ parathyroid tests **NIPE:** If *Benicar* does not control BP, a diuretic can be added or *Benicar HCT* used; titrate at 2–4-wk intervals

Olmesartan, Amlodipine, & Hydrochlorothiazide (Tribenzor) [Antihypertensive/Angiotensin II Receptor Blocker + Calcium Channel Blocker + Hydrochlorothiazide] Uses: *Hypertension* **Action:** Combo ARB, CCB, thiazide diuretic **Dose:** begin w/ 20/5/12.5 olmesartan/amlodipine/HCTZ, ↑ to max 40/10/25 mg **Caution:** [C, (1st tri; D 2nd/3rd tri); –] **CI:** Anuria; sulfa allergy; PRG, neonate exposure, CrCl < 30 mg/min, age > 75 y, severe liver dx **Disp:** Tabs: (olmesartan mg/amlodipine mg/HCTZ mg) 20/5/12.5; 40/5/12.5; 40/5/25; 40/10/12.5 mg; 40/10/25 mg **SE:** Edema, HA, fatigue, N/D, muscle spasms, Jt swelling, hyperuricemia, URI, UTI, syncope) **Interactions:** ↑ Risk of digitalis, Li tox; ↑ Risk of hypokalemia W/ ACTH, amphotericin B, corticosteroids; ↑ risk of hyperkalemia W/ K+ supls, K+- sparing diuretics or K+-containing salt substitutes; ↓ effects W/ NSAIDs; ↓ effect OF norepinephrine **Labs:** Monitor lytes, uric acid **NIPE:** Avoid w/ vol depletion; thiazide diuretics may exacerbate SLE, associated NA glaucoma; titrate at 2 wk intervals

Olopatadine Nasal (Patanase) [Antihistamine (H₁-Blocker)] Uses: *Seasonal allergic rhinitis* **Action:** H₁-receptor antagonist **Dose:** 2 sprays each nostril bid **Caution:** [C, ?] **Disp:** 0.6% 240-spray bottle **SE:** Epistaxis, bitter taste somnolence, HA, rhinitis **Interaction:** ↑ Effects OF CNS depressants; ↑ CNS depression W/ EtOH **NIPE:** Avoid eyes; monitor for nasal changes

Olopatadine Ophthalmic (Patanol, Pataday) [Ophthalmic Antihistamine] Uses: *Allergic conjunctivitis* **Action:** H₁-receptor antagonist **Dose:** *Patanol:* 1–2 gtt in eye(s) bid; *Pataday:* 1 gtt in eye(s) qd **Caution:** [C, ?] **Disp:** *Patanol:* Soln 0.1% 5 mL *Pataday:* 0.2% 2.5 mL **SE:** Local irritation, HA, rhinitis **NIPE:** ⊗ In children < 3 y; may reinsert contacts 10 min later if eye not red

Olsalazine (Dipentum) [Anti-Inflammatory/Aminosalicylic Acid Derivative] Uses: *Maint remission in UC* **Action:** Topical anti-inflammatory **Dose:** 500 mg PO bid (w/ food) **Caution:** [C, –] **CI:** Salicylate sensitivity **Disp:** Caps 250 mg **SE:** D, HA, blood dyscrasias, hep **Interaction:** ↑ Effects OF anticoagulants **Labs:** ↑ LFTs **NIPE:** Food ↓ GI upset

Omalizumab (Xolair) [Antiasthmatic/Monoclonal Antibody] **WARNING:** Reports of anaphylaxis 2–24 h after administration, even in previously

treated pts **Uses:** *Mod–severe asthma in ≥ 12 y w/ reactivity to an allergen & when Sxs inadequately controlled w/ inhaled steroids* **Action:** Anti-IgE Ab **Dose:** 150–375 mg SQ q2–4wk (dose/frequency based on serum IgE level & body wgt; see package insert) **Caution:** [B, ?/–] **CI:** Component allergy, acute bronchospasm **Disp:** 150-mg single-use 5-mL vial **SE:** Site Rxn, sinusitis, PRG, anaphylaxis reported in 3 pts **Interactions:** No drug interaction studies done **NIPE:** ⊘ D/C abruptly; not for acute bronchospasm; administration w/in 8 h of reconstitution & store in refrigerator; continue other asthma meds as indicated

Omega-3 Fatty Acid (Fish Oil) (Lovaza) [Lipid Regulator/Ethyl Ester]
Uses: *Rx hypertriglyceridemia* **Action:** Omega-3 acid ethyl esters, ↓ thrombus inflammation & triglycerides **Dose:** *Hypertriglyceridemia:* 4 g/d ÷ in 1–2 doses **Caution:** Fish hypersensitivity; PRG risk factor [C, –], w/ anticoagulant use, w/ bleeding risk **CI:** Hypersensitivity to components **Disp:** 1000-mg gel caps **SE:** Dyspepsia, N, GI pain, rash, flu-like synd **Interactions:** ↑ Effects *OF* anticoagulants **Labs:** Monitor triglycerides, LDL, ALT **NIPE:** Only FDA-approved fish oil supl; not for exogenous hypertriglyceridemia (type 1 hyperchylomicronemia); many OTC products. D/C after 2 mo if triglyceride levels do not ↓; previously called "Omacor"

Omeprazole (Prilosec, Prilosec OTC) [Anti-Ulcer Agent/Proton Pump Inhibitor]
Uses: *Duodenal/gastric ulcers (adults), GERD, & erosive gastritis (adults & children),* *prevent NSAID ulcers, ZE synd, H pylori Infxns* **Action:** PPI **Dose:** *Adults.* 20–40 mg PO daily–bid × 4–8 wk; *H pylori* 20 mg PO bid × 10 d w/ amoxicillin & clarithromycin or 40 mg PO × 14 d w/ clarithromycin; pathologic hypersecretory condition 60 mg/d (varies); 80 mg/d max *Peds 1–16 y.* *5–10 kg.* *5 mg/d* **10–20 kg.** 10 mg PO qd *> 20 kg.* 20 mg PO qd; 40 mg/d max **Caution:** [C, +/–] **Disp:** OTC tabs 20 mg; Prilosec DR caps 10, 20, 40 mg; Prilosec DR susp 2.5, 10 mg **SE:** HA, D **Interactions:** ↑ Effects *OF* clarithromycin, digoxin, phenytoin, warfarin; ↓ effects *W/* sucralfate; ↓ effects *OF* ampicillin, cyanocobalamin, ketoconazole **Labs:** ↑ LFTs; risk of hypomagnesemia w/ long-term use, monitor **NIPE:** Combo w/ antibiotic Rx for *H pylori*, ? ↑ risk of fxs w/ all PPIs

Omeprazole & Sodium Bicarbonate (Zegerid, Zegerid OTC) [Anti-Ulcer Agent/Proton Pump Inhibitor]
Uses: *Duodenal/gastric ulcers, GERD, & erosive gastritis, (↓ GI bleed in critically ill pts)* *prevent NSAID ulcers, ZE synd, H. pylori Infxns* **Action:** PPI w/ NaHCO₃ **Dose:** *Duodenal ulcer:* 20 PO daily–bid × 4 PO *Gastric ulcer:* 40 PO daily–bid × 4 PO *GERD no erosions* 20 mg PO daily × 4 wk, *w/ erosions* treat 4ons ily *UGI bleed prevention:* 40 mg q6 prevention 40 mg/d × 14 d **Caution:** [C, +/–] w/ Drugs that rely on gastric acid (eg, ampicillin); response does not R/O malignancy **Disp:** omeprazole mg/NaHCO₃ mg: Zegerid OTC caps 20/1100; Zegerid 20/1100, mg 40/1100; *Zegerid powder packet* for oral susp 20/1680, 40/1680 **SE:** HA, Abd pain, N/V/D, flatulence **Interactions:** Avoid w/ atazanavir & nelfinavir; ↑ effects *OF* clarithromycin, digoxin,

diazepam, phenytoin, warfarin; ↓ effects *W/* sucralfate; ↓ effects *OF* ampicillin, clopidogrel, cyanocobalamin, ketoconazole) **Labs:**↑ LFTs; risk of hypomagnesemia w/ long-term use, monitor **NIPE:** Not approved in Peds; take 1 h ac; mix powder in small cup w/ 2 tbsp H_2O (not food or other Liq) refill & drink; do not open caps; possible ↑ risk of fxs w/ all PPIs

Omeprazole, Sodium Bicarbonate, & Magnesium Hydroxide (Zegerid with Magnesium Hydroxide) [Anti-Ulcer Agent/Proton Pump Inhibitor] Uses: *Duodenal or gastric ulcer, GERD, maintenance esophagitis* **Action:** PPI w/ acid buffering **Dose:** 20–40 mg omeprazole daily, empty stomach 1 h pc *Duodenal ulcer, GERD:* 20 mg 4–8 wk *Gastric ulcer:* 40 mg 4–8 wk *Esophagitis maint:* 20 mg **Caution:** [C; ?/–] w/ resp alkalosis; may ↓ absorption drugs requiring acid environment **CI:** ↓ Renal Fxn **Disp:** Chew tabs, 20, 40 mg omeprazole; w/ 600 mg $NaHCO_3$; 700 mg $MgOH_2$ **SE:** N, V, D, Abd pain, HA **Interactions:** ↑ Drug levels metabolized by cytochrome P450; ↑ effects *OF* diazepam, phenytoin, warfarin tacrolimus, clarithromycin **Labs:** ↓ K^+, ↓ Ca^{2+}, monitor INR w/ warfarin **NIPE:** Atrophic gastritis w/ long-term PPI; ?; ↑ risk of fxs w/ all PPI; long-term use + Ca^{2+} → milk-alkali synd

Ondansetron (Zofran, Zofran ODT) [Antiemetic/5-HT Antagonist] Uses: *Prevent chemotherapy-associated & post-op N/V* **Action:** Serotonin receptor (5-HT_3) antagonist **Dose:** *Adults & Peds. Chemotherapy:* 0.15 mg/kg/dose IV prior to chemotherapy, then 4 & 8 h after 1st dose or 4–8 mg PO tid; 1st dose 30 min prior to chemotherapy & give on schedule, not PRN *Adults. Post-op:* 4 mg IV stat preanesthesia or post-op *Peds. Post-op: < 40 kg.* 0.1 mg/kg *> 40 kg.* 4 mg IV; ↓ w/ hepatic impair **Caution:** [B, +/–] **Disp:** Tabs 4, 8, 24 mg, soln 4 mg/5 mL, Inj 2 mg/mL, 32 mg/50 mL; Zofran ODT tabs 4, 8 mg **SE:** D, HA, constipation, dizziness **Interactions:** ↓ Effects *W/* cimetidine, phenobarbital, rifampin **Labs:** ↑ LFTs **NIPE:** Food ↑ absorption

Ondansetron, Oral Soluble Film (Zuplenz) [Antiemetic/5-HT Antagonist] Uses: *Prevent chemotherapy/RT-associated & post-op N/V* **Action:** Serotonin receptor (5-HT_3) antagonist **Dose:** *Adults. Highly emetogenic chemotherapy:* 24 mg (8-mg film × 3) 30 min prechemotherapy *Adults. RTN & V:* 8 mg film tid *Adults & Peds > 12 y. Mod emetogenic chemotherapy:* 8-mg film 30 min prechemotherapy, then 8 mg in 8 h; 8 mg film bid × 1–2 d after chemotherapy *Adults. Post-op:*16 mg (8-mg film × 2) 1 h pre-op; ↓ w/ hepatic impair **Caution:** [B, +/–] **CI:** w/ Apomorphine (↓ BP, LOC) **Disp:** Oral soluble film 4, 8 mg **SE:** HA, malaise/fatigue, constipation, D **Interactions:** ↓ Effects *W/* potent CYP3A4 inducers (eg, phenytoin, carbamazepine, rifampicin) ; may ↓ analgesia of tramadol **NIPE:** Use w/ dry hands, do not chew/swallow; place on tongue, dissolves in 4–20 s

Oprelvekin (Neumega) [Thrombopoietic Growth Factor] WARNING: Allergic Rxn w/ anaphylaxis reported; D/C w/ any allergic Rxn Uses: *Prevent ↓ plt w/ chemotherapy* **Action:** ↑ Proliferation & maturation of megakaryocytes (IL-11) **Dose:** *Adults.* 50 mcg/kg/d SQ for 10–21 d *Peds > 12 y.* 75–100 mcg/

kg/d SQ for 10–21 d *< 12 y.* Use only in clinical trials; ↓ w/ CrCl < 30 mL/min 25 mcg/kg **Caution:** [C, ?/–] **Disp:** 5 mg powder for Inj **SE:** Tachycardia, palpitations, arrhythmias, edema, HA, dizziness, visual disturbances, papilledema, insomnia, fatigue, fever, N, anemia, dyspnea, allergic Rxns including anaphylaxis **Interactions:** None noted **Labs:** ↓ HMG, albumin; monitor lytes; obtain CBCs before & during therapy; monitor plt counts **NIPE:** Monitor for peripheral edema; use med w/in 3 h of reconstitution; initiate 6–24 h after chemotherapy completion

Oral Contraceptives, Biphasic, Monophasic, Triphasic, Progestin-Only (Table 5) [Progestin/Hormone] WARNING: Cigarette smoking ↑ risk of serious CV SE; ↑ risk w/ > 15 cigarette/d, > 35 y; strongly advise women on OCP to not smoke. Pts should be counseled that these products do not protect against HIV & other STD **Uses:** *Birth control; regulation of anovulatory bleeding; dysmenorrhea; endometriosis; polycystic ovaries; acne*(Note: FDA approvals vary widely, see package insert) **Action:** *Birth control:* Suppresses LH surge, prevents ovulation; progestins thicken cervical mucus; ↓ fallopian tubule cilia, ↓ endometrial thickness to ↓ chances of fertilization *Anovulatory bleeding:* Cyclic hormones mimic body's natural cycle & regulate endometrial lining, results in regular bleeding q28d; may ↓ uterine bleeding & dysmenorrhea **Dose:** Start d 1 menstrual cycle or 1st Sunday after onset of menses; 28-d cycle pills take daily; 21-d cycle pills take daily, no pills during last 7 d of cycle (during menses); some available as transdermal patch **Caution:** [X, +] Migraine, HTN, DM, sickle cell Dz, gallbladder Dz; monitor for breast Dz, ; w/ drosperinone-containing OCP, ✓ K+ if taking drugs w/ ↑ K+ risk; drosperinone implicated in ↑ VTE risk **CI:** AUB, PRG, estrogen-dependent malignancy, ↑ hypercoagulation/liver Dz, hemiplegic migraine, smokers > 35 y; drosperinone has mineralocortocoid effect; do not use w/ renal/liver/adrenal problems **Disp:** See Table 5; 28-d cycle pills (21 active pills + 7 placebo or Fe or folate supl); 21-d cycle pills (21 active pills) **SE:** Intramenstrual bleeding, oligomenorrhea, amenorrhea, ↑ appetite/wgt gain, ↓ libido, fatigue, depression, mood swings, mastalgia, HA, melasma, ↑ Vag discharge, acne/greasy skin, corneal edema, N **NIPE:** Taken correctly, up to 99.9% effective for contraception; no STDs prevention—instruct in use to reduce STDs, use additional barrier contraceptive; long term, can ↓ risk of ectopic PRG, benign breast Dz, ovarian & uterine CA. Suggestions for OCP prescribing and/or regimen changes are noted below. Listing of other forms of Rx birth control can be found in Table 5

Criteria for Specific OTC Choices:
• *Rx menstrual cycle control:* Start w/ monophasic × 3 mo before switching to another brand; w/ continued bleeding change to pill w/ ↑ estrogen
• *Rx birth control:* Choose pill w/ lowest SE profile for particular pt; SEs numerous; d/t estrogenic excess or progesterone deficiency; each pill's SE profile can be unique (see package insert); newer extended-cycle combos have shorter/fewer hormone-free intervals; ? ↓ PRG risk; OCP troubleshooting SE w/ suggested OCP

- *Absent menstrual flow:* ↑ Estrogen, ↓ progestin: Brevicon, Necon 1/35, Norinyl 1/35, Modicon, Necon 1/50, Norinyl 1/50, Ortho-Cyclen, Ortho-Novum 1/50, Ortho-Novum 1/35, Ovcon 35
- *Acne:* Use ↑ estrogen, ↓ androgenic: Brevicon, Ortho-Cyclen, Demulen 1/50, Estrostep, Ortho Tri-Cyclen, Mircette, Modicon, Necon, Ortho Evra, Yasmin, Yaz
- *Breakthrough bleed:* ↑ Estrogen, ↑ progestin, ↓ androgenic: Demulen 1/50, Desogen, Estrostep, Loestrin 1/20, Ortho-Cept, Ovcon 50, Yasmin, Zovia 1/50E
- *Breast tenderness or* ↑ *wgt:* ↓ progestin: Use ↓ estrogen pill rather than current; Alesse, Levlite, Loestrin 1/20 Fe, Ortho Evra, Yasmin, Yaz
- *Depression:* ↓ Progestin: Alesse, Brevicon, Levlite, Modicon, Necon, Ortho Evra, Ovcon 35, Ortho-Cyclen, Ortho Tri-Cyclen Tri-Levlen, Triphasil, Trivora
- *Endometriosis:* ↓ Estrogen, ↑ progestin: Demulen 1/35, Loestrin 1.5/30, Loestrin 1/20 Fe, Lo Ovral, Levlen, Levora, Nordette, Zovia 1/35; cont w/o placebo pills or w/ 4 d of placebo pills
- *HA:* ↓ Estrogen, ↓ progestin: Alesse, Levlite, Ortho Evra
- *Moodiness and/or irritability:* ↓ Progestin: Alesse, Brevicon, Levlite, Modicon, Necon 1/35, Ortho Evra, Ortho-Cyclen, Ortho Tri-Cyclen, Ovcon 35, Tri-Levlen, Triphasil, Trivora
- *Severe menstrual cramping:* ↑ Progestin: Demulen 1/50, Desogen, Loestrin 1.5/30, Mircette, Ortho-Cept, Yasmin, Yaz, Zovia 1/50E, Zovia 1/35E

Orlistat (Xenical, Alli [OTC]) [Obesity Management/GI Lipase Inhibitor] Uses: *Manage obesity w/ BMI ≥ 30 kg/m² or ≥ 27 kg/m² w/ other risk factors; type 2 DM, dyslipidemia* **Action:** Reversible Inhib of gastric & pancreatic lipases **Dose:** 120 mg PO tid w/ a fat-containing meal; Alli (OTC) 60 mg PO tid w/ fat-containing meals **Caution:** [B, ?] May ↓ cyclosporine & warfarin dose requirements **CI:** Cholestasis, malabsorption, organ transplant **Disp:** Caps Xenical 120 mg; Alli OTC 60-mg caps **SE:** Abd pain/discomfort, fatty stools, fecal urgency **Interactions:** ↑ Effects *OF* pravastatin; ↓ effects *OF* cyclosporine, fat-soluble vits **Labs:** Monitor INR if taking warfarin, ↓ serum glucose, total cholesterol, LDL **NIPE:** Do not use if meal contains no fat; GI effects ↑ w/ high-fat meals; supl w/ fat-soluble vits

Orphenadrine (Norflex) [Skeletal Muscle Relaxant] Uses: *Discomfort associated w/ painful musculoskeletal conditions* **Action:** Central atropine-like effect; indirect skeletal muscle relaxation, euphoria, analgesia **Dose:** 100 mg PO bid, 60 mg IM/IV q12h **Caution:** [C, +/−] **CI:** NAG, GI or bladder obst, cardiospasm, MyG **Disp:** SR tabs 100 mg; Inj 30 mg/mL **SE:** Drowsiness, dizziness, blurred vision, flushing, tachycardia, constipation **Interactions:** ↑ CNS depression *W/* anxiolytics, butorphanol, hypnotics, MAOIs, nalbuphine, opioids, pentazocine, phenothiazine, tramadol, TCAs, kava kava, valerian, EtOH; ↑ effects *W/* anticholinergics **NIPE:** Impaired body temperature regulation

Oseltamivir (Tamiflu) [Antiviral/Neuraminidase Inhibitor] Uses: *Prevention & Rx influenza A & B* **Action:** ↓ Viral neuraminidase **Dose:** Adults.

Tx: 75 mg PO bid for 5 d *Prophylaxis:* 75 mg PO daily × 10 d *Peds. Tx:* Dose bid × 5 d.:= *33 lb 30 mg; 33–51 lb 45 mg; 51–88 lb 60 mg;* > *88 lb 75 mg all dosing is PO bid. Prophylaxis: Same dosing but once per d for 10 d;* ↓ w/ renal impair **Caution:** [C, ?/–] **CI:** Component allergy **Disp:** Caps 30, 45, 75 mg, powder 12 mg/mL **SE:** N/V, insomnia, reports of neuropsychological events in children (self-injury, confusion, delirium) **Interactions:** ↑ Effects W/ probenecid **NIPE:** Take w/o regard to food; initiate w/in 48 h of Sx onset or exposure; 2009 H1N1 strains susceptible; ✓ CDC updates http://www.cdc.gov/h1n1flu/guidance/

Oxacillin (Prostaphlin) [Antibiotic/Penicillin] Uses: *Infxns d/t susceptible *S aureus* & *Streptococcus** Action: Bactericidal; ↓ cell wall synth *Spectrum:* Excellent gram(+), poor gram(−) **Dose:** *Adults.* 250–500 mg (2 g severe) IM/IV q4–6h *Peds.* 150–200 mg/kg/d IV ÷ q4–6h **Caution:** [B, M] **CI:** PCN sensitivity **Disp:** Powder for Inj 500 mg, 1, 2, 10 g **SE:** GI upset, interstitial nephritis, blood dyscrasias **Interactions:** ↑ Effects W/ disulfiram, probenecid; ↑ effects OF anticoagulants, MTX; ↑ effects W/ chloramphenicol, tetracyclines, carbonated drinks, fruit juice, food; ↑ effects OF OCPs **NIPE:** Take w/o food

Oxaliplatin (Eloxatin) [Antineoplastic/Alkylating Agent] WARNING: Administer w/ supervision of physician experienced in chemotherapy. Appropriate management is possible only w/ adequate diagnostic & Rx facilities. Anaphylactic-like Rxns reported Uses: *Adjuvant Rx stage III colon CA (primary resected) & met colon CA w/ 5-FU* **Action:** Metabolized to platinum derivatives, cross-links DNA **Dose:** Per protocol; see package insert *Premedicate:* Antiemetic w/ or w/o dexamethasone **Caution:** [D, –] See Warning **CI:** Allergy to components or platinum **Disp:** Inj 50, 100 mg **SE:** Anaphylaxis, granulocytopenia, paresthesia, N/V/D, stomatitis, fatigue, neuropathy, hepatotox, pulm tox **Interactions:** ↑ Effects OF nephrotoxic drugs **Labs:** ↑ Bilirubin, Cr, LFTs; ↓ HMG, K+, neutrophils, plts, WBC; monitor CBC, plts, LFTs, BUN, & Cr before each chemotherapy cycle **NIPE:** ↑ Acute neurologic Sxs w/ cold exposure/cold Liq; 5-FU & Leucovorin are given in combo; epi, corticosteroids, & antihistamines alleviate severe Rxns

Oxandrolone (Oxandrin) [C-III] [Anabolic Steroid] WARNING: Risk of peliosis hepatis, liver cell tumors, may ↑ risk atherosclerosis Uses: *Wgt ↑ after wgt loss from severe trauma, extensive surgery* **Action:** Anabolic steroid; ↑ lean body mass **Dose:** *Adults.* 2.5–20 mg/d PO ÷ bid-qid *Peds.* ≤ 0.1 mg/kg/d ÷ bid–qid **Caution:** [X; ?/–] ↑ INR w/ warfarin **CI:** PRG, prostate CA, male breast CA, breast CA w/ hypercalcemia, nephrosis **Disp:** Tabs 2.5, 10 mg **SE:** Acne, hepatotox, dyslipidemia **Interactions:** ↑ Effects OF oral anticoagulants, oxyphenbutazone; ↑ risk of edema W/ ACTH, corticosteroids **Labs:** ✓ Lipids & LFTS **NIPE:** Use intermittently, 2–4 wk typical

Oxaprozin (Daypro, Daypro ALTA) [Analgesic, Anti-Inflammatory, Antipyretic/NSAID] WARNING: May ↑ risk of CV events & GI bleeding Uses: *Arthritis & pain* **Action:** NSAID; ↓ prostaglandin synth **Dose:**

Adults. 600–1200 mg/daily (÷ dose helps GI tolerance); ↓ w/ renal/hepatic impair **Peds.** *JRA (Daypro):* **22–31 kg.** 600 mg/d **32–54 kg.** 900 mg/d **Caution:** [C (D in 3rd tri), ?] Peptic ulcer, bleeding disorders **CI:** ASA/NSAID sensitivity perioperative pain w/ CABG **Disp:** Daypro ALTA tabs 600 mg; caplets 600 mg **SE:** CNS inhibition, sleep disturbance, rash, GI upset, peptic ulcer, edema, renal failure, anaphylactoid Rxn w/ ASA triad (asthmatic w/ rhinitis, nasal polyps & bronchospasm w/ NSAID use) **Interactions:** ↑ Effects *OF* aminoglycosides, anticoagulants, ASA, Li, MTX, ↓ effects *OF* antihypertensives, diuretics **NIPE:** ↑ Risk of photosensitivity—use sunblock; take w/ food

Oxazepam [C-IV] [Anxiolytic/Benzodiazepines] Uses: *Anxiety, acute EtOH withdrawal*, anxiety w/ depressive Sxs **Action:** Benzodiazepine; diazepam metabolite **Dose:** *Adults.* 10–15 mg PO tid–qid; severe anxiety & EtOH withdrawal may require up to 30 mg qid **Peds.** 1 mg/kg/d ÷ doses **Caution:** [D, ?/–] **CI:** Component allergy, NAG **Disp:** Caps 10, 15, 30 mg; tabs 15 mg **SE:** Sedation, ataxia, dizziness, rash, blood dyscrasias, dependence **Interactions:** ↑ CNS effects *W/* anticonvulsants, antidepressants, antihistamines, barbiturates, MAOIs, opioids, phenothiazine, kava kava, lemon balm, sassafras, valerian, EtOH; ↑ effects *W/* cimetidine; ↓ effects *W/* OCPs, phenytoin, theophylline, tobacco; ↓ effects *OF* levodopa **Labs:** False ↑ serum glucose **NIPE:** ⊘ D/C abruptly

Oxcarbazepine (Trileptal) [Anticonvulsant/Carbamazepine] Uses: *Partial Szs*, bipolar disorders **Action:** Blocks voltage-sensitive Na⁺ channels, stabilization of hyperexcited neural membranes **Dose:** *Adults.* 300 mg PO bid, ↑ weekly to target maint 1200–2400 mg/d **Peds.** 8–10 mg/kg bid, 600 mg max, ↑ weekly to target maint dose; ↓ w/ renal Insuff **Caution:** [C, –] Carbamazepine sensitivity **CI:** Components sensitivity **Disp:** Tabs 150, 300, 600 mg; susp 300 mg/5 mL **SE:** ↓ Na⁺, HA, dizziness, fatigue, somnolence, GI upset, diplopia, conc difficulties, fatal skin/multiorgan hypersensitivity Rxns **Interactions:** ↑ Effects *W/* benzodiazepines, EtOH; ↑ effects *OF* phenobarbital, phenytoin; ↓ effects *W/* barbiturates, carbamazepine, phenobarbital, valproic acid, verapamil; ↓ effects *OF* CCBs, OCPs **Labs:** ↓ Thyroid levels, serum Na; ✓ Na⁺ if fatigued **NIPE:** Take w/o regard to food; use barrier contraception; do not abruptly D/C; advise about SJS & topic epidermal necrolysis

Oxiconazole (Oxistat) [Azole Antifungal] Uses: *Tinea cruris, tinea corporis, tinea pedis, tinea versicolor* **Action:** ? ↓ Ergosterols in fungal cell membrane *Spectrum:* Most *E floccosum, T mentagrophytes, T rubrum, M furfur* **Dose:** Apply thin layer daily bid **Caution:** [B, M] **CI:** Component allergy **Disp:** Cream, lotion 1% **SE:** Local irritation **NIPE:** Avoid eyes, nose, mouth, mucous membranes

Oxybutynin (Ditropan, Ditropan XL) [GU Antispasmodic/Anticholinergic] Uses: *Symptomatic relief of urgency, nocturia, incontinence w/ neurogenic or reflex neurogenic bladder* **Action:** Anticholinergic, relaxes bladder smooth muscle, ↑ bladder capacity **Dose:** *Adults.* 5 mg bid–tid, 5 mg qid max. XL 5–10 mg/d, 30 mg/d max **Peds.** *> 5 y.* 5 mg PO bid–tid, 15 mg/d max *1–5.* 0.2 mg/kg/

dose bid–qid (syrup 5 mg/5 mL); 15 mg/d max; ↓ in elderly; periodic drug holidays OK **Caution:** [B, ?] **CI:** NAG, MyG, GI/GU obst, UC, megacolon **Disp:** Tabs 5 mg; XL tabs 5, 10, 15 mg; syrup 5 mg/5 mL **SE:** Anticholinergic (drowsiness, xerostomia, constipation, tachycardia) **Interactions:** ↑ Effects W/ CNS depressants, EtOH; ↑ effects OF atenolol, digoxin, nitrofurantoin; ↑ anticholinergic effects W/ antihistamines, anticholinergics; ↓ effects OF haloperidol, levodopa **NIPE:** ↓ Temperature regulation; ↑ photosensitivity—use sunscreen; ER form empty shell expelled in stool; ↑ QT interval—monitor ECG; memory impair

Oxybutynin, Topical (Gelnique) [GU Antispasmodic/Anticholinergic]

Uses: *OAB* **Action:** Anticholinergic, relaxes bladder smooth muscle, ↑ bladder capacity **Dose:** 1-g sachet qd to dry skin (Abd/shoulders/thighs/upper arms) **Caution:** [B; ?/–] **CI:** Gastric or urinary retention; NAG **Disp:** Gel 10%, 1-g sachets (100 mg oxybutynin) **SE:** Anticholinergic (lethargy, xerostomia, constipation, blurred vision, ↑ HR); rash, pruritus, redness, pain at site; UTI **Interactions:** CNS depression W/ EtOH, other CNS depressants; additive effect W/ other anticholinergics **NIPE:** Cover w/ clothing, skin-to-skin transfer can occur; gel is flammable; after applying wait 1 h before showering

Oxybutynin Transdermal System (Oxytrol) [GU Antispasmodic/Anticholinergic]

Uses: *Rx OAB* **Action:** Anticholinergic, relaxes bladder smooth muscle, ↑ bladder capacity ↑ **Dose:** One 3.9 mg/d system apply 2 × /wk (q3–4d) to abdomen, hip, or buttock **Caution:** [B, ?/–] **CI:** GI/GU obst, NAG **Disp:** 3.9-mg/d transdermal patch **SE:** Anticholinergic, itching/redness at site **Interactions:** ↑ Effects W/ anticholinergics; CNS depression W/ EtOH, other CNS depressants; metabolized by the cytochrome P450 CYP3A4 enzyme system **NIPE:** do not apply to same site w/in 7 d

Oxycodone [Dihydrohydroxycodeinone] (OxyContin, Roxicodone) [C-II] [Opioid Analgesic]

WARNING: High abuse potential; CR only for extended chronic pain, not for PRN use; 60-, 80-mg tabs for opioid-tolerant pts; do not crush, break or chew **Uses:** *Mod–severe pain, usually in combo w/ nonnarcotic analgesics* **Action:** Narcotic analgesic **Dose:** *Adults.* 5 mg PO q6h PRN (IR). *Mod–severe chronic pain:* 10–160 mg PO q12h (ER) *Peds 6–12 y.* 1.25 mg PO q6h PRN > *12 y.* 2.5 mg q6h PRN; ↓ w/ severe liver/renal Dz, elderly; w/ food **Caution:** [B D if prolonged use/near term], M] **CI:** Allergy, resp depression, acute asthma, ileus w/ microsomal morphine **Disp:** CR Roxicodone tabs 15, 30 mg; ER (OxyContin) 10, 15, 20, 30, 40,60, 80 mg; Liq 5 mg/5 mL; soln conc 20 mg/mL **SE:** ↓ BP, sedation, resp depression, dizziness, GI upset, constipation, risk of abuse **Interactions:** ↑ CNS & resp depression W/ amitriptyline, barbiturates, cimetidine, clomipramine, MAOIs, nortriptyline, protease Inhibs, TCAs **Labs:** ↑ Serum amylase, lipase **NIPE:** Take w/ food; OxyContin for chronic CA pain; do not crush/chew/cut ER product; sought after as drug of abuse; reformulated *OxyContin* is intended to prevent the opioid medication from being cut, broken, chewed, crushed, or dissolved to release more medication

Oxycodone & Acetaminophen (Percocet, Tylox) [C-II] [Opioid + Analgesic] Uses: *Mod–severe pain* Action: Narcotic analgesic Dose: *Adults.* 1–2 tabs/caps PO q4–6h PRN *Peds.* Oxycodone 0.05–0.15 mg/kg/dose q4–6h PRN, 5 mg/dose max Caution: [C (D prolonged use or near term), M] CI: Allergy, paralytic ileus, resp depression Disp: Percocet tabs (oxycodone mg/APAP mg): 2.5/325, 5/325, 7.5/325, 10/325, 7.5/500, 10/650; Tylox caps 5 mg oxycodone & 500 mg APAP; soln 5 mg oxycodone & 325 mg APAP/5 mL SE: ↓ BP, sedation, dizziness, GI upset, constipation Interactions: ↑ CNS & resp depression W/amitriptylline, barbiturates, cimetidine, clomipramine, MAOIs, nortriptylline, protease Inhibs, TCAs Labs: False ↑ serum amylase, lipase NIPE: Take w/ food

Oxycodone & Aspirin (Percodan) [C-II] [Narcotic Analgesic/Nonsteroidal Analgesic] Uses: *Mod–modly severe pain* Action: Narcotic analgesic w/ NSAID Dose: *Adults.* 1–2 tabs/caps PO q4–6h PRN *Peds.* Oxycodone 0.05–0.15 mg/kg/dose q4–6h PRN, up to 5 mg/dose; ↓ in severe hepatic failure Caution: [D, –] Peptic ulcer CI: Component allergy, children (< 16 y) w/ viral Infxn (Reyes synd), resp depression, ileus, hemophilia Disp: *Generics:* 4.83 mg oxycodone hydrochloride, 0.38 mg oxycodone terephthalate, 325 mg ASA; *Percodan* 4.83 mg oxycodone hydrochloride, 325 mg ASA SE: Sedation, dizziness, GI upset/ulcer, constipation, allergy Interactions: ↑ CNS & resp depression W/ amitriptyline, barbiturates, cimetidine, clomipramine, MAOIs, nortriptyline, protease Inhibs, TCAs; ↑ effects OF anticoagulants Labs: ↑ Serum amylase, lipase NIPE: Take w/ food; monitor for possible drug abuse

Oxycodone/Ibuprofen (Combunox) [C-II] [Narcotic Analgesic/NSAID] WARNING: May ↑ risk of serious CV events; CI in perioperative CABG pain; ↑ risk of GI events such as bleeding Uses: *Short-term (not > 7 d) management of acute mod–severe pain* Action: Narcotic w/ NSAID Dose: 1 tab q6h PRN 4 tabs max/24 h; 7 d max Caution: [C, –] w/ impaired renal/hepatic Fxn; COPD, CNS depression, avoid in PRG CI: Paralytic ileus, 3rd tri PRG, allergy to ASA or NSAIDs, where opioids are CI Disp: Tabs 5 mg oxycodone/400 mg ibuprofen SE: N/V, somnolence, dizziness, sweating, flatulence Interactions: ↑ CNS & resp depression W/ amitriptyline, barbiturates, cimetidine, clomipramine, MAOIs, nortriptyline, protease Inhibs, TCAs; ↑ effects W/ ASA, corticosteroids, probenecid, EtOH; ↑ effects OF aminoglycosides, anticoagulants, digoxin, hypoglycemics, Li, MTX; ↑ risks of bleeding W/ abciximab, cefotetan, valproic acid, thrombolytic drugs, warfarin, ticlopidine, garlic, ginger, ginkgo; ↓ effects W/ feverfew; ↑ effects OF antihypertensives Labs: ↑ Serum amylase, lipase, LFTs, BUN, Cr; ✓ renal Fxn NIPE: Take w/ food; abuse potential w/ oxycodone

Oxymorphone (Opana, Opana ER) [C-II] [Opioid Analgesic] WARNING: (Opana ER) Abuse potential, CR only for chronic pain; do not consume EtOH-containing beverages, may cause fatal OD Uses: *Mod/severe pain, sedative* Action: Narcotic analgesic Dose: 10–20 mg PO q4–6h PRN if opioid-naïve or

1–1.5 mg SQ/IM q4–6h PRN or 0.5 mg IV q4–6h PRN; start 20 mg/dose max PO
Chronic pain: ER 5 mg PO q12h; if opioid-naïve ↑ PRN 5–10 mg PO q12h q3–7d;
take 1 h pc or 2 h ac; ↓ dose w/ elderly, renal/hepatic impair **Caution:** [B, ?] **CI:** ↑
ICP, severe resp depression, w/ EtOH or liposomal morphine, severe hepatic impair
Disp: Tabs 5, 10 mg; ER 5, 10, 20, 40 mg **SE:** ↓ BP, sedation, GI upset, constipa-
tion, histamine release **Interactions:** ↑ Effects *W/* CNS depressants, cimetidine,
neuroleptics, EtOH; ↓ effects *W/* phenothiazines **Labs:** ↑ Amylase, lipase **NIPE:**
Related to hydromorphone

Oxytocin (Pitocin) [Oxytocic/Hormone] Uses: *Induce labor, control
postpartum hemorrhage* **Action:** Stimulate muscular contractions of the uterus
Dose: 0.0005–0.001 units/min IV Inf; titrate 0.001–0.002 units/min q30–60min
Caution: [Uncategorized, +/–] **CI:** Where Vag delivery not favorable, fetal distress
Disp: Inj 10 units/mL **SE:** Uterine rupture, fetal death; arrhythmias, anaphylaxis,
H_2O intoxication **Interactions:** ↑ Pressor effects *W/* sympathomimetics **NIPE:**
Monitor vital signs; nasal form for breast-feeding only

Paclitaxel (Taxol, Abraxane) [Antineoplastic/Antimitotic]
WARNING: Administer only by healthcare provider experienced in chemotherapy; fatal anaphylaxis & hypersensitivity possible; severe myelosuppression possible Uses: *Ovarian & breast CA, PCa*, Kaposi sarcoma, NSCLC **Action:** Mitotic
spindle poison; promotes microtubule assembly & stabilization against depolymer-
ization **Dose:** Per protocols; use glass or polyolefin containers (eg, nitroglycerin
tubing set); PVC sets leach plasticizer; ↓ in hepatic failure **Caution:** [D, –] **CI:**
Neutropenia < 1500 WBC/mm^3; solid tumors, component allergy **Disp:** Inj 5 mg/
mL, 6 mg/mL albumin-bound (Abraxane) **SE:** ↓ BM, peripheral neuropathy, transient ileus, myalgia, bradycardia, ↓ BP, mucositis, N/V/D, fever, rash, HA, phlebitis; hematologic tox schedule-dependent; leukopenia dose-limiting by 24-h Inf;
neurotox limited w/ short (1–3 h) Inf; allergic Rxns (dyspnea, ↓ BP, urticaria, rash)
Interactions: ↑ Effects *W/* cyclosporine, dexamethasone, diazepam, ketoconazole,
midazolam, quinidine, teniposide, verapamil, vincristine; ↑ risk of bleeding *W/*
anticoagulants, plt Inhibs, thrombolytics; ↑ myelosuppression when cisplatin is
administered before paclitaxel; ↓ effects *W/* carbamazepine, phenobarbital; ↓
effects of live virus vaccines **Labs:** ↑ AST, alk phos, triglycerides **NIPE:** ⊘ PRG,
breast-feeding, live virus vaccines; use barrier contraception; maint hydration;
monitor for S/Sxs of Infx: If allergic Rxn occurs, usually w/in 10 min of Inf; minimize w/ corticosteroid, antihistamine preTx; localized skin Rxns may occur up to
10 d after Inf; may cause profound BM suppression, mucous membrane irritation,
& peripheral neurotox

Paliperidone (Invega, Invega Sustenna) [Benzisoxazole] WARNING:
Not for dementia-related psychosis Uses: *Schizophrenia* **Action:** Risperidone
metabolite, antagonizes DA, & serotonin receptors **Dose:** *Invega:* 6 mg PO qAM,
12 mg/d max *CrCl 50–79 mL/min:* 6 mg/d max *CrCl 10–49 mL/min:* 3 mg/d max
Invega Sustenna: 234 mg d 1, 156 mg 1 wk later IM (deltoid), then 117 mg monthly

(deltoid or gluteal); range 39–234 mg/mo **Caution:** [C, ?/–] w/ ↓ HR, ↓ K+/Mg2+, renal/hepatic impair; w/ phenothiazines, ranolazine, ziprasidone, prolonged QT, Hx arrhythmia **CI:** Risperidone/ paliperidone hypersensitivity **Disp:** *Invega* ER tabs 1.5, 3, 6, 9 mg; *Invega Sustenna* prefilled syringes 39, 78, 117, 156, 234 mg **SE:** Impaired temperature regulation, ↑ QT & HR, HA, anxiety, dizziness, N, dry mouth, fatigue, EPS **Interactions:** ↑ Risk of prolongation of QT *W/* Class Ia & Class III antiarrhythmics, chlorpromazine, thioridazine, gatifloxacin, moxifloxacine, EtOH; ↑ risk of orthostatic hypotension *W/* CNS drugs; ↑ effects *W/* divalproex Na; ↓ effects *W/* carbamazepine; ↓ effects *OF* levodopa & other DA agonists **Labs:** ↑ Serum glucose, LFTs **NIPE:** Do not chew/cut/crush pill; determine tolerability to oral risperidone or paliperidone before using injectable; monitor for orthostatic effects & renal Fxn esp in elderly; may cause tachycardia, light-headedness, & muscle tremors

Palivizumab (Synagis) [Antiviral/Monoclonal Antibody] Uses: *Prevent RSV Infxn* **Action:** MoAb **Dose:** *Peds.* 15 mg/kg IM monthly, typically Nov–Apr **Caution:** [C, ?] Renal/hepatic dysfunction **CI:** Component allergy **Disp:** Vials 50, 100 mg **SE:** Hypersensitivity Rxn, URI, rhinitis, cough, local irritation **Labs:** ↑ LFT **NIPE:** Infrequent nonfatal anaphylaxis has occurred w/ subsequent doses; use drug w/in 6 h after reconstitution; ⊘ Inj in gluteal site; use only for RSV prophylaxis

Palifermin (Kepivance) [Growth Factor/Keratinocyte Growth Factor] Uses: *Oral mucositis w/ BMT* **Action:** Synthetic keratinocyte GF **Dose:** *Phase 1:* 60 mcg/kg IV daily × 3, 3rd dose 24–48 h before chemotherapy *Phase 2:* 60 mcg/kg IV daily × 3, stat after stem cell Inf **Caution:** [C, ?/–] **CI:** N/A **Disp:** Inj 6.25 mg **SE:** Unusual mouth sensations, tongue thickening, rash **Labs:** ↑ Amylase, lipase **NIPE:** Eval for rash & taste alterations; may cause severe HA; *E coli*–derived; separate phases by 4 d; safety unknown w/ nonhematologic malignancies

Palonosetron (Aloxi) [Antiemetic/5-HT3 Receptor Antagonist] **WARNING:** May ↑ QTc interval **Uses:** *Prevention acute & delayed N/V w/ emetogenic chemotherapy; prevent post-op N/V* **Action:** 5-HT3 receptor antagonist **Dose:** *Chemotherapy:* 0.25 mg IV 30 min prior to chemotherapy *Post-op N/V:* 0.75 mg stat before induction **Caution:** [B, ?] **CI:** Component allergy **Disp:** 0.25 mg/5 mL vial **SE:** HA, constipation, dizziness, Abd pain, anxiety **Interactions:** Potential for drug interactions low **Labs:** Monitor ECG **NIPE:** Not recommended for < 18 y; may ↑ QTc interval esp in pts taking diuretics & antiarrhythmics

Pamidronate (Aredia) [Antihypercalcemic/Bisphosphonate] Uses: *Hypercalcemia of malignancy, Paget Dz, palliate symptomatic bone metastases* **Action:** Bisphosphonate; ↓ nl & abnormal bone resorption **Dose:** *Hypercalcemia* 60–90 mg IV over 2–24 h or 90 mg IV over 24 h if severe; may repeat in 7 d. *Paget Dz:* 30 mg/d IV slow Inf over 4 h × 3 d *Osteolytic bone mets in myeloma:* 90 mg IV over 4 h qmo *Osteolytic bone mets breast CA:* 90 mg IV over 2 h q3–4wk;

90 mg/max single dose **Caution:** [D, ?/–] Avoid invasive dental procedures w/ use **CI:** PRG, bisphosphonate sensitivity **Disp:** Inj 30, 60, 90 mg **SE:** Fever, malaise, fever, convulsions, Inj site Rxn, uveitis, fluid overload, HTN, Abd pain, N/V, constipation, UTI, bone pain, hypophosphatemia; jaw osteonecrosis (mostly CA pts; avoid dental work), renal tox **Interactions:** ↓ Serum Ca levels W/ foscarnet; ↓ effects W/ Ca, vit D **Labs:** ↓ K+, Ca²⁺, Mg²⁺; follow Cr, hold dose if Cr ↑ by 0.5 mg/dL w/ nl baseline or by 1 mg/dL w/ abnormal baseline; restart when Cr returns w/in 10% of baseline; may cause profound hypocalcemia—monitor Ca **NIPE:** ⊘ Ingest food w/ Ca or vits w/ minerals before or 2–3 h after administration of drug; may cause fever 24 h post-Inj; perform dental exam pretherapy; ↑ risk of jaw fx; may ↑ atypical subtrochanteric femur fxs

Pancrelipase (Pancrease, Cotazym, Creon, Ultrase) [Pancreatic Enzyme] Uses: *Exocrine pancreatic secretion deficiency (eg, CF, chronic pancreatitis, pancreatic Insuff), steatorrhea of malabsorption* **Action:** Pancreatic enzyme supl **Dose:** 1–3 caps (tabs) w/ meals & snacks; ↑ to 8 caps (tabs); do not crush or chew EC products; dose dependent on digestive requirements of pt; avoid antacids **Caution:** [C, ?/–] **CI:** Pork product allergy, acute pancreatitis **Disp:** Caps, tabs **SE:** N/V, Abd cramps **Interactions:** ↓ Effects W/ antacids w/ Ca or Mg; ↓ effects OF Fe **Labs:** ↑ Serum & urine uric acid **NIPE:** Take w/ food; stress adherence to diet (usually low fat, high protein, high calorie); maint adequate hydration; monitor for GI obst; individualize therapy

Pancuronium (Pavulon) [Skeletal Muscle Relaxant/Nondepolarizing Neuromuscular Blocking Agent] WARNING: Should only be administered by adequately trained individuals Uses: *Paralysis w/ mechanical ventilation* **Action:** Nondepolarizing neuromuscular blocker **Dose:** *Adults & Peds > 1 mo.* Initial 0.06–0.1 mg/kg; maint 0.01 mg/kg 60–100 min after, then 0.01 mg/kg q25–60min PRN; ↓ w/ renal/hepatic impair; intubate pt & keep on controlled ventilation; use adequate sedation or analgesia **Caution:** [C, ?/–] **CI:** Component or bromide sensitivity **Disp:** Inj 1, 2 mg/mL **SE:** Tachycardia, HTN, pruritus, other histamine Rxns **Interactions:** ↑ Effects W/ amikacin, clindamycin, Li, quinidine, succinylcholine, gentamicin, streptomycin, verapamil; ↓ effects W/ carbamazepine, phenytoin, theophylline **NIPE:** Neuromuscular blocker does not alter pain, use analgesics for pain

Panitumumab (Vectibix) [Human Epidermal Growth Factor Receptor (EGFR) Inhibitor] WARNING: Derm tox common (89%) & severe in 12%; can be associated w/ Infxn (sepsis, abscesses requiring I&D); w/ severe derm tox, hold or D/C & monitor for Infxns; severe Inf Rxns (anaphylactic Rxn, bronchospasm, fever, chills, hypotension) in 1%; w/ severe Rxns, stat D/C Inf & possibly permanent discontinuation Uses: *Rx EGFR-expressing met colon CA* **Action:** Anti-EGFR MoAb **Dose:** 6 mg/kg IV Inf over 60 min q14d; doses > 1000 mg over 90 min ↓ Inf rate by 50% w/ grade 1–2 Inf Rxn, D/C permanently w/ grade 3–4 Rxn. For derm tox, hold until < grade 2 tox. If improves < 1 mo, restart

50% original dose. If tox recurs or resolution > 1 mo permanently D/C. If ↓ dose tolerated, ↑ dose by 25% **Caution:** [C, −] D/C nursing during, 2 mo after **Disp:** Vial 20 mg/mL **SE:** Rash, acneiform dermatitis, pruritus, paronychia, Abd pain, N/V/D, constipation, fatigue, dehydration, photosensitivity, conjunctivitis, ocular hyperemia, ↑ lacrimation, stomatitis, mucositis, pulm fibrosis, severe derm tox, Inf Rxns **Labs:** ✓ lytes, ↓ Mg²⁺, ✓ lytes **NIPE:** May impair female fertility; wear sunscreen/hats, limit sun exposure; monitor for S/Sxs of Infxn/sepsis

Pantoprazole (Protonix) [Gastric Acid Suppressant/Proton Pump Inhibitor] **Uses:** *GERD, erosive gastritis*, ZE synd, PUD **Action:** PPI **Dose:** 40 mg/d PO; do not crush/chew tabs; 40 mg IV/d (not > 3 mg/min, use Protonix filter) **Caution:** [B, ?/−] **Disp:** Tabs, DR 20, 40 mg; 40 mg powder for oral susp (mix in applesauce or juice, give stat) Inj 40 mg **SE:** CP, anxiety, GI upset **Interactions:** ↑ Effects *OF* warfarin; ↑ effects of photosensitivity *W/* St. John's wort; ↓ effects *OF* ketoconazole **Labs:** ↑ Serum glucose, lipids, LFTs; monitor PT, INR **NIPE:** ⊘ Sun exposure—use sunblock; take w/o regard to food; antacids will not affect drug absorption; risk of hypomagnesemia w/ long-term use, monitor

Paregoric [Camphorated Tincture of Opium] [C-III] [Narcotic Antidiarrheal] **Uses:** *D*, pain & neonatal opiate withdrawal synd **Action:** Narcotic **Dose:** *Adults.* 5–10 mL PO daily–qid PRN *Peds.* 0.25–0.5 mL/kg daily–qid *Neonatal Withdrawal.* 3–6 gtt PO q3–6h PRN to relieve Sxs × 3–5 d, then taper over 2–4 wk **Caution:** [B (D w/ prolonged use/high dose near term, +] **CI:** Toxic D; convulsive disorder, morphine sensitivity **Disp:** Liq 2 mg morphine = 20 mg opium/5 mL **SE:** ↓ BP, sedation, constipation **Interactions:** ↓ Effects *OF* ampicillin esters, azole antifungals, Fe salts **Labs:** ↑ LFTs, SCr **NIPE:** Take w/o regard to food; contains anhydrous morphine from opium; short-term use only; may cause constipation & CNS depression

Paroxetine (Paxil, Paxil CR, Pexeva) [Antidepressant/SSRI] **WARNING:** Closely monitor for worsening depression or emergence of suicidality, particularly in children, adolescents, & young adults; not for use in peds **Uses:** *Depression, obsessive-compulsive disorder, panic disorder, SAD*, PMDD **Action:** SSRI **Dose:** 10–60 mg PO single daily dose in AM; CR 25 mg/d PO; ↑ 12.5 mg/wk (max range 26–62.5 mg/d) **Caution:** [D, ?] ↑ Bleeding risk **CI:** w/ MAOI, thioridazine, pimozide **Disp:** Tabs 10, 20, 30, 40 mg; susp 10 mg/5 mL; CR 12.5, 25, 37.5 mg **SE:** HA, somnolence, dizziness, GI upset, N/D, ↓ appetite, sweating, xerostomia, tachycardia, ↓ libido **Interactions:** ↑ Risk of QT prolongation *W/* pimozide, thioridazine; ↑ effects *W/* cimetidine; ↑ effects *OF* BBs, dexfenfluramine, dextromethorphan, fenfluramine, haloperidol, MAOIs, theophylline, TCAs, warfarin, St. John's wort, EtOH; ↓ effects *W/* cyproheptadine, phenobarbital, phenytoin; ↓ effects *OF* digoxin, phenytoin **Labs:** ↑ Alk phos, bilirubin, glucose **NIPE:** Take w/o regard to food; may take up to 4 wk for full effect; ⊘ D/C abruptly

Pazopanib Hydrochloride (Votrient) [Kinase Inhibitor] **WARNING:** Administer only by physician experienced in chemotherapy. Severe & fatal hepatotox

Peginterferon Alfa-2b

observed **Uses:** *Rx advanced RCC* **Action:** TKI **Dose:** *Adults.* 800 mg PO once daily, ↓ to 200 mg daily if mod hepatic impair, not recommended in severe hepatic Dz (bilirubin > 3 × ULN) **Caution:** [D, –] Avoid w/ CYP 3A4 inducers/Inhib & QTc prolonging drugs, all SSRI **CI:** Severe hepatic Dz **Disp:** 200-mg tab **SE:** ↑ BP, N/V/D, GI perforation, anorexia, hair depigmentation, ↑ bleeding, CP, ↑ QT **Interactions:** ↑ Effects *W/* strong CYP3A4 Inhibs (eg, ketoconazole, ritonavir, clarithromycin), grapefruit juice; ↓ effects *W/* strong CYP3A4 inducers (eg, rifampin) **Labs:**↑ AST/ALT/bilirubin;↓ WBC, ↓ Na,↓ plt; monitor LFTs before starting drug & at least once q4wk for at least 1st 4 mo of Tx & then periodically **NIPE:** Hold for surgical procedures 7 d before; D/C w/ wound dehiscence; take on empty stomach; swallow whole; monitor ECG

Pegfilgrastim (Neulasta) [Colony Stimulating Factor] Uses: *↓ Frequency of Infxn in pts w/ nonmyeloid malignancies receiving myelosuppressive anti-CA drugs that cause febrile neutropenia* **Action:** Granulocyte- & macrophage-stimulating factor **Dose:** *Adults.* 6 mg SQ × 1/chemotherapy cycle **Caution:** [C, M] w/ Sickle cell **CI:** Allergy to *E coli*–derived proteins or filgrastim **Disp:** Syringes: 6 mg/0.6 mL **SE:** Splenic rupture, HA, fever, weakness, fatigue, dizziness, insomnia, edema, N/V/D, stomatitis, anorexia, constipation, taste perversion, dyspepsia, Abd pain, granulocytopenia, neutropenic fever, ↑ LFTs & uric acid, arthralgia, myalgia, bone pain, ARDS, sickle cell Dz **Interactions:** ↑ Effects *W/* Li **Labs:** ↑ LFTs, uric acid, alk phos, LDH **NIPE:** ⊘ Exposure to Infxn; never give between 14 d before & 24 h after dose of cytotoxic chemotherapy; monitor for S/Sxs of Infxn; monitor for Kehr sign (Abd pain & referred left shoulder pain) associated w/ splenic rupture

Peginterferon Alfa-2a [Pegylated Interferon] (Pegasys) [Antiviral/ Immunomodulator] WARNING: Can cause or aggravate fatal or life-threatening neuropsychological, autoimmune, ischemic, & infectious disorders. Monitor pts closely **Uses:** *Chronic hep C w/ compensated liver Dz* **Action:** Immune modulator **Dose:** 180 mcg (1 mL) SQ qwk ↓ 48 wk; ↓ in renal impair **Caution:** [C, ?/–] w/ NRITs **CI:** Autoimmune hep, decompensated liver Dz **Disp:** 180 mcg/mL Inj **SE:** Depression, insomnia, suicidal behavior,GI upset, alopecia, pruritus **Interactions:** ↑ Effects *OF* methadone, theophylline **Labs:** ↑ ALTs; ↓ WBC & plt; monitor CBC, TFTs, LFTs, before & during therapy **NIPE:** Contra in PRG & men w/ pregnant partners; may have abortifacient effects

Peginterferon Alfa-2b (PEG-Intron) [Antiviral/Immunomodulator] WARNING: Can cause or aggravate fatal or life-threatening neuropsychological, autoimmune, ischemic, & infectious disorders; monitor pts closely **Uses:** *Rx hep C* **Action:** Immune modulator **Dose:** 1 mcg/kg/wk SQ; 1.5 mcg/kg/wk combo w/ ribavirin; w/ depression **Caution:** [C, ?/–] w/ Psychological disorder h/o **CI:** Autoimmune hep, decompensated liver Dz, hemoglobinopathy **Disp:** Vials 50, 80, 120, 150 mcg/0.5 mL; redipen 50, 80, 120, 150 mcg/5 mL; reconstitute w/ 0.7 mL w/ sterile H_2O **SE:** Depression, insomnia, suicidal behavior, GI upset, neutropenia,

↓ plt, alopecia, pruritus **Interactions:** ↑ Myelosuppression *W/* antineoplastics; ↑ effects *OF* doxorubicin, theophylline; ↑ neurotox *W/* vinblastine **Labs:** ↑ ALT, ↓ neutrophils, plts; monitor CBC/plts **NIPE:** Maint hydration; monitor for S/Sxs of Infxn; may exacerbate depression, autoimmune, ischemic & infectious disorder; use barrier contraception; give hs or w/ APAP to ↓ flu-like Sxs; use stat or store in refrigerator × 24 h; do not freeze

Pegloticase (Krystexxa) [PEGylated Uric Acid Specific Enzyme]
WARNING: Anaphylaxis/Inf Rxn reported; administration in settings prepared to manage these Rxns; premed w/ antihistamines & corticosteroids **Uses:** *Refractory gout* **Action:** PEGylated recombinant urate–oxidase enzyme **Dose:** 8 mg IV q2wk (in 250 mL NS/1/2 NS over 120 min) premed w/ antihistamines & corticosteroids **Caution:** [C; –] **CI:** G6PD Deficiency **Disp:** Inj **SE:** Inf Rxn (anaphylaxis), urticaria, pruritis, erythema, chest pain, dyspnea); may cause gout flare, N **Labs:** ✓ uric acid level before each Inf, consider D/C if 2 consecutive levels > 6 mg/dL **NIPE:** Do not IV push; monitor closely for anaphylaxis/Inf Rxns; observe at least 1 h post-Inf

Pemetrexed (Alimta) [Antineoplastic/Folate Antagonist] **Uses:** *w/ Cisplatin in nonresectable mesothelioma*, NSCLC **Action:** Antifolate antineoplastic **Dose:** 500 mg/m² IV over 10 min q3wk; hold if CrCl < 45 mL/min; give w/ vit B₁₂ (1000 mcg IM q9wk) & folic acid (350–1000 mcg PO daily); start 1 wk before; dexamethasone 4 mg PO bid × 3, start 1 d before each Rx **Caution:** [D, –] w/ Renal/hepatic/BM impair **CI:** Component sensitivity **Disp:** 500-mg vial **SE:** Neutropenia, ↓ plt, N/V/D, anorexia, stomatitis, renal failure, neuropathy, fever, fatigue, mood changes, dyspnea, anaphylactic Rxns **Interactions:** ↑ Effects *W/* NSAIDs, probenecid d/t ↓ pemetrexed clearance **Labs:** ↑ Cr, LFTs; ↓ HMG, Hct; monitor CBC/plts **NIPE:** ⊘ PRG & lactation; ⊘ use NSAIDs 5 d before, during, or 5 d after Tx; ↓ dose w/ grade 3–4 mucositis; may cause serious BM suppression & mucous membrane irritation

Pemirolast (Alamast) [Mast Cell Stabilizer] **Uses:** *Allergic conjunctivitis* **Action:** Mast cell stabilizer **Dose:** 1–2 gtt in each eye qid **Caution:** [C, ?/–] **Disp:** 0.1% (1 mg/mL) in 10-mL bottles **SE:** HA, rhinitis, cold/flu Sxs, local irritation **NIPE:** Wait 10 min before inserting contacts

Penbutolol (Levatol) [Antihypertensive/Beta-Blockers] **Uses:** *HTN* **Action:** β-Adrenergic receptor blocker, β₁, β₂ **Dose:** 20–40 mg/d; ↓ in hepatic Insuff **Caution:** [C 1st tri; D if 2nd/3rd tri, M] **CI:** Asthma, cardiogenic shock, cardiac failure, heart block, bradycardia, COPD, pulm edema **Disp:** Tabs 20 mg **SE:** Flushing, ↓ BP, fatigue, hyperglycemia, GI upset, sexual dysfunction, bronchospasm **Interactions:** ↑ Effects *W/* CCBs, fluoroquinolones; ↑ bradycardia *W/* adenosine, amiodarone, digitalis, dipyridamole, epinephrine, neuroleptics, phenylephrine, physostigmine, tacrine; ↑ effects *OF* lidocaine, verapamil; ↓ effects *W/* antacids, NSAIDs; ↓ effects *OF* insulin, hypoglycemics, theophylline **Labs:** ↑ Serum glucose, BUN, K⁺, lipoprotein, triglycerides, uric acid **NIPE:** ↑ Cold sensitivity; D/C abruptly can lead to ↑ angina; may cause severe hypotension & bradycardia.

Penciclovir (Denavir) [Antiviral/Nucleoside Analogue] Uses: *Herpes simplex (herpes labialis/ cold sores)* **Action:** Competitive Inhib of DNA polymerase **Dose:** Apply at 1st sign of lesions, then q2h while awake × 4 d **Caution:** [B, ?/–] **CI:** Allergy, previous Rxn to famciclovir **Disp:** Cream 1% **SE:** Erythema, HA **NIPE:** ⊘ Recommended in lactation or in children; ⊘ do not apply to mucous membranes or near eyes

Penicillin G, Aqueous (Potassium or Sodium) (Pfizerpen, Pentids) [Antibiotic/Penicillin] Uses: *Bacteremia, endocarditis, pericarditis, resp tract Infxns, meningitis, neurosyphilis, skin/skin structure Infxns* **Action:** Bactericidal; ↓ cell wall synth *Spectrum:* Most gram(+) (not staphylococci), streptococci, *N meningitidis*, syphilis, clostridia, & anaerobes (not *Bacteroides*) **Dose:** *Adults.* Based on indication range 0.6–24 mill units/d in ÷ doses q4h *Peds. Newborns < 1 wk.* 25,000–50,000 units/kg/dose IV q12h *Infants 1 wk–< 1 mo.* 25,000–50,000 units/kg/dose IV q8h *Children.* 100,000–300,000 units/kg/24h IV ÷ q4h; ↓ in renal impair **Caution:** [B, M] **CI:** Allergy **Disp:** Powder for Inj **SE:** Allergic Rxns; interstitial nephritis, D, Szs **Notes:** Contains 1.7 mEq of K⁺/MU **Interactions:** ↑ Effects *W/* probenecid; ↑ effects *OF* MTX; ↑ risk of bleeding *W/* anticoagulants; ↓ effects *W/* chloramphenicol, macrolides, tetracyclines; ↓ effects *OF* OCPs **Labs:** ↑ K⁺ (monitor ECG for peaked T waves), ↑ eosinophils; ↓ serum albumin **NIPE:** Monitor for super Infxn, & hypovolemia d/t D; use barrier contraception

Penicillin G Benzathine (Bicillin) [Antibiotic/Penicillin] Uses: *Single-dose regimen for streptococcal pharyngitis, rheumatic fever, glomerulonephritis prophylaxis, & syphilis* **Action:** Bactericidal; ↓ cell wall synth. *Spectrum:* See Penicillin G **Dose:** *Adults.* 1.2–2.4 MU deep IM Inj q2–4wk *Peds.* 50,000 units/kg/dose, 2.4 MU/dose max; deep IM Inj q2–4 wk **Caution:** [B, M] **CI:** Allergy **Disp:** Inj 300,000, 600,000 units/mL; Bicillin L-A benzathine salt only; Bicillin C-R combo of benzathine & procaine (300,000 units procaine w/ 300,000 units benzathine/mL or 900,000 units benzathine w/ 300,000 units procaine/2 mL) **SE:** Inj site pain, acute interstitial nephritis, anaphylaxis **Interactions:** ↑ Effects *W/* probenecid; ↑ PCN 1/2-life *W/* ASA, furosemide, indomethacin, sulfonamides, thiazide diuretics; ↑ risk of bleeding *W/* anticoagulants; ↓ effects *W/* chloramphenicol, macrolides, tetracyclines; ↓ effects *OF* OCPs **Labs:** ↑ Eosinophils; ↓ serum albumin **NIPE:** Monitor for super Infxn; use barrier contraception; IM use only; sustained action, w/ detectable levels up to 4 wk; drug of choice for noncongenital syphilis

Penicillin G Procaine (Wycillin, Others) [Antibiotic/Penicillin] Uses: *Infxns of resp tract, skin/soft tissue, scarlet fever, syphilis* **Action:** Bactericidal; ↓ cell wall synth *Spectrum:* PCN G-sensitive organisms that respond to low, persistent serum levels **Dose:** *Adults.* 0.6–4.8 MU/d in ÷ doses q12–24h; give probenecid at least 30 min prior to PCN to prolong action *Peds.* 25,000–50,000 units/kg/d IM ÷ daily–bid **Caution:** [B, M] **CI:** Allergy **Disp:** Inj 300,000, 500,000, 600,000 units/mL **SE:** Pain at Inj site, interstitial nephritis, anaphylaxis **Interactions:** ↑ Effects W/ probenecid; ↑ penicillin 1/2-life W/ ASA, furosemide, indomethacin, sulfonamides, thiazide diuretics; ↑ risk of bleeding W/ anticoagulants; ↓ effects W/ chloramphenicol, macrolides, tetracyclines; ↓ effects OF OCPs **Labs:** ↑ Eosinophils; ↓ serum albumin **NIPE:** Monitor for super Infxn; use barrier contraception; LA parenteral PCN; levels up to 15 h

Penicillin V (Pen-Vee K, Veetids, Others) [Antibiotic/Penicillin] Uses: Susceptible streptococci Infxns, otitis media, URIs, skin/soft-tissue Infxns (PCN-sensitive staphylococci) **Action:** Bactericidal; ↓ cell wall synth. *Spectrum:* Most gram(+), including streptococci **Dose:** *Adults.* 250–500 mg PO q6h, q8h, q12h *Peds.* 25–50 mg/kg/25h PO in 4 doses; ↓ in renal impair; take on empty stomach **Caution:** [B, M] **CI:** Allergy **Disp:** Tabs 125, 250, 500 mg; susp 125, 250 mg/5 mL **SE:** GI upset, interstitial nephritis, anaphylaxis, convulsions **Interactions:** ↓ Effects W/ ASA, probenecid; ↑ effects OF MTX & anticoagulants; ↑ risk of anaphylaxes W/ BB; ↓ effects W/ chloramphenicol, macrolides, tetracyclines; ↓ effects OF OCPs **Labs:** ↓ Eosinophils; ↓ serum albumin, WBC **NIPE:** Monitor for super Infxn; monitor for signs hypovolemia d/t D; use barrier contraception; well-tolerated PO PCN; 250 mg = 400,000 units of PCN G

Pentamidine (Pentam 300, NebuPent) [Antiprotozoal] Uses: *Rx & prevention of PCP* **Action:** ↓ DNA, RNA, phospholipid, & protein synth **Dose:** *Rx: Adults & Peds.* 4 mg/kg/24 h IV daily × 14–21 d. *Prevention: Adults & Peds > 5 y.* 300 mg once q4wk, give via Respirgard II nebulizer; ↓ IV w/ renal impair **Caution:** [C, ?] **CI:** Component allergy, use w/ didanosine **Disp:** Inj 300 mg/vial; aerosol 300 mg **SE:** Pancreatic cell necrosis w/ hyperglycemia; pancreatitis, CP, fatigue, dizziness, rash, GI upset, renal impair, blood dyscrasias (leukopenia, ↓ plt) **Interactions:** ↑ Nephrotoxic effects W/ aminoglycosides, amphotericin B, capreomycin, cidofovir, cisplatin, cyclosporine, colistin, ganciclovir, methoxyflurane, polymyxin B, vancomycin; ↑ BM suppression W/ antineoplastics, radiation therapy **Labs:** ↑ LFTs, serum K+ (monitor ECG for peaked T waves), ↓ HMG, Hct, plts, WBCs; ↑/↓ glucose; monitor CBC, glucose, pancreatic Fxn monthly for 1st 3 mo **NIPE:** Reconstitute w/ sterile H2O only, Inh may cause metallic taste; ↑ fluids to 2–3 L/d; monitor for ↓ BP following IV dose; prolonged use may ↑ Infxn risk; risk of ventricular arrhythmias

Pentazocine (Talwin, Talwin Compound, Talwin NX) [C-IV] [Narcotic Analgesic] WARNING: Oral use only; severe & potentially lethal Rxns from misuse by Inj Uses: *Mod–severe pain* **Action:** Partial narcotic agonist–antagonist **Dose:** *Adults.* 30 mg IM or IV; 50–100 mg PO q3–4h PRN *Peds 5–8 y.* 15 mg IM q4h PRN *8–14 y.* 30 mg IM q4h PRN; ↓ in renal/hepatic impair **Caution:** [C (1st tri, D w/ prolonged use/high dose near term), +/−] **CI:** Allergy, ↑ ICP (unless ventilated) **Disp:** *Talwin Compound* tabs 12.5 mg + 325 mg ASA; *Talwin NX* 50 mg + 0.5 mg naloxone; Inj 30 mg/mL **SE:** Considerable dysphoria; drowsiness, GI upset, xerostomia, Szs **Notes:** 30–60 mg IM = 10 mg of morphine IM

Interactions: ↑ CNS depression *W/* antihistamines, barbiturates, hypnotics, phenothiazine, EtOH; ↑ effects *W/* cimetidine; ↑ effects *OF* digitoxin, phenytoin, rifampin; ↓ effects *OF* opioids **Labs:** ↑ Serum amylase, lipase **NIPE:** May cause withdrawal in pts using opioids; Talwin NX has naloxone to curb abuse by nonoral route; 30 y cause IM = 10 mg of morphine IM

Pentobarbital (Nembutal, Others) [C-II] [Anticonvulsant, Sedative/ Hypnotic/Barbiturate] **Uses:** *Insomnia (short-term), convulsions*, sedation, induce coma w/ severe head injury **Action:** Barbiturate **Dose:** *Adults.* *Sedative:* 150–200 mg IM × 1100 mg IV, repeat PRN to 500 mg/max *Hypnotic:* 100–200 mg PO or PR hs PRN *Induced coma:* Load 5–10 mg/kg IV, w/ maint 1–3 mg/kg/h IV *Peds.* *Induced coma:* As adult dose **Caution:** [D, +/−] Severe hepatic impair **CI:** Allergy **Disp:** Caps 50, 100 mg; elixir 18.2 mg/5 mL (= 20 mg pentobarbital); supp 30, 60, 120, 200 mg; Inj 50 mg/mL **SE:** Resp depression, ↓ BP w/ aggressive IV use for cerebral edema; bradycardia, ↓ BP, sedation, lethargy, resp ↓, hangover, rash, SJS, blood dyscrasias **Interactions:** ↑ Effects *W/* MAOIs, narcotic analgesics, EtOH; ↓ effects *OF* anticoagulants, BBs, corticosteroids, cyclosporine, digoxin, doxycycline, griseofulvin, neuroleptics, OCPs, quinidine, theophylline, verapamil **NIPE:** Tolerance to sedative–hypnotic effect w/in 1–2 wk; monitor for drowsiness, resp depression, hypotension

Pentosan Polysulfate Sodium (Elmiron) [Urinary Analgesic] **Uses:** *Relieve pain/discomfort w/ interstitial cystitis* **Action:** Bladder wall buffer **Dose:** 100 mg PO tid; on empty stomach w/ H$_2$O 1 h ac or 2 h pc **Caution:** [B, ?/−] **CI:** Allergy **Disp:** Caps 100 mg **SE:** Alopecia, N/D, HA, anticoagulant effects, rectal bleeding **Interactions:** Risk of ↑ anticoagulation *W/* anticoagulants, ASA, thrombolytics **Labs:** ↑ LFTs, ↓ plts **NIPE:** Reassess after 3 mo

Pentoxifylline (Trental) [Hemorheologic/Xanthine Derivative] **Uses:** *Rx Sxs of peripheral vascular Dz* **Action:** ↓ Blood cell viscosity, restores RBC flexibility **Dose:** *Adults.* 400 mg PO tid pc; Rx min 8 wk for effect; ↓ to bid w/ GI/CNS SEs **Caution:** [C, +/−] **CI:** Cerebral/retinal hemorrhage, methylxanthine (caffeine) intolerance **Disp:** Tabs CR 400 mg; tabs ER 400 mg **SE:** Dizziness, HA, GI upset **Interactions:** ↑ Risk of bleeding *W/* anticoagulants, NSAIDs; ↑ effects *OF* antihypertensives, theophylline **NIPE:** Take w/ food to < GI upset

Perindopril Erbumine (Aceon) [Antihypertensive/ACEI] **WARNING:** ACE Inhibs can cause death to developing fetus; D/C stat w/ PRG **Uses:** *HTN*, CHF, DN, post-MI **Action:** ACE Inhib **Dose:** 4–8 mg/d ÷ dose; 16 mg/d max; avoid w/ food; ↓ w/ elderly/renal impair **Caution:** [C (1st tri, D 2nd & 3rd tri), ?/−] ACE-Inhib–induced angioedema **CI:** Bilateral RAS, primary hyperaldosteronism **Disp:** Tabs 2, 4, 8 mg **SE:** Weakness, HA, ↓ BP, dizziness, GI upset, cough **Interactions:** ↑ Effects *W/* antihypertensives, diuretics; ↑ effects *OF* cyclosporine, insulin, Li, sulfonylureas, tacrolimus; ↓ effects *W/* NSAIDs **Labs:** ↑ Serum K$^+$, LFTs, uric acid, cholesterol, Cr **NIPE:** ↓ Effects if taken w/ food; risk of persistent cough; OK w/ diuretics; monitor ECG for hyperkalemia (peaked T waves)

Permethrin (Nix, Elimite) [OTC] [Scabicides/Pediculicides] Uses: *Rx lice/scabies* **Action:** Pediculicide **Dose:** *Adults & Peds.* *Lice:* Saturate hair & scalp; allow 10 min before rinsing. *Scabies:* Apply cream head to toe; leave for 8–14 h, wash w/ H_2O **Caution:** [B, ?/–] **CI:** Allergy **Disp:** Topical lotion 1%; cream 5% **SE:** Local irritation **NIPE:** Drug remains on hair up to 2 wk, reapply in 1 wk if live lice; sprays available (Rid, A200, Nix) to disinfect clothing, bedding, combs, & brushes; lotion not OK in peds < 2 y; may repeat after 7 d

Perphenazine (Trilafon) [Antipsychotic, Antiemetic/Phenothiazine] Uses: *Psychotic disorders, severe N*, intractable hiccups **Action:** Phenothiazine, blocks brain dopaminergic receptors **Dose:** *Adults. Antipsychotic:* 4–16 mg PO tid; max 64 mg/d *Hiccups:* 5 mg IM q6h PRN or 1 mg IV at intervals not < 1–2 mg/ min, 5 mg max *Peds. 1–6 y.* 4–6 mg/d PO in ÷ doses *6–12 y.* 6 mg/d PO in ÷ doses *> 12 y.* 4–16 mg PO bid–qid; ↓ in hepatic Insuff **Caution:** [C, ?/–] NAG, severe ↑/↓ BP **CI:** Phenothiazine sensitivity, BM depression, severe liver or cardiac Dz **Disp:** Tabs 2, 4, 8, 16 mg; PO conc 16 mg/5 mL; Inj 5 mg/mL **SE:** ↑ BP, tachycardia, bradycardia, EPS, drowsiness, Szs, photosensitivity, skin discoloration, blood dyscrasias, constipation **Interactions:** ↑ Effects *W/* antidepressants; ↑ effects *OF* anticholinergics, antidepressants, propranolol, phenytoin; ↓ CNS effects *W/* CNS depressants, EtOH; ↓ effects *W/* antacids, Li, phenobarbital, caffeine, tobacco; ↓ effects *OF* levodopa, Li **Labs:** ↑ Serum cholesterol, glucose, LFTs; ↓ HMG, plts, WBCs **NIPE:** Take oral dose w/ food; risk of photosensitivity—use sunblock

Phenazopyridine (Pyridium, Azo-Standard, Urogesic, Many Others) [Urinary Analgesic] Uses: *Lower urinary tract irritation* **Action:** Anesthetic on urinary tract mucosa **Dose:** *Adults.* 100–200 mg PO tid; 2 d max w/ antibiotics for UTI; ↓ w/ renal Insuff **Caution:** [B, ?] Hepatic Dz **CI:** Renal failure **Disp:** Tabs 100, 200 mg **SE:** GI disturbances, HA, dizziness, ARF, methemoglobinemia **Labs:** Interferes *W/* urinary tests for glucose, ketones, bilirubin, protein, steroids **NIPE:** Tinting of sclera/skin; urine may turn red-orange in color & can stain clothing & contacts; take w/ food

Phenelzine (Nardil) [Antidepressant/MAOI] WARNING: Antidepressants ↑ the risk of suicidal thinking & behavior in children & adolescents w/ MDD & other psychological disorders; not for peds use Uses: *Depression*, bulimia **Action:** MAOI **Dose:** *Adults.* 15 mg PO tid, ↑ to 60–90 mg/d ÷ doses *Elderly:* 15–60 mg/d ÷ doses **Caution:** [C, –] Interacts w/ SSRI, ergots, triptans **CI:** CHF, h/o liver Dz, Pheo **Disp:** Tabs 15 mg **SE:** Postural ↓ BP; edema, dizziness, sedation, rash, sexual dysfunction, xerostomia, constipation, urinary retention **Interactions:** ↑ HTN Rxn *W/* amphetamines, fluoxetine, levodopa, metaraminol, phenylephrine, phenylpropanolamine, pseudoephedrine, reserpine, sertraline, tyramine, EtOH, foods *W/* tyramine, caffeine, tryptophan; ↑ effects *OF* barbiturates, narcotics, sedatives, sumatriptan, TCAs, ephedra, ginseng **Labs:** ↓ Glucose, false(+) ↑ in bilirubin & uric acid **NIPE:** 2–4 wk for effect; avoid tyramine-containing foods (eg, beer, red wine, aged cheeses/meats, overripe & dried fruits) d/t risk of HTN; monitor for ↑ suicidal ideations, depression, hypoglycemia

Phenobarbital [C-IV] [Anticonvulsant, Sedative/Hypnotic/Barbiturate] Uses: *Sz disorders*, insomnia, anxiety **Action:** Barbiturate **Dose:** *Adults. Sedative–hypnotic:* 30–120 mg/d PO or IM PRN *Anticonvulsant:* Load 10–12 mg/kg in 3 ÷ doses, then 1–3 mg/kg/24 h PO, IM, or IV *Peds. Sedative–hypnotic:* 2–3 mg/kg/24 h PO or IM hs PRN *Anticonvulsant:* Load 15–20 mg/kg ÷ in 2 equal doses 4 h apart, then 3–5 mg/kg/24 h PO ÷ in 2–3 doses; ↓ w/ CrCl < 10 mL/min **Caution:** [D, M] CI: Porphyria, hepatic impair, dyspnea, airway obst **Disp:** Tabs 15, 16, 30, 32, 60, 65, 100 mg; elixir 15, 20 mg/5 mL; Inj 30, 60, 65, 130 mg/mL **SE:** Bradycardia, ↓ BP, hangover, SJS, blood dyscrasias, resp depression **Notes:** Levels: *Trough:* Just before next dose *Therapeutic trough:* 15–40 mcg/mL *Toxic trough:* > 40 mcg/mL *1/2-life:* 40–120 h **Interactions:** ↑ CNS depression **W/** CNS depressants, anesthetics, antianxiety meds, antihistamines, narcotic analgesics, EtOH, Indian snakeroot, kava kava; ↑ effects **W/** chloramphenicol, MAOIs, procarbazine, valproic acid; ↓ effects **W/** rifampin; ↓ effects **OF** anticoagulants, BBs, carbamazepine, clozapine, corticosteroids, doxorubicin, doxycycline, estrogens, felodipine, griseofulvin, haloperidol, methadone, metronidazole, OCPs, phenothiazine, quinidine, TCAs, theophylline, verapamil **Labs:** ↓ Bilirubin **NIPE:** May take 2–3 wk for full effects; ⊘ D/C abruptly; tolerance develops to sedation; paradoxic hyperactivity seen in aged pts; long 1/2-life allows single daily dosing

Phenylephrine, Nasal (Neo-Synephrine Nasal) (OTC) [Vasopressor/Decongestant] WARNING: Not for use in Peds < 2 y Uses: *Nasal congestion* **Action:** α-Adrenergic agonist **Dose:** *Adults.* 1–2 sprays/nostril q4h (usual 0.25%) PRN *Peds. 2–6 y.* 0.125% 1 gt/nostril q2–4h *6–12 y.* 1–2 sprays/nostril q4h 0.25% 2–3 gtt **Caution:** [C, +/−] HTN, acute pancreatitis, hep, coronary Dz, NAG, hyperthyroidism CI: Bradycardia, arrhythmias **Disp:** Nasal soln 0.125%, 0.25%, 0.5%, 1%; Liq 7.5 mg/5 mL; gtt 2.5 mg/mL **SE:** Arrhythmias, HTN, nasal irritation, dryness, sneezing, rebound congestion w/ prolonged use, HA **NIPE:** Do not use > 3 d; use prior to nasal intubation & NG tube insertion to ↓ bleeding

Phenylephrine, Ophthalmic (Neo-Synephrine Ophthalmic, AK-Dilate, Zincfrin [OTC]) [Vasopressor] Uses: *Mydriasis, ocular redness [OTC], perioperative mydriasis, posterior synechiae, uveitis w/ posterior synechiae* **Action:** α-Adrenergic agonist **Dose:** *Adults. Redness:* 1 gt 0.12% q3–4h PRN *Exam mydriasis:* 1 gt 2.5% (15 min–1 h for effect). *Pre-op:* 1 gt 2.5–10% 30–60 min pre-op *Ocular disorders:* 1 gt 2.5–10% daily–tid *Peds.* As adult, only use 2.5% for exam, pre-op, & ocular conditions **Caution:** [C, May cause late-term fetal anoxia/bradycardia, +/−] HTN, w/ elderly w/ CAD CI: NAG **Disp:** Ophthal soln 0.12% (Zincfrin OTC), 2.5%, 10% **SE:** Tearing, HA, irritation, eye pain, photophobia, arrhythmia, tremor

Phenylephrine, Oral (Sudafed PE, SudoGest PE, Nasop, Lusonal, AH-Chew D, Sudafed PE Quick Dissolve) (OTC) [Vasopressor/Decongestant] WARNING: Not for use in peds < 2 y Uses: *Nasal congestion*

Action: α-Adrenergic agonist **Dose:** *Adults.* 10–20 mg PO q4h PRN, max 60 mg/d *Peds.* 5 mg PO q4h PRN, max 60 mg/d **Caution:** [C, +/−] HTN, acute pancreatitis, hep, coronary Dz, NAG, hyperthyroidism **CI:** MAOI w/in 14 d, NAG, severe ↑ BP or CAD, urinary retention **Disp:** Liq 7.5 mg/5 mL; gtt 2.5 mg/mL; tabs 5, 10 mg; chew tabs 10 mg; tabs once daily 10 mg; strips 10 mg **SE:** Arrhythmias, HTN, HA, agitation, anxiety, tremor, palpitations **Interactions:** ↑ Risk of HTN crisis *W* / MAOIs; ↑ risk of pressor effects *W*/ BB; ↑ risk of arrhythmias *W*/ epinephrine, isoproterenol; ↓ effects *OF* guanethidine, methyldopa, reserpine **NIPE:** Use w/ BB may cause severe HTN & cause intracranial bleed/ischemia

Phenylephrine, Systemic (Neo-Synephrine) [Vasopressor/ Adrenergic]: WARNING: Prescribers should be aware of full prescribing info before use **Uses:** *Vascular failure in shock, allergy, or drug-induced ↓ BP* **Action:** α-Adrenergic agonist **Dose:** *Adults. Mild–mod ↓ BP:* 2–5 mg IM or SQ ↑ BP for 2 h; 0.1–0.5 mg IV elevates BP for 15 min *Severe ↓ BP/shock:* Cont Inf at 100–180 mcg/min; after BP stable, maint 40–60 mcg/min *Peds. ↓ BP:* 5–20 mcg/ kg/dose IV q10–15 min or 0.1–0.5 mcg/kg/min IV Inf, titrate to effect **Caution:** [C, +/−] HTN, acute pancreatitis, hep, coronary Dz, NAG, hyperthyroidism **CI:** Bradycardia, arrhythmias **Disp:** Inj 10 mg/mL **SE:** Arrhythmias, HTN, peripheral vasoconstriction ↑ w/ oxytocin, MAOIs, & TCAs; HA, weakness, necrosis, ↓ renal perfusion **Interactions:** ↑ HTN *W*/ BBs, MAOIs; ↑ pressor response *W*/ guanethidine, methyldopa, reserpine, TCAs **NIPE:** Restore blood vol if loss has occurred; use large veins to avoid extrav; phentolamine 10 mg in 10–15 mL of NS for local Inj to Rx extrav; monitor ECG for arrhythmias

Phenytoin (Dilantin) [Anticonvulsant/Hydantoin] **Uses:** *Sz disorders* **Action:** ↓ Sz spread in the motor cortex **Dose:** *Adults & Peds. Load:* 15–20 mg/kg IV, 50 mg/min max or PO in 400-mg doses at 4-h intervals *Adults. Maint:* Initial 200 mg PO or IV bid or 300 mg hs then follow levels; alternately 5–7 mg/ kg/d based on IDW ÷ daily–tid *Peds. Maint:* 4–7 mg/kg/24h PO or IV ÷ daily–bid; avoid PO susp (erratic absorption) **Caution:** [D, +] **CI:** Heart block, sinus bradycardia **Disp:** *Dilantin Infatab:* Chew tabs 50 mg *Dilantin/Phenytek:* Caps 100 mg; caps ER 30, 100, 200, 300 mg; susp 125 mg/5 mL; Inj 50 mg/mL **SE:** Nystagmus/ ataxia early signs of tox; gum hyperplasia w/ long-term use. *IV:* ↓ BP, bradycardia, arrhythmias, phlebitis; peripheral neuropathy, rash, blood dyscrasias, SJS **Notes:** *Levels: Trough:* Just before next dose *Therapeutic:* 10–20 mcg/mL *Toxic:* > 20 mcg/mL. Phenytoin albumin bound, levels = bound & free phenytoin; w/ ↓ albumin & azotemia, low levels may be therapeutic (nl free levels) **Interactions:** ↑ Effects *W*/ amiodarone, allopurinol, chloramphenicol, disulfiram, INH, omeprazole, sulfonamides, quinolones, TMP; ↑ effects *OF* Li; ↓ effects *W*/ cimetidine, cisplatin, diazoxide, folate, pyridoxine, rifampin; ↓ effects *OF* azole antifungals, benzodiazepines, carbamazepine, corticosteroids, cyclosporine, digitalis glycosides, doxycycline, furosemide, levodopa, OCPs, quinidine, tacrolimus, theophylline, thyroid meds, valproic acid **Labs:** ↑ Serum cholesterol, glucose, alk phos

NIPE: Take w/ food; may alter urine color; use barrier contraception; ⊘ D/C abruptly; do not change dosage at intervals < 7–10 d; hold tube feeds 1 h before & after dose if using oral susp; avoid large dose ↑

Physostigmine (Antilirium) [Antimuscarinic Antidote/Reversible Cholinesterase Inhibitor] Uses: *Antidote for TCA, atropine, & scopolamine OD; glaucoma* Action: Reversible cholinesterase Inhib Dose: *Adults.* 0.5–2 mg IV or IM q20min *Peds.* 0.01–0.03 mg/kg/dose IV q5–10min up to 2 mg total PRN Caution: [C, ?] CI: GI/GU disord; CV Dz, asthma Disp: Inj 1 mg/mL SE: Rapid IV administration associated w/ Szs; cholinergic SE; sweating, salivation, lacrimation, GI upset, asystole, changes in HR Interactions: ↑ Resp depression W/ succinylcholine, ↑ effects W/ cholinergics, jaborandi tree, pill-bearing spurge Labs: ↑ ALT, AST, serum amylase NIPE: Excessive readministration can result in cholinergic crisis; crisis reversed w/ atropine

Phytonadione [Vitamin K] (AquaMEPHYTON, Others) [Blood Modifier/Vitamin K] Uses: *Coagulation disorders d/t faulty formation of factors II, VII, IX, X*; hyperalimentation Action: Cofactor for production of factors II, VII, IX, & X Dose: *Adults & Peds. Anticoagulant-induced prothrombin deficiency:* 1–10 mg PO or IV slowly *Hyperalimentation:* 10 mg IM or IV qwk *Peds Infants.* 0.5–1 mg/dose IM, SQ, or PO Caution: [C, +] CI: Allergy Disp: Tabs 5 mg; Inj 2, 10 mg/mL SE: Anaphylaxis from IV dosage; give IV slowly; GI upset (PO), Inj site Rxns Interactions: ↓ Effects W/ antibiotics, cholestyramine, colestipol, salicylates, sucralfate; ↓ effects OF oral anticoagulants Labs: Falsely ↑ urine steroids NIPE: w/ parenteral Rx, 1st change in PT/INR usually seen in 12–24 h; use makes rewarfarinization more difficult; may cause ↑ clotting risk.

Pimecrolimus (Elidel) [Topical Immunomodulator] WARNING: Associated w/ rare skin malignancies & lymphoma, limit to area, not for age < 2 y Uses: *Atopic dermatitis* refractory, severe perianal itching Action: Inhibits T-lymphocytes Dose: *Adults & Peds > 2 y.* Apply bid; use at least 1 wk following resolution Caution: [C, ?/–] w/ local Infxn, lymphadenopathy; immunocompromise; avoid in pts < 2 y CI: Allergy component, < 2 y Disp: Cream 1% SE: Phototox, local irritation/burning, flu-like Sxs, may ↑ malignancy NIPE: Use on dry skin only; wash hands after; 2nd-line/short-term use only

Pimozide (Orap) [Antipsychotic/Dopamine Antagonist] WARNING: ↑ Mortality in elderly w/ dementia-related psychosis Uses: * Tourette Dz *agitation, psychosis Action: Typical antipsychotic, DA antagonist Dose: 10 mg PO qd, ↓ to 5 mg w/ SE or hepatic impair Caution: [D, –] NAG, elderly, hepatic impair, neurologic Dzs CI: Compound hypersensitivity, coma, dysrhythmia, ↑ QT synd, w/ QT prolonging drugs, ↓ K+, ↓ mg, w/ CYP3A4 Inhib (Table 10) Disp: Tabs 1, 2 mg SE: CNS (somnolence, agitation, others), rash, xerostomia, weakness, rigidity, visual changes, constipation, ↑ salivation, akathisia, tardive dyskinesia, neuroleptic malignant synd, ↑ QT Interactions: ↑ Effects OF CYP1A2 Inhibs; eg; amiodarone, amprenavir, clarithromycin, diltiazem, ketoconazole, verapamil, grapefruit juice (Table 10); ↑ risk of CNS depression W/ analgesics, other CNS depressants, EtOH Labs: ↓ K+, ↑ glu, monitor CBC—D/C w/ low WBCs NIPE: Monitor ECG for ↑ QT synd ✓ & hypokalemia (flattened T waves), ⊘ D/C abruptly

Pindolol (Visken) [Antihypertensive/Beta-Blocker] Uses: *HTN* Action: β-Adrenergic receptor blocker, β₁, β₂, ISA Dose: 5–10 mg bid, 60 mg/d max; ↓ in hepatic/renal failure Caution: [B (1st tri, D if 2nd or 3rd tri), +/−] CI: Uncompensated CHF, cardiogenic shock, bradycardia, heart block, asthma, COPD Disp: Tabs 5, 10 mg SE: Insomnia, dizziness, fatigue, edema, GI upset, dyspnea; fluid retention may exacerbate CHF Interactions: ↑ HTN & bradycardia W/ amphetamines, ephedrine, phenylephrine; ↑ effects W/ antihypertensives, diuretics; ↓ effects W/ NSAIDs; ↓ effect OF hypoglycemics Labs: ↑ LFTs, uric acid NIPE: ⊘ D/C abruptly—can cause angina; ↑ cold sensitivity; monitor for hyperglycemia

Pioglitazone (Actos) [Hypoglycemic/Thiazolidinedione] WARNING: May cause or worsen CHF; use for > 1y, may be associated with ↑ risk of bladder CA Uses: *Type 2 DM as adjunct to diet & exercise* Action: ↑ Insulin sensitivity Dose: 15–45 mg/d PO; start 15–30 mg OD; increase by 15 mg OD to a max 45 mg OD Caution: [C, −] CI: CHF, hepatic impair; NYHA Class III or IV HF Disp: Tabs 15, 30, 45 mg SE: Wgt gain, myalgia, URI, HA, hypoglycemia, edema Interactions: ↑ Effects W/ CYP2C8 Inhibs (eg, gemfibrozil); ↓ effects W/ CYP2C8 inducers (eg, rifampin); ↓ effects OF OC, midazolam; monitor for HF W/ insulin; monitor glycemic control W/ ketoconazole Labs: ↑ LFTs—monitor NIPE: Take w/o regard to food; use barrier contraception; ↑ fx risk in women; ↑ risk of fluid retention leading to CHF

Pioglitazone HCl/Glimepiride (Duetact) [Hypoglycemic/Thiazolidinedione & Sulfonylurea] WARNING: Pioglitazone may cause or worsen CHF; use of pioglitazone for > 1 y may be associated w/ ↑ risk of bladder CA Uses: Type 2 DM as adjunct to diet & exercise Action: Combined ↑ insulin resistance, ↑ pancreatic insulin secretion, ↓ hepatic glucose output & production Dose: Initially 1 tab PO OD w/ the 1st main meal Caution: [C, −] CI: Hepatic impair, DKA; NYHA Class III or IV HF Disp: Tabs (pioglitazone HCL mg/ glimepiride mg): 30/2, 30/4 SE: ↑ Risk of CV mortality, hypoglycemia, wgt gain, HA, edema, N, URI Interactions: ↑ Effects W/ ASA, BB, chloramphenicol, ketoconazole, MAOIs, NSAIDs, probenecid, salicylates, sulfonamides; ↓ effects W/ corticosteroids, diuretics, estrogens, INH, phenothiazine, phenytoin, sympathomimetics, thyroid drugs; ↓ effects OF OCPs; monitor for HF W/ insulin Labs: ↑ LFTs—monitor t NIPE: Take w/ 1st main meal of the d; use barrier contraception; ⊘ use in type 1 DM; ↑ fx risk in women receiving pioglitazone; if currently on pioglitazone and glimepiride separately, may start on 30/2 or 30/4; if switching from different sulfonylurea then starting dose is 30/2 OD

Pioglitazone/Metformin (Actoplus Met) [Hypoglycemic/Thiazolidinedione & Biguanide] WARNING: Metformin can cause lactic acidosis, fatal in 50% of cases; pioglitazone may cause or worsen CHF & use for > 1y may be associated w/ ↑ risk of bladder CA **Uses:** *Type 2 DM as adjunct to diet & exercise* **Action:** Combined ↑ insulin sensitivity w/ ↓ hepatic glucose release **Dose:** Initial 1 tab PO daily or bid, titrate; XR: 1 tab PO daily w/ evening meal; max daily pioglitazone 45 mg & metformin 2550 mg; metformin ER 2000 mg; give w/ meals **Caution:** [C, –] D/C w/ radiologic IV contrast agents during & 48 h > use **CI:** CHF—NYHA Class III or IV HF; renal impair, acidosis **Disp:** Tabs (pioglitazone mg/metformin mg): 15/500, 15/850, tabs XR (pioglitazone mg/metformin ER mg): 15/1000, 30/1000 **SE:** Lactic acidosis, CHF, ↓ glucose, edema, wgt gain, myalgia, URI, HA, GI upset, liver damage **Interactions:** ↑ Effects of metformin on lactate **W/** EtOH; ↑ Effects **W/** amiloride, cimetidine, digoxin, furosemide, ketoconazole, MAOIs, morphine, procainamide, quinidine, quinine, ranitidine, triamterene, TMP, vancomycin; ↓ effects **OF** OCPs; ↓ effects **W/** corticosteroids, CCBs, diuretics, estrogens, INH, OCPs, phenothiazine, phenytoin, sympathomimetics, thyroid drugs, tobacco; monitor for HF **W/** insulin; BB may mask hypoglycemia **Labs:** ↑ LFTs, monitor serum glucose & LFTs **NIPE:** Take w/o regard to food; use barrier contraception; ⊘ dehydration, EtOH; ↑ fx risk in women receiving pioglitazone

Piperacillin (Pipracil) [Antibiotic/Penicillin-4th Generation] **Uses:** *Infxns of skin, bone, resp, & urinary tract, abdomen, sepsis* **Action:** 4th-gen PCN; bactericidal; ↓ cell wall synth *Spectrum:* Primarily gram(+), better *Enterococcus, H influenzae,* not staphylococci; gram(−) *E coli, Proteus, Shigella, Pseudomonas,* not β-lactamase producers **Dose:** *Adults.* 2–4 g IV q4–6h *Peds.* 200–300 mg/kg/d IV ÷ q4–6h; ↓ in renal Insuff **Caution:** [B, M] **CI:** PCN/β-lactam sensitivity **Disp:** Powder for Inj: 2, 3, 4, 40 g **SE:** ↓ Plt aggregation, interstitial nephritis, renal failure, anaphylaxis, hemolytic anemia **Interactions:** ↑ Effects **W/** probenecid; ↑ effects **OF** anticoagulants, MTX; ↓ effects **W/** macrolides, tetracyclines; ↓ effects **OF** OCPs **Labs:** ↑ LFTs, BUN, Cr, + direct Coombs test, ↓ K⁺ **NIPE:** Inactivation of aminoglycosides if drugs given together—administration at least 1 h apart; often used w/ aminoglycoside; monitor for hypovolemia d/t D

Piperacillin–Tazobactam (Zosyn) [Antibiotic/Extended Spectrum Penicillin, Beta-Lactamase Inhibitor] **Uses:** *Infxns of skin, bone, resp & urinary tract, abdomen, sepsis* **Action:** 4th-gen PCN plus β-lactamase Inhib; bactericidal; ↓ cell wall synth *Spectrum:* Good, excellent gram(−); anaerobes & β-lactamase producers **Dose:** *Adults.* 3.375–4.5 g IV q6h; ↓ in renal Insuff **Caution:** [B, M] **CI:** PCN or β-lactam sensitivity **Disp:** Powder for Inj: Frozen, premix Inj 3.25, 3.375, 4.5 g **SE:** D, HA, insomnia, GI upset, serum sickness-like Rxn, pseudomembranous colitis **Interactions:** ↑ Effects **W/** probenecid; ↑ effects **OF** anticoagulants, MTX; ↓ effects **W/** macrolides, tetracyclines; ↓ effects **OF** OCPs **Labs:** ↑ LFTs, BUN, Cr, (+) direct Coombs test, ↓ K⁺ **NIPE:** Inactivation of aminoglycosides if drugs given together—administration at least 1 h apart; often used in combo w/ aminoglycoside; monitor for hypovolemia d/t D

Pirbuterol (Maxair) [Bronchodilator/Sympathomimetic] Uses: *Prevention & Rx reversible bronchospasm* **Action:** β_2-Adrenergic agonist **Dose:** 2 Inh q4–6h; max 12 Inh/d **Caution:** [C, ?/–] **Disp:** Aerosol 0.2 mg/actuation **SE:** Nervousness, restlessness, trembling, HA, taste changes, tachycardia **Interactions:** ↑ Effects W/ epinephrine, sympathomimetics; ↑ vascular effects W/ MAOIs, TCAs; ↓ effects W/ BB **NIPE:** Rinse mouth after use; shake well before use; teach pt proper inhaler technique; monitor for hyperglycemia

Piroxicam (Feldene) [Bronchodilator/Beta-Adrenergic Agonist]: WARNING: May ↑ risk of CV events & GI bleeding Uses: *Arthritis & pain* **Action:** NSAID; ↓ prostaglandins **Dose:** 10–20 mg/d **Caution:** [B (1st tri, D if 3rd tri or near term), +] GI bleeding **CI:** ASA/NSAID sensitivity **Disp:** Caps 10, 20 mg **SE:** Dizziness, rash, GI upset, edema, ARF, peptic ulcer **Interactions:** ↑ Effects W/ probenecid; ↑ effects OF aminoglycosides, anticoagulants, hypoglycemics, Li, MTX; ↑ risk of bleeding W/ ASA, corticosteroids, NSAIDs, feverfew, garlic, ginger, ginkgo, EtOH; ↓ effect W/ ASA, antacids, cholestyramine; ↓ effect OF BBs, diuretics **Labs:** ↑ BUN, Cr, LFTs **NIPE:** Take w/ food, full effect after 2 wk administration, ↑ risk of photosensitivity—use sunblock

Pitavastatin (Livalo) [HMG-CoA Reductase Inhibitor] Uses: *Reduce elevated total cholesterol* **Action:** Statin, inhibits HMG-CoA reductase **Dose:** 1–4 mg once/d w/o regard to meals; CrCl 30–60 mg/min start 1 mg w/ 2 mg max **Caution:** [X, –] May cause myopathy & rhabdomyolysis **CI:** Active liver Dz,w/ lopinavir/ritonavir/cyclosporine, severe renal impair not on dialysis **Disp:** Tabs 1, 2, 4 mg **SE:** Muscle pain, back pain, Jt pain, & constipation **Interactions:** ↑ Effects W/ cyclosporine, erythromycin, lopinavir, rifampin, ritonavir; ↑ risk of myopathy W/ fibrates, niacin; ↑ effects OF warfarin **Labs:** ↑ Glucose, LFTs— monitor < therapy & 12 wk > start of drug & periodically **NIPE:** OK w/ grapefruit

Plasma Protein Fraction (Plasmanate, Others) [Plasma Volume Expander] Uses: *Shock & ↓ BP* **Action:** Plasma vol expander **Dose:** Adults. Initial: 250–500 mL IV (not > 10 mL/min); subsequent Inf based on response Peds. 10–15 mL/kg/dose IV; subsequent Inf based on response **Caution:** [C, +] **CI:** Renal Insuff, CHF, cardiopulmonary bypass **Disp:** Inj 5% **SE:** ↓ BP w/ rapid Inf; hypocoagulability, metabolic acidosis, PE **NIPE:** 130–160 mEq Na^{2+}/L; not substitute for RBC

Plerixafor (Mozobil) [Hematopoietic Stem Cell Mobilizer] Uses: *Mobilize stem cells for ABMT in lymphoma & myeloma in combo w/ G-CSF* **Action:** Hematopoietic stem cell mobilizer **Dose:** 0.24 mg/kg SQ daily; max 40 mg/d; CrCl < 50 mL/min: 0.16 mg/kg, max 27 mg/d **Caution:** [D, ?] **Contra:** Not for use in leukemia **Disp:** IV 20 mg/mL (1.2 mL) **SE:** HA, N/V, D, Inj site Rxns **Interactions:** ↑ Effects W/ reduce renal Fxn or compete for active tubular secretion **Labs:** ↑ WBC, neutrophils ↓ plt **NIPE:** Give w/ filgrastim 10 mcg/kg; monitor for splenic rupture (LUQ pain, left scapular or shoulder pain)

Pneumococcal 13-Valent Conjugate Vaccine (Prevnar 13) [Vaccine] Uses: *Immunization against pneumococcal Infxns in infants & children* **Action:**

Active immunization **Dose:** 0.5 mL IM/dose; series of 4 doses; 1st dose age 2 mo; then 4 mo, 6 mo, & 12–15 mo; if previous *Prevnar* switch to *Prevnar 13*; if completed *Prevnar* series, supplemental dose *Prevnar 13* at least 8 wk after last *Prevnar* dose **Caution:** [C, +] w/ ↓ plt **CI:** Sensitivity to components/diphtheria toxoid, febrile illness **Disp:** Inj **SE:** Local Rxns, anorexia, fever, irritability, ↓/↑ sleep, V, D; **Interactions:** May ↓ response *W/* immunosuppressant (radiation, chemotherapy, high-dose steroids) **NIPE:** Keep epi (1:1000) available for Rxns; replaces *Prevnar* (has additional spectrum); does not replace *Pneumovax-23* in age > 24 mo w/ immunosuppression

Pneumococcal Vaccine, Polyvalent (Pneumovax-23) [Vaccine/Inactive Bacteria]
Uses: *Immunization against pneumococcal Infxns in pts at high risk (eg, all pts > 65 y, also asplenia, sickle cell, Dz, HIV & other immunocompromised & w/ chronic illness)* **Action:** Active immunization **Dose:** 0.5 mL IM or SQ **Caution:** [C, ?] **CI:** Do not vaccinate during immunosuppressive therapy **Disp:** Inj 0.5 mL **SE:** Fever, Inj site Rxn, hemolytic anemia w/ other heme conditions, ↓ plt w/ stable ITP, anaphylaxis, Guillain-Barré synd **Interactions:** ↓ Effects *W/* corticosteroids, immunosuppressants **NIPE:** Keep epi (1:1000) available for Rxns. Revaccinate q3–5y if very high risk (eg, asplenia, nephrotic synd), consider revaccination if > 6 y since initial or if previously vaccinated w/ 14-valent vaccine

Podophyllin (Podocon-25, Condylox Gel 0.5%, Condylox) [Antimitotic Effect]
Uses: *Topical therapy of benign growths (genital & perianal warts [condylomata acuminata]*, papillomas, fibromas) **Action:** Direct antimitotic effect; exact mechanism unknown **Dose:** *Condylox gel & Condylox:* Apply bid for 3 consecutive d/wk for 4 wk; 0.5 mL/d max; *Podocon-25:* Use sparingly on the lesion, leave on for 1–4 h, thoroughly wash off **Caution:** [X, ?] Immunosuppression **CI:** DM, bleeding lesions **Disp:** Podocon-25 (w/ benzoin) 15-mL bottles; Condylox gel 0.5% 35-g clear gel; Condylox soln 0.5% 35-g clear gel **SE:** Local Rxns, anemias, tachycardia, paresthesias, GI upset, renal/hepatic damage **NIPE:** Podocon-25 applied by the clinician; do not dispense directly to pt; ⊘ use on warts on mucous membranes; ⊘ use near eyes

Polyethylene Glycol [PEG]-Electrolyte Soln (GoLYTELY, CoLyte) [Laxative]
Uses: *Bowel prep prior to exam or surgery* **Action:** Osmotic cathartic **Dose:** *Adults.* Following 3–4-h fast, drink 240 mL of soln q10 min until 4 L consumed or until BMs are clear *Peds.* 25–40 mL/kg/h for 4–10 h **Caution:** [C, ?] **CI:** GI obst, bowel perforation, megacolon, UC **Disp:** Powder for recons to 4 L **SE:** Cramping or N, bloating **NIPE:** Instruct pt to drink Sol rapidly q10min until finished; 1st BM should occur in approximately 1 h; chilled soln more palatable

Polyethylene Glycol [PEG] 3350 (MiraLAX) [Osmotic Laxative]
Uses: *Occasional constipation* **Action:** Osmotic laxative **Dose:** 17-g powder (1 heaping tbsp) in 8 oz (1 cup) of H_2O & drink; max 14 d **Caution:** [C, ?] Rule out bowel obst before use **CI:** GI obst, allergy to PEG **Disp:** Powder for reconstitution; bottle cap holds 17 g **SE:** Upset stomach, bloating, cramping, gas, severe D, hives **NIPE:** May take 2–4 d for BM; can add to H_2O, juice, soda, coffee, or tea

Polymyxin B & Hydrocortisone (Otobiotic Otic) [Antibiotic/Anti-Inflammatory] Uses: *Superficial bacterial Infxns of external ear canal* **Action:** Antibiotic/anti-inflammatory combo **Dose:** 4 gtt in ear(s) tid–qid **Caution:** [B, ?] **Disp:** Soln polymyxin B 10,000 units/hydrocortisone 0.5%/mL **SE:** Local irritation **NIPE:** Clean ear before instillation of gtts; ⊘ use w/ perforated eardrum; useful in neomycin allergy

Posaconazole (Noxafil) [Anti-Infective/Antifungal] Uses: *Prevent Aspergillus & Candida Infxns in severely immunocompromised; Rx oropharyngeal Candida* **Action:** ↓ Cell membrane ergosterol synth **Dose:** *Adults. Invasive fungal prophylaxis:* 200 mg PO tid *Oropharyngeal candidiasis:* 100 mg PO daily × 13 d, if refractory 40 mg PO bid *Peds > 13 y.* 200 mg PO tid; take w/ meal **Caution:** [C, ?] Multiple drug interactions; ↑ QT, cardiac Dzs, severe renal/liver impair **CI:** Component hypersensitivity; w/ many drugs including alfuzosin, astemizole, alprazolam, phenothiazine, terfenadine, triazolam, others **Disp:** Soln 40 mg/mL **SE:** ↑ QT, hepatic failure, fever, N/V/D, HA, Abd pain, anemia, rash, dyspnea, cough, anorexia, fatigue **Interactions:** ↑ Effects *OF* CCB, cyclosporine, midazolam, sirolimus, statins, tacrolimus, vinca alkaloids; ↓ effects *W/* cimetidine, phenytoin, rifabutin **Labs:** ↑ LFTs; ↓ K⁺, plts; monitor LFTs, lytes, CBC **NIPE:** Monitor for breakthrough fungal Infxns; ⊘ for children < 13 y

Potassium Citrate (Urocit-K) [Urinary Alkalinizer] Uses: *Alkalinize urine, prevention of urinary stones (uric acid, Ca stones if hypocitraturic)* **Action:** Urinary alkalinizer **Dose:** 1 packet dissolved in H₂O or 15–30 mL after meals & hs 10–20 mEq PO tid w/ meals, max 100 mEq/d **Caution:** [A, +] **CI:** Severe renal impair, dehydration, ↑ K⁺, peptic ulcer; w/ K⁺-sparing diuretics, salt substitutes **Disp:** 540-, 1080-mg tabs **SE:** GI upset, metabolic alkalosis **Interactions:** ↑ Risk of hyperkalemia *W/* ACEIs, K⁺-sparing diuretics **Labs:** ↑ K⁺, ↓ Ca²⁺ **NIPE:** Take w/in 30 min of meals or hs snack; tabs 540 mg = 5 mEq, 1080 mg = 10 mEq; monitor ECG for hyperkalemia (peaked T waves)

Potassium Citrate & Citric Acid (Polycitra-K) [Urinary Alkalinizer] Uses: *Alkalinize urine, prevent urinary stones (uric acid, CA stones if hypocitraturic)* **Action:** Urinary alkalinizer **Dose:** 10–20 mEq PO tid w/ meals, max 100 mEq/d **Caution:** [A, +] **CI:** Severe renal impair, dehydration, ↑ K⁺, peptic ulcer; w/ use of K⁺-sparing diuretics or salt substitutes **Disp:** Soln 10 mEq/5 mL; powder 30 mEq/packet **SE:** GI upset, metabolic alkalosis **Interactions:** ↑ Risk *OF* hyperkalemia *W/* ACEIs, K⁺-sparing diuretics **Labs:** ↑ K⁺, ↓ Ca²⁺

Potassium Iodide [Lugol Soln] (Iosat, SSKI, Thyro-Block, ThyroSafe, ThyroShield) [OTC] [Iodine Supplement] Uses: *Thyroid storm*, ↓ vascularity before thyroid surgery, block thyroid uptake of radioactive iodine (nuclear scans or nuclear emergency), thin bronchial secretions **Action:** Iodine supl **Dose:** *Adults & Peds > 2 y. Pre-op thyroidectomy:* 50–250 mg PO tid (2–6 gtt strong iodine soln); give 10 d pre-op *Protection:* 130 mg/d **Peds.** *Protection: < 1 y.* 16.25 mg qd *1 mo–3 y.* 32.5 mg qd *3–12 y.* 1/2 adult dose **Caution:** [D, +] ↑ K⁺,

TB, PE, bronchitis, renal impair **CI:** Iodine sensitivity **Disp:** Tabs 65, 130 mg; soln (saturated soln of potassium iodide [SSKI]) 1 g/mL; Lugol soln, strong iodine 100 mg/mL; syrup 325 mg/5 mL **SE:** Fever, HA, urticaria, angioedema, goiter, GI upset, eosinophilia **Interactions:** ↑ Risk of hypothyroidism **W/** antithyroid drugs & Li; ↑ risk of hyperkalemia **W/** ACEIs, K⁺-sparing diuretics, K⁺ supls **Labs:** May alter TFTs **NIPE:** Take pc w/ food or milk; w/ nuclear radiation emergency, give until radiation exposure no longer exists; monitor for hyperkalemia (peaked T waves)

Potassium Supplements (Kaon, Kaochlor, K-Lor, Slow-K, Micro-K, Klorvess, Others) [Potassium Supplement/Electrolyte] Uses: *Prevention or Rx of ↓ K⁺* (eg, diuretic use) **Action:** K⁺ supl **Dose:** *Adults.* 20–100 mEq/d PO ÷ daily–bid; IV 10–20 mEq/h, max 40 mEq/h & 150 mEq/d (monitor K⁺ levels frequently w/ high-dose IV) *Peds.* Calculate K⁺ deficit; 1–3 mEq/kg/d PO ÷ daily–qid; IV max dose 0.5–1 mEq/kg × 1–2 h **Caution:** [A, +] Renal Insuff, use w/ NSAIDs & ACE Inhibs **CI:** ↑ K⁺ **Disp:** PO forms (Table 6); Inj **SE:** GI irritation; bradycardia, heart block **Interactions:** ↑ Effects **W/** ACEI, K⁺-sparing diuretics, salt substitutes **Labs:** ↑ K⁺, monitor K⁺, monitor ECG for hyperkalemia (peaked T waves) **NIPE:** Take w/ food; mix powder & Liq w/ beverage (unsalted tomato juice, etc); swallow SR tabs whole; Cl⁻ salt OK w/ alkalosis ; w/ acidosis use acetate, bicarbonate, citrate, or gluconate salt; do not administer IV K⁺ undiluted

Pralatrexate (Folotyn) [Folate Analogue Inhibitor] WARNING: Administer only by healthcare provider experienced in chemotherapy Uses: *Tx refractory T-cell lymphoma* **Action:** Folate analogue metabolic Inhib; ↓ dihydrofolate reductase **Dose:** *Adults.* IV push over 3 reducta 30 mg/m² once weekly for 6 wk **Caution:** [D, –] **Disp:** Inj 20 mg/mL (1 mL, 2 mL) **SE:** Anemia, mucositis, N/V/D, edema, fever, fatigue, rash **Interactions:** ↑ Effects **W/** probenecid, NSAIDs, TMP/sulfamethoxazole **Labs:** ↓ Plt, ↓ WBC; monitor CBC weekly; monitor renal & hepatic Fxn < the 1st & 4th dose per cycle **NIPE:** Give folic acid supls prior to & during therapy

Pramipexole (Mirapex, Mirapex ER) [Antiparkinson Agent/Dopamine Agonist] Uses: *Parkinson Dz (Mirapex, Mirapex ER), RLS (Mirapex)* **Action:** DA agonist **Dose:** *Mirapex* 1.5–4.5 mg/d PO, initial 0.375 mg/d in 3 ÷ doses; titrate slowly; *Mirapex ER* start 0.375 PO daily, may ↑ dose every 5–7 d to 0.75, then by 0.75 mg to max 4.5 mg/d **Caution:** [C, ?/] Daytime falling asleep, ↓ BP **CI:** None **Disp:** *Mirapex* tabs 0.125, 0.25, 0.5, 1, 1.5 mg; *Mirapex ER* 0.375, 0.75, 1.5, 3,4.5 mg **SE:** Somnolence, N, constipation, dizziness, fatigue, hallucinations, dry mouth, muscle spasms, edema **Interactions:** ↑ Drug levels & effects **W/** cimetidine, diltiazem, ranitidine, triamterene, verapamil, quinidine, quinine; ↑ effects **OF** levodopa; ↑ CNS depression **W/** CNS depressants, EtOH; ↓ effects **W/** antipsychotics, butyrophenones, metoclopramide, phenothiazine, thioxanthenes; ↓ effects **W/** DA antagonists (eg, neuroleptics, metoclopramide) **NIPE:** Avoid abrupt cessation/withdraw over 1 wk; ↑ risk of hallucinations in elderly

Pramoxine (Anusol Ointment, ProctoFoam-NS, Others) [Topical Anesthetic] Uses: *Relief of pain & itching from hemorrhoids, anorectal surgery*; topical for burns & dermatosis **Action:** Topical anesthetic **Dose:** Apply freely to anal area q3h **Caution:** [C, ?] **Disp:** [OTC] All 1%; foam (Procto-Foam-NS), cream, oint, lotion, gel, pads, spray **SE:** Contact dermatitis, mucosal thinning w/ chronic use **NIPE:** ⊘ Use on large areas

Pramoxine + Hydrocortisone (Enzone, ProctoFoam-HC) [Topical Anesthetic/Anti-Inflammatory] Uses: *Relief of pain & itching from hemorrhoids* & anti-inflammatory **Action:** Topical anesthetic, anti-inflammatory **Dose:** Apply freely to anal area tid–qid **Caution:** [C, ?/–] **Disp:** *Cream:* Pramoxine 1%, acetate 0.5%/1% *Foam:* Pramoxine 1%, hydrocortisone 1% *Lotion:* Pramoxine 1%, hydrocortisone 0.25%/1%/2.5%, pramoxine 2.5%, & hydrocortisone 1% **SE:** Contact dermatitis, mucosal thinning w/ chronic use **NIPE:** ⊘ Use on large areas

Prasugrel Hydrochloride (Effient) [Platelet Inhibitor] WARNING: Can cause sig, sometimes fatal, bleeding; do not use w/ planned CABG w/ active-bleeding, Hx TIA or stroke or pts > 75 y Uses: *↓ Thrombotic CV events (eg, stent thrombosis)* administer ASAP in ECC setting w/ high-risk ST depression or T-wave inversion w/ planned PCI **Action:** ↓ Plt aggregation **Dose:** 10 mg/d; wgt < 60 kg, consider 5 mg/d; 60 mg PO loading dose in ECC 2009, ACCF/AHA/SCAI Jt STEMI/PCI guidelines: Use at least 12 mo w/ cardiac stent (bare or drug eluting); consider > 15 mo w/ drug eluting stent **Caution:** [B, ?] Active bleeding; ↑ bleeding risk; w/ CYP3A4 substrates **CI:** Coagulation disorders, active intracranial bleeding or PUD; Hx TIA/stroke **Disp:** Tabs 5, 10 mg **SE:** ↑ Bleeding time, ↑ BP, GI intolerance, HA, dizziness, rash **Interactions:**↑ Risk of bleeding *W/* heparin, warfarin, fibrinolytics, chronic NSAIDs use **Labs:** ↓ WBC **NIPE:** Plt aggregation to baseline ~ 7 d after D/C, plt transfusion reverses acutely

Pravastatin (Pravachol) [Antilipemic/HMG-CoA Reductase Inhibitor] Uses: *↓ Cholesterol* **Action:** HMG-CoA reductase Inhib **Dose:** 10–80 mg PO hs; ↓ in sig renal/hepatic impair **Caution:** [X, –] w/ gemfibrozil **CI:** Liver Dz or persistent LFTs ↑ **Disp:** Tabs 10, 20, 40, 80 mg **SE:** Use caution w/ concurrent gemfibrozil; HA, GI upset, hep, myopathy, renal failure **Interactions:** ↑ Risk of myopathy & rhabdomyolysis *W/* clarithromycin, clofibrate, cyclosporine, danazol, erythromycin, fluoxetine, gemfibrozil, niacin, nefazodone, troleandomycin; ↑ effects *W/* azole antifungals, cimetidine, grapefruit juice; ↑ effects *OF* warfarin; ↑ CNS effects & liver tox w/ concurrent EtOH use; ↓ effects *W/* cholestyramine, isradipine **Labs:** ↑ LFTs **NIPE:** ⊘ PRG, breast-feeding; take w/o regard to food; full effect may take up to 4 wk; ↑ risk of photosensitivity—use sunblock

Prazosin (Minipress) [Antihypertensive/Alpha-Blocker] Uses: *HTN* **Action:** Peripherally acting α-adrenergic blocker **Dose:** *Adults.* 1 mg PO tid; can ↑ to 20 mg/d max PRN *Peds.* 0.05–0.1 mg/kg/d in 3 ÷ doses; max 0.5 mg/

kg/d **Caution:** [C, ?] Use w/ PDE5 Inhib (eg, sildenafil) can cause ↓ BP **CI:** Component allergy, concurrent use of PDE5 Inhibs **Disp:** Caps 1, 2, 5 mg; tabs ER 2.5, 5 mg **SE:** Dizziness, edema, palpitations, fatigue, GI upset **Interactions:** ↑ Hypotension *W/* antihypertensives, diuretics, verapamil, nitrates, EtOH; ↓ effects *W/* NSAIDs, butcher's broom **Labs:** ↑ Serum Na levels; alters test for Pheo **NIPE:** ⊘ D/C abruptly; can cause orthostatic ↓ BP, take the 1st dose hs; tolerance develops to this effect; tachyphylaxis may result; concurrent use w/ Viagra-type drugs can cause life-threatening hypotension

Prednisolone [See Steroids Table 2]

Prednisone [See Steroids Table 2]

Pregabalin (Lyrica) [Antinociceptive/Antiseizure] **Uses:** *DM peripheral neuropathy pain; postherpetic neuralgia; fibromyalgia; adjunct w/ adult partial onset Szs* **Action:** Nerve transmission modulator, antinociceptive, antiSz effect; mechanism ?; related to gabapentin **Dose:** *Neuropathic pain:* 50 mg tid, ↑ to 300 mg/d w/in 1 wk based on response, 300 mg/d max *Postherpetic neuralgia:* 75–150 mg bid, or 50–100 mg tid; start 75 mg bid or 50 mg tid; ↑ to 300 mg/d w/in 1 wk PRN; if pain persists after 2–4 wk, ↑ to 600 mg/d *Epilepsy:* start 150 mg/d (75 mg bid or 50 mg tid) may ↑ to max 600 mg/d; ↓ w/ CrCl < 60; w/ or w/o food **Caution:** [C, –] w/ sig renal impair (see package insert), w/ elderly & severe CHF avoid abrupt D/C **CI:** PRG **Disp:** Caps 25, 50, 75, 100, 150, 200, 225, 300 mg; soln 20 mg/mL; **SE:** Dizziness, drowsiness, xerostomia, edema, blurred vision, wgt gain, difficulty concentrating; suicidal ideation **NIPE:** Avoid abrupt D/C—can cause Szs; taper over at least 1 wk

Probenecid (Benemid, Others) [Uricosuric/Analgesic] **Uses:** *Prevent gout & hyperuricemia; extends levels of PCNs & cephalosporins* **Action:** Uricosuric, renal tubular blocker of organic anions **Dose:** *Adults. Gout:* 250 mg bid × 1 wk, then 0.5 g PO bid; can ↑ by 500 mg/mo up to 2–3 g/d *Antibiotic effect:* 1–2 g PO 30 min before dose *Peds > 2 y.* 25 mg/kg, then 40 mg/kg/d PO ÷ qid **Caution:** [B, ?] **CI:** High-dose ASA, mod–severe renal impair, age < 2 y **Disp:** Tabs 500 mg **SE:** HA, GI upset, rash, pruritus, dizziness, blood dyscrasias **Interactions:** ↑ Effects *OF* acyclovir, allopurinol; ↑ effects *OF* benzodiazepines, cephalosporins, ciprofloxacin, clofibrate, dapsone, dyphylline, MTX, NSAIDs, olanzapine, rifampin, sulfonamides, sulfonylureas zidovudine; ↓ effects *W/* niacin, EtOH; ↑ effects *OF* penicillamine **Labs:** False(+) urine glucose; false ↑ level of theophylline **NIPE:** Take w/ food, ↑ fluids to 2–3 L/d; do not use during acute gout attack; caution when used concurrently w/ benzodiazepines

Procainamide (Pronestyl, Pronestyl SR, Procanbid) [Antiarrhythmic] **WARNING: Positive ANA titer or SLE w/ prolonged use; only use in life-threatening arrhythmias; hematologic tox can be severe, follow CBC** **Uses:** *Supraventricular/ventricular arrhythmias* **Action:** Class Ia antiarrhythmic (Table 9) **Dose:** *Adults. Recurrent VF/VT:* 20 mg/min IV (total 17 mg/kg max) *Maint:* 1–4 mg/min *Stable wide-complex tachycardia of unknown origin, AF w/ rapid rate in*

WPW: 20 mg/min IV until arrhythmia suppression, ↓ BP, or QRS widens > 50%, then 1–4 mg/min *Chronic dosing:* 50 mg/kg/d PO in ÷ doses q4–6h *Recurrent VF/VT:* 20–50 mg/min IV; max total 17 mg/kg *ECC 2010:* Stable monomorphic VT, **refractory reentry SVT, stable wide-complex tachycardia, AF w/ WPW:** 20 mg/min IV until 1 of these: Arrhythmia stopped, hypotension, QRS widens > 50%, total 17 mg/kg; then maintenance Inf of 1–4 mg/min *Peds. Chronic maint:* 15–50 mg/kg/24 h PO ÷ q3–6h *ECC 2010:* **SVT, aflutter, VT (w/ pulses):** 15 mg/kg IV/IO over 30–60 min **Caution:** [C, +] ↑ In renal/hepatic impair **CI:** Complete heart block, 2nd-/3rd-degree heart block w/o pacemaker, torsades de pointes, SLE **Disp:** Tabs & caps 250, 500 mg; SR tabs 500, 750, 1000 mg; Inj 100, 500 mg/mL **SE:** ↓BP, lupus-like synd, GI upset, taste perversion, arrhythmias, tachycardia, heart block, angioneurotic edema, blood dyscrasias **Notes:** *Levels:Trough:* Just before next dose *Therapeutic:* 4–10 mcg/mL; *N*-acetyl procainamide (NAPA) + procaine 5–30 mcg/mL *Toxic:* > 10 mcg/mL; NAPA + procaine > 30 mcg/mL *1/2-life:* Procaine 3–5 h, NAPA 6–10 h **Interactions:** ↑ Effects *W/* acetazolamide, amiodarone, cimetidine, ranitidine, TMP; ↑ effects *OF* anticholinergics, antihypertensives; ↓ effects *W/* procaine, EtOH **Labs:** ↑ LFTs **NIPE:** Take w/ food if GI upset; ⊘ crush SR tab; may cause severe hematologic tox

Procarbazine (Matulane) [Antineoplastic/Alkylating Agent]
WARNING: Highly toxic; handle w/ care **Uses:** *Hodgkin Dz*, NHL, brain & lung tumors **Action:** Alkylating agent; ↓ DNA & RNA synth **Dose:** Per protocol **Caution:** [D, ?] w/ EtOH ingestion **CI:** Inadequate BM reserve **Disp:** Caps 50 mg **SE:** ↓ BM, hemolytic Rxns (w/ G6PD deficiency), N/V/D; disulfiram-like Rxn; cutaneous & constitutional Sxs, myalgia, arthralgia, CNS effects, azoospermia, cessation of menses **Interactions:** ↑ CNS depression *W/* antihistamines, barbiturates, CNS depressants, narcotics, phenothiazine; ↑ risk of HTN *W/* guanethidine, levodopa, MAOIs, methyldopa, sympathomimetics, TCAs, caffeine, tyramine-containing foods (aged cheese/meats, red wine, beer, dried fruits); ↓ effects *OF* digoxin **NIPE:** Disulfiram-like Rxn w/ EtOH (tachycardia, N/V, sweating, flushing, HA, blurred vision, confusion); ↑ fluids to 2–3 L/d; ↑ risk of photosensitivity—use sunblock; ⊘ exposure to Infxn

Prochlorperazine (Compazine) [Antiemetic, Antipsychotic/Phenothiazine] **Uses:** *N/V, agitation, & psychotic disorders* **Action:** Phenothiazine; blocks postsynaptic dopaminergic CNS receptors **Dose:** *Adults. Antiemetic:* 5–10 mg PO tid–qid or 25 mg PR bid or 5–10 mg deep IM q4–6h *Antipsychotic:* 10–20 mg IM acutely or 5–10 mg PO tid–qid for maint; ↑ doses may be required for antipsychotic effect *Peds.* 0.1–0.15 mg/kg/dose IM q4–6h or 0.4 mg/kg/24 h PO ÷ tid–qid **Caution:** [C, +/–] NAG, severe liver/cardiac Dz **CI:** Phenothiazine sensitivity, BM suppression; age < 2 y or wgt < 9 kg **Disp:** Tabs 5, 10, 25 mg; SR caps 10, 15 mg; syrup 5 mg/5 mL; supp 2.5, 5, 25 mg; Inj 5 mg/mL **SE:** EPS common; Rx w/ diphenhydramine or benztropine **Interactions:** ↑ Effects *W/* chloroquine, indomethacin, narcotics, procarbazine, SSRIs, pyrimethamine; ↑ effect *OF* antidepressants, BBs, EtOH; ↓ effects *W/* antacids, anticholinergics, barbiturates, tobacco; ↓ effects *OF* anticoagulants, guanethidine, levodopa, Li **Labs:** False(+) urine bilirubin, amylase, PKU, ↑ serum prolactin **NIPE:** ⊘ D/C abruptly; risk of photosensitivity—use sunblock; urine may turn pink/red; over sedation w/ anticholinergics, CNS depressants & EtOH

Promethazine (Phenergan) [Antihistamine, Antiemetic, Sedative/Phenothiazine]
WARNING: Do not use in pts < 2 y; resp depression risk; tissue damage, including gangrene w/ extrav **Uses:** *N/V, motion sickness, adjunct to post-op analgesics, sedation, rhinitis* **Action:** Phenothiazine; blocks CNS postsynaptic mesolimbic dopaminergic receptors **Dose: Adults.** 12.5–50 mg PO, PR, or IM bid–qid PRN **Peds > 2 y.** 0.1–0.5 mg/kg/dose PO or IM q2–6h PRN **Caution:** [C, +/–] Use w/ agents w/ resp depressant effects **CI:** Component allergy, NAG, age < 2 y **Disp:** Tabs 12.5, 25, 50 mg; syrup 6.25, 25 mg/5 mL; supp 12.5, 25, 50 mg; Inj 25, 50 mg/mL **SE:** Drowsiness, tardive dyskinesia, EPS, lowered Sz threshold, ↓ BP, GI upset, blood dyscrasias, photosensitivity, resp depression in children **Interactions:** ↑ Effects *W/* CNS depressants, MAOIs, EtOH; ↑ effects *OF* antihypertensives; ↓ effects *W/* anticholinergics, barbiturates, tobacco; ↓ effect *OF* levodopa **Labs:** Effects skin allergy tests **NIPE:** IM/PO preferred route; not SQ or intra-arterial; use sunblock for photosensitivity; may lower Sz threshold

Propafenone (Rythmol) [Antiarrhythmic]
WARNING: Excess mortality or nonfatal cardiac arrest possible; avoid in asymptomatic & symptomatic non–life-threatening ventricular arrhythmias **Uses:** *Life-threatening ventricular arrhythmias, AF* **Action:** Class Ic antiarrhythmic (Table 9) **Dose: Adults.** 150–300 mg PO q8h **Peds.** 8–10 mg/kg/d ÷ in 3–4 doses; may ↑ 2 mg/kg/d, 20 mg/kg/d max **Caution:** [C, ?] w/ Fosamprenavir, ritonavir, MI w/in 2 y, w/ liver/renal impair **CI:** Uncontrolled CHF, bronchospasm, cardiogenic shock, AV block w/o pacer **Disp:** Tabs 150, 225, 300 mg; ER caps 225, 325, 425 mg **SE:** Dizziness, unusual taste, 1st-degree heart block, arrhythmias, prolongs QRS & QT intervals; fatigue, GI upset, blood dyscrasias **Interactions:** ↑ Effects *W/* cimetidine, quinidine; ↑ effects *OF* anticoagulants, BBs, digitalis glycosides, theophylline; ↓ effects *W/* rifampin, phenobarbital, rifabutin **Labs:** ↑ ANA titers; monitor ECG for ↑ QT interval **NIPE:** Take w/o regard to food; associated w/ a high cardiac arrest rate & mortality

Propantheline (Pro-Banthine) [Antimuscarinic]
Uses: *PUD*, symptomatic Rx of small intestine hypermotility, spastic colon, ureteral spasm, bladder spasm, pylorospasm* **Action:** Antimuscarinic **Dose: Adults.** 15 mg PO ac & 30 mg PO hs; ↓ in elderly **Peds.** 2–3 mg/kg/24 h PO ÷ tid–qid **Caution:** [C, ?] **CI:** NAG, UC, toxic megacolon, GI/GU obst **Disp:** Tabs 7.5, 15 mg **SE:** Anticholinergic (eg, xerostomia, blurred vision) **Interactions:** ↑ Anticholinergic effects *W/* antihistamines, antidepressants, atropine, haloperidol, phenothiazines, quinidine, TCAs; ↑ effects *OF* atenolol, digoxin (monitor ECG); ↑ adverse effects when used w/ procainamide; ↓ effects *W/* antacids **NIPE:** May cause heat intolerance—avoid exposure to high temperatures; ↑ risk of photosensitivity—use sunblock

Propofol (Diprivan) [Anesthetic]   Uses: *Induction & maint of anesthesia; sedation in intubated pts* **Action:** Sedative–hypnotic; mechanism unknown; acts in 40 s **Dose:** *Adults. Anesthesia:* 2–2.5 mg/kg (also *ECC 2005*), then 0.1–0.2 mg/kg/min Inf *ICU sedation:* 5 mcg/kg/min IV × 5 min, ↑ PRN 5–10 mcg/kg/min q5–10min, 5–50 mcg/kg/min cont Inf *Peds. Anesthesia:* 2.5–3.5 mg/kg induction; then 125–300 mcg/kg/min; ↓ in elderly, debilitated, ASA II/IV pts **Caution:** [B, +] **CI:** If general anesthesia CI, sensitivity to egg, egg products, soybeans, soybean products **Disp:** Inj 10 mg/mL **SE:** ↓ BP, pain at site, apnea, anaphylaxis **Interactions:** ↑ Effects *W/* antihistamines, opioids, hypnotics, EtOH **Labs:** ↑ Serum cortisol levels; may ↑ triglycerides w/ extended dosing **NIPE:** 1 mL has 0.1 g fat; ⊘ if h/o allergy to egg/soybean products; monitor BP for hypotension; monitor for resp depression

Propoxyphene (Darvon); Propoxyphene & Acetaminophen (Darvocet); Propoxyphene & Aspirin (Darvon Compound-65, Darvon-N w/ Aspirin) [C-IV] [Opioid + Analgesic]   In November 2010 the FDA banned all products containing propoxyphene d/t the ↑ risk of abnormal & potentially fatal heart rhythm disturbances

Propranolol (Inderal) [Antihypertensive, Antianginal, Antiarrhythmic/Beta-Blocker]   Uses: *HTN, angina, MI, hyperthyroidism, essential tremor, hypertrophic subaortic stenosis, Pheo; prevents migraines & atrial arrhythmias* **Action:** β-Adrenergic receptor blocker, β₁, β₂; only BB to block conversion of T_4 to T_3 **Dose:** *Adults. Angina:* 80–320 mg/d PO ÷ bid–qid or 80–160 mg/d SR *Arrhythmia:* 10–80 mg PO tid–qid or 1 mg IV slowly, repeat q5min, 5 mg max *HTN:* 40 mg PO bid or 60–80 mg/d SR, ↑ weekly to max 640 mg/d PO *Hypertrophic subaortic stenosis:* 20–40 mg PO tid–qid *MI:* 180–240 mg PO ÷ tid–qid *Migraine prophylaxis:* 80 mg/d ÷ qid–tid, ↑ weekly 160–240 mg/d ÷ tid–qid max; wean if no response in 6 wk *Pheo:* 30–60 mg/d ÷ tid–qid *Thyrotoxicosis:* 1–3 mg IV × 1; 10–40 mg PO q6h *Tremor:* 40 mg PO bid, ↑ PRN 320 mg/d max *ECC 2010:* SVT: 0.5–1 mg IV given over 1 min; repeat PRN up to 0.1 mg/kg *Peds. Arrhythmia:* 0.5–1.0 mg/kg/d ÷ tid–qid, ↑ PRN q3–7d to 60 mg/d max; 0.01–0.1 mg/kg IV over 10 min, 1 mg max *HTN:* 0.5–1.0 mg/kg ÷ bid–qid, ↑ PRN q3–7d to 2 mg/kg/d max; ↓ in renal impair **Caution:** [C (1st tri, D if 2nd or 3rd tri), +] **CI:** Uncompensated CHF, cardiogenic shock, bradycardia, heart block, PE, severe resp Dz **Disp:** Tabs 10, 20, 40, 80 mg; SR caps 60, 80, 120, 160 mg; oral soln 4, 8, mg/mL; Inj 1 mg/mL **SE:** Bradycardia, ↓ BP, fatigue, GI upset, ED **Interactions:** ↑ Effects *W/* antihypertensives, cimetidine, hydralazine, neuroleptics, nitrates, propylthiouracil, theophylline, EtOH; ↑ effects *OF* benzodiazepines, CCB, digitalis, glycosides, hypoglycemics, hydralazine, lidocaine, neuroleptics; ↓ effects *W/* NSAIDs, phenobarbital, phenytoin, rifampin, tobacco **Labs:** ↑ LFTs, BUN; ↑/↓ serum glucose; ↓ plts, thyroxine **NIPE:** ⊘ D/C abruptly—may ↑ angina; concurrent use of epi may cause severe HTN/bradycardia; ↑ cold sensitivity

Propylthiouracil [PTU] [Antithyroid Agent/Thyroid Hormone Antagonist] WARNING: Severe liver failure reported; use only if pt cannot tolerate methimazole; d/t fetal anomalies w/ methimazole, PTU may be DOC in 1st tri Uses: *Hyperthyroidism* Action: ↓ Production of T3 & T4 & conversion of T4 to T3 Dose: Adults. Initial: 100 mg PO q8h (may need up to 1200 mg/d); after pt euthyroid (6–8 wk), taper dose by 1/2 q4–6wk to maint, 50–150 mg/24 h; can usually D/C in 2–3 y; ↓ in elderly Peds. Initial: 5–7 mg/kg/24 h PO ÷ q8h Maint: 1/3–2/3 of initial dose Caution: [D, –] See Warning CI: Allergy Disp: Tabs 50 mg SE: Fever, rash, leukopenia, dizziness, GI upset, taste perversion, SLE-like synd Interactions: ↑ Effects W/ iodinated glycerol, Li, KI, NaI Labs: ↑ LFTs, PT; ↑ effects of anticoagulants; monitor TFT & LFT NIPE: Take w/ food for GI upset; omit dietary sources of I; full effects take 6–12 wk; monitor pt clinically

Protamine (Generic) [Heparin Antagonist] Uses: *Reverse heparin effect* Action: Neutralize heparin by forming a stable complex Dose: Based on degree of heparin reversal; give IV slowly; 1 mg reverses ~ 100 units of heparin given in the preceding 3–4 h, 50 mg max Caution: [C, ?] CI: Allergy Disp: Inj 10 mg/mL SE: Follow coagulants; anticoagulant effect if given w/o heparin; ↓ BP, bradycardia, dyspnea, hemorrhage Interactions: Incompatible W/ many penicillins & cephalosporins—⊘ mix Labs: ✓ aPTT ~ 15 min after use to assess response NIPE: Give by slow IV Inj over 10 min; antidote for heparin tox

Pseudoephedrine (Sudafed, Novafed, Afrinol, Others) [OTC] [Decongestant/Sympathomimetic] WARNING: Not for use in peds < 2 y Uses: *Decongestant* Action: Stimulates α-adrenergic receptors w/ vasoconstriction Dose: Adults. 30–60 mg PO q6–8h Peds 2–5 y. 15 mg q4–6h, 60 mg/24 h max 6–12 y. 30 mg q4–6h, 120 mg/24 h max; ↓ w/ renal Insuff Caution: [C, +] CI: Poorly controlled HTN or CAD, w/ MAOIs Disp: Tabs 30, 60 mg; caps 60 mg; SR tabs 120, 240 mg; Liq 7.5 mg/0.8 mL, 15, 30 mg/5 mL SE: HTN, insomnia, tachycardia, arrhythmias, nervousness, tremor Interactions: ↑ Risk of HTN crisis W/ MAOIs; ↑ effects W/ BBs, sympathomimetics; ↓ effects W/ TCAs; ↓ effect OF methyldopa, reserpine NIPE: Found in many OTC cough/cold preps; OTC restricted distribution

Psyllium (Metamucil, Serutan, Effer-Syllium) [Laxative] Uses: *Constipation & colonic diverticular Dz* Action: Bulk laxative Dose: 1 tsp (7 g) in glass of H_2O PO daily–tid Caution: [B, ?] Effer-Syllium (effervescent psyllium) usually contains K^+, caution w/ renal failure; PKU (in products w/ aspartame) CI: Suspected bowel obst Disp: Granules 4, 25 g/tsp; powder 3.5 g/packet, caps 0.52g (3 g/6 caps), wafers 3.4 g/dose SE: D, Abd cramps, bowel obst, constipation, bronchospasm Interactions: ↓ Effects OF digitalis glycosides, K^+-sparing diuretics, nitrofurantoin, salicylates, tetracyclines, warfarin NIPE: Psyllium dust Inh may cause wheezing, runny nose, watery eyes

Pyrazinamide (Generic) [Antitubercular] Uses: *Active TB in combo w/ other agents* Action: Bacteriostatic; unknown mechanism Dose: Adults. 15–30

mg/kg/24 h PO ÷ tid–qid; max 2 g/d; dosing based on lean body wgt; ↓ dose in renal/hepatic impair **Peds.** 15–30 mg/kg/d PO ÷ daily–bid; ↓ w/ renal/hepatic impair **Caution:** [C, +/–] **CI:** Severe hepatic damage, acute gout **Disp:** Tabs 500 mg **SE:** Hepatotox, malaise, GI upset, arthralgia, myalgia, gout **Interactions:** ↓ Effects *OF* probenecid **Labs:** ↑ Uric acid **NIPE:** ↑ Risk of photosensitivity—use sunblock; ↑ fluids to 2 L/d; use in combo w/ other antiTB drugs; consult *MMWR* for latest TB recommendations; dosage regimen differs for "directly observed" therapy

Pyridoxine [Vitamin B₆] [Vitamin B₆ Supplement] Uses: *Rx & prevention of vit B₆ deficiency* Action: Vit B₆ supl Dose: **Adults. Deficiency:** 10–20 mg/d PO. *Drug-induced neuritis:* 100–200 mg/d; 25–100 mg/d prophylaxis **Peds.** 5–25 mg/d × 3 wk **Caution:** [A (C if doses exceed RDA), +] **CI:** Component allergy **Disp:** Tabs 25, 50, 100 mg; Inj 100 mg/mL **SE:** Allergic Rxns, HA, N **Interactions:** ↓ Effects *OF* levodopa, phenobarbital, phenytoin **Labs:** ↑ AST; ↓ folic acid **NIPE:** Antidote for INH poisoning; risk of sensory nerve damage (numbness, tingling, ↓ sensation)—usually reversed when drug D/C

Quadrivalent Human Papillomavirus (HPV Types 6, 11, 16, 18) Recombinant Vaccine (Gardasil) [Vaccine] Uses: Prevent cervical CA, genital warts, cervical adenocarcinoma in situ, cervical intraepithelial neoplasia grades 2 & 3, vulvar intraepithelial neoplasia grades 2 & 3, Vag intraepithelial neoplasia grades 2 & 3, cervical intraepithelial neoplasia grade 1 caused by HPV types 6, 11, 16, 18 Dose: 0.5-mL IM Inj in deltoid or upper thigh **Peds < 9 y.** Not recommended **Females 9–26 y.** Give 1st, 2nd dose 2 mo > 1st, 3rd dose 6 mo > 1st dose **Caution:** [B, –] **CI:** Yeast allergies **Disp:** 0.5 mL for IM Inj **SE:** Inj site Rxn, fever **Interactions:** ↓ Response *W/* immunosuppressants **NIPE:** May not protect all recipients; not a substitute for routine cervical screening; give IM Inj in deltoid or upper thigh

Quazepam (Doral) [C-IV] [Sedative/Hypnotic/Benzodiazempine] Uses: *Insomnia* Action: Benzodiazepine Dose: 7.5–15 mg PO hs PRN; ↓ in elderly & hepatic failure **Caution:** [X, ?/–] NA glaucoma **Contra:** PRG, sleep apnea **Disp:** Tabs 7.5, 15 mg **SE:** Sedation, hangover, somnolence, resp depression **Interactions:** ↑ Risk of CNS depression *W/* antihistamines, benzodiazepines, opioids, verapamil, grapefruit juice, EtOH; ↑ effects *W/* azole antifungals, cimetidine, digoxin, disulfiram, INH, levodopa, macrolides, neuroleptics, phenytoin, quinolones, SSRIs, verapamil, grapefruit juice, EtOH; ↓ effects *W/* carbamazepine, rifampin, rifabutin, tobacco **NIPE:** ⊘ Breast-feed, PRG; ⊘ D/C abruptly; use barrier contraception

Quetiapine (Seroquel, Seroquel XR) [Antipsychotic] WARNING: Closely monitor pts for worsening depression or emergence of suicidality, particularly in ped pts; not for use in peds; ↑ mortality in elderly w/ dementia-related psychosis Uses: *Acute exacerbations of schizophrenia* Action: Serotonin & DA antagonism Dose: 150–750 mg/d; initiate at 25–100 mg bid–tid; slowly ↑ dose; XR:

400–800 mg PO qPM; start 300 mg/d, ↑ 300 mg/d, 800 mg/d max ↓ dose w/ hepatic & geriatric pts **Caution:** [C, –] **CI:** Component allergy **Disp:** Tabs 25, 50, 100, 200, 300, 400 mg; tabs XR 200, 300, 400 mg **SE:** Confusion w/ nefazodone; HA, somnolence, ↑ wgt, ↓ BP, dizziness, cataracts, neuroleptic malignant synd, tardive dyskinesia **Interactions:** ↑ Effects *W/* azole antifungals, cimetidine, macrolides, EtOH; ↑ effects *OF* antihypertensives, lorazepam; ↓ effects *W/* barbiturates, carbamazepine, glucocorticoids, phenytoin, rifampin, thioridazine; ↓ effects *OF* DA antagonists, levodopa **Labs:** ↑ LFTs, cholesterol, triglycerides, glucose **NIPE:** ↑ Risk of cataract formation, tardive dyskinesia; take w/o regard to food; ↓ body temperature regulation ability; ↑ risk of depression/suicide tendencies, esp in peds; risk of ↑ QT internal—monitor ECG

Quinapril (Accupril) [Antihypertensive/ACEI] WARNING: ACE Inhibs used during PRG can cause fetal injury & death **Uses:** *HTN, CHF, DN, post-MI* **Action:** ACE Inhib **Dose:** 10–80 mg PO daily; ↓ in renal impair **Caution:** [D, +] w/ RAS, vol depletion **CI:** ACE Inhib sensitivity, angioedema, PRG **Disp:** Tabs 5, 10, 20, 40 mg **SE:** Dizziness, HA, ↓ BP, impaired renal Fxn, angioedema, taste perversion, cough **Interactions:** ↑ Effects *W/* diuretics, antihypertensives; ↑ effects *OF* insulin, Li; ↓ effects *W/* ASA, NSAIDs; ↓ effects *OF* quinolones, tetracyclines **Labs:** ↑ K⁺, ↓ LFTs, glucose **NIPE:** ↓ Absorption *W/* high-fat foods; ↑ risk of cough; risk of hyperkalemia—monitor ECG (peaked T waves), EtOH ↑ risk of adverse effects

Quinidine (Quinidex, Quinaglute) [Antiarrhythmic/Antimalarial] WARNING: Mortality rates ↑ when used to treat non-life-threatening arrhythmias **Uses:** *Prevention of tachydysrhythmias, malaria* **Action:** Class Ia antiarrhythmic **Dose:** *Adults. AF/aflutter conversion:* After digitalization, 200 mg q2–3h × 8 doses; ↑ daily to 3–4 g max or nl rhythm *Peds.* 15–60 mg/kg/24 h PO in 4–5 ÷ doses; ↓ in renal impair **Caution:** [C, +] w/ Ritonavir **CI:** Digitalis tox & AV block; conduction disorders **Disp:** *Sulfate:* Tabs 200, 300 mg; SR tabs 300 mg *Gluconate:* SR tabs 324 mg; Inj 80 mg/mL **SE:** Extreme ↓ BP w/ IV use; syncope, QT prolongation, GI upset, arrhythmias, fatigue, cinchonism (tinnitus, hearing loss, delirium, visual changes), fever, hemolytic anemia, ↓ plt, rash **Notes:** *Levels: Trough:* Just before next dose *Therapeutic:* 2–5 mcg/mL *Toxic:* > 10 mcg/mL *1/2-life:* 6–8 h; sulfate salt 83% quinidine; gluconate salt 62% quinidine **Interactions:** ↑ Effects *W/* acetazolamide, antacids, amiodarone, azole antifungals, cimetidine, K⁺, macrolides, NaHCO₃, thiazide diuretics, lily of the valley, pheasant's eye herb, scopolia root, squill; ↑ effects *OF* anticoagulants, anticholinergics, dextromethorphan, digitalis glycosides, disopyramide, haloperidol, metoprolol, nifedipine, procainamide, propafenone, propranolol, TCAs, verapamil; ↓ effects *W/* barbiturates, disopyramide, nifedipine, phenobarbital, phenytoin, rifampin, sucralfate **NIPE:** Take w/ food, ↑ risk of photosensitivity—use sunblock; use w/ drug that slows AV conduction (eg, digoxin, diltiazem, BB), QT prolongation—monitor ECG

Quinupristin–Dalfopristin (Synercid) [Antibiotic/Streptogramin]
Uses: *Vancomycin-resistant Infxns d/t *E faecium* & other gram(+)* **Action:** ↓ Ribosomal protein synth *Spectrum:* Vancomycin-resistant *E faecium,* methicillin-susceptible *S aureus, S pyogenes;* not against *E faecalis* **Dose:** *Adults & Peds.* 7.5 mg/kg IV q8–12h (central line preferred); incompatible w/ NS or heparin; flush IV w/ dextrose; ↓ w/ hepatic failure **Caution:** [B, M] Multiple drug interactions w/ drugs metabolized by CYP3A4 (eg, cyclosporine) **CI:** Component allergy **Disp:** Inj 500 mg (150 mg quinupristin/350 mg dalfopristin), 600 mg (180 mg quinupristin/420 mg dalfopristin) **SE:** Hyperbilirubinemia, Inf site Rxns & pain, arthralgia, myalgia **Interactions:** ↑ Effects *OF* CCBs, carbamazepine, cyclosporine, diazepam, disopyramide, docetaxel, lovastatin, methylprednisolone, midazolam, paclitaxel, tacrolimus, quinidine, vinblastine **Labs:** ↑ ALT, AST, bilirubin **NIPE:** Inf site Rxns & pain; if D—monitor for signs of lytes disturbance/hypovolemia

Rabeprazole (AcipHex) [Antiulcer Agent/Proton Pump Inhibitor] **Uses:** *PUD, GERD, ZE* *H pylori* **Action:** PPI **Dose:** 20 mg/d; may ↑ to 60 mg/d; *H pylori* 20 mg PO bid × 7 d (w/ amoxicillin & clarithromycin); do not crush/chew tabs; do not use clopidogrel **Caution:** [B, ?/−] **Disp:** Tabs 20 mg ER **SE:** HA, fatigue, GI upset **Interactions:** ↑ Effects *OF* cyclosporine, digoxin; ↓ effects *OF* ketoconazole **Labs:** ↑ LFTs, TSH **NIPE:** Take w/o regard to food; ↑ risk of photosensitivity—use sunblock; risk of hypomagnesemia w/ long-term use, monitor; ? ↑ risk of fxs w/ all PPI

Raloxifene (Evista) [Selective Estrogen Receptor Modulator]
WARNING: ↑ Risk of venous thromboembolism & death from stroke **Uses:** *Prevent osteoporosis, breast CA prevention* **Action:** Partial antagonist of estrogen, behaves like estrogen **Dose:** 60 mg/d **Caution:** [X, −] **CI:** Thromboembolism, PRG **Disp:** Tabs 60 mg **SE:** CP, insomnia, rash, hot flashes, GI upset, hepatic dysfunction, leg cramps **Interactions:** ↓ Effects *W/* ampicillin, cholestyramine **NIPE:** ⊘ PRG, breast-feeding; take w/o regard to food; ↑ risk of venous thromboembolic effects—esp w/ prolonged immobilization

Raltegravir (Isentress) [HIV-1 Integrase Strand Transfer Inhibitor]
WARNING: Development of immune reconstitution synd: ↑ CK, myopathy & rhabdomyolysis **Uses:** *HIV in combo w/ other agents* **Action:** HIV-integrase strand transfer Inhib **Dose:** 400 mg PO bid, 800 mg PO bid w/ rifampin; w/ or w/o food **Caution:** [C, −] **CI:** None **Disp:** Tabs 400 mg **SE:** N/D, HA, fever, paranoia, anxiety **Interactions:** ↑ Effects *W/* UGT1A1 Inhibs; ↓ effects *W/* rifampine **Labs:** ↑ Cholesterol, mono lipids **NIPE:** Caution w/ drugs that cause myopathy such as statins; ✓ dose before dialysis sessions; initial therapy may cause immune reconstitution synd (inflammatory response to residual opportunistic Infxns (eg, *M avium, PCP*)

Ramelteon (Rozerem) [Hypnotic-Melatonin Receptor Agonist]
Uses: Short-term Rx of insomnia esp w/ difficulty of sleep onset **Action:** Hypnotic agent; melatonin receptor agonist; **Dose:** 8-mg tabs PO w/in 30 min of bedtime **Caution:** [C, −] **CI:** Severe hepatic impair; concurrent use of fluvoxamine; hypersensitivity **Disp:** 8-mg

tabs **SE:** HA, N, somnolence, fatigue, dizziness, URI, depression, D, myalgia, arthralgia **Interactions:** ↑ Effects W/ CYP1A2 Inhibs (fluvoxamine), CYP3A4 Inhibs (ketoconazole), & CYP2C9 Inhibs (fluconazole); ↑ risk of CNS depression w/ EtOH & CNS depressants; ↓ effects W/ CYP450 inducers (rifampin) **Labs:** ↓ Testosterone levels & ↑ prolactin levels noted **NIPE:** High-fat foods delay effect; ⊘ use in pts w/ severe sleep apnea & severe COPD

Ramipril (Altace) [Antihypertensive/ACEI]   WARNING: ACE Inhibs used during PRG can cause fetal injury & death **Uses:** *HTN, CHF, DN, post-MI* **Action:** ACE Inhib **Dose:** 2.5–20 mg/d PO ÷ daily–bid; ↓ in renal failure **Caution:** [D, +] **CI:** ACE-Inhib-induced angioedema **Disp:** Caps 1.25, 2.5, 5, 10 mg **SE:** Cough, HA, dizziness, ↓ BP, renal impair, angioedema **Interactions:** ↑ Effects W/ α-adrenergic blockers, loop diuretics; ↑ effects OF insulin, Li; ↑ risk of hyperkalemia W/ K+, K+-sparing diuretics, K+ salt substitutes (monitor ECG for peaked T waves), TMP, ↓ effects W/ ASA, NSAIDs, Ca **Labs:** ↑ BUN, Cr, K+, HMG, Hct, cholesterol, glucose **NIPE:** ↑ Risk of photosensitivity—use sunscreen; ↑ risk of cough esp w/ capsaicin; take w/o food; OK in combo w/ diuretics

Ranibizumab (Lucentis) [Vascular Endothelial GF Inhibitor] **Uses:** *Neovascular "wet" macular degeneration* **Action:** VEGF Inhib **Dose:** 0.5 mg intravitreal Inj qmo **Caution:** [C, ?] h/o thromboembolism **CI:** Periocular Infxn **Disp:** Inj **SE:** Endophthalmitis, retinal detachment/hemorrhage, cataract, intraocular inflammation, conjunctival hemorrhage, eye pain, floaters, eye pain

Ranitidine Hydrochloride (Zantac, Zantac OTC, Zantac EFFER Dose) [Antiulcer Agent/H₂-Receptor Antagonist] **Uses:** *Duodenal ulcer, active benign ulcers, hypersecretory conditions, & GERD* **Action:** H₂-receptor antagonist **Dose:** **Adults.** *Ulcer:* 150 mg PO bid, 300 mg PO hs, or 50 mg IV q6–8h; or 400 mg IV/d cont Inf, then maint of 150 mg PO hs *Hypersecretion:* 150 mg PO bid, up to 600 mg/d *GERD:* 300 mg PO bid; maint 300 mg PO hs *Dyspepsia:* 75 mg PO daily–bid *Peds.* 0.75–1.5 mg/kg/dose IV q6–8h or 1.25–2.5 mg/kg/dose PO q12h; ↓ in renal Insuff/failure **Caution:** [B, +] **CI:** Component allergy **Disp:** Tabs 75 [OTC], 150, 300 mg; caps 150, 300 mg; effervescent tabs 150 mg; syrup 15 mg/mL; Inj 25 mg/mL **SE:** Dizziness, sedation, rash, GI upset **Interactions:** ↑ Effects OF glipizide, glyburide, procainamide, warfarin; ↓ effects W/ antacids, tobacco; ↓ effects OF diazepam **Labs:** ↑ SCr, ALT **NIPE:** ASA, NSAIDs, EtOH, caffeine ↑ stomach acid production; PO & parenteral doses differ

Ranolazine (Ranexa) [Antianginal] **Uses:** *Chronic angina* **Action:** ↓ Ischemia-related Na+ entry into myocardium **Dose:** **Adults.** 500 mg bid–1000 mg PO bid **CI:** w/ Hepatic impair, CYP3A Inhibs (Table 10); w/ agents that ↑ QT interval; ↓ K+ **Caution:** [C, ?/–] HTN may develop w/ renal impair **Disp:** SR tabs 500 mg **SE:** Dizziness, HA, constipation, arrhythmias **Interactions:** Risk of ↑ QT interval W/ diltiazem, verapamil, grapefruit juice **Labs:** ↓ K+—monitor ECG (flattened T waves) **NIPE:** Not 1st-line; use w/ amlodipine, nitrates, BB

Rasagiline Mesylate (Azilect) [Anti-Parkinson Agent/MAO B Inhibitor] Uses: *Early Parkinson Dz monotherapy; levodopa adjunct w/ advanced Dz* Action: MAO B Inhib Dose: *Adults. Early Dz:* 1 mg PO daily, start 0.5 mg PO daily w/ levodopa; ↓ w/ CYP1A2 Inhibs or hepatic impair CI: MAOIs, sympathomimetic amines, meperidine, methadone, tramadol, propoxyphene, dextromethorphan, mirtazapine, cyclobenzaprine, St. John's wort, sympathomimetic vasoconstrictors, general anesthetics, SSRIs Caution: [C, ?] Avoid tyramine-containing foods; mod/severe hepatic impair Disp: Tabs 0.5, 1 mg SE: Arthralgia, indigestion, dyskinesia, hallucinations, ↓ wgt, postural ↓ BP, N/V, constipation, xerostomia, rash, sedation, CV conduction disturbances Interactions: ↑ Risk of HTN crisis W/ tyramine-containing foods (beer, red wine, aged cheese/meat, dried fruit); ↑ effects W/ ciprofloxacin; ↑ CNS tox/death W/ TCA, SSRIs, MAOIs Labs: Monitor LFTs NIPE: Rare melanoma reported; do periodic skin exams (skin CA risk); D/C 14 d prior to elective surgery; D/C fluoxetine 5 wk before starting rasagiline; initial ↓ levodopa dose OK; allow at least 14 d after discontinuing rasagiline before starting SSRI, tricyclic, or SNRI

Rasburicase (Elitek) [Antigout Agent/Antimetabolite] WARNING: Anaphylaxis possible; do not use in G6PD deficiency & hemolysis; can cause methemoglobinemia; can interfere w/ uric acid assays; collect blood samples & store on ice Uses: *Reduce ↑ uric acid d/t tumor lysis (peds)* Action: Catalyzes uric acid Dose: *Adult & Peds.* 0.20 mg/kg IV over 30 min, daily × 5; do not bolus Caution: [C, ?/–] CI: Anaphylaxis, screen for G6PD deficiency to avoid hemolysis, methemoglobinemia Disp: 1.5, 7.5 mg powder Inj SE: Fever, neutropenia, GI upset, HA, rash Labs: Falsely ↓ uric acid values; ↑ neutrophils NIPE: Place blood test tube for uric acid level on ice to D/C enzymatic Rxn; removed by dialysis

Repaglinide (Prandin) [Hypoglycemic/Meglitinide] Action: ↑ Pancreatic insulin release Dose: 0.5–4 mg ac, PO start 1–2 mg, to 16 mg/d max; take pc Caution: [C, ?/–] CI: DKA, type 1 DM Disp: Tabs 0.5, 1, 2 mg SE: HA, hyper-/hypoglycemia, GI upset Interactions: BB use may mask hypoglycemia NIPE: Take 15 min ac; skip drug if meal skipped

Repaglinide & Metformin (PrandiMet) [Hypoglycemic/Meglitinide + Biguanide] WARNING: Associated w/ lactic acidosis, risk ↑ w/ sepsis, dehydration, renal/hepatic impair, ↑ alcohol, acute CHF; Sxs include myalgias, malaise, resp distress, Abd pain, somnolence & death: ↓ pH, ↑ anion gap, ↑ blood lactate; D/C stat & hospitalize if suspected Uses: *Type 2 DM* Action: Meglitinide & biguanide (see Metformin) Dose: *Adults.* 1/500 mg bid w/in 15 min pc (skip dose w/ skipped meal); max 10/2500 mg/d or 4/1000 mg/meal Caution:[C,–] CI: SCr > 1.4 mg/dL (females) or > 1.5 mg/dL (males); metabolic acidosis; w/ gemfibrozil Disp: Tabs (repaglinide mg/metformin mg) 1/500, 2/500 SE: Hypoglycemia, HA, N/V/D, anorexia, weakness, myalgia, rash, ↓ vit B_{12} Interactions: Suspend use w/ iodinated contrast, do not use w/ NPH insulin, use w/ cationic drugs & CYP2C8 & CYP3A4 Inhibs; BB use may mask hypoglycemia,

↑ effects *W/* amiloride, cimetidine, digoxin, furosemide, MAOIs, morphine, procainamide, quinidine, quinine, ranitidine, triamterene, TMP, vancomycin; ↓ effects *W/* corticosteroids, CCBs, diuretics, estrogens, INH, OCPs, phenothiazine, phenytoin, sympathomimetics, thyroid drugs, tobacco **Labs:** Monitor LFTs, BUN/Cr, serum to B$_{12}$ **NIPE:** Take w/ food; avoid dehydration, EtOH, before surgery

Retapamulin (Altabax) [Pleuromutilin Antibiotic] Uses: *Topical Rx impetigo in pts > 9 mo* **Action:** Pleuromutilin antibiotic, bacteriostatic, ↓ bacteria protein synth *Spectrum: S aureus* (not MRSA), *S pyogenes* **Dose:** Apply bid × 5 d **Caution:** [B, ?] **Disp:** 10 mg/1 g **SE:** Local irritation **NIPE:** Prolonged use may result in super Infxn

Reteplase (Retavase) [Tissue Plasminogen Activator] Uses: *Post-AMI* **Action:** Thrombolytic **Dose:** 10 units IV over 2 min, 2nd dose in 30 min, 10 units IV over 2 min *ECC 2010:* 10 units IV bolus over 2 min; 30 min later, 10 units IV bolus over 2 min w/ NS flush before & after each dose. **Caution:** [C, ?/–] **CI:** Internal bleeding, spinal surgery/trauma, h/o CNS AVM/CVA, bleeding diathesis, severe uncontrolled ↑ BP, sensitivity to thrombolytics **Disp:** Inj 10.8 units/2 mL **SE:** Bleeding including CNS, allergic Rxns **Interactions:** ↑ Risk of bleeding *W/* ASA, abciximab, dipyridamole, heparin, NSAIDs, anticoagulants, vit K antagonists **Labs:** ↓ Fibrinogen, plasminogen **NIPE:** Monitor ECG during Rx for ↑ risk of reperfusion arrhythmias; minimize or avoid invasive testing (venipuncture, Inj) d/t ↑ risk of bleeding

Ribavirin (Virazole, Copegus) [Antiviral/Nucleoside Analogue]
WARNING: Monotherapy for chronic hep C ineffective; hemolytic anemia possible, teratogenic & embryocidal; use 2 forms birth control for up to 6 mo after D/C drug; ↓ in resp Fxn when used in infants as Inh Uses: *RSV Infxn in infants [Virazole]; hep C (in combo w/ interferon α$_{2b}$ [Copegus])* **Action:** Unknown **Dose:** *RSV:* 6 g in 300 mL sterile H$_2$O, inhale over 12–18 h *Hep C:* 600 mg PO bid in combo w/ interferon α$_{2b}$, alfa-2b (use Rebetron) [X, ?] May accumulate on soft contact lenses **CI:** PRG, autoimmune hep, CrCl < 50 mL/min **Disp:** Powder for aerosol 6 g; tabs 200, 400, 600 mg, caps 200 mg, soln 40 mg/mL **SE:** Fatigue, HA, GI upset, anemia, myalgia, alopecia, bronchospasm **Interactions:** ↓ Effects *W/* Al, Mg, simethicone; ↓ effect *OF* zidovudine **Labs:** ↑ LFTs; ↓ HMG, Hct, plts, WBC; monitor Labs; PRG test monthly **NIPE:** ⊘ PRG, breast-feeding; PRG test monthly—2 forms birth control; ↑ risk of photosensitivity—use sunblock; take w/o regard to food; Virazole aerosolized by a SPAG; monitor resp Fxn closely; hep C viral genotyping may modify dose

Rifabutin (Mycobutin) [Antibiotic/Antitubercular] Uses: *Prevent MAC Infxn in AIDS pts w/ CD4 count < 100* **Action:** ↓ DNA-dependent RNA polymerase activity **Dose:** *Adults.* 150–300 mg/d PO *Peds 1 y.* 15–25 mg/kg/d PO *2–10 y.* 4.4–18.8 mg/kg/d PO *14–16 y.* 2.8–5.4 mg/kg/d PO **Caution:** [B, ?/–] WBC < 1000 cells/mm^3 or plts < 50,000 cells/mm^3; ritonavir **CI:** Allergy **Disp:** Caps 150 mg **SE:** Discolored urine, rash, neutropenia, leukopenia, myalgia **Interactions:** ↑ Effects *W/* ritonavir; ↓ effects *OF* anticoagulants, anticonvulsants, barbiturates, benzodiazepines, BBs, corticosteroids, methadone, morphine, OCPs, quinidine, theophylline, TCAs **Labs:** ↑ LFTs **NIPE:** Urine & body fluids may turn reddish brown in color, discoloration of soft contact lenses, use barrier contraception, take w/o food; SE/interactions similar to rifampin

Rifampin (Rifadin) [Antibiotic/Antitubercular] Uses: *TB & Rx & prophylaxis of *N meningitidis, H influenzae,* or *S aureus* carriers*; adjunct w/ severe *S aureus* **Action:** ↓ DNA-dependent RNA polymerase **Dose:** *Adults. N meningitidis* & *H influenzae carrier:* 600 mg PO for 4 d *TB:* 600 mg PO or IV daily or 2 × /wk w/ combo regimen *Peds.* 10–20 mg/kg/dose PO or IV daily–bid; ↓ in hepatic failure **Caution:** [C, +] w/ fosamprenavir, multiple drug interactions **CI:** Allergy, active *N meningitidis* Infxn, w/ saquinavir/ritonavir **Disp:** Caps 150, 300 mg; Inj 600 mg **SE:** Red-orange colored bodily fluids, flushing, HA **Interactions:** ↓ Effects *W/* aminosalicylic acid; ↓ effects *OF* APAP, aminophylline, amiodarone, anticoagulants, barbiturates, BBs, CCBs, chloramphenicol, clofibrate, delavirdine, digoxin, disopyramide, doxycycline, enalapril, estrogens, haloperidol, hypoglycemics, hydantoins, methadone, morphine, nifedipine, ondansetron, OCPs, phenytoin, protease Inhibs, quinidine, repaglinide, sertraline, sulfapyridine, sulfones, tacrolimus, theophylline, thyroid drugs, tocainide, TCAs, theophylline, verapamil, zidovudine, zolpidem **Labs:** ↑ LFTs, uric acid **NIPE:** Use barrier contraception; take w/o food; reddish brown color in urine & body fluids; stains soft contact lenses; never use as single agent w/ active TB

Rifapentine (Priftin) [Antibiotic/Antitubercular] Uses: *Pulm TB* **Action:** ↓ DNA-dependent RNA polymerase *Spectrum: M tuberculosis* **Dose:** *Intensive phase:* 600 mg PO 2 × /wk for 2 mo; separate doses by > 3 d *Continuation phase:* 600 mg/wk for 4 mo; part of 3–4 drug regimen **Caution:** [C, red-orange breast milk] Strong CYP450 inducer, ↓ protease Inhib efficacy, antiepileptics, BBs, CCBs **CI:** Rifamycins allergy **Disp:** 150-mg tabs **SE:** Neutropenia, hyperuricemia, HTN, HA, dizziness, rash, GI upset, blood dyscrasias, hematuria, discolored secretions **Interactions:** ↓ Effects *OF* anticoagulants, BBs, CCBs, corticosteroids, cyclosporine, digoxin, fluoroquinolones, methadone, metoprolol, OCPs, phenytoin, propranolol, protease Inhibs, rifampin, sulfonylureas, TCAs, theophylline, verapamil, warfarin **Labs:** ↑ LFTs—monitor; plts, uric acid; ↓ HMG, neutrophil, WBCs **NIPE:** May take w/ food; body fluids, teeth, tongue, feces may become orange-red; may permanently discolor soft contact lenses; use barrier contraception

Rifaximin (Xifaxan, Xifaxan 550) [Antibiotic/Rifamycin Antibacterial] Uses: *Traveler's D (noninvasive strains of *E coli* in pts > 12 y* (*Xifaxan*); hepatic encephalopathy (*Xifaxan 550*) > 18 y* **Action:** Not absorbed, derivative of rifamycin *Spectrum: E coli* **Dose:** D (*Xifaxan*): 1 tab PO daily × 3 d; encephalopathy (*Xifaxan 550*) 500 mg PO bid; w/ or w/o food 1 tab PO daily × 3 d **Caution:** [C, ?/–] Hx allergy; pseudomembranous colitis; w/ severe (Child–Pugh C) hepatic impair **CI:** Allergy to rifamycins **Disp:** Tabs: *Xifaxan* 200 mg; *Xifaxan 550:* 550 mg **SE:** *Xifaxan:* Flatulence, HA, Abd pain, rectal tenesmus & urgency,

N **Xifaxan 550**: Edema, N, dizziness, fatigue, ascites, flatulence, HA **Interactions:** None sig **Labs:** None noted **NIPE:** May be taken w/o regard to food; ⊘ crush/ chew tabs—swallow whole; D/C if D Sx worsen or persist > 24–48 h, or w/ fever or blood in stool

Rimantadine (Flumadine) [Antiviral] Uses: *Prophylaxis & Rx of influenza A viral Infxns* **Action:** Antiviral **Dose:** *Adults & Peds > 9 y.* 100 mg PO bid *Peds 1–9 y.* 5 mg/kg/d PO, 150 mg/d max; daily w/ severe renal/hepatic impair & elderly; initiate w/in 48 h of Sx onset **Caution:** [C, –] w/ cimetidine; avoid w/ PRG, breast-feeding **CI:** Component & amantadine allergy **Disp:** Tabs 100 mg; syrup 50 mg/5 mL **SE:** Orthostatic ↓ BP, edema, dizziness, GI upset, ↓ Sz threshold **Interactions:** ↑ Effects *W/* cimetidine; ↓ effects *W/* APAP, ASA; concurrent use w/ EtOH may cause confusion, syncope, light-headedness or hypotension **NIPE:** See CDC (*MMWR*) for current influenza A guidelines

Rimexolone (Vexol Ophthalmic) [Steroid] Uses: *Post-op inflammation & uveitis* **Action:** Steroid **Dose:** *Adults & Peds > 2 y. Uveitis:* 1–2 gtt/h daytime & q2h at night, taper to 1 gt q4h *Post-op:* 1–2 gtt qid × 2 wk **Caution:** [C, ?/–] Ocular Infxns **Disp:** Susp 1% **SE:** Blurred vision, local irritation **NIPE:** Shake well, ⊘ touch eye w/ dppr; taper dose

Risedronate (Actonel, Actonel w/ Calcium) [Biphosphonate/Hormone] Uses: *Paget Dz; Rx/prevention glucocorticoid-induced/postmenopausal osteoporosis; ↑ bone mass in osteoporotic men; w/ Ca only FDA approved for female osteoporosis* **Action:** Bisphosphonate; ↓ osteoclast-mediated bone resorption **Dose:** *Paget Dz:* 30 mg/d PO for 2 mo *Osteoporosis Rx/prevention:* 5 mg daily or 35 mg qwk; 30 min before 1st food/drink of the d; stay upright for at least 30 min after dose **Caution:** [C, ?/–] CA supls & antacids ↓ absorption **CI:** Component allergy, esophageal abnormalities, unable to stand/sit for 30 min, CrCl < 30 mL/ min **Disp:** Tabs 5, 30, 35, 75 mg; risedronate 35 mg (4 tabs)/calcium carbonate 1250 mg (24 tabs) **SE:** HA, D, Abd pain, arthralgia; flu-like Sxs, rash, esophagitis, bone pain **Interactions:** ↓ Effects *W/* antacids, ASA, Ca²⁺, food **Labs:** ↓ Ca²⁺, monitor LFTs, Ca²⁺, PO³⁺, K⁺; interference w/ bone-imaging agents **NIPE:** EtOH intake & cigarette smoking promote osteoporosis; ↑ risk of jaw fx; jaw osteonecrosis, avoid dental work; may ↑ atypical subtrochantericfemur fxs

Risedronate, Delayed Release (Atelvia) [Biphosphonate/ Hormone] Uses: *Postmenopausal osteoporosis* **Action:** See Risedronate **Dose:** One 35-mg tab 1 × wk; in AM following breakfast w/ 4-oz H₂O; do not lie down for 30 min **Caution:** [C, ?/–] **CI:** Component allergy, Ca²⁺, esophageal abnormalities, unable to stand/sit for 30 min **Disp:** DR tabs 35 mg **SE:** D, influenza, arthralgia, back/Abd pain; rare hypersensitivity, eye inflammation **Interactions:** ↓ Absorption *W/* Ca or Mg-based supls, antacids, laxatives, or Fe Prep **Labs:** Correct ↓ Ca²⁺ before use; ✓ Ca²⁺ **NIPE:** Do not use w/ Actonel or CrCl < 30 mL/ min; jaw osteonecrosis reported, avoid dental work; may ↑ subtrochanteric femur fxs; severe bone/Jt pain; may interfere *W/* bone imaging agents

Risperidone, Oral (Risperdal, Risperdal M-Tab) [Antipsychotic]
WARNING: ↑ Mortality in elderly w/ dementia-related psychosis **Uses:** *Psychotic disorders (schizophrenia)*, dementia of the elderly, bipolar disorder, mania, Tourette disorder, autism **Action:** Benzisoxazole antipsychotic **Dose:** *Adults.* 0.5–6 mg PO bid *M-Tab:* 1–6 mg/d start 1–2 mg/d, titrate q3–7d *Peds.* 0.25 mg PO bid, ↑ q5–7d; ↓ start dose w/ elderly, renal/hepatic impair **Caution:** [C, –], ↑ BP w/ antihypertensives, clozapine **CI:** Component allergy **Disp:** Tabs 0.25, 0.5, 1, 2, 3, 4 mg; soln 1 mg/mL, M-Tab (ODT) tabs 0.5, 1, 2, 3, 4 mg **SE:** Orthostatic ↓ BP, EPS w/ high dose, tachycardia, arrhythmias, sedation, dystonias, neuroleptic malignant synd, sexual dysfunction, constipation, xerostomia, blood dyscrasias, neutropenia, agranulocytosis, cholestatic jaundice **Interactions:** ↑ Effects *W/*clozapine, CNS depressants, EtOH; ↑ effects *OF* antihypertensives; ↑ effects *W/* carbamazepine; ↓ effects *OF* levodopa **Labs:** ↑ LFTs, serum prolactin, glucose; ↓ WBC **NIPE:** ↑ Risk photosensitivity—use sunblock, extrapyramidal effects; may alter body temperature regulation; several wk to see effect; risk ↑ QT interval—monitor ECG

Risperidone, Parenteral (Risperdal Consta) [Antipsychotic]
WARNING: Not approved for dementia-related psychosis; ↑ mortality risk in elderly dementia pts on atypical antipsychotics; most deaths d/t CV or infectious events **Uses:** Schizophrenia **Action:** Benzisoxazole antipsychotic **Dose:** 25 mg q2wk IM may ↑ to max 50 mg q2wk; w/ renal/hepatic impair start PO Risperdal 0.5 mg PO bid × 1 wk titrate weekly **Caution:** [C, –], ↑ BP w/ antihypertensives, clozapine **CI:** Component allergy **Disp:** Inj 25, 37.5, 50 mg/vial **SE:** See Risperidone Oral **Interactions:** ↑ Effects *W/* clozapine, CNS depressants, EtOH; ↑ effects *OF* antihypertensives; ↓ effects *W/* carbamazepine; ↓ effects *OF* levodopa **Labs:** ↑ LFTs, serum prolactin **NIPE:** ↑ Risk of photosensitivity—use sunscreen, extrapyramidal effects; may alter body temperature regulation; several wk to see effect; LA Inj

Ritonavir (Norvir) [Antiretroviral/Protease Inhibitor] **WARNING:** Life-threatening adverse events when used w/ certain nonsedating antihistamines, sedative hypnotics, antiarrhythmics, or ergot alkaloids d/t inhibited drug metabolism **Uses:** *HIV* **Actions:** Protease Inhib; ↓ maturation of immature noninfectious virions to mature infectious virus **Dose:** *Adults.* Initial 300 mg PO bid, titrate over 1 wk to 600 mg PO bid (titration will ↓ GI SE) *Peds > 1 mo.* 250 mg/m² titrate to 400 mg bid (adjust w/ fosamprenavir, indinavir, nelfinavir, & saquinavir); take w/ food **Caution:** [B, +] w/ ergotamine, amiodarone, bepridil, flecainide, propafenone, quinidine, pimozide, midazolam, triazolam **CI:** Component allergy **Disp:** Caps & tabs 100 mg; soln 80 mg/mL **SE:** N/V/D/C, Abd pain, taste perversion, anemia, weakness, HA, fever, malaise, rash, paresthesias **Interactions:** ↑ Effects *W/* erythromycin, ILs, grapefruit juice, food; ↑ effects *OF* amiodarone, astemizole, atorvastatin, barbiturates, bepridil, bupropion, cerivastatin, cisapride, clorazepate, clozapine, clarithromycin, desipramine, diazepam, encainide, ergot alkaloids, estazolam, flecainide, flurazepam, indinavir, ketoconazole, lovastatin, meperidine, midazolam, nelfinavir, phenytoin, pimozide, piroxicam, propafenone, propoxyphene, quinidine, rifabutin, saquinavir, sildenafil, simvastatin, SSRIs, TCAs, terfenadine, triazolam, troleandomycin, zolpidem; ↑ risk of hypotension W/ concurrent use of Viagra-type drugs; ↑ SEs W/ EtOH; ↓ effects W/ barbiturates, carbamazepine, phenytoin, rifabutin, rifampin, St. John's wort, tobacco; ↓ effects OF didanosine, hypnotics, methadone, OCPs, sedatives, theophylline, warfarin **Labs:** ↑ Serum glucose, LFTs, triglycerides, uric acid **NIPE:** Food ↑ absorption; use barrier contraception; disulfiram-like Rxn w/ disulfiram, metronidazole; refrigerate

Rivastigmine (Exelon) [Cholinesterase Inhibitor/Anti-Alzheimer Agent] Uses: *Mild–mod dementia in Alzheimer Dz* Action: Enhances cholinergic activity Dose: 1.5 mg bid; ↑ to 6 mg bid, w/ ↑ at 2-wk intervals (take w/ food) Caution: [B, ?] w/ BBs, CCBs, smoking, neuromuscular blockade, digoxin CI: Rivastigmine or carbamate allergy Disp: Caps 1.5, 3, 4.5, 6 mg; soln 2 mg/mL SE: Dose-related GI effects, N/V/D, dizziness, insomnia, fatigue, tremor, diaphoresis, HA, wgt loss (in 18–26%) Interactions: ↑ Risk OF GI bleed W/ NSAIDs; ↓ effects W/ nicotine; ↓ effects OF anticholinergics NIPE: Take w/ food; swallow caps whole, do not break/chew/crush; avoid EtOH; risk of severe emesis w/ stopping & restarting drug

Rivastigmine Transdermal (Exelon Patch) [Cholinesterase Inhibitor/ Anti-Alzheimer Agent] Uses: *Mild/mod Alzheimer & Parkinson Dz dementia* Action: Acetylcholinesterase Inhib Dose: Initial: 4.6-mg patch/d applied to back, chest, upper arm, ↑ 9.5 mg after 4 wk if tolerated Caution: [B, ?] SSS, conduction defects, asthma, COPD, urinary obst, Szs; death from multiple patches at same time reported CI: Hypersensitivity to rivastigmine, other carbamates Disp: Transdermal patch 5 cm² (4.6 mg/24 h), 10 cm² (9.5 mg/24 h) SE: N/V/D Interactions: ↑ Risk of GI bleed W/ NSAIDs; ↓ effects W/ nicotine; ↓ effects OF anticholinergics NIPE: Risk of severe emesis w/ stopping & restarting drug

Rizatriptan (Maxalt, Maxalt MLT) [Antimigraine Agent/5-HT₁ Agonist] Uses: *Rx acute migraine* Action: Vascular serotonin receptor agonist Dose: 5–10 mg PO, repeat in 2 h, PRN, 30 mg/d max Caution: [C, M] CI: Angina, ischemic heart Dz, ischemic bowel Dz, hemiplegic/basilar migraine, uncontrolled HTN, ergot or serotonin 5-HT₁ agonist use w/in 24 h, MAOI use w/in 14 d Disp: Tab 5, 10 mg; Maxalt MLT: OD tabs 5, 10 mg SE: CP, palpitations, N, V, asthenia, dizziness, somnolence, fatigue Interactions: ↑ Vasospastic effects W/ ergots, 5-HT agonists; ↓ effects W/ MAOIs, propranolol NIPE: Tx for migraines—not for prophylaxis; acute MIs & arrhythmias have occurred after taking 5-HT₁ drugs

Rocuronium (Zemuron) [Skeletal Muscle Relaxant] Uses: *Skeletal muscle relaxation during rapid-sequence intubation, surgery, or mechanical ventilation* Action: Nondepolarizing neuromuscular blocker Dose: Rapid-sequence intubation: 0.6–1.2 mg/kg IV Cont Inf: 5–12.5 mcg/kg/min IV; adjust/titrate based on monitoring; ↓ in hepatic impair **Caution:** [C, ?] Aminoglycosides, vancomycin, tetracycline, polymyxins enhance blockade **CI:** Component or pancuronium allergy **Disp:** Inj preservative-free 10 mg/mL **SE:** BP changes, tachycardia **Interactions:** ↑ Effects *W*/ MAOIs, propranolol; ↑ vasospastic Rxn *W*/ ergot-containing drugs; ↑ risk of hyperreflexia, incoordination, weakness *W*/ SSRIs **NIPE:** Food delays drug action; ⊘ take > 30 mg/24 h

Romidepsin (Istodax) [Histone Deacetylase Inhibitor] Uses: *Rx cutaneous T-cell lymphoma in pts who have received at least 1 prior systemic therapy * **Action:** Histone deacetylase (HDAC) Inhib **Dose:** 14 mg/m² IV over 4 h d 1, 8, & 15 of a 28-d cycle;repeat cycles every 28 d if tolerated; Tx D/C or interruption w/ or w/o dose reduction to 10 mg/m² to manage adverse drug Rxns **Caution:** [D, ?] Risk of ↑ QT, hematologic tox **Disp:** Inj 10 mg **SE:** N, V, fatigue, Infxn, anorexia **Interactions:** May ↑ conc *W*/ strong CYP3A4 Inhibs (eg, azole antifungals, protease Inhibs, clarithromycin, nefazodone; caution w/ mod CYP3A4 Inhibs; ↓ *W*/ strong CYP3A4 inducers (eg, carbamazepine, phenytoin, phenobarbital, rifampin, avoid) **Labs:** ↓ α Plt; monitor PT/INR *W*/ warfarin; monitor lytes, CBC w/ differential **NIPE:** Hazardous agent, precautions for handling & disposal; ⊘ St. John's wort

Romiplostim (Nplate) [Thrombopoietin Receptor Agonist] **WARNING:** ↑ Risk for heme malignancies & thromboembolism. D/C may worsen ↓ plt **Uses:** *↓ Plt d/t ITP* **Action:** Thrombopoietic, colony-stimulating factor **Dose:** *Adults.* 1 mcg/kg SQ weekly, adjust 1 mcg/kg/wk to plt count > 50,000 cells/mm³ max 10 mcg/kg/wk **Caution:** [C, ?] **Contra:** None **Disp:** 500 mcg/mL(250-mcg vial) **SE:** HA, fatigue, dizziness, N/V/D, myalgia, epistaxis **Interactions:** ↑ Risk of bleeding *W*/ anticoagulants & antiplt drugs **Labs:** Monitor CBC, plts, & peripheral smears before & weekly while adjustment of dose & monthly w/ stable dose & weekly for 2 wk after D/C drug **NIPE:** D/C if no ↑ plt after 4 wk max dose; ↓ dose w/ plt count > 200,000 cells/mm³ risk of hematological malignancies; risk of renal or hepatic impair

Ropinirole (Requip) [Dopamine Agonist/Anti-Parkinson Agent] **Uses:** *Rx of Parkinson Dz, RLS* **Action:** DA agonist **Dose:** Initial 0.25 mg PO tid, weekly ↑ 0.25 mg/dose, to 3 mg max, max 4 mg RLS **Caution:** [C, ?/–] Severe CV, renal, or hepatic impair **CI:** Component allergy **Disp:** Tabs 0.25, 0.5, 1, 2, 3, 4, 5 mg **SE:** Syncope, postural ↓ BP, N/V, HA, somnolence, dose-related hallucinations, dyskinesias, dizziness **Interactions:** ↑ Risk of bleeding *W*/ ASA, NSAIDs, feverfew, garlic, ginger, horse chestnut, red clover, EtOH, tobacco); ↑ effects *OF* amitriptyline, Li, MTX, theophylline, warfarin; ↑ risk of photosensitivity *W*/ dong quai—use sunscreen, St. John's wort; ↓ effects *W*/ antacids, rifampin; ↓ effects *OF* ACEIs, diuretics **Labs:** ↑ ALT, AST **NIPE:** Take *W*/ food; D/C w/ 7-d taper

Rosiglitazone (Avandia) [Hypoglycemic/Thiazolidinedione] **WARNING:** May cause or worsen CHF; may ↑ myocardial ischemia **Uses:** *Type

2 DM* **Action:** Thiazolidinedione; ↑ insulin sensitivity **Dose:** 4–8 mg/d PO or in 2 ÷ doses (w/o regard to meals) **Caution:** [C, –] w/ ESRD, CHF, edema **CI:** DKA, severe CHF (NYHA Class III), ALT > 2.5 ULN **Disp:** Tabs 2, 4, 8 mg **SE:** May ↑ CV, CHF & ? CA risk; wgt gain, hyperlipidemia, HA, edema, fluid retention, worsen CHF, hyper-/hypoglycemia, hepatic damage w/ ↑ LFTs **Interactions:** ↑ Risk of hypoglycemia *W/* insulin, ketoconazole, oral hypoglycemics, fenugreek, garlic, ginseng, glucomannan; ↓ effects *OF* OCPs **Labs:** ↑ LFTs, total cholesterol, LDL, HDL, ↓ HMG, Hct **NIPE:** Use barrier contraception; not recommended in Class III, IV heart Dz; ? ↑ MI risk, now requires REMS restricted distribution program; BB may mask hypoglycemia; after November 18, 2011, Avandia (rosiglitazone), Avandamet (rosiglitazone/metformin), & Avandaryl (rosiglitazone/glimepiride) will be withdrawn from retail pharmacies. To order/prescribe/receive drugs, healthcare providers & pts must enroll in the Avandia-Rosiglitazone Medicines Access Program

Rosiglitazone/Metformin (Avandamet) [Hypoglycemic/Thiazoli-dinedione & Biguanide]

WARNING: Associated w/ lactic acidosis; may cause or worsen CHF; may ↑ myocardial ischemia **Uses:** Type 2 DM **Action:** ↓ Hepatic glucose production & intestinal absorption of glucose; ↑ insulin sensitivity **Dose:** *Adults. Initial:* 2 mg/500 mg PO OD or bid w/ AM & PM meal; ↑ by 2 mg/500 mg/d after 4 wk; max 8 mg/2000 mg/d *Peds.* Not recommended **Caution:** [C, –] Hold dose before & 48 h after ionic contrast; not for DKA; w/ ESRD (renal elimination), CHF, edema **CI:** SCr > 1.4 mg/dL in females or > 1.5 mg/dL in males; hypoxemic conditions (eg, acute CHF/sepsis); active liver Dz; metabolic acidosis; DKA, severe CHF (NYHA Class III), ALT > 2.5 ULN **Disp:** Tabs (rosiglitazone mg/metformin mg): 2/500, 4/500, 2/1000, 4/1000 **SE:** Wgt gain, hyperlipidemia, HA, edema, fluid retention, exacerbated CHF, hyper-/hypoglycemia, hepatic damage, anorexia, N/V, rash, lactic acidosis (rare, but serious) **Interactions:** ↑ Risk of hypoglycemia *W/* insulin, ketoconazole, fenugreek, garlic, ginseng, glucomannan; ↑ effects *W/* amiloride, cimetidine, digoxin, furosemide, MAOIs, morphine, procainamide, quinidine, quinine, ranitidine, triamterene, TMP, vancomycin; ↓ effects *W/* corticosteroids, CCBs, diuretics, estrogens, INH, OCPs, phenothiazine, phenytoin, sympathomimetics, thyroid drugs, tobacco; ↓ effects *OF* OCPs **Labs:** ↑ LFTs, lipids, SCr ↓ HMG, Hct; monitor LFTs, SCr baseline & periodically **NIPE:** Use barrier contraception; take w/ food; ⊘ dehydration, EtOH, before surgery; not recommended in Class III, IV heart Dz; ? ↑ MI risk, now requires REMS restricted distribution program; after November 18, 2011, Avandia (rosiglitazone), Avandamet (rosiglitazone/metformin), & Avandaryl (rosiglitazone/glimepiride) will be withdrawn from retail pharmacies. To order/prescribe/receive drugs, healthcare providers & pts must enroll in the Avandia-Rosiglitazone Medicines Access Program

Rosuvastatin (Crestor) [Antilipemic/HMG-CoA Reductase Inhibitor]

Uses: *Rx primary hypercholesterolemia & mixed dyslipidemia* **Action:** HMG-CoA reductase Inhib **Dose:** 5–40 mg PO daily; max 5 mg/d w/ cyclosporine, 10 mg/d w/ gemfibrozil or CrCl < 30 mL/min (avoid Al-/Mg-based antacids for 2 h after) **Caution:** [X, ?/–] **CI:** Active liver Dz, unexplained ↑ LFTs **Disp:** Tabs 5, 10, 20, 40 mg **SE:** Myalgia, constipation, asthenia, Abd pain, N, myopathy, rarely rhabdomyolysis **Interactions:** ↑ Effects *OF* warfarin; ↑ risk of myopathy *W/* cyclosporine, fibrates, niacin, statins **Labs:** ↑ LFTs; monitor LFTs at baseline, 12 wk, then q6mo; ↑ urine protein, HMG **NIPE:** ⊘ PRG or breast-feeding; ↓ dose in Asian pts; OK w/ grapefruit

Rotavirus Vaccine, Live, Oral, Attenuated (Rotarix) [Live Attenuated Human G1P[8] Rotavirus Vaccine] **Uses:** *Prevent rotavirus gastroenteritis in peds* **Action:** Active immunization w/ live attenuated rotavirus **Dose:** *Peds 6–14 wk.* 1st dose PO at 6 wk of age, wait at least 4 wk, then a 2nd dose by 24 wk of age **Caution:** [C, ?] **CI:** Component sensitivity; uncorrected congenital GI malformation; chronic GI illness, acute mod–severe D illness, fever **Disp:** SDV **SE:** Irritability, cough, runny nose, fever, ↓ appetite, V **Interactions:** ↓ Response if given *W/* immunosuppressants such as irradiation, chemotherapy, high-dose steroids **NIPE:** May give w/ concomitant vaccines such as DTaP, hep B, inactivated poliovirus vaccine combined, Hib conjugated; begin series by age 12 wk, conclude by age 24 wk; can be given to infant in house w/ immunosuppressed family member or mother who is breast-feeding. Safety & effectiveness not studied in immunocompromised infants

Rotavirus Vaccine, Live, Oral, Pentavalent (RotaTeq) [Vaccine] **Uses:** *Prevent rotavirus gastroenteritis* **Action:** Active immunization w/ live attenuated rotavirus; **Dose:** *Peds 6–14 wk.* Single dose PO at 2, 4, & 6 mo **Caution:** [?, ?] **CI:** Uncorrected congenital GI malformation, chronic GI illness, acute mod–severe D illness, fever **Disp:** Oral susp 2-mL single-use tubes **SE:** Fever, D, V **Interactions:** ↓ Effects *W/* immunosuppressants such as irradiation, chemotherapy or high-dose steroids **NIPE:** Begin series by 12 wk & conclude by 32 wk of age; ⊘ take w/ oral polio vaccine; begin series by age 12 wk & conclude by age 32 wk; can be given to infant in house w/ immunosuppressed family member or mother who is breast-feeding. Safety & effectiveness not studied in immunocompromised infants

Rufinamide (Banzel) [Antiepileptic] **WARNING:** Antiepileptics associated w/ ↑ risk of suicide ideation. Severe hypersensitivity Rxns reported **Uses:** *Adjunct Lennox–Gastaut Szs* **Action:** Anticonvulsant **Dose:** *Adults. Initial:* 400–800 mg/d ÷ bid (max 3200 mg/d ÷ bid) *Peds ≥ 4 y. Initial:* 10 mg/kg/d ÷ bid, target 45 mg/kg/d ÷ bid; 3200 mg/d max **Caution:** [C, –] **Contra:** Familial short QT synd **Disp:** Tab 200, 400 mg **SE:** ↑ QT, HA, somnolence, N/V, ataxia, rash **Interactions:** ↑ CNS depression *W/* EtOH & other CNS depressants; ↑ effects *OF* phenobarbital, phenytoin, triazolam; ↑ effects *W/* valproate ↓ effects *OF* carbamazepine, lamotrigine, phenytoin; ↓ effects *W/* carbamazepine, phenobarbital, primidone, phenytoin **NIPE:** Monitor for rash; use w/ OC may lead to contraceptive failure—use barrier contraception; ↑ QT—monitor ECG; take w/ food in 2 equal ÷ doses; monitor for depression or suicidal ideation

Salmeterol (Serevent Diskus) [Bronchodilator/Sympathomimetic]
WARNING: LA β_2-agonists, such as salmeterol, may ↑ the risk of asthma-related death. Do not use alone, only as additional therapy for pts not controlled on other asthma meds **Uses:** *Asthma, exercise-induced asthma, COPD* **Action:** Sympathomimetic bronchodilator, LA β_2-agonist **Dose:** *Adults & Peds > 12 y.* 1 Diskus-dose inhaled bid **Caution:** [C, ?/–] **CI:** Acute asthma; w/in 14 d of MAOI; w/o concomitant use of inhaled steroid **Disp:** 50 mcg/dose, dry powder discus, metered-dose inhaler, 21 mcg/activation **SE:** HA, pharyngitis, tachycardia, arrhythmias, nervousness, GI upset, tremors **Interactions:** ↑ CV effects *W*/ MAOIs, TCAs; ↓ effects *W*/ BBs **Labs:** ↑ Glucose; ↓ serum K⁺—monitor ECG for hypokalemia (flattened T waves) **NIPE:** Shake canister before use, inhale q12h; not for acute attacks; must use w/ steroid or short-acting β-agonist

Saquinavir (Fortovase, Invirase) [Antiretroviral/Protease Inhibitor]
WARNING: Invirase & Fortovase not bioequivalent/interchangeable; must use Invirase in combo w/ ritonavir, which provides saquinavir plasma levels = to those w/ Fortovase **Uses:** *HIV Infxn* **Action:** HIV protease Inhib **Dose:** 1200 mg PO tid w/in 2 h pc (dose adjust w/ ritonavir, delavirdine, lopinavir, & nelfinavir) **Caution:** [B, +] w/ ketoconazole, statins, sildenafil **CI:** w/ rifampin, severe hepatic impair, allergy, sun exposure w/o sunscreen/clothing, triazolam, midazolam, ergots **Disp:** Caps 200 mg, tabs 500 mg **SE:** Dyslipidemia, lipodystrophy, rash, hyperglycemia, GI upset, weakness **Interactions:** ↑ Risk of life-threatening arrhythmias *W*/ amiodarone, astemizole, bepridil, cisapride, flecainide, propafenone, pimozide, quinidine, terfenadine; ↑ risk of myopathy *W*/ HMG-CoA reductase Inhibs; ↑ risk of peripheral vasospasm & ischemia *W*/ ergot derivatives; ↑ effects *W*/ delavirdine, indinavir, ketoconazole, macrolide antibiotics, nelfinavir, ritonavir, grapefruit juice, garlic, St. John's wort, food; ↑ effects *OF* amitriptyline, benzodiazepines, CCB, lovastatin, macrolide antibiotics, phenytoin, sildenafil, simvastatin, terfenadine, TCAs, verapamil; ↓ effects *W*/ barbiturates, carbamazepine, dexamethasone, efavirenz, phenytoin, rifabutin, rifampin, St. John's wort; ↓ effects *OF* OCPs **Labs:** ↑ LFTs, ↓ neutrophils **NIPE:** Take 2 h after meal; use barrier contraception; ↑ risk of photosensitivity—avoid direct sunlight

Sargramostim [GM-CSF] (Leukine) [Hematopoietic Drug/Colony-Stimulating Factor] **Uses:** *Myeloid recovery following BMT or chemotherapy* **Action:** Recombinant GF, activates mature granulocytes & macrophages **Dose:** *Adults & Peds.* 250 mcg/m²/d IV for 21 d (BMT) **Caution:** [C, ?/–] Li, corticosteroids **CI:** > 10% blasts, allergy to yeast, concurrent chemotherapy/RT **Disp:** Inj 250, 500 mcg **SE:** Bone pain, fever, ↓ BP, tachycardia, flushing, GI upset, myalgia **Interactions:** ↑ Effects *W*/ corticosteroids, Li **Labs:** ↑ BUN, LFTs **NIPE:** ⊘ Exposure to Infxn; rotate Inj sites; use APAP PRN for pain

Saxagliptin (Onglyza) [Dipeptidyl Peptidase-4 Inhibitor] **Uses:** *Monotherapy or combo for type 2 DM* **Action:** Dipeptidyl peptidase-4 (DDP-4) Inhib, ↑ insulin synth/release **Dose:** 2.5 or 5 mg once/d w/o regard to meals;

2.5 mg once/d w/ CrCl < 50 mL/min or w/ strong CYP3A4/5 Inhib (eg, atazanavir, clarithromycin, indinavir, itraconazole, ketoconazole, nefazodone, nelfinavir, ritonavir, saquinavir, & telithromycin) **Caution:** [B, ?] May cause ↓ BS when used w/ insulin secretagogues such as sulfonylureas **CI:** w/ Insulin or to treat DKA **Disp:** Tabs 2.5, 5 mg **SE:** URI, nasopharyngitis, UTI, HA **Interactions:** ↑ Effects W/ strong CYP3A4/5 Inhibs: atazanavir, clarithromycin, indinavir, itraconazole, ketoconazole, nefazodone, nelfinavir, ritonavir, saquinavir, telithromycin; sulfonylurea **Labs:** Monitor BUN/Cr **NIPE:** No evidence for ↑ CV risk

Saxagliptin & Metformin (Kombiglyze XR) [Dipeptidyl Peptidase-4 Inhibitor + Biguanide] WARNING: Lactic acidosis can occur w/ metformin accumulation; ↑ risk w/ sepsis, vol depletion, CHF, renal/hepatic impair, excess alcohol; if lactic acidosis suspected D/C med & hospitalize Uses: *Type 2 DM* **Action:** Dipeptidyl peptidase-4 (DDP-4) Inhib, ↑ insulin synth/release & biguanide; ↓ hepatic glucose production & intestinal absorption of glucose; ↑ insulin sensitivity **Dose:** 5/500 mg–5/2000 mg saxagliptin/metformin HCl XR PO daily w/ evening meal **Caution:** [B; ?/–] **CI:** SCr > 1.4 mg/dL (females) or > 1.5 mg/dL (males); met acidosis; radiologic tests w/ iodinated contrast; w/insulin or to Rx type 1 DM or DKA; B$_{12}$ deficiency; hypoxic states (acute MI, acute CHF, sepsis) **Disp:** Tabs mg saxagliptin/mg metformin 5 mg/500 mg XR; 5/1000, 2.5/1000 **SE:** Lactic acidosis; ↓ B$_{12}$ levels; ↓ glu w/ insulin secretagogue; N/V/D, anorexia, HA, URI, UTI, urticaria, myalgia **Interactions:** ↑ Effects W/ strong CYP3A4/5 Inhibs: atazanavir, clarithromycin, indinavir, itraconazole, ketoconazole, nefazodone, nelfinavir, ritonavir, saquinavir, telithromycin; sulfonylurea; **Labs:** Monitor BUN/Cr **NIPE:** Do not exceed 5 mg/2000 mg saxagliptin/metformin HCl XR/d; do not crush or chew; w/ strong CYP3A4/5 Inhibs do not exceed 2.5 mg saxagliptin/d

Scopolamine, Scopolamine Transdermal & Ophthalmic (Scopace, Transderm-Scop) [Antiemetic/Antivertigo/Anticholinergic] Uses: *Prevent N/V associated w/ motion sickness, anesthesia, opiates; mydriatic*, cycloplegic, Rx uveitis & iridocyclitis **Action:** Anticholinergic, inhibits iris & ciliary bodies, antiemetic **Dose:** 1 mg/72 h, 1 patch behind ear q3d; apply > 4 h before exposure; cycloplegic 1–2 gtt 1 h preprocedure, uveitis 1–2 gtt up to qid max; ↓ in elderly **Caution:** [C, +] w/ APAP, levodopa, ketoconazole, digitalis, KCl **CI:** NAG, GI or GU obst, thyrotoxicosis, paralytic ileus **Disp:** Patch 1.5 mg (releases 1 mg over 72 h), ophthal 0.25% **SE:** Xerostomia, drowsiness, blurred vision, tachycardia, constipation **Interactions:** ↑ Effects W/ antihistamines, antidepressants, disopyramide, opioids, phenothiazine, quinidine, TCAs, EtOH **NIPE:** Do not blink excessively after dose, wait 5 min before dosing other eye; antiemetic activity w/ patch requires several h; ⊘ D/C abruptly; wash hands after applying patch; may cause heat intolerance, may cause stroke

Secobarbital (Seconal) [C-II] [Anticonvulsant, Sedative/Hypnotic/ Barbiturate] Uses: *Insomnia, short-term use*, preanesthetic agent **Action:** Rapid-acting barbiturate **Dose:** *Adults.* 100–200 mg hs, 100–300 mg pre-op *Peds.*

2–6 mg/kg/dose, 100 mg/max, ↓ in elderly **Caution:** [D, +] w/ CYP2C9, 3A3/4, 3A5/7 inducer (Table 10); ↑ tox w/ other CNS depressants **CI:** Porphyria, w/ voriconazole, PRG **Disp:** Caps 50, 100 mg **SE:** Tolerance in 1–2 wk; resp depression, CNS depression, porphyria, photosensitivity **Interactions:** ↑ Effects **W/** MAOIs, valproic acid, EtOH, kava kava, valerian; ↑ effects **OF** meperidine; ↓ effects **OF** anticoagulants, BBs, CCBs, CNS depressants, chloramphenicol, corticosteroids, cyclosporine, digitoxin, disopyramide, doxycycline, estrogen, griseofulvin, methadone, neuroleptics, OCPs, propafenone, quinidine, tacrolimus, theophylline **NIPE:** Tolerance in 1–2 wk; photosensitivity; ⊘ PRG, breast-feeding; use barrier contraception; do not D/C abruptly—may cause withdrawal

Selegiline, Oral (Eldepryl, Zelapar) [Anti-Parkinson Agent/MAOI]
WARNING: Closely monitor pts for worsening depression or emergence of suicidality, particularly in ped pts **Uses:** *Parkinson Dz* **Action:** MAOI **Dose:** 5 mg PO bid; 1.25–2.5 once-daily tabs PO qAM (before breakfast w/o Liq) 2.5 mg/d max; ↓ in elderly **Caution:** [C, ?] w/ Drugs that induce CYP3A4 (Table 10) (eg, phenytoin, carbamazepine, nafcillin, phenobarbital, & rifampin); avoid w/ antidepressants **CI:** w/ Meperidine, MAOI, dextromethorphan, general anesthesia w/in 10 d, Pheo **Disp:** Tabs/caps 5 mg; once-daily tabs 1.25 mg **SE:** N, dizziness, orthostatic ↓ BP, arrhythmias, tachycardia, edema, confusion, xerostomia **Interactions:** ↑ Risk of serotonin synd **W/** dextroamphetamine, dextromethorphan, fenfluramine, meperidine, methylphenidate, sibutramine, venlafaxine; ↑ risk of hypertension **W/** dextroamphetamine, levodopa, methylphenidate, SSRIs, tyramine-containing foods (beer, red wine, aged cheese/meat, dried fruits), EtOH, ephedra, ginseng, ma huang, St. John's wort **Labs:** + for amphetamine on urine drug screen **NIPE:** ↓ Carbidopa/levodopa if used in combo; see transdermal form

Selegiline, Transdermal (Emsam) [Anti-Parkinson Agent/MAO B Inhibitor] **WARNING:** May ↑ risk of suicidal thinking & behavior in children & adolescents w/ major depression disorder **Uses:** *Depression* **Action:** MAOI **Dose:** *Adults.* Apply patch daily to upper torso, upper thigh, or outer upper arm **CI:** Tyramine-containing foods w/ 9- or 12-mg doses; serotonin-sparing agents **Caution:** [C, –] ↑ Carbamazepine & oxcarbazepine levels **Disp:** ER Patches 6, 9, 12 mg **SE:** Local Rxns requiring topical steroids; HA, insomnia, orthostatic, ↓ BP, serotonin synd, suicide risk **Interactions:** ↑ Risk of serotonin synd **W/** dextroamphetamine, dextromethorphan, fenfluramine, meperidine, methylphenidate, sibutramine, venlafaxine; ↑ risk of hypertension **W/** dextroamphetamine, levodopa, methylphenidate, SSRIs, tyramine-containing foods (beer, red wine, aged cheese/meat, dried fruits), EtOH, ephedra, ginseng, ma huang, St. John's wort **NIPE:** ⊘ EtOH & tyramine-containing foods; rotate site; see oral form

Selenium Sulfide (Exsel Shampoo, Selsun Blue Shampoo, Selsun Shampoo) [Antiseborrheic] **Uses:** *Scalp seborrheic dermatitis*, scalp itching & flaking d/t *dandruff*; tinea versicolor **Action:** Antiseborrheic **Dose:** *Dandruff, seborrhea:* Massage 5–10 mL into wet scalp, leave on 2–3 min, rinse, repeat; use 2 × /wk, then once q1–4wk PRN *Tinea versicolor:* Apply 2.5% daily on area & lateral w/ small amounts of H₂O; leave on 10 min, then rinse **Caution:** [C, ?] **CI:** Open wounds **Disp:** Shampoo [OTC]; 2.5% lotion **SE:** Dry or oily scalp, lethargy, hair discoloration, local irritation **NIPE:** ⊘ Use on excoriated skin; may cause reversible hair loss; rinse thoroughly after use; do not use more than 2 × /wk

Sertaconazole (Ertaczo) [Antifungal] Uses: *Topical Rx interdigital tinea pedis* **Action:** Imidazole antifungal *Spectrum: T rubrum, T mentagrophytes, E floccosum* **Dose:** *Adults & Peds > 12.* Apply between toes & immediate surrounding healthy skin bid × 4 wk **Caution:** [C, ?] **CI:** Component allergy **Disp:** 2% Cream **SE:** Contact dermatitis, dry/burning skin, tenderness **NIPE:** Use in immunocompetent pts; not for oral, intravag, ophthal use; avoid occlusive dressings; avoid contact w/ mucous membranes

Sertraline (Zoloft) [Antidepressant/SSRI] **WARNING:** Closely monitor pts for worsening depression or emergence of suicidality, particularly in ped pts Uses: *Depression, panic disorders, obsessive-compulsive disorder (OCD), post-traumatic stress disorder (PTSD)*, social anxiety disorder, eating disorders, premenstrual disorders **Action:** ↓ Neuronal uptake of serotonin **Dose:** *Adults. Depression:* 50–200 mg/d PO *PTSD:* 25 mg PO daily × 1 wk, then 50 mg PO daily, 200 mg/d max *Peds. 6–12 y.* 25 mg PO daily *13–17 y.* 50 mg PO daily **Caution:** [C, ?/–] w/ Haloperidol (serotonin synd), sumatriptan, linezolid, hepatic impair **CI:** MAOI use w/in 14 d; concomitant pimozide **Disp:** Tabs 25, 50, 100, 150, 200 mg; 20 mg/mL oral **SE:** Activate manic/hypomanic state, ↓ wgt, insomnia, somnolence, fatigue, tremor, xerostomia, N/D, dyspepsia, ejaculatory dysfunction, ↓ libido, hepatotox **Interactions:** ↑ Effects W/ cimetidine, tryptophan, St. John's wort; ↑ effects OF benzodiazepines, phenytoin, TCAs, warfarin, EtOH; ↑ risk of serotonin synd W/ MAOIs **Labs:** ↓ LFTs, triglycerides, ↓ uric acid **NIPE:** ⊘ D/C abruptly; take w/o regard to food; may trigger manic or hypomanic condition in susceptible pts

Sevelamer Carbonate (Renvela) [Phosphate Binder] Uses: *Control ↑ PO₄³⁻ in ESRD* **Action:** Phosphate binder **Dose:** *Initial:* PO₄³⁻ > 5.5 & < 7.5 mg/dL: 800 mg PO; ≥ 7.5 mg/dL: 1600 mg PO tid *Switching from sevelamer HCl:* g/g basis; titrate ↑/↓ 1 tab/meal 2-wk intervals PRN; take w/ food **Caution:** [C, ?] w/ swallow disorders, bowel problems, may ↓ absorption of vits D, E, K **CI:** ↓ PO₄, bowel obst **Disp:** Tab 800 mg **SE:** N/V/D, dyspepsia, Abd pain, flatulence, constipation **Interactions:** ↓ Effects OF ciprofloxacin. Monitor narrow therapeutic index drugs esp antiarrhythmics & antiepileptics **Labs:** Monitor serum bicarbonate, chloride levels **NIPE:** Separate other meds (esp narrow therapeutic index drugs) 1 h before or 3 h after sevelamer carbonate

Sevelamer HCl (Renagel) [Phosphate Binder] Uses: *↓ PO₄³⁻ in ESRD* **Action:** Binds intestinal PO₄³⁻ **Dose:** 2–4 caps PO tid w/ meals; adjust based on PO₄³⁻; max 4 g/dose **Caution:** [C, ?] May ↓ absorption of vits D, E, K, ↓ ciprofloxacin & other meds levels **CI:** ↓ PO₄³⁻, bowel obst **Disp:** Tab 400, 800 mg **SE:** BP changes, N/V/D, dyspepsia, thrombosis **Interactions:** ↓ Effects OF antiarrhythmics, anticonvulsants, ciprofloxacin when given W/ sevelamer **Labs:** ↑ Alk phos **NIPE:** Must be administer w/ meals; take daily multivit, may ↓ fat-soluble vit absorption; take 1 h before or 3 h after other meds; do not open or chew caps; 800 mg sevelamer = 667 mg Ca acetate

Sildenafil (Viagra, Revatio) [Vasodilator/PDE5 Inhibitor] **Uses:** *Viagra:* *ED*; *Revatio:* *Pulm artery HTN* **Action:** ↓ PDE5 (responsible for cyclic guanosine monophosphate [cGMP] breakdown); ↑ cGMP activity to relax smooth muscles & ↑ flow to corpus cavernosum & pulm vasculature; ↑ antiproliferative on pulm artery smooth muscle **Dose:** *ED:* 25–100 mg PO 1 h before sexual activity, max 1/d; ↓ if > 65 y; avoid fatty foods w/ dose; *Revatio:* Pulm HTN: 20 mg PO tid **Caution:** [B, ?] w/ CYP3A4 Inhibs (Table10), ↓ dose w/ ritonavir; retinitis pigmentosa; hepatic/severe renal impair; w/ sig hypo-/hypertension **CI:** w/ Nitrates or if sex not advised **Disp:** Tabs *Viagra* 25, 50, 100 mg, tabs *Revatio* 20 mg **SE:** HA; flushing; dizziness; blue haze visual change, hearing loss, priapism **Interactions:** ↑ Effects W/ amlodipine, cimetidine, erythromycin, indinavir, itraconazole, ketoconazole, nelfinavir, protease Inhibs, ritonavir, saquinavir, grapefruit juice; ↑ risk of hypotension W/ amlodipine, antihypertensives, nitrates; ↓ effects W/ rifampin **NIPE:** High-fat food delays absorption; ↑ risk of cardiac arrest if used w/ nitrates; cardiac events in absence of nitrates debatable; transient global amnesia reports; do not use nitrogen w/in 24 h of this drug

Silodosin (Rapaflo) [Selective Alpha-1 Adrenergic Receptor Antagonist] **Uses:** *BPH* **Action:** Antagonist of prostatic α_1-receptors (mostly α_{1a}) **Dose:** 8 mg/d; 4 mg/d w/ CrCl 30–50 mL/min; take w/ food **Caution:** [B, ?] Not for use in females; do not use w/ other α-blockers or w/ cyclosporine; R/O PCa before use; IFIS possible w/ cataract surgery; avoid **CI:** Severe hepatic/renal impair (CrCl < 30 mL/min), w/ CYP3A4 Inhibs (eg, ketoconazole, clarithromycin, itraconazole, ritonavir) **Disp:** Caps 4, 8 mg **SE:** Retrograde ejaculation, dizziness, D, syncope, somnolence, orthostatic ↓ BP, nasopharyngitis, nasal congestion **Interactions:** ↑ Risk of hepatic/renal impair W/ CYP3A4 Inhibs (eg, ketoconazole, clarithromycin, itraconazole, ritonavir) **NIPE:** Not for use as antihypertensive; no effect on QT interval

Silver Nitrate (Dey-Drop, Others) [Antiseptic/Astringent] **Uses:** *Removal of granulation tissue & warts; prophylaxis in burns* **Action:** Topical antiseptic & astringent **Dose:** *Adults & Peds.* Apply to moist surface 2–3 × /wk for several wk or until effect **Caution:** [C, ?] **CI:** Do not use on broken skin **Disp:** Topical impregnated applicator sticks, soln 0.5%, 10%, 25%, 50%; ophthal 1% amp; topical ointment 10% **SE:** May stain tissue black, usually resolves; local irritation, methemoglobinemia **NIPE:** D/C if redness or irritation develops; no longer used in US for newborn prevention of gonococcus conjunctivitis

Silver Sulfadiazine (Silvadene, Others) [Antibiotic] **Uses:** *Prevention & Rx of Infxn in 2nd- & 3rd-degree burns* **Action:** Bactericidal **Dose:** *Adults & Peds.* Aseptically cover the area w/ 1/16-in coating bid **Caution:** [B unless near term, ?/−] **CI:** Infants < 2 mo, PRG near term **Disp:** Cream 1% **SE:** Itching, rash, skin discoloration, blood dyscrasias, hep, allergy **Interactions:** May inactivate topical proteolytic enzymes **Labs:** ↓ WBCs; monitor LFTs, BUN, Cr **NIPE:** Photosensitivity—use sunscreen; systemic absorption w/ extensive application

Simethicone (Mylicon, Others) [OTC] [Antiflatulent] Uses: Flatulence **Action:** Defoaming, alters gas bubble surface tension action **Dose: *Adults & Peds > 12 y.*** 40–125 mg PO pc & hs PRN; 500 mg/d max ***Peds < 2 y.*** 20 mg PO qid PRN ***2–12 y.*** 40 mg PO qid PRN **Caution:** [C, ?] **CI:** GI perforation or obst **Disp:** [OTC] Tabs 80, 125 mg; caps 125 mg; softgels 125, 166, 180 mg; susp 40 mg/0.6 mL; chew tabs 80, 125 mg **SE:** N/D **Interactions:** ↑ Effects *OF* topical proteolytic enzymes **NIPE:** Available in combo products OTC

Simvastatin (Zocor) [Antilipemic/HMG-CoA Reductase Inhibitor] Uses: ↓ Cholesterol **Action:** HMG-CoA reductase Inhib **Dose: *Adults.*** 5–80 mg PO; w/ meals; ↓ in renal Insuff ***Peds 10–17 y.*** 10 mg, 40 mg/d max **Caution:** [X, −] Avoid concurrent use of gemfibrozil **CI:** PRG, liver Dz **Disp:** Tabs 5, 10, 20, 40, 80 mg **SE:** HA, GI upset, myalgia, myopathy (muscle pain, tenderness or weakness w/ CK 10× ULN), hep **Interactions:** ↑ Effects *OF* digoxin, warfarin; ↑ risk of myopathy/rhabdomyolysis *W/* amiodarone, cyclosporine, CYP3A4 Inhibs, fibrates, HIV protease Inhibs, macrolides, niacin, verapamil, grapefruit juice; ↓ effects *W/* cholestyramine, colestipol, fluvastatin, isradipine, propranolol **Labs:** ↑ LFTs, monitor **NIPE:** Take w/ food & in the evening; ⊘ PRG, breastfeeding; combo w/ ezetimibe/simvastatin; pt to report muscle pain

Sipuleucel-T (Provenge) [Autologous cellular Immunotherapy] Uses: * Asymptomatic/minimally symptomatic metastatic castrate resistant PCa* **Action:** Autologous (pt specific) cellular immunotherapy **Dose:** 3 IV doses q2 wk; premedicate w/ APAP & diphenhydramine **Caution:** [N/A, N/A] Confirm identity/ expiry date before Inf; acute transfusion Rxn possible; not tested for transmissible Dz **CI:** None **Disp:** 50 MU autologous CD54 + cells activated w/ PAP GM-CSF, in 250 mL LR **SE:** Chills, fatigue, fever, back pain, N, Jt ache, HA **Interactions:** ↓ Effects *W/* concomitant chemotherapy or immunosuppressive therapy **NIPE:** Pt must undergo leukophoresis, w/ shipping & autologous cell processing at manufacturing facility before each Inf

Sirolimus [Rapamycin] (Rapamune) [Immunosuppressant] **WARNING:** Use only by healthcare providers experienced in immunosuppression; immunosuppression associated w/ lymphoma, ↑ Infxn risk; do not use in lung transplant (fatal bronchial anastomotic dehiscence) Uses: *Prevent organ rejection in new Tx pts* **Action:** ↓ T-lymphocyte activation **Dose: *Adults > 40 kg.*** 6 mg PO on d 1, then 2 mg/d PO ***Peds < 40 kg & > 13 y.*** 3 mg/m² load, then 1 mg/m²/d (in H₂O/ OJ; no grapefruit juice w/ sirolimus); take 4 h after cyclosporine; ↓ in hepatic impair **Caution:** [C, ?/−] Grapefruit juice, ketoconazole **CI:** Component allergy **Disp:** Soln 1 mg/mL, tabs 1, 2 mg **SE:** HTN, edema, CP, fever, HA, insomnia, acne, rash, GI upset, Infxns, blood dyscrasias, arthralgia, tachycardia, renal impair, hepatic artery thrombosis, graft loss & death in de novo liver transplant (↑ hepatic artery thrombosis), delayed wound healing Notes: Levels: *Trough:* 4–20 ng/mL; can vary based on assay & use of other immunosuppression agents **Interactions:** ↑ Effects *W/* azole antifungals, cimetidine, cyclosporine, diltiazem, macrolides, nicardipine, protease Inhibs, verapamil, grapefruit juice; ↓ effects *W/* carbamazepine, phenobarbital, phenytoin, rifabutin, rifapentine, rifampin; ↓ effects *OF* live virus vaccines **Labs:** ↑ LFTs, BUN, Cr, cholesterol, triglycerides; ↑/↓ K+, **NIPE:** Take w/o regard to food; ⊘ PRG while taking drug & for 12 wk after drug D/C

Sitagliptin (Januvia) [Hypoglycemic/DPP-4 Inhibitor] Uses: *Monotherapy or combo for Type 2 DM* **Action:** Dipeptidyl peptidase-4 (DDP-4) Inhib, ↑ insulin synth/release **Dose:** Renal impair: CrCl ≥ 30–50 mL/min: 50 mg once daily; CrCl < 30 mL/min or on dialysis: 25mg once daily **Caution:** [B, ?] Use w/ sulfonylurea may ↑ hypoglycemic risk **CI:** DKA, type 1 DM **Disp:** Tabs 25, 50, 100 mg **SE:** URI, HA, D, Abd pain, arthralgia, severe pancreatitis **Interactions:** ↑ Risk of hypoglycemia *W/* sulfonylureas **Labs:** Monitor LFTs, BUN/Cr **NIPE:** ⊘ Children < 18 y; monitor renal Fxn before starting therapy; start drug at low dose & periodically ↑; monitor for severe pancreatitis; no evidence for ↑ CV risk

Sitagliptin/Metformin (Janumet) [Hypoglycemic/DPP-4 Inhibitor/Biguanide] **WARNING:** Associated w/ lactic acidosis Uses: *Adjunct to diet & exercise in type 2 DM* **Action:** See individual agents **Dose:** 1 tab PO bid, titrate; 100 mg sitagliptin & 2000 mg metformin/d max; take w/ meals **Caution:** [B, ?/–] **CI:** Type 1 DM, DKA, male SCr > 1.5 mg/dL; female SCr > 1.4 mg/dL **Disp:** Tabs (mg/mg) 50/500, 50/1000 **SE:** Nasopharyngitis, N/V/D, flatulence, Abd discomfort, dyspepsia, asthenia, HA, severe pancreatitis (monitor closely) **Interactions:** ↑ Effects *W/* amiloride, cimetidine, digoxin, furosemide, MAOIs, morphine, procainamide, quinidine, quinine, ranitidine, triamterene, TMP, vancomycin; ↓ effects *W/* corticosteroids, CCBs, diuretics, estrogens, INH, OCPs, phenothiazine, phenytoin, sympathomimetics, thyroid drugs, tobacco; monitor digoxin levels **Labs:** Monitor LFTs, BUN/Cr, CBC **NIPE:** ⊘ Children < 18 y; monitor renal Fxn; start drug at low dose & periodically ↑; hold w/ contrast study; monitor for severe pancreatitis; BB may mask hypoglycemia

Smallpox Vaccine (Dryvax) [Vaccine] **WARNING:** Acute myocarditis & other infectious complications possible **CI** in immunocompromised, eczema or exfoliative skin conditions, infants < 1 y Uses: Immunization against smallpox (variola virus) **Action:** Active immunization w/ live attenuated cowpox (vaccinia) virus **Dose:** *Adults (routine nonemergency) or all ages (emergency).* 2–3 Punctures w/ bifurcated needle dipped in vaccine into deltoid, posterior triceps muscle trace blood should be seen, if not 3 more needle insertions; ✓ site for Rxn in 6–8 d; if major Rxn, site scabs, & heals, leaving scar; if mild/equivocal Rxn, repeat w/ 15 punctures **Caution:** [X, N/A] **CI:** *Nonemergency use:* In febrile illness, immunosuppression, h/o eczema & their household contacts *Emergency:* No absolute CI, if nonemergent, CI include PRG, eczema or other exfoliative skin Dz, severe immunosuppression **Disp:** Vial for reconstitution: 100 mill pock-forming units/mL **SE:** Inj site edema, erythema, pain, pruritus; erythema/rash, fatigue, fever, malaise, arthralgias/myalgias, N/D, lymphadenopathy, encephalopathy, rashes, spread of inoculation to other sites (including eye); SLS, eczema vaccinatum w/ severe disability **NIPE:** Virus transmission possible until scab separates from skin (14–21 d); avoid infant contact or household contacts w/ PRG for 14 d; avoid PRG w/in 4 wk; intradermal use only; restricted distribution

Sodium Bicarbonate [NaHCO₃] [Antacid/Alkalinizing Agent]

Uses: *Alkalinization of urine*, RTA, *metabolic acidosis, ↑ K+, TCA OD* **Action:** Alkalinizing agent **Dose:** *Adults. ECC 2010:* Cardiac arrest w/ good ventilation, hyperkalemia, OD of TCAs, ASA, cocaine, diphenhydramine: 1 mEq/kg IV bolus; repeat 1/2 dose q10min PRN. If rapidly available, use ABG to guide therapy (ABG results unreliable in cardiac arrest) *Metabolic acidosis:* 2–5 mEq/kg IV over 8 h & PRN based on acid–base status. *Hyperkalemia:* 1 mg/kg IV over 5 min *Alkalinize urine:* 4 g (48 mEq) PO, then 1–2 g q4h; adjust based on urine pH; 2 amp (100 mEq/1 L D₅W at 100–250 mL/h) IV, monitor urine pH & serum bicarbonate *CRF:* 1–3 mEq/kg/d *Distal RTA:* 1 mEq/kg/d PO **Peds.** NaHCO₃ *ECC 2010:* Severe metabolic acidosis, hyperkalemia: 1 mEq/kg slow bolus; 4.2% conc in infants < 1 mo **Sodium channel blocker OD:** 1–2 mEq/kg IV/IO bolus until pH > 7.45 (7.50–7.55 severe OD), then Inf 150 mEq NaHCO₃/L soln to maint alkalosis *CRF:* See Adult dosage *Distal RTA:* 2–3 mEq/kg/d PO *Proximal RTA:* 5–10 mEq/kg/d; titrate based on serum bicarbonate *Urine alkalinization:* 84–840 mg/kg/d (1–10 mEq/kg/d) in ÷ doses; adjust based on urine pH **Caution:** [C, ?] **CI:** Alkalosis, ↑ Na+, severe pulm edema, ↓ Ca²+ **Disp:** Powder, tabs; 300 mg = 3.6 mEq; 325 mg = 3.8 mEq; 520 mg = 6.3 mEq; 600 mg = 7.3 mEq; 650 mg = 7.6 mEq; Inj 1 mEq/1 mL, 4.2% (5 mEq/10 mL), 7.5% (8.92 mEq/mL), 8.4% (10 mEq/10 mL) vial or amp **SE:** Belching, edema, flatulence, metabolic alkalosis **Interactions:** ↑ Effects *OF* anorexiants, amphetamines, ephedrine, flecainide, mecamylamine, pseudoephedrine, quinidine, sympathomimetics; ↓ effects *OF* Li, MTX, salicylates, tetracyclines **Labs:** ↑ K+, Na+, lactate **NIPE:** 1 g Neutralizes 12 mEq of acid; 50 mEq bicarbonate = 50 mEq Na; can make 3 amps in 1 L D₅W to = D₅NS w/ 150 mEq bicarbonate; ⊘ Take w/in 2 h of other drugs; ↑ risk of milk-alkali synd w/ long-term use or when taken w/ milk

Sodium Citrate/Citric Acid (Bicitra, Oracit) [Alkalinizing Agent]

Uses: *Chronic metabolic acidosis, alkalinize urine; dissolve uric acid & cysteine stones* **Action:** Urinary alkalinizer **Dose:** *Adults.* 10–30 mL in 1–3 oz H₂O pc & hs **Peds.** 5–15 mL in 1–3 oz H₂O pc & hs; best after meals **Caution:** [C, +] **CI:** Al-based antacids; severe renal impair or Na-restricted diets **Disp:** 15- or 30-mL units **Dose:** 16 (473 mL) or 4 (118 mL) fl oz **SE:** Tetany, metabolic alkalosis, GI upset; avoid use of multiple 50-mL amps; can cause ↑ Na+/hyperosmolality **Interactions:** ↑ Effects *OF* amphetamines, ephedrine, flecainide, pseudoephedrine, quinidine; ↓

effects *OF* barbiturates, chlorpropamide, Li, salicylates **Labs:** ↑ K$^+$, monitor ECG for hyperkalemia (peaked T waves) **NIPE:** 1 mL = 1 mEq Na & 1 mEq bicarbonate; dilute w/ H$_2$O

Sodium Oxybate (Xyrem) [C-III] [Inhibitory Neurotransmitter]
WARNING: Known drug of abuse even at recommended doses; confusion, depression, resp depression may occur **Uses:** *Narcolepsy-associated cataplexy* **Action:** Inhibitory neurotransmitter **Dose:** *Adults & Peds > 16 y.* 2.25 g PO qhs, 2nd dose 2.5–4 h later; may ↑ 9 g/d max **Caution:** [B, ?/–] **CI:** Succinic semialdehyde dehydrogenase deficiency; potentiates EtOH **Disp:** 500-mg/mL (180-mL) PO soln **SE:** Confusion, depression, ↓ diminished level of consciousness, incontinence, sig V, resp depression, psychological Sxs **Interactions:** ↑ Risk of CNS depression *W/* sedatives, hypnotics, EtOH **NIPE:** Dilute w/ 2 oz H$_2$O, ⊘ eat before 2 h of taking this drug; may lead to dependence; synonym for hydroxybutyrate (GHB), abused as a "date rape drug"; controlled distribution (prescriber & pt registration); must be administered when pt in bed

Sodium Phosphate (Visicol) [Laxative] **Uses:** *Bowel prep prior to colonoscopy*, short-term constipation **Action:** Hyperosmotic laxative **Dose:** 3 tabs PO w/ at least 8 oz clear Liq q15 min (20 tabs total night before procedure); 3–5 h before colonoscopy, repeat) **Caution:** [C, ?] Renal impair, lytes disturbances **CI:** Megacolon, bowel obst, CHF, ascites, unstable angina, gastric retention, bowel perforation, colitis, hypomotility **Disp:** Tabs 0.398, 1.102 g **SE:** D, flatulence, cramps, Abd bloating/pain **Interactions:** May bind w/ Al- & Mg-containing antacids & sucralfate; ↑ risk of hypoglycemia *W/* bisphosphonates; ↓ absorption *OF* other meds **Labs:** Monitor lytes—↑ PO^3, ↓ K$^+$, Na; ↑ QT—monitor ECG **NIPE:** Drink clear Liq 12 h before start of this med; ⊘ take w/ drugs that prolong QT interval, ⊘ take other laxatives

Sodium Polystyrene Sulfonate (Kayexalate) [Potassium Removing Resin] **Uses:** *Rx of ↑ K* **Action:** Na$^+$/K$^+$ ion-exchange resin **Dose:** *Adults.* 15–60 g PO or 30–60 g PR q6h based on serum K$^+$ *Peds.* 1 g/kg/ dose PO or PR q6h based on serum K$^+$ (given w/ agent, eg, sorbitol, to promote movement through the bowel) **Caution:** [C, M] **CI:** ↑ Na$^+$ **Disp:** Powder; susp 15 g/60 mL sorbitol **SE:** Na retention, GI upset, fecal impaction **Interactions:** ↑ Risk of systemic alkalosis *W/* Ca- or Mg-containing antacids **Labs:** ↑ Na$^+$, ↓ K$^+$ **NIPE:** Mix w/ chilled fluid other than OJ; enema acts more quickly than PO; PO most effective; onset of action > 2 h; monitor ECG for hypokalemia (flattened T waves)

Solifenacin (Vesicare) [Antispasmodic/Muscarinic Receptor Antagonist] **Uses:** *OAB* **Action:** Antimuscarinic, ↓ detrusor contractions **Dose:** 5 mg PO daily, 10 mg/d max; ↓ w/ renal/hepatic impair **Caution:** [C, ?/–] BOO or GI obst, UC, MyG, renal/hepatic impair, QT prolongation risk **CI:** NAG, urinary/gastric retention **Disp:** Tabs 5, 10 mg **SE:** Constipation, xerostomia, dyspepsia, blurred vision, drowsiness **Interactions:** ↑ Effects *OF* azole antifungals & other CYP3A4 Inhibs; ↑ risk of prolonged QT interval *W/* amiodarone, amitriptyline, bepridil, disopyramide, erythromycin, gatifloxacin, haloperidol, imipramine, moxifloxacin, quinidine, pimozide, procainamide, sparfloxacin, thioridazine; other drugs that prolong QT **Labs:** Monitor BUN, CR, LFTs **NIPE:** Take w/ or w/o food, swallow whole w/ H$_2$O; do not ↑ dose w/ severe renal/mod hepatic impair; recent concern over cytogenic effects; monitor ECG for ↑ QT interval

Somatropin (Serostim) [Growth Hormone] **Uses:** *HIV-associated wasting/cachexia* **Action:** Anabolic peptide hormone **Dose:** 0.1 mg/kg SQ hs **Caution:** [B; ?] **CI:** Active neoplasm; acute critical illness post-op; benzyl alcohol sensitivity; hypersensitivity **Disp:** Powder for Inj **SE:** Arthralgia, edema, pancreatitis **Labs:** ↑ blood glucose **NIPE:** Use under guidance of healthcare provider trained in AIDs management

Sorafenib (Nexavar) [Antineoplastic/Kinase Inhibitor] **Uses:** *Advanced RCC* metastatic liver CA **Action:** Kinase Inhib **Dose:** **Adults.** 400 mg PO bid on empty stomach **Caution:** [D, –] w/ Irinotecan, doxorubicin, warfarin; avoid conception (male/female) **Disp:** Tabs 200 mg **SE:** Hand–foot synd; Tx-emergent hypertension; bleeding, ↑ INR, cardiac infarction/ischemia; ↑ pancreatic enzymes, hypophosphatemia, lymphopenia, anemia, fatigue, alopecia, pruritus, D, GI upset, HA, neuropathy **Interactions:** ↑ Effects *OF* warfarin **NIPE:** Monitor BP 1st 6 wk; may require ↓ dose (daily or qod); impaired metabolism in pt of Asian descent; unknown effect on wound healing, D/C before major surgery

Sorbitol (Generic) [Laxative] **Uses:** *Constipation* **Action:** Laxative **Dose:** 30–60 mL PO of a 20–70% soln PRN **Caution:** [B, +] **CI:** Anuria **Disp:** Liq 70% **SE:** Edema, lytes loss, lactic acidosis, GI upset, xerostomia **NIPE:** ⊘ Use unless soln clear; may be vehicle for many Liq formulations (eg, zinc, Kayexalate)

Sotalol (Betapace) [Antiarrhythmic, Antihypertensive/Beta-Blocker] **WARNING:** To minimize risk of induced arrhythmia, pts initiated/reinitiated on Betapace AF should be placed for a minimum of 3 d (on their maint) in a facility that can provide cardiac resuscitation, cont ECG monitoring, & calculations of CrCl. Betapace should not be substituted for Betapace AF because of labeling **Uses:** *Ventricular arrhythmias, AF* **Action:** β-Adrenergic blocker **Dose:** **Adults.** *CrCl > 60 mL/min:* 80 mg PO bid, may ↑ to 240–320 mg/d *CrCl 30–60 mL/min:* 80 mg q24h *CrCl 10–30 mL/min:* Dose q36–48h 80 mg PO bid *ECC 2010:* SVT & ventricular arrhythmias: 1–1.5 mg/kg IV over 5 min *Peds.* **Neonates.** 9 mg/m^2 tid *1–19 mo.* 20.4 mg/m^2 tid *20–23 mo.* 29.1 mg/m^2 tid = *2 y.* 30 mg/m^2 tid; to max dose of 90 mg/m^2 tid; ↓ w/ renal impair **Caution:** [B (1st tri) (D if 2nd or 3rd tri), +] **CI:** Asthma, COPD, bradycardia, ↑ prolonged QT interval, 2nd-/3rd-degree heart block w/o pacemaker, cardiogenic shock, uncontrolled CHF **Disp:** Tabs 80, 120, 160, 240 mg **SE:** Bradycardia, CP, palpitations, fatigue, dizziness, weakness, dyspnea **Interactions:** ↑ Effects *W/* ASA, antihypertensives, nitrates, OCPs, fluoxetine, prazosin, sulfinpyrazone, verapamil, EtOH; ↑ risk of prolonged QT interval *W/* amiodarone, amitriptyline, bepridil, disopyramide, erythromycin, gatifloxacin, haloperidol, imipramine, moxifloxacin, quinidine, pimozide, procainamide, sparfloxacin, thioridazine; ↑ effects *OF* lidocaine; ↓ effects *W/* antacids, clonidine, NSAIDs, thyroid drugs; ↓ effects *OF* hypoglycemics, terbutaline, theophylline **Labs:** ↑ BUN, serum glucose, triglycerides, K+, uric acid **NIPE:** May ↑ sensitivity to cold; D/C MAOIs 14 d before drug; take w/o food; Betapace should not be substituted for Betapace AF because of differences in labeling

Sotalol (Betapace AF) [Antiarrhythmic, Antihypertensive/Beta-Blocker] WARNING: See Sotalol (Betapace)

Uses: *Maint sinus rhythm for symptomatic AF/flutter* **Action:** β-Adrenergic blocker **Dose: Adults.** *CrCl > 60 mL/min:* 80 mg PO q12h *CrCl 40–60 mL/min:* 80 mg PO q24h; ↑ to 120 mg during hospitalization; monitor QT interval 2–4 h after each dose, dose reduction or D/C if QT interval = 500 ms. **Peds. Neonates.** 9 mg/m² tid *1–19 mo.* 20 mg/m² tid *20–23 mo.* 29.1 mg/m² tid = *2 y.* 30 mg/m² tid; can double all doses as max daily dose; allow 36 h between changes **Caution:** [B (1st tri, D if 2nd or 3rd tri), +] If converting from previous antiarrhythmic **CI:** Asthma, bradycardia, ↑ QT interval, 2nd-/3rd-degree heart block w/o pacemaker, cardiogenic shock, uncontrolled CHF, CrCl < 40 mL/min **Disp:** Tabs 80, 120, 160 mg **SE:** Bradycardia, CP, palpitations, fatigue, dizziness, weakness, dyspnea **Interactions:** ↑ Risk of prolonged QT interval *W/* amiodarone, amitriptyline, bepridil, disopyramide, erythromycin, gatifloxacin, haloperidol, imipramine, moxifloxacin, quinidine, pimozide, procainamide, sparfloxacin, TCAs, thioridazine; ↑ effects *W/* general anesthesia, phenytoin administered *W/* verapamil ↑ effects *OF* insulin, oral hypoglycemics; ↑ risk of hypotension *W/* antihypertensives, ASA, bismuth subsalicylate, Mg salicylate, sulfinpyrazone, nitrates, OCPs, EtOH; ↑ CV Rxns CCB, digoxin; ↑ risk *OF* severe HTN if used w/in 14 d of MAOIs; ↓ effects *W/* antacids; ↑ effects *OF* β-adrenergic bronchodilators, DA, dobutamine, theophylline **Labs:** ↑ ANA titers, BUN, K+, serum glucose, LFTs, triglycerides, uric acid; monitor QT interval; follow renal Fxn **NIPE:** ⊘ D/C abruptly after long-term use; take w/o food; administer antacids 2 h < or > sotalol; Betapace should not be substituted for Betapace AF because of differences in labeling

Spinosad [Natroba] [Pediculicide]

Uses: *Head lice* **Action:** Neuronal excitation of lice, w/ paralysis & death **Dose:** Cover dry scalp w/ susp, then apply to dry hair; rinse off in 10 min **Caution:** [B; ?/–] **CI:** < 6 mo old **Disp:** 0.9% Topical susp **SE:** Scalp/ocular erythema **NIPE:** Shake well before use; use w/ overall lice management program; in benzyl alcohol, serious Rxns in neonates, in breast milk, pump, & discard milk for 8 h after use; wash hands after application

Spironolactone (Aldactone) [Potassium-Sparing Diuretic] WARNING: Tumorogenic in animal studies; avoid unnecessary use

Uses: *Hyperaldosteronism, HTN, ascites from cirrhosis* **Action:** Aldosterone antagonist; K+-sparing diuretic **Dose: Adults.** *CHF (NYHA Class III–IV)* 12.5–25 mg/d (w/ ACE & loop diuretic); *HTN* 25–50 mg/d *Ascites:* 100–400 mg qAM w/ 40–(IV) 12.5–25 mg/d (w/ ACE & loop diuretic); wait at least 3 d before ↑ dose **Peds.** 1–3.3 mg/kg/24 h PO ÷ bid–qid **Neonates.** 0.5–1 mg/kg/dose q8h; take w/ food **Caution:** [D, +] **CI:**

↑ K+, ARF, anuria **Disp:** Tabs 25, 50, 100 mg **SE:** ↑ K+ & gynecomastia, arrhythmia, sexual dysfunction, confusion, dizziness, D/N/V, abnormal menstruation **Interactions:** ↑ Risk of hyperkalemia *W/* ACEIs, K+ supls, K+-sparing diuretics, ↑ K+ diet; ↑ effects *OF* Li; ↓ effects *W/* salicylates; ↓ effects *OF* anticoagulants **Labs:** ↑ K+ **BUN NIPE:** Take w/ food; ↑ risk of gynecomastia; max effects of drug may take 2–3 wk; monitor ECG for hyperkalemia (peaked T waves)

Starch, Topical, Rectal (Tucks Suppositories [OTC]) [Protectant]
Uses: *Temporary relief of anorectal disorders (itching, etc)* **Action:** Topical protectant **Dose:** *Adults & Peds ≥ 12 y.* Cleanse, rinse, & dry, insert 1 supp rectally 6 × /d × 7 d max **Caution:** [?, ?] **CI:** None **Disp:** Supp **NIPE:** D/C w/ or if rectal bleeding occurs or if condition worsens or does not improve w/n 7 d

Stavudine (Zerit) [Antiretroviral/Reverse Transcriptase Inhibitor]
WARNING: Lactic acidosis & severe hepatomegaly w/ steatosis & pancreatitis reported **Uses:** *HIV in combo w/ other antiretrovirals* **Action:** RT Inhib **Dose:** *Adults* > 60 kg. 40 mg bid < 60 kg. 30 mg bid *Peds Birth–13 d.* 0.5 mg/kg q12h > 14 d & < 30 kg. 1 mg/kg q12h ≥ 30 kg. Adult dose; ↓ w/ renal Insuff **Caution:** [C, +] **CI:** Allergy **Disp:** Caps 15, 20, 30, 40 mg; soln 1 mg/mL **SE:** Peripheral neuropathy, HA, chills, fever, malaise, rash, GI upset, anemias, lactic acidosis, ↑ LFTs, pancreatitis **Interactions:** ↑ Risk of pancreatitis w/ didanosine; ↑ effects *W/* probenecid; ↓ effects *W/* zidovudine **Labs:** ↑ LFTs **NIPE:** Take w/o regard to food; take w/ plenty of H2O; monitor for S/Sxs of lactic acidosis (tachypnea, altered breathing, lethargy); may cause peripheral neuropathy (numbness, tingling in extremities)

Steroids, Systemic [Glucocorticoid] (See Also Table 2) The following relates only to the commonly used systemic glucocorticoids
Uses: *Endocrine disorders* (adrenal Insuff), *rheumatoid disorders*, collagenvascular Dzs, derm Dzs, allergic states, cerebral edema*, nephritis, nephrotic synd, immunosuppression for transplantation, ↑ Ca2+, malignancies (breast, lymphomas), pre-op (in any pt who has been on steroids in the previous year, known hypoadrenalism, pre-op for adrenalectomy); Inj into Jts/tissue **Action:** Glucocorticoid **Dose:** Varies w/ use & institutional protocols: *Adrenal Insuff, acute: Adults.* Hydrocortisone: 100 mg IV, then 300 mg/d ÷ q6h; convert to 50 mg PO q8h × 6 doses, taper to 30–50 mg/d ÷ bid *Peds.* Hydrocortisone: 1–2 mg/kg IV, then 150–250 mg/d ÷ tid

- *Adrenal Insuff, chronic (physiologic replacement):* May need mineralocorticoid supl such as Florinef *Adults.* Hydrocortisone 20 mg PO qAM, 10 mg PO qPM; *cortisone* 0.5–0.75 mg/kg/d ÷ bid; *cortisone* 0.25–0.35 mg/kg/d IM; *dexamethasone* 0.03–0.15 mg/kg/d or 0.6–0.75 mg/m2/d ÷ q6–12h PO, IM, IV *Peds.* Hydrocortisone 0.5–0.75 mg/kg/d PO tid; *hydrocortisone succinate* 0.25–0.35 mg/kg/d IM

- *Asthma, acute: Adults.* Methylprednisolone: 60 mg PO/IV q6h or *dexamethasone* 12 mg IV q6h *Peds.* Prednisolone 1–2 mg/kg/d or *prednisone* 1–2 mg/kg/d ÷

daily–bid for up to 5 d; *methylprednisolone* 2–4 mg/kg/d IV ÷ tid; *dexamethasone* 0.1–0.3 mg/kg/d ÷ q6h

- *Congenital adrenal hyperplasia:* **Peds.** Initial *hydrocortisone* 30–36 mg/m²/d PO ÷ 1/3 dose qAM, 2/3 dose qPM; maint 20–25 mg/m²/d ÷ bid
- *Extubation/airway edema:* **Adults.** *Dexamethasone* 0.5–1 mg/kg/d IM/IV ÷ q6h (start 24 h prior to extubation; continue × 4 more doses) **Peds.** *Dexamethasone* 0.1–0.3 mg/kg/d ÷ q6h × 3–5 d (start 48–72 h before extubation)
- *Immunosuppressive/anti-inflammatory:* **Adults & Older Peds.** *Hydrocortisone* 15–240 mg PO, IM, IV q12h; *methylprednisolone* 4–48 mg/d PO, taper to lowest effective dose; *methylprednisolone Na succinate* 10–80 mg/d IM **Adults.** *Prednisone* or *prednisolone* 5–60 mg/d PO ÷ daily–qid **Infants & Younger Children.** *Hydrocortisone* 2.5–10 mg/kg/d PO ÷ q6–8h; 1–5 mg/kg/d IM/IV ÷ bid
- *Nephrotic synd:* **Peds.** *Prednisolone* or *prednisone:* 2 mg/kg/d PO tid–qid until urine is protein-free for 5 d, use up to 28 d; for persistent proteinuria, 4 mg/kg/dose PO qod max 120 mg/d for an additional 28 d; maint 2 mg/kg/dose qod for 28 d; taper over 4–6 wk (max 80 mg/d)
- *Septic shock (controversial):* **Adults.** *Hydrocortisone* 500 mg–1 g IM/IV q2–6h **Peds.** *Hydrocortisone* 50 mg/kg IM/IV, repeat q4–24 h PRN
- *Status asthmaticus:* **Adults & Peds.** *Hydrocortisone* 1–2 mg/kg/dose IV q6h; then ↓ by 0.5–1 mg/kg q6h
- *Rheumatic Dz:* **Adults.** *Intra-articular:* *Hydrocortisone* acetate 25–37.5 mg large Jt, 10–25 mg small Jt; *methylprednisolone* acetate 20–80 mg large Jt, 4–10 mg small Jt *Intrabursal:* *Hydrocortisone* acetate 25–37.5 mg *Intraganglial:* *Hydrocortisone* acetate 25–37.5 mg *Tendon sheath:* *Hydrocortisone* acetate 5–12.5 mg
- *Perioperative steroid coverage:* *Hydrocortisone* 100 mg IV night before surgery, 1 h pre-op, intraoperative, & 4, 8, & 12 h post-op; post-op d 1 100 mg IV q6h; post-op d 2 100 mg IV q8h; post-op d 3 100 mg IV q12h; post-op d 4 50 mg IV q12h; post-op d 5 25 mg IV q12h; resume prior PO dosing if chronic use or D/C if only perioperative coverage required
- *Cerebral edema:* *Dexamethasone* 10 mg IV; then 4 mg IV q4–6h

Caution: [C, ?/–] **CI:** Active varicella Infxn, serious Infxn except TB, fungal Infxns **Disp:** Table 2 **SE:** ↑ Appetite, hyperglycemia, osteoporosis, nervousness, insomnia, "steroid psychosis," adrenal suppression **Labs:** ↓ K⁺ ↑ glucose **NIPE:** Hydrocortisone succinate for systemic, acetate for intra-articular; never abruptly D/C steroids, taper dose; also used for bacterial & TB meningitis; can ↑ Infxn risk & fx risk from osteoporosis; risk of GI perforation w/ chronic use

Steroids, Topical [Glucocorticoid] (See Also Table 3) **Uses:** *Steroid-responsive dermatoses (seborrheic/atopic dermatitis, neurodermatitis, anogenital pruritus, psoriasis)* **Action:** Glucocorticoid; ↓ capillary permeability, stabilizes lysosomes to control inflammation; controls protein synth; ↓ migration of leukocytes, fibroblasts **Dose:** Use lowest potency produce for shortest period for effect (See Table 3) **Caution:** [C, +] Do not use occlusive dressings; high potency topical products not for rosacea, perioral dermatitis; not for use on face, groin, axillae; none for use in a diapered area **CI:** Component hypersensitivity **Disp:** See Table 3 **SE:** Skin atrophy w/ chronic use; chronic administration or application over large area may cause adrenal suppression or hyperglycemia

Streptokinase (Streptase, Kabikinase) [Plasminogen Activator/ Thrombolytic Enzyme] Uses: *Coronary artery thrombosis, acute massive PE, DVT, & some occluded vascular grafts* **Action:** Activates plasminogen to plasmin that degrades fibrin **Dose:** *Adults. PE:* Load 250,000 units peripheral IV over 30 min, then 100,000 units/h IV for 24–72 h *Coronary artery thrombosis:* 1.5 MU IV over 60 min *DVT or arterial embolism:* Load as w/ PE, then 100,000 units/h for 72 h *ECC 2010:* **AMI:** 1.5 MU over 1 h **Peds.** 3500–4000 units/kg over 30 min, then 1000–1500 units/kg/h *Occluded catheter (controversial):* 10,000–25,000 units in NS to final vol of catheter (leave in for 1 h, aspirate & flush w/ NS) **Caution:** [C, +] **CI:** Streptococcal Infxn or streptokinase in last 6 mo, active bleeding, CVA, TIA, spinal surgery/trauma in last mo, vascular anomalies, severe hepatic/renal Dz, endocarditis, pericarditis, severe uncontrolled HTN **Disp:** Powder for Inj 250,000, 750,000, 1,500,000 units **SE:** Bleeding, ↓ BP, fever, bruising, rash, GI upset, hemorrhage, anaphylaxis **Interactions:** ↑ Risk of bleeding **W/** anticoagulants, ASA, heparin, indomethacin, NSAIDs, dong quai, feverfew, garlic, ginger, horse chestnut, red clover **Labs:** ↑ PT, PTT **NIPE:** If Inf inadequate to keep clotting time 2–5 × control, see package insert for adjustments; Abs remain 3–6 mo following dose; reconstitute w/ NS & roll (not shake) to mix; most effective w/ AMI w/in 4 h; most effective for PE/DVT w/in 1 d; monitor for bleeding

Streptomycin [Antibiotic/Aminoglycoside] WARNING: Neuro-/oto-/ renal tox possible; neuromuscular blockage w/ resp paralysis possible Uses: *TB combo therapy* streptococcal or enterococcal endocarditis **Action:** Aminoglycoside; ↓ protein synth **Dose:** *Adults.* Endocarditis: 1 g q12h 1–2 wk, then 500 mg q12h 1–4 wk; *TB:* 15 mg/kg/d (up to 1 g), DOT 2 ×/wk 20–30 mg/kg/dose (max 1.5 g), DOT 3 ×/wk 25–30 mg/kg/dose (max 1 g) **Peds.** 15 mg/kg/d; DOT 2 ×/wk 20–40 mg/kg/dose (max 1 g); DOT 3 ×/wk 25–30 mg/kg/dose (max 1 g); w/ renal Insuff, either IM or IV over 30–60 min **Caution:** [D, +] **CI:** PRG **Disp:** Inj 400 mg/mL (1-g vial) **SE:** ↑ Incidence of vestibular & auditory tox, ↑ neurotox risk in pts w/ impaired renal Fxn Notes: Monitor levels: *Peak:* 20–30 mcg/mL *Trough:* < 5 mcg/mL *Toxic peak:* > 50 mcg/mL *Trough:* > 10 mcg/mL IV over 30–60 min **Interactions:** ↑ Risk of nephrotox **W/** amphotericin B, cephalosporins, cisplatin, methoxyflurane, polymyxin B, vancomycin; ↑ risk of ototox **W/** carboplatin, furosemide, mannitol, urea; ↑ effects **OF** anticoagulants **Labs:** False(+) urine glucose, false ↑ urine protein **NIPE:** ↑ Fluid intake

Streptozocin (Zanosar) [Alkylating Agent/Nitrosourea] Uses: *Pancreatic islet cell tumors* & carcinoid tumors **Action:** DNA–DNA (interstrand) cross-linking; DNA, RNA, & protein synth Inhib **Dose:** Per protocol; ↓ in renal failure **Caution:** w/ renal failure [D, ?/–] **CI:** w/ rotavirus vaccine, PRG **Disp:** Inj

1 g SE: N/V/D, duodenal ulcers, depression, ↓ BM rare (20%) & mild; nephrotox (proteinuria & azotemia dose related), hypophosphatemia dose limiting; hypo-/hyperglycemia; Inj site Rxns **Interactions:** ↑ Risk of nephrotox *W/* aminoglycosides, amphotericin B, cisplatin, vancomycin; ↑ effects *OF* doxorubicin; ↓ effects *W/* phenytoin **Labs:** Monitor Cr **NIPE:** ⊘ PRG, breast-feeding; ↑ fluid intake to 2–3 L/d

Succimer (Chemet) [Chelating Agent] Uses: *Lead poisoning (levels > 45 mcg/mL)* **Action:** Heavy-metal chelating agent **Dose:** *Adults & Peds.* 10 mg/kg/dose q8h × 5 d, then 10 mg/kg/dose q12h for 14 d; ↓ in renal Insuff **Caution:** [C, ?] **CI:** Allergy **Disp:** Caps 100 mg **SE:** Rash, fever, GI upset, hemorrhoids, metallic taste, drowsiness **Labs:** ↑ LFTs; monitor lead levels **NIPE:** ⊘ Take w/ other chelating agents; ↑ fluid intake to 2–3 L/d; may open caps

Succinylcholine (Anectine, Quelicin, Sucostrin, Others) [Skeletal Muscle Relaxant] **WARNING:** Risk of cardiac arrest from hyperkalemic rhabdomyolysis Uses: *Adjunct to general anesthesia, facilitates ET intubation; induce skeletal muscle relaxation during surgery or mechanical ventilation* **Action:** Depolarizing neuromuscular blocker; rapid onset, short duration (3–5 min) **Dose:** *Adults.* Rapid sequence intubation 1–2 mg/kg IV over 10–30 s or 2–4 mg/kg IM *(ECC 2005) Peds.* 1–2 mg/kg/dose IV, then by 0.3–0.6 mg/kg/dose q5min; ↓ w/ severe renal/hepatic impair **Caution:** see Warning [C, M] **CI:** w/ Malignant hyperthermia risk, myopathy, recent major burn, multiple trauma, extensive skeletal muscle denervation, NAG, pseudocholinesterase deficiency **Disp:** Inj 20, 50, 100 mg/mL **SE:** Fasciculations, ↑ intraocular, intragastric, & ICP, salivation, myoglobinuria, malignant hyperthermia, resp depression, or prolonged apnea; multiple drugs potentiate; CV effects (arrhythmias, ↓ BP, brady-/tachycardia) **Interactions:** ↑ Effects *W/* amikacin, gentamicin, neomycin, streptomycin, Li, MAOIs, opiates; ↓ effect *W/* diazepam **Labs:** ↑ Serum K+ **NIPE:** May be given IV push/Inf/IM deltoid; hyperkalemic rhabdomyolysis in children w/ undiagnosed myopathy such as Duchenne muscular dystrophy

Sucralfate (Carafate) [Antiulcer Agent/Pepsin Inhibitor] Uses: *Duodenal ulcers*, gastric ulcers, stomatitis, GERD, preventing stress ulcers, esophagitis **Action:** Forms ulcer-adherent complex that protects against acid, pepsin, & bile acid **Dose:** *Adults.* 1 g PO qid, 1 h prior to meals & hs *Peds* 40–80 mg/kg/d ÷ q6h; continue 4–8 wk unless healing demonstrated by x-ray or endoscopy; separate from other drugs by 2 h; take on empty stomach ac **Caution:** [B, +] **CI:** Component allergy **Disp:** Tabs 1 g; susp 1 g/10 mL **SE:** Constipation, D, dizziness, xerostomia **Interactions:** ↓ Effects *OF* cimetidine, digoxin, levothyroxine, phenytoin, quinolones, quinidine, ranitidine, tetracyclines, theophylline, warfarin **NIPE:** Take w/o food; AI may accumulate in renal failure

Sulfacetamide (Bleph-10, Cetamide, Sodium Sulamyd) [Antibiotic/ Sulfonamide] Uses: *Conjunctival Infxns* **Action:** Sulfonamide antibiotic **Dose:** 10% oint apply qid & hs; soln for keratitis apply q2–3h based on severity

Caution: [C, M] **CI:** Sulfonamide sensitivity; age < 2 mo **Disp:** Oint 10%; soln 10%, 15%, 30%; topical cream 10%; foam, gel, lotion, pad all 10% **SE:** Irritation, burning; blurred vision, brow ache, SJS, photosensitivity **Interactions:** ↓ Effects *W/* tetracyclines **NIPE:** Not compatible w/ Ag-containing preps; purulent exudate inactivates drug; ↑ risk of photosensitivity—use sunblock

Sulfacetamide & Prednisolone (Blephamide, Others) [Antibiotic, Anti-Inflammatory]
Uses: *Steroid-responsive inflammatory ocular conditions w/ Infxn or a risk of Infxn* **Action:** Antibiotic & anti-inflammatory **Dose:** *Adults & Peds > 2 y.* Apply oint lower conjunctival sac daily–qid; soln 1–3 gtt 2–3 h while awake **Caution:** [C, ?/–] Sulfonamide sensitivity; age < 2 mo **Disp:** *Oint:* sulfacetamide 10%/prednisolone 0.5%, sulfacetamide 10%/prednisolone 0.2%, sulfacetamide 10%/ prednisolone 0.25% *Susp:* sulfacetamide 10%/prednisolone 0.25%, sulfacetamide 10%/ prednisolone 0.5%, sulfacetamide 10%/prednisolone 0.2% **SE:** Irritation, burning, blurred vision, brow ache, SJS, photosensitivity **Interactions:** ↑ Effects *W/* tetracyclines **NIPE:** Not compatible w/ Ag-containing preps; purulent exudate inactivates drug; ↑ risk of sensitivity to light; ⊘ D/C abruptly; OK ophthal susp use as otic agent

Sulfasalazine (Azulfidine, Azulfidine EN) [Anti-Inflammatory, Antirheumatic (DMARD)/Sulfonamide]
Uses: *UC, RA, JRA*, active Crohn Dz, ankylosing spondylitis, psoriasis **Action:** Sulfonamide; actions unclear **Dose:** *Adults.* UC: Initial, 1 g PO tid–qid; ↑ to a max of 8 g/d in 3–4 ÷ doses; maint 500 mg PO qid *RA:* (EC tab) 0.5–1 g/d, ↑ weekly to maint 2 g ÷ bid *Peds.* UC: Initial, 40–60 mg/kg/24 h PO ÷ q4–6h; maint 20–30 mg/kg/24 h PO ÷ q6h *RA > 6 y:* 30–50 mg/kg/d in 2 doses, start w/ 1/4–1/3 maint dose, ↑ weekly until dose reached at 1 mo, 2 g/d max; ↓ w/ renal Insuff **Caution:** [B (D if near term), M] **CI:** Sulfonamide or salicylate sensitivity, porphyria, GI or GU obstr; avoid in hepatic impair **Disp:** Tabs 500 mg; EC DR tabs 500 mg **SE:** GI upset; discolors urine; dizziness, HA, photosensitivity, oligospermia, anemias, Stevens–Johnson synd **Interactions:** ↑ Effects *OF* oral anticoagulants, oral hypoglycemics, MTX, phenytoin, zidovudine; ↓ effects *W/* antibiotics; ↓ effects *OF* digoxin, folic acid, Fe, procaine, proparacaine, sulfonylureas, tetracaine **Labs:** ↑ LFTs, BUN, Cr; ↓ plts, WBCs **NIPE:** Take pc; ↑ fluids to 2–3 L/d; ↑ risk of photosensitivity—use sunblock & avoid sunlight exposure; may cause yellow-orange skin/contact lens discoloration

Sulfinpyrazone (Anturane) [Uricosuric/Antigout Agent]
Uses: *Acute & chronic gout* **Action:** ↓ Renal tubular absorption of uric acid **Dose:** 100–200 mg PO bid for 1 wk, ↑ PRN to maint of 200–400 mg bid; max 800 mg/d; take w/ food or antacids, & plenty of fluids; avoid salicylates **Caution:** [C (D if near term), ?/–] **CI:** Renal impair, avoid salicylates; peptic ulcer; blood dyscrasias, near-term PRG, allergy **Disp:** Tabs 100 mg; caps 200 mg **SE:** N/V, stomach pain, urolithiasis, leucopenia **Interactions:** ↑ Effects *OF* oral anticoagulants, oral hypoglycemics, MTX; ↓ effects *W/* ASA, cholestyramine, niacin, salicylates, EtOH; ↓

effects *OF* APAP, theophylline, verapamil **Labs:** ↑ BUN, Cr; ↓ plts, WBCs **NIPE:** Take w/ food; ↑ fluids to 2–3 L/d

Sulindac (Clinoril) [Analgesic, Anti-Inflammatory, Antipyretic/NSAID]
WARNING: May ↑ risk of CV events & GI bleeding; do not use for post CABG pain control **Uses:** *Arthritis & pain* **Action:** NSAID; ↓ prostaglandins **Dose:** 150–200 mg bid, 400 mg/d max; w/ food **Caution:** [B (D if 3rd tri or near term), ?] **CI:** NSAID or ASA sensitivity, w/ ketorolac, ulcer, GI bleeding, post-op pain in CABG **Disp:** Tabs 150, 200 mg **SE:** Dizziness, rash, GI upset, pruritus, edema, ↓ renal blood flow, renal failure (? fewer renal effects than other NSAIDs), peptic ulcer, GI bleeding **Interactions:** ↑ Effects *W/* NSAIDs, probenecid; ↑ effects *OF* aminoglycosides, anticoagulants, cyclosporine, digoxin, Li, MTX, K⁺-sparing diuretics; ↑ risk of bleeding *W/* ASA, anticoagulants, NSAIDs, thrombolytics, EtOH, dong quai, feverfew, garlic, ginger, horse chestnut, red clover; ↓ effects *W/* antacids, ASA; ↓ effects *OF* antihypertensives, diuretics, hydralazine **Labs:** ↑ LFTs, BUN, Cr, K⁺ **NIPE:** Take w/ food; ↑ risk of photosensitivity—use sunblock; may take several wk for full drug effect; monitor ECG for hyperkalemia (peaked T waves)

Sumatriptan (Alsuma, Imitrex Injection, Imitrex Nasal Spray, Imitrex Oral) [Antimigraine Agent/Selective 5-HT₁ Receptor Agonist]
Uses: *Rx acute migraine & cluster HA* **Action:** Vascular serotonin receptor agonist **Dose:** *Adults.* *SQ:* 6 mg SQ as a single dose PRN; repeat PRN in 1 h to a max of 12 mg/24 h *PO:* 25 mg, repeat in 2 h, PRN, 100 mg/d max PO dose; max 300 mg/d *Nasal spray:* 1 spray into 1 nostril, repeat in 2 h to 40 mg/24 h max *Peds. Nasal spray:* 6–9 y. 5–20 mg/d *12–17 y.* 5–20 mg, up to 40 mg/d **Caution:** [C, M] **CI:** IV use, angina, ischemic heart Dz, CV synds, uncontrolled HTN, severe hepatic impair, ergot use, MAOI use w/in 14 d, hemiplegic or basilar migraine **Disp:** *Imitrex Oral* OD tabs 25, 50, 100 mg; *Imitrex Inj* 6, 8, 12 mg/mL; *ODTs* 25, 50, 100 mg; *Imitrex nasal spray* 5, 10, 20 mg/spray; *Alsuma Auto-Injector* 6 mg/0.5 mL **SE:** Pain & bruising at Inj site; dizziness, hot flashes, paresthesias, CP, weakness, numbness, coronary vasospasm, HTN **Interactions:** ↑ Effects of weakness, incoordination & hyperreflexia *W/* ergots, MAOIs & SSRIs, horehound, St. John's wort **Labs:** ↑ LFTs **NIPE:** Administer drug as soon as possible after onset of migraine

Sumatriptan & Naproxen Sodium (Treximet) [Selective 5-HT₁ᵦ/₁ᴅ Receptor Agonist + NSAID]
WARNING: ↑ Risk of serious CV (MI, stroke) serious GI events (bleeding, ulceration, perforation) of the stomach or intestines **Uses:** *Prevent migraines* **Action:** Anti-inflammatory NSAID w/ 5-HT₁ receptor agonist, constricts CNS vessels **Dose:** *Adults.* 1 tab PO; repeat PRN after 2 h; max 2 tabs/24 h, w/ or w/o food **Caution:** [C, −] **CI:** Sig CV Dz, severe hepatic impair, severe ↑ BP **Disp:** Tab (naproxen mg/sumatriptan mg) 500/85 **SE:** Dizziness, somnolence, paresthesia, N, dyspepsia, dry mouth, chest/neck/throat/jaw pain, tightness, pressure **Interactions:** ↑ Risk of serotonin synd *W/* SSRIs (citalopram, escitalopram, fluoxetine, fluvoxamine) & SNRIs (eg, duloxetine, venlafaxine);

↑ effects **OF** methotrexate, Li; ↑ risk of renal tox **W/** ACEIs, diuretics; ↑ risk of GI bleed **W/** oral corticosteroids, anticoagulants, smoking, EtOH; ↓ effects **OF** diuretics, antihypertensives **Labs:** May interfere w/ tests for 17-ketogenic steroids, 5-HIAA **NIPE:** Do not split/crush/chew; ⊘ take w/in 24 h of ergot-type drugs or other 5-HT₁ agonists; ⊘ take during or w/in 2 wk after discontinuing MAO-type A Inhibs

Sumatriptan Needleless System (Sumavel DosePro) [Antimigraine Agent/Selective 5-HT₁ Receptor Agonist] **Uses:** *Rx acute migraine & cluster HA* **Action:** Vascular serotonin receptor agonist **Dose:** *Adults.* **SQ:** 6 mg SQ as a single dose PRN; repeat PRN in 1 h to a max of 12 mg/24 h; administer in abdomen/thigh. **Caution:** [C, M] **CI:** See Sumatriptan **Disp:** Needle free SQ Injector 6 mg/0.5 mL **SE:** Inj site Rxn, tingling, warm/hot/burning sensation, feeling of heaviness/pressure/tightness/ numbness, feeling strange, light-headedness, flushing, tightness in chest, discomfort in nasal cavity/sinuses/jaw, dizziness/vertigo, drowsiness/sedation, HA **Interactions:** ↑ risk of serotonin synd **W/** SSRIs (eg, citalopram, escitalopram, fluoxetine, fluvoxamine, paroxetine, sertraline) or SNRIs (eg, duloxetine, venlafaxine) **NIPE:** Do not give during or w/in 2 wk after D/C MAOIs; supervise 1st dose & consider ECG monitoring in pts w/ unrecognized CAD (postmenopausal women, hypercholesterolemia, men > 40 y, HTN, obesity, DM, smokers, strong family Hx

Sunitinib (Sutent) [Kinase Inhibitor] **Uses:** *Advanced GI stromal tumor (GIST) refractory/intolerant to imatinib; advanced RCC; well-differentiated pancreatic neuroendocrine tumors unresectable, locally advanced, metastatic* **Action:** Multi TKI **Dose:** *Adults.* 50 mg PO daily × 4 wk, followed by 2 wk holiday = 1 cycle; ↓ to 37.5 mg w/ CYP3A4 Inhibs (Table 10), to ↑ 87.5 mg w/ CYP3A4 inducers **CI:** w/ Atazanavir **Caution:** [D, –] Multiple interactions require dose modification (eg, St. John's wort) **Disp:** Caps 12.5, 25, 50 mg **SE:** Bleeding, ↑ BP, ↓ ejection fraction, ↑ QT interval, pancreatitis, DVT, Szs, adrenal Insuff, N/V/D, skin discoloration, oral ulcers, taste perversion, hypothyroidism **Labs:** ↓ WBC & plt, monitor CBC, plts, chemistries at cycle onset; baseline cardiac Fxn OK; monitor LVEF, ECG, CBC/plts, chemistries (K⁺/Mg²⁺/phosphate), TFT & LFTs periodically **NIPE:** ↓ Dose in 12.5-mg increments if not tolerated

Tacrine (Cognex) [Anti-Alzheimer Agent/Centrally Acting Reversible Cholinesterase Inhibitor] **Uses:** *Mild–mod Alzheimer dementia* **Action:** Cholinesterase Inhib **Dose:** 10–40 mg PO qid to 160 mg/d; separate doses from food **Caution:** [C, ?] **CI:** Previous tacrine-induced jaundice **Disp:** Caps 10, 20, 30, 40 mg **SE:** LFTs, HA, dizziness, GI upset, flushing, confusion, ataxia, myalgia, bradycardia **Interactions:** ↑ Effects **W/** cimetidine, quinolones; ↑ effects **OF** cholinesterase Inhibs, succinylcholine, theophylline; ↓ effects **W/** tobacco, food; ↓ effects **OF** anticholinergics **Labs:** ↑ LFTs **NIPE:** If taken w/ food ↓ drug plasma levels by 30%; may take up to 6 wk for ALT elevations—monitor LFTs; serum conc > 20 ng/mL have more SE

Tacrolimus [FK506] (Prograf, Protopic) [Immunosuppressant/ Macrolide] WARNING: ↑ Risk of Infxn & lymphoma Uses: *Prevent organ rejection*, eczema Action: Macrolide immunosuppressant Dose: *Adults. IV:* 0.05–0.1 mg/kg/d cont Inf *PO:* 0.1–0.2 mg/kg/d ÷ 2 doses *Peds. IV:* 0.03–0.05 mg/kg/d as cont Inf *PO:* 0.15–0.2 mg/kg/d PO ÷ q12h *Adults & Peds.* Eczema: Apply bid, continue 1 wk after clearing; take on empty stomach; ↓ w/ hepatic/renal impair Caution: [C, –] w/ Cyclosporine; avoid topical if < 2 y of age CI: Component allergy, castor oil allergy w/ IV Disp: Caps 0.5, 1, 5 mg; Inj 5 mg/mL; oint 0.03, 0.1% SE: Neuro- & nephrotox, HTN, edema, HA, insomnia, fever, pruritus, (↓/↑) K⁺, hyperglycemia, GI upset, anemia, leukocytosis, tremors, paresthesias, PE, Szs, lymphoma Lab: Monitor drug levels; trough 5–20 ng/mL based on indication & time since transplant NIPE: Reports of ↑ CA risk; topical use for short term & 2nd line

Tadalafil (Cialis) [Anti-Impotence Agent/PDE5] Uses: *ED* Action: PDE5 Inhib, ↑ cyclic guanosine monophosphate & NO levels; relaxes smooth muscles, dilates cavernosal arteries Dose: *Adults. PRN:* 10 mg PO before sexual activity (5–20 mg max) 1 dose/72 h *Daily dosing:* 2.5 mg qd w/o regard to timing of sex, may ↑ to 5 mg qd; w/o regard to meals; 5 mg (10 mg max) w/ renal/hepatic Insuff Caution: [B, –] w/ α-blockers (except tamsulosin); use w/ CYP3A4 Inhib (Table 10) (eg, ritonavir, ketoconazole, itraconazole) 2.5 mg/daily dose or 5 mg PRN dose; CrCl < 30 mL/min/HD/severe hepatic impair Disp: Tabs 5-, 10-, 20-mg SE: HA, flushing, dyspepsia, back/limb pain, myalgia, nasal congestion, urticaria, Stevens–Johnson synd, dermatitis, visual field defect, NIAON, sudden ↓/loss of hearing, tinnitus Interactions: ↑ Effects *W/* ketoconazole, ritonavir, & other cytochrome P450 CYP3A4 Inhibs; ↑ hypotension *W/* antihypertensives, nitrates, EtOH; ↓ effects *W/* P450 CYP3A4 inducers such as rifampin, antacids; daily dosing may ↑ drug interactions NIPE: ↑ Risk of priapism; use barrier contraception to prevent STDs; longest acting of class (36 h); daily dosing may ↑ drug interactions; excessive EtOH may ↑ orthostasis; transient global amnesia reports

Tadalafil (Adcirca) [Phosphodiesterase Type 5 Inhibitor] Uses: *Pulm artery hypertension* Action: PDE5 Inhib; ↑ cyclic guanosine monophosphate (cGMP) concs; relaxes pulm artery smooth muscles Dose: 40 mg/ 1 × d w/o regard to meals; ↓ w/ renal/hepatic Insuff Caution: [B, –] w/ CV Dz, impaired autonomic control of BP, AS, α-blockers (except tamsulosin); use w/ CYP3A4 Inhib/inducers (eg, ritonavir, ketoconazole); monitor for sudden ↓/loss of hearing or vision (NAION), tinnitus, priapism CI: w/ Nitrates, component hypersensitivity Disp: Tabs 20 mg SE: HA Interactions: ↑ Risk of hypotension *W/* α-blockers, antihypertensives, EtOH NIPE: D/C therapy at least 24 h prior to starting ritonavir; D/C therapy 48 h before taking nitrates; use Tadalafil (Cialis) for ED

Talc (Sterile Talc Powder) [Sclerosing Agent] Uses: *↓ Recurrence of malignant PE (pleurodesis)* Action: Sclerosing agent Dose: *Mix slurry:* 50 mL

NS w/ 5-g vial, mix, distribute 25 mL into two 60-mL syringes, vol to 50 mL/ syringe w/ NS. Infuse each into chest tube, flush w/ 25 mL NS. Keep tube clamped; have pt change positions q15min for 2 h, unclamp tube **Caution:** [X, −] **CI:** Planned further surgery on site **Disp:** 5-g Powder **SE:** Pain, Infxn **NIPE:** May add 10–20 mL 1% lidocaine/syringe); must have chest tube placed, monitor closely while tube clamped (tension pneumothorax), not antineoplastic; monitor for MI, PE, resp distress

Tamoxifen (Generic) [Antineoplastic/Antiestrogen] WARNING:
CA of the uterus, stroke, & blood clots can occur **Uses:** *Breast CA [postmeno-pausal, estrogen receptor (+)], ↓ reduction of breast CA in high-risk women, met male breast CA*, ductal carcinoma in situ, mastalgia, pancreatic CA, gynecomastia, ovulation induction **Action:** Nonsteroidal antiestrogen; mixed agonist–antagonist effect **Dose:** 20–40 mg/d; doses > 20 mg ÷ bid *Prevention:* 20 mg PO/d for 5 y **Caution:** [D, −] w/ hyperlipidemia **CI:** PRG, undiagnosed Vag bleeding, h/o thromboembolism **Disp:** Tabs 10, 20 mg; oral soln 10 mg/5 mL **SE:** Uterine malignancy & thrombotic events noted in breast CA prevention trials; menopausal Sxs (hot flashes, N/V) in premenopausal pts; Vag bleeding & menstrual irregularities; skin rash, pruritus vulvae, dizziness, HA, peripheral edema; acute flare of bone metastasis pain & Ca^{2+}; retinopathy reported (high dose) **Interactions:** ↑ Effects W/ bromocriptine, grapefruit juice; ↑ effects OF cyclosporine, warfarin; ↓ effects W/ antacids, aminoglutethimide, estrogens **Labs:** ↑ Ca^{2+}, BUN, Cr, LFTs; ↓ WBC, ↓ plts **NIPE:** ⊘ PRG or breast-feeding; use barrier contraception; ↑ risk of photo-sensitivity—use sunscreen; ↑ risk of PRG in premenopausal women (induces ovulation); brand Nolvadex suspended in United State

Tamsulosin (Flomax, Generic) [Smooth Muscle Relaxant/ Antiadrenergic] **Uses:** *BPH* **Action:** Antagonist of prostatic a receptors **Dose:** 0.4 mg/d, may ↑ to 0.8 mg PO daily **Caution:** [B, ?] **CI:** Female gender **Disp:** Caps 0.4 mg **SE:** HA, dizziness, syncope, somnolence, ↓ libido, GI upset, retrograde ejaculation, rhinitis, rash, angioedema, IFIS **Interactions:** ↑ Effects W/ cimetidine; ↑ hypotension W/ doxazosin, prazosin, terazosin **NIPE:** Not for use as antihypertensive; do not open/crush/chew; approved for use w/ dutasteride for BPH

Tapentadol (Nucynta) [Opioid] [C-II] **Uses:** *Mod/severe acute pain* **Action:** Mu-opioid agonist & norepinephrine reuptake Inhib **Dose:** 50–100 mg PO q4–6h PRN (max 600 mg/d); w/ mod hepatic impair: 50 mg q8h PRN (max 3 doses/24 h) **Caution:** [C, −] h/o Szs, CNS depression; ↑ ICP, severe renal impair, biliary tract Dz, elderly, serotonin synd w/ concomitant serotonergic agents **CI:** ↓ Pulm Fxn, use w/ or w/in 14 d of MAOI **Disp:** Tabs 50, 75, 100 mg **SE:** N/V, dizziness, somnolence, HA **Interactions:** ↑ CNS depression W/ general anesthetics, hypnotics, phenothiazines, sedatives, EtOH; ↑ risk of serotonin synd W/ MAOIs, SNRIs, SSRIs, TCA, triptans **NIPE:** Taper dose w/ D/C; ⊘ during or w/in 14 d of MAOI; up↑ risk of Szs

Tazarotene (Tazorac, Avage) [Keratolytic/Retinoid] Uses: *Facial acne vulgaris; stable plaque psoriasis up to 20% BSA* **Action:** Keratolytic **Dose:** *Adults & Peds > 12 y. Acne:* Cleanse face, dry, apply thin film qhs lesions. *Psoriasis:* Apply qhs **Caution:** [X, ?/−] **CI:** Retinoid sensitivity **Disp:** Gel 0.05%, 0.1%; cream 0.05%, 0.1% **SE:** Burning, erythema, irritation, rash, photosensitivity, desquamation, bleeding, skin discoloration **Interactions:** ↑ Risk of photosensitivity *W/* quinolones, phenothiazine, sulfonamides, tetracyclines, thiazide diuretics **NIPE:** ⊘ PRG or breast-feeding; use contraception; use sunscreen for ↑ photosensitivity risk; D/C w/ excessive pruritus, burning, skin redness, or peeling until Sxs resolve

Telavancin (Vibativ) [Antibacterial/Lipoglycopeptide] WARNING: Fetal risk; must have PRG test prior to use in childbearing age Uses: *Comp skin/ skin structure Infxns d/t susceptible gram(+) bacteria* **Action:** Lipoglycopeptide antibacterial *Spectrum:* Good gram(±) aerobic & anaerobic incl MRSA, MSSA, some VRE; poor gram(−) **Dose:** 10 mg/kg IV q24h; 7.5 mg/kg q24h w/ CrCl 30–50 mL/min; 10 mg/kg q48h w/ CrCl 10–30 mL/min **Caution:** [C, ?/] Nephrotox; *C difficile*–associated Dz, ↑ α QTc, interferes w/ coagulation tests **CI:** PRG **Disp:** Inj 250, 750 mg **SE:** Taste disturbance, N, V, foamy urine **Interactions:** ↑ Risk of renal tox *W/* NSAIDs, ACEI, loop diuretics **Labs:** May interfere w/ coagulation tests (eg, PT/INR, aPTT, ACT, coagulation-based factor Xa tests) & some urine protein tests **NIPE:** ↓ Efficacy w/ mod/severe renal impair

Telbivudine (Tyzeka) [Antiretroviral, NRTI] WARNING: May cause lactic acidosis & severe hepatomegaly w/ steatosis when used alone or w/ antiretrovirals; D/C of the drug may lead to exacerbations of hep B; monitor LFTs Uses: *Rx chronic hep B* **Action:** Nucleoside RT Inhib **Dose:** *CrCl > 50 mL/min:* 600 mg PO daily *CrCl 30–49 mL/min:* 600 mg q48h *CrCl < 30 mL/min:* 600 mg q72h *ESRD:* 600 mg q96h; dose after HD **Caution:** [B, ?/−]; may cause myopathy; follow closely w/ other myopathy-causing drugs **Disp:** Tabs 600 mg **SE:** Fatigue, Abd pain, N/V/D, HA, URI, nasopharyngitis, LFTs/CPK, myalgia/myopathy, flu-like Sxs, dizziness, insomnia, dyspepsia **Interactions:** Use w/ PEG-interferon may ↑ peripheral neuropathy risk; ↑ risk of myopathy *W/* azole antifungals, chloroquine, corticosteroids, cyclosporine, erythromycin, fibrates, hydroxychloroquine, niacin, penicillamine, statins, zidovudine; ↑ risk of renal impair *W/* cyclosporine, tacrolimus **Labs:** ↑ LFTs, CPK **NIPE:** Not a cure for hep B, does not reduce transmission of hep B by sexual contact or blood contamination; monitor for liver tox/hep (jaundice, rash, hepatomegaly, fatigue)

Telithromycin (Ketek) [Antibiotic/Macrolide Derivative] WARNING: CI in MyG Uses: *Mild–mod CAP* **Action:** Unique macrolide, blocks protein synth; bactericidal *Spectrum: S aureus, S pneumoniae, H influenzae, M catarrhalis, C pneumoniae, M pneumoniae* **Dose:** *Caps:* 800 mg (2 tabs) PO daily for 7–10 d **Caution:** [C, M] Pseudomembranous colitis, ↑ QTc interval, visual disturbances, hepatic dysfunction; dosing in renal impair unknown **CI:** Macrolide allergy, w/

pimozide, cisapride; w/ MyG **Disp:** Tabs 300, 400 mg **SE:** N/V/D, dizziness, blurred vision **Interactions:** A CYP450 Inhib = multiple drug interactions; hold statins d/t ↑ risk of myopathy; avoid rifampin, ergots, simvastatin, lovastatin, atorvastatin (suspend during therapy). Do not use w/ Class Ia (eg, quinidine, procainamide) or Class III (eg, dofetilide) antiarrhythmics; ↑ QTc interval & arrhythmias **W/** antiarrhythmics, mesoridazine, quinolone antibiotics, thioridazine; ↑ effects **OF** alprazolam, atorvastatin, benzodiazepines, CCBs, carbamazepine, cisapride, colchicine, cyclosporine, digoxin, ergot alkaloids, felodipine, fentanyl, mirtazapine, midazolam, nateglinide, nefazodone, pimozide, sildenafil, simvastatin, sirolimus, tacrolimus, tadalafil, triazolam, vardenafil, venlafaxine, verapamil, warfarin; ↓ effects **W/** azole antifungals, ciprofloxin, clarithromycin, diclofenac, doxycycline, erythromycin, imatinib, INH, nefazodone, nicardipine, propofol, protease Inhibs, quinidine; ↑ effect **W/** aminoglutethimide, carbamazepine, nafcillin, nevirapine, phenobarbital, phenytoin, rifabutin, rifamycins **Labs:** ↑ LFTs, plts **NIPE:** Take w/o regard to food; ⊘ chew/crush tabs, monitor ECG; hold statins d/t ↑ risk of myopathy

Telmisartan (Micardis) [Antihypertensive/ARB]
Uses: *HTN, CHF* **Action:** Angiotensin II receptor antagonist **Dose:** 40–80 mg/d **Caution:** [C (1st tri; D 2nd & 3rd tri), ?/–] **CI:** Angiotensin II receptor antagonist sensitivity **Disp:** Tabs 20, 40, 80 mg **SE:** Edema, GI upset, HA, angioedema, renal impair, orthostatic ↓ BP **Interactions:** ↑ Risk of hyperkalemia **W/** K⁺ supls, K⁺-sparing diuretics, K⁺-containing salt substitutes; ↑ effects **W/** EtOH; ↑ effects **OF** digoxin; ↓ effects **OF** warfarin **Labs:** ↑ Cr, ↓ HMG **NIPE:** Take w/o regard to food; ⊘ PRG; use barrier contraception

Telmisartan & Amlodipine (Twynsta) [Angiotensin II Receptor Blocker + Calcium Channel Blocker]
WARNING: Use of renin-angiotensin agents in PRG can cause fetal injury & death, D/C stat when PRG detected **Uses:** *Hypertension* **Action:** CCB; relaxes coronary vascular smooth muscle & angiotensin II receptor antagonist **Dose:** Start 40/5-mg telmisartan/amlodipine; max 80/10 mg PO/d; ↑ dose after 2 wk **W/P:** [C (1st); D 2nd/3rd tri), ?/–] **CI:** PRG **Disp:** Tabs mg telmisartan/mg amlodipine 40/5; 40/10; 80/5; 80/10 mg **SE:** HA, edema, dizziness, N, ↓ BP **Interactions:** ↑ Effects **OF** digoxin, Li; CCB w/ CAD may cause ACS **NIPE:** Slow titrate w/ hepatic/renal impair; avoid w/ ACE/other ARBs; correct hypovolemia before; w/CHF monitor

Temazepam (Restoril) [C-IV] [Sedative/Hypnotic/Benzodiazepine]
Uses: *Insomnia*, anxiety, depression, panic attacks **Action:** Benzodiazepine **Dose:** 15–30 mg PO hs PRN; ↓ in elderly **Caution:** [X, ?/–] Potentiates CNS depressive effects of opioids, barbs, EtOH, antihistamines, MAOIs, TCAs **CI:** NAG **Disp:** Caps 7.5, 15, 22.5, 30 mg **SE:** Confusion, dizziness, drowsiness, hangover **Interactions:** ↑ Effects **W/** cimetidine, disulfiram, kava kava, valerian; ↑ CNS depression **W/** anticonvulsants, CNS depressants, EtOH; ↑ effects **OF** haloperidol, phenytoin; ↓ effects **W/** aminophylline, dyphylline, OCPs, oxtriphylline, rifampin,

theophylline, tobacco; ↓ effects *OF* levodopa **NIPE:** Abrupt D/C after > 10 d use may cause withdrawal; ⊘ use in PRG or breast-feeding

Temozolomide (Temodar) [Alkylating agent] Uses: *GBM, refractory anaplastic astrocytoma* **Action:** Alkylating agent **Dose:** *GBM New:* 75 mg/m^2 PO/IV/d × 42 d W/ RT, maint 150 mg/m^2/d d 1–5 of 28-d cycle × 6 cycles; may ↑ to 200 mg/m^2/d × 5 d q28d in cycle 2 *Refractory astrocytoma:* 150 mg/m^2 PO/IV/d × 5 d/28-d cycle; adjust dose based on ANC & plt count (see label & use local protocols) **Caution:** [D, ?/–] severe renal/hepatic impair, myelosuppression (monitor ANC & plt), myelodysplastic synd, secondary malignancies, PCP pneumonia (PCP prophylaxis required) **CI:** Hypersensitivity to components or dacarbazine **Disp:** Caps 5, 20, 100, 140, 180, 250 mg; powder for Inj 100 mg **SE:** N/V/D, fatigue, HA, asthenia, Sz, hemiparesis, fever, dizziness, coordination abnormality, alopecia, rash, constipation, anorexia, amnesia, insomnia, viral Infxn **Interactions:** ↑ Effects W/ valproic acid **Labs:** ↓ WBC, plt; monitor CBC—dl CBC on 22nd d of each cycle & weekly until recovery if ANC or plts below nl limits **NIPE:** Inf over 90 min; swallow caps whole w/ H$_2$O; if caps open avoid Inh & contact w/ skin/mucous membranes; to reduce N—take on empty stomach at hs, take antiemetics before dosing

Temsirolimus (Torisel) [mTOR Kinase Inhibitor] Uses: *Advanced RCC* **Action:** Multikinase Inhib, ↓ mTOR (mammalian target of rapamycin), ↓ hypoxic-induced factors, ↓ VEGF **Dose:** 25 mg IV 30–60 min 1 × /wk. Hold w/ ANC < 1000 cells/mm^3, plt < 75,000 cells/mm^3, or National Cancer Institute (NCI) grade 3 tox. Resume when tox grade 2 or less, restart w/ dose ↓ 5 mg/wk not < 15 mg/wk w/ *CYP3A4 Inhibs:* ↓ 12.5 mg/wk *w/ CYP3A4 inducers:* ↑ 50 mg/wk **Caution:** [D, –] Avoid live vaccines, ↓ wound healing, avoid perioperatively **CI:** None **Disp:** Inj 25 mg/mL w/ 250 mL diluent **SE:** Rash, asthenia, mucositis, N, bowel perforation, anorexia, edema **Interactions:** ↑ Effects W/ strong CYP3A4 Inhibs such as ketoconazole, itraconazole, clarithromycin, atazanavir, indinavir, nefazodone, nelfinavir, ritonavir, saquinavir, telithromycin, voriconazole, grapefruit juice; ↓ effects W/ strong CYP3A 4 inducers such as dexamethasone, phenytoin, carbamazepine, rifampin, rifabutin, rifampicin, phenobarbital, St. John's wort **Labs:** ↑ Lipids, ↑ glucose, ↑ triglycerides, ↑ LFTs, ↑ Cr, ↓ WBC, ↓ HCT, ↓ plt, ↓ PO$_4$; monitor Cr, CBC, plts, lipids, glucose **NIPE:** Combine only w/ provided diluent for IV administration; premedicate w/ antihistamine; w/ sunitinib & anticoagulants dose-limiting tox likely; females use w/ contraception; ⊘ live vaccines or people recently immunized w/ live vaccines

Tenecteplase (TNKase) [Thrombolytic/Recombinant Tissue Plasminogen Activator] Uses: *Restore perfusion & ↓ mortality w/ AMI* **Action:** Thrombolytic; TPA **Dose:** 30–50 mg; see the table below **Caution:** [C, ?], Bleeding w/ NSAIDs, ticlopidine, clopidogrel, GP IIb/IIIa antagonists **CI:** Bleeding, CVA, CNS neoplasm, uncontrolled ↑ BP, major surgery (intracranial, intraspinal) or trauma w/in 2 mo **Disp:** Inj 50 mg, reconstitute w/ 10 mL sterile H$_2$O only **SE:** Bleeding, allergy **Interactions:** ↑ Risk of bleeding W/ heparin, ASA, clopidogrel,

dipyridamole, indomethacin, vit K antagonists GP IIb/IIIa Inhibs; ↓ effects **W/** aminocaproic acid **Labs:** ↑ PT, PTT, INR **NIPE:** Eval for S/Sxs bleeding; do not shake w/ reconstitution; start ASA ASAP, IV heparin ASAP w/ aPTT 50–70
Tenecteplase Dosing (From one vial of reconstituted TNKase)

Wgt (kg)	TNKase (mg)	TNKase[a] Vol (mL)
< 60	30	6
60–69	35	7
70–79	40	8
80–89	45	9
≥ 90	50	10

Tenofovir (Viread) [Antiretroviral/NRTI]   WARNING: Lactic acidosis & severe hepatomegaly w/ steatosis, including fatal cases, have been reported w/ the use of nucleoside analogues alone or in combo w/ other antiretrovirals. Not OK w/ chronic hep; effects in pts coinfected w/ hep B & HIV unknown **Uses:** *HIV Infxn* **Action:** Nucleotide RT Inhib **Dose:** 300 mg PO daily w/ or w/o meal; CrCl ≥ 50 mL/min q24h, CrCl 30–49 mL/min q48h, CrCl 10–29 mL/min 2 × /wk **Caution:** [B, ?/–] Didanosine (separate administration times), lopinavir, ritonavir w/ known risk factors for liver Dz **CI:** Hypersensitivity **Disp:** Tabs 300 mg **SE:** GI upset, metabolic synd, hepatotox; separate didanosine doses by 2 h **Interactions:** ↑ Effects **W/** acyclovir, cidofovir, ganciclovir, indinavir, lopinavir, ritonavir, valacyclovir, food **Labs:** ↑ LFTs, triglycerides **NIPE:** Take w/ food, take 2 h before or 1 h after didanosine, lopinavir/ritonavir; combo product w/ emtricitabine is Truvada
Tenofovir/Emtricitabine (Truvada) [Antiretroviral, Dual NRTI] WARNING: Lactic acidosis & severe hepatomegaly w/ steatosis, including fatal cases, have been reported w/ the use of nucleoside analogues alone or in combo w/ other antiretrovirals. Not OK w/ chronic hep; effects in pts coinfected w/ hep B & HIV unknown **Uses:** *HIV Infxn* **Action:** Dual nucleotide RT Inhib **Dose:** 300 mg PO daily w/ or w/o a meal; adjust w/ renal impair **Caution:** [B, ?/–] known risk factors for liver Dz **CI:** CrCl < 30 mL/min **Disp:** Tabs 200 mg emtricitabine/300 mg tenofovir **SE:** GI upset, rash, metabolic synd, hepatotox **Interactions:** ↑ Effects **W/** acyclovir, cidofovir, ganciclovir, indinavir, lopinavir, ritonavir, valacyclovir, food; ↓ effects **OF** didanosine, lamivudine, ritonavir **Labs:** ↑ LFTs, triglycerides **NIPE:** Take w/ food, take 2 h before or 1 h after didanosine, lopinavir/ritonavir; causes redistribution & accumulation of body fat; take w/ other antiretrovirals; not a cure for HIV or prevention of opportunistic Infxns
Terazosin (Hytrin) [Antihypertensive/Peripherally Acting Antiadrenergic] **Uses:** *BPH & HTN* **Action:** α_1-Blocker (blood vessel & bladder neck/prostate) **Dose:** Initial, 1 mg PO hs; ↑ 20 mg/d max; may ↓ w/ diuretic or

Teriparatide **339**

other BP meds **Caution:** [C, ?] w/ BB, CCB, ACE Inhib **CI:** α-Antagonist sensitivity **Disp:** Tabs 1, 2, 5, 10 mg; caps 1, 2, 5, 10 mg **SE:** ↓ BP, & syncope following 1st dose or w/PDE5 Inhib; dizziness, weakness, nasal congestion, edema, palpitations, GI upset **Interactions:** ↑ Effects *W/* antihypertensives, diuretics; ↑ effects *OF* finasteride; ↓ effects *W/* NSAIDs, α-blockers, ephedra, garlic, ginseng, saw palmetto, yohimbe; ↓ effects *OF* clonidine; use w/ PDE5 Inhib (eg, sildenafil) can cause ↓ BP **Labs:** ↓ Albumin, HMG, Hct, WBCs **NIPE:** Take w/o regard to food, ⊘ D/C abruptly; caution w/ 1st dose syncope; if for HTN, combine w/ thiazide diuretic

Terbinafine (Lamisil, Lamisil AT, Others [OTC]) [Antifungal] **Uses:** *Onychomycosis, athlete's foot, jock itch, ringworm*, cutaneous candidiasis, pityriasis versicolor **Action:** ↓ Squalene epoxidase resulting in fungal death **Dose:** *PO:* 250 mg/d PO for 6–12 wk. *Topical:* Apply to area tinea pedis bid, tinea cruris, & corporus qd–bid, tinea versicolor soln bid; ↓ PO in renal/hepatic impair **Caution:** [B, –] PO ↑ effects of drug metabolism by CYP2D6, w/ hepatic/renal impair **CI:** CrCl < 50 mL/min, WBC < 1000 cells/mm³, severe liver Dz **Disp:** Tabs 250 mg; Lamisil AT [OTC] cream, gel, soln 1% **SE:** HA, dizziness, rash, pruritus, alopecia, GI upset, taste perversion, neutropenia, retinal damage, Stevens–Johnson syndr **Interactions:** ↑ Effects *W/* cimetidine; ↑ effects *OF* dextromethorphan, theophylline, caffeine; ↓ effects *W/* rifampin; ↓ effects *OF* cyclosporine **Labs:** ↑ LFTs; follow CBC/LFTs w/ oral med **NIPE:** Effect may take mo d/t need for new nail growth; do not use occlusive dressings; topical not for nails; rare reports of liver failure

Terbutaline (Brethine, Bricanyl) [Bronchodilator/Sympathomimetic] **Uses:** *Reversible bronchospasm (asthma, COPD); inhibit labor* **Action:** Sympathomimetic; tocolytic **Dose:** *Adults. Bronchodilator:* 2.5–5 mg PO qid or 0.25 mg SQ; repeat in 15 min PRN; max 0.5 mg in 4 h *Metered-dose inhaler:* 2 Inh q4–6h. *Premature labor:* Acutely 2.5–10 mg/min/IV, gradually ↑ as tolerated q10–20 min; maint 2.5–5 mg PO q4–6h until term *Peds. PO:* 0.05–0.15 mg/kg/dose PO tid; max 5 mg/24h; ↓ in renal failure **Caution:** [B, +] Tox w/ MAOIs, TCAs; DM, HTN, hyperthyroidism, CV Dz, DM, convulsive disorders **CI:** Component allergy **Disp:** Tabs 2.5, 5 mg; Inj 1 mg/mL; metered-dose inhaler **SE:** HTN, hyperthyroidism, β₁-adrenergic effects w/ high dose, nervousness, trembling, tachycardia, HTN, dizziness **Interactions:** ↑ Effects *W/* MAOIs, TCAs; ↓ effects *W/* BBs **Labs:** ↑ LFTs, serum glucose; ↓ K⁺—monitor labs **NIPE:** Take oral dose w/ food; monitor ECG for hypokalemia (flattened T waves)

Terconazole (Terazol 7) [Antifungal] **Uses:** *Vag fungal Infxns* **Action:** Topical triazole antifungal **Dose:** 1 applicator-full or 1 supp intravag hs × 3–7 d **Caution:** [C, ?] **CI:** Component allergy **Disp:** Vag cream 0.4%, 0.8%, Vag supp 80 mg **SE:** Vulvar/Vag burning **NIPE:** Insert cream or supp high into Vag, complete full course of Rx, ⊘ intercourse during drug Rx, ↑ risk of breakdown of latex condoms & diaphragms w/ drug

Teriparatide (Forteo) [Antiosteoporotic/Parathyroid Hormone] **WARNING:** ↑ Osteosarcoma risk in animals, where potential benefits outweigh risks **Uses:** *Severe/refractory osteoporosis* **Action:** PTH (recombinant) **Dose:** 20 mcg SQ daily in thigh or abdomen **Caution:** [C, ?/–] Caution in urolithiasis **CI:** w/ Paget Dz, prior radiation, bone metastases; Ca²⁺ **Disp:** 3-mL prefilled device (discard after 28 d) **SE:** Orthostatic ↓ BP on administration, N/D, leg cramps **Labs:** ↑ Serum Ca²⁺, uric acid, urine Ca²⁺ **NIPE:** ⊘ Take if h/o Paget Dz, bone mets or malignancy, or h/o radiation therapy; take w/o regard to food; not used to prevent osteoporosis; 2 y max use; monitor ECG for cardiac conduction changes related to ↑ Ca²⁺

Tesamorelin (Egrifta) [Growth Hormone-Releasing Factor Analog]

Uses: *↓ Excess Abd fat in HIV-infected pts w/ lipodystrophy* **Action:** Binds/stimulates GH-releasing factor receptors **Dose:** 2 mg SQ/d **Caution:** [X; HIV-infected mothers should not breast-feed] **CI:** Hypothalamic-pituitary axis disorders; head radiation/trauma; malignancy; PRG; child w/ open epiphyses **Disp:** Vial 1 mg **SE:** Arthralgias, Inj site Rxn, edema, myalgia, N, V **Labs:** ↑ Glucose, ✓ glucose **NIPE:** ? ↑ Mortality w/ acute critical illness; ↑ IGF

Testosterone (AndroGel, 1%, AndroGel 1.62% Androderm, Axiron, Fortesta, Striant, Testim) [CIII] [Androgen Replacement]

WARNING: Virilization in children reported exposed to topical testosterone products. Children to avoid contact w/ unwashed or unclothed application sites **Uses:** *Male hypogonadism (congenital/acquired)* **Action:** Testosterone replacement; ↑ lean body mass, libido **Dose:** All daily applications AndroGel 1% 50 mg (4 pumps); AndroGel 1.62% (italics) 40.5 mg (2 pumps) apply to clean skin on upper body only *Androderm:* Two 2.5-mg or one 5-mg patch daily *Axiron:* 60 mg (1 pump = 30 mg each axilla) qAM *Fortesta:* 40 mg (4 pumps)on clean dry thighs; adjust form 1–7 pumps based on blood test 2 h after (d 14 & 35) *Striant:* 30-mg Buccal tabs bid *Testim:* One 5-g gel tube *Testopel:* 150–450 mg (2–6 pellets) SQ implant q3–6mo (implant 2 75-mg pellets for each 25-mg testosterone required weekly; eg, for 75 mg/wk, implant 450 mg (6 pellets) **Caution:**[X, –] May cause polycythemia, worsening of BPH Sx **CI:** PCa, male breast CA, pregnant or breast-feeding women **Disp:** AndroGel 1% 12.5 mg/pump; AndroGel 1.62% 20.25 mg/pump Androderm: 2.5-, 5-mg patches; *Axiron* metered-dose pump 30 mg/pump *Fortesta:* Metered-dose gel pump 10 mg/pump *Striant:* 30-mg Buccal tab *Testopel* 75 mg/implant **SE:** Site Rxns, acne, edema, wgt gain, gynecomastia, HTN, sleep apnea, prostate enlargement, ↑ PSA **Interactions:** ↑ Effects *OF* anticoagulants, cyclosporine, insulin, hypoglycemics, oxyphenbutazone; ↑ effects *W/* grapefruit juice; ↓ effects *W/* St. John's wort **Labs:** ↑ AST, Cr, Hgb, Hct, LDL, serum alk phos, bilirubin, Ca, K⁺, & Na; ✓ thyroid hormones **NIPE:** IM testosterone enanthate (*Delatestryl;* *Testro-L.A.*)& cypionate (*Depo-Testosterone*) dose q14–28d w/ variable serum levels; PO agents (methyltestosterone & oxandrolone) associated w/ hepatic tumors; transdermal/mucosal forms preferred; wash hands stat after topical applications, *Andro-Gel* formulations not equivalent; ✓ levels & adjust PRN (300–1000 ng/dL nl testosterone range)

Tetanus Immune Globulin [Tetanus Prophylaxis/Immune Serum]
Uses: Prophylaxis;*Passive tetanus immunization* (suspected contaminated wound w/ unknown immunization status, see also Table 7), or Tx of tetanus **Action:** Passive immunization **Dose:** *Adults & Peds.* 250–500 units IM (< 7 y 4 unit/kg) 500 units if Tx delayed *Tx:* Children 500–3000 units, adults 3000–6000 unit **Caution:** [C, ?] **CI:** Thimerosal sensitivity **Disp:** Inj 250-unit vial/syringe **SE:** Pain, tenderness, erythema at site; fever, angioedema, anaphylaxis **Interactions:** ↓ Immune response when administration **W/ Td NIPE:** Drug does not cause AIDS or hep; may begin active immunization series at different Inj site if required

Tetanus Toxoid (TT) [Tetanus Prophylaxis/Vaccine] Uses: *Tetanus prophylaxis* **Action:** Active immunization **Dose:** Based on previous immunization, see Table 7 **Caution:** [C, ?] **CI:** Chloramphenicol use, neurologic Sxs w/ previous use, active Infxn w/ routine primary immunization **Disp:** Inj tetanus toxoid, fluid, 4–5 Lf units/0.5 mL; tetanus toxoid, adsorbed, 5, 10 Lf units/0.5 mL **SE:** Inj site erythema, induration, sterile abscess, chills, fever, malaise, neurologic disturbances **Interactions:** Delay of active immunity if given **W/** tetanus immune globulin; ↓ immune response if given to pts taking corticosteroids or immunosuppressive drugs **NIPE:** Stress the need of timely completion of immunization series; DTaP rather than TT or Td all adults 19–64 y who have not previously received 1 dose of DTaP (protection adult pertussis); also use DT or Td instead of TT to maintain diphtheria immunity; if IM, use only preservative-free Inj; do not confuse Td (for adults) w/ DT (for children)

Tetrabenazine (Xenazine) [Monoamine Depletory]   WARNING: ↑ Risk of depression, suicide w/ Huntington Dz Uses: * Rx chorea in Huntington Dz* **Action:** Monoamine depleter **Dose:** 25–100 mg/d ÷ doses; 12.5 mg PO/d × 1 wk, ↑ to 12.5 mg bid, may ↑ to 12.5 mg tid after 1 wk; if > 50 mg needed, ✓ for CYP2D6 gene;if poor metabolizer, 25 mg max; 50 mg/d max; extensive/indeterminate metabolizer 37.5 mg dose max, 100 mg/d max **Caution:** [C; ?/–] 1/2 dose w/ strong CYP2D6 Inhib (paroxetine, fluoxetine); wait 20 d after reserpine D/C before use **CI:** Suicidality, untreated, or inadequately treated depression; hepatic impair; w/ MOAI or reserpine **Disp:** Tabs 12.5, 25 mg **SE:** Sedation, insomnia, depression, anxiety, irritability, akathisia, Parkinsonism, balance difficulties, neuroleptic malignant synd, fatigue, N, V, dysphagia, ↑ QT **Interactions:** ↑ Risk of QT prolongation **W/** chlorpromazine, thioridazine, ziprasidone, moxifloxacin, quinidine, procainamide, amiodarone, sotalol; ↑ effects **W/** CYP2D6 Inhibs (eg, paroxetine, fluoxetine); ↑ risks of neuroleptic malignant synd & extrapyramidal synd **W/** neuroleptics, DA antagonists; ↑ CNS depression **W/** EtOH & other CNS depressants

Tetracycline (Achromycin V, Sumycin) [Antibiotic/Tetracycline]
Uses: *Broad-spectrum antibiotic* **Action:** Bacteriostatic; ↓ protein synth *Spectrum:* Gram(+): *Staphylococcus, Streptococcus.* Gram(–): *H pylori.* Others: *Chlamydia, Rickettsia, & Mycoplasma* **Dose:** *Adults.* 250–500 mg PO bid–qid *Peds > 8 y.* 25–50 mg/kg/24 h PO q6–12h; ↓ w/ renal/hepatic impair, w/o food

preferred **Caution:** [D, +] **CI:** PRG, antacids, w/ dairy products, children < 8 y **Disp:** Caps 100, 250, 500 mg; tabs 250, 500 mg; PO susp 250 mg/5 mL **SE:** Photosensitivity, GI upset, renal failure, pseudotumor cerebri, hepatic impair **Interactions:** ↑ Effects *OF* anticoagulants, digoxin; ↓ effects *W/* antacids, cimetidine, laxatives, penicillin, Fe supl, dairy products; ↓ effects *OF* OCPs **Labs:** False(−) of urinary glucose, serum folate; false ↑ serum glucose **NIPE:** ⊘ Take w/ dairy products; take w/o food; use barrier contraception; can stain tooth enamel & depress bone formation in children

Thalidomide (Thalomid) [Immunomodulatory Agent] WARNING:
Restricted use; use associated w/ severe birth defects & ↑ risk of venous thromboembolism **Uses:** *Erythema nodosum leprosum (ENL)*, GVHD, aphthous ulceration in HIV(+) **Action:** ↓ Neutrophil chemotaxis, ↓ monocyte phagocytosis **Dose:** *GVHD:* 100–1600 mg PO daily *Stomatitis:* 200 mg bid for 5 d, then 200 mg daily up to 8 wk *Erythema nodosum leprosum:* 100–300 mg PO qhs Cautions: [X, −] May ↑ HIV viral load; h/o Szs **CI:** PRG; sexually active males not using latex condoms, or females not using 2 forms of contraception **Disp:** Caps 50, 100, 200 mg **SE:** Dizziness, drowsiness, rash, fever, orthostasis, SJS, peripheral neuropathy, Szs **Interactions:** ↑ Effects *OF* barbiturates, CNS depressants, chlorpromazine, reserpine, EtOH; ↑ peripheral neuropathy *W/* INH, Li, metronidazole, phenytoin **Labs:** Monitor LFTs, WBC, differential, PRG test before start of therapy & monthly during therapy **NIPE:** If also taking drugs that ↓ hormonal contraceptives (carbamazepine, griseofulvin, phenytoin, rifabutin, rifampin) use 2 other contraceptive methods; take 1 h pc—food will affect absorption; photosensitivity—use sunblock; ⊘ PRG & breast-feeding; healthcare provider must register w/ STEPS risk management program; informed consent necessary; stat D/C if rash develops

Theophylline (Theo24, Theochron) [Bronchodilator/Xanthine Derivative]
Uses: *Asthma, bronchospasm* **Action:** Relaxes smooth muscle of the bronchi & pulm blood vessels **Dose:** *Adults.* 900 mg PO ÷ q6h; SR products may be ÷ q8–12h (maint) *Peds.* 16–22 mg/kg/24 h PO ÷ q6h; SR products may be ÷ q8–12h (maint); ↓ in hepatic failure **Caution:** [C, +] Multiple interactions (eg, caffeine, smoking, carbamazepine, barbiturates, BBs, ciprofloxacin, E-mycin, INH, loop diuretics) **CI:** Arrhythmia, hyperthyroidism, uncontrolled Szs **Disp:** Elixir 80, 15 mL; soln 80 mg/15 mL; syrup 80, 150 mg/15 mL; caps 100, 200, 250 mg; tabs 100, 125, 200, 250, 300 mg; SR caps 100, 125, 200, 260, 300 mg; SR tabs 100, 200, 300, 400, 450, 600 mg **SE:** N/V, tachycardia, Szs, nervousness, arrhythmias Notes: *Levels IV:* Sample 12–24 h after Inf started *Therapeutic:* 5–15 mcg/mL *Toxic:*> 20 mcg/mL *Levels PO:* Trough just before next dose *Therapeutic:* 5–15 mcg/mL **Interactions:** ↑ Effects *W/* allopurinol, BBs, CCBs, cimetidine, corticosteroids, macrolide antibiotics, OCPs, quinolones, rifampin, tacrine, tetracyclines, verapamil, zileuton; ↑ effects *OF* digitalis; ↓ effects *W/* barbiturates, loop diuretics, thyroid hormones, tobacco, St. John's wort; ↓ effects *OF* benzodiazepines, Li,

phenytoin **Labs:** ↑ Glucose **NIPE:** Use barrier contraception; take w/ food if GI upset; caffeine foods ↑ drug effects; smoking ↓ drug effects

Thiamine [Vitamin B₁] [Vitamin] **Uses:** *Thiamine deficiency (beriberi), alcoholic neuritis, Wernicke encephalopathy* **Action:** Dietary supl **Dose:** *Adults. Deficiency:* 100 mg/d IM for 2 wk, then 5–10 mg/d PO for 1 mo *Wernicke encephalopathy:* 100 mg IV single dose, then 100 mg/d IM for 2 wk **Peds.** 10–25 mg/d IM for 2 wk, then 5–10 mg/24 h PO for 1 mo **Caution:** [A (C if doses exceed RDA), +] **CI:** Component allergy **Disp:** Tabs 5, 10, 25, 50, 100, 250, 500 mg; Inj 100, 200 mg/mL **SE:** Angioedema, paresthesias, rash, anaphylaxis w/ rapid IV **Interactions:** ↑ Effects *OF* neuromuscular blocking drugs **Labs:** Interference w/ theophylline levels **NIPE:** IV use associated w/ anaphylactic Rxn; give IV slowly

Thiethylperazine (Torecan) [Antiemetic] **Uses:** *N/V* **Action:** Antidopaminergic antiemetic **Dose:** 10 mg PO, PR, or IM daily–tid; ↓ in hepatic failure **Caution:** [X, ?] **CI:** Phenothiazine & sulfite sensitivity, PRG **Disp:** Tabs 10 mg; supp 10 mg; Inj 5 mg/mL **SE:** EPS, xerostomia, drowsiness, orthostatic ↓ BP, tachycardia, confusion **Interactions:** ↑ Effects *W/* atropine, CNS depressants, epinephrine, Li, MAOIs, TCAs, EtOH; ↑ effects *OF* antihypertensives, phenytoin; ↓ effects *OF* bromocriptine, cabergoline, levodopa **Labs:** ↑ Serum prolactin level, interferes w/ PRG test **NIPE:** May cause tardive dyskinesia; ↑ risk of photosensitivity—use sunblock

6-Thioguanine [6-TG] (Tabloid) [Purine Antimetabolite] **Uses:** *AML, ALL, CML* **Action:** Purine-based antimetabolite (substitutes for natural purines interfering w/ nucleotide synth) **Dose:** 2–3 mg/kg/d; ↓ in severe renal/hepatic impair **Caution:** [D, −] **CI:** Resistance to mercaptopurine **Disp:** Tabs 40 mg **SE:** ↓ BM (leucopenia/thrombocytopenia), N/V/D, anorexia, stomatitis, rash, hyperuricemia, rare hepatotox **Interactions:** ↑ Bleeding *W/* anticoagulants, NSAIDs, salicylates, thrombolytics **Labs:** ↑ Serum & urine uric acid **NIPE:** Take w/o food; ↑ fluids to 2–3 L/d; ⊘ exposure to Infxn

Thiopental Sodium (Pentothal) [C-III] [Thiobarbiturate] **Uses:** *General anesthesia, short procedure anesthesia; Sz control after anesthesia, neurosurg pts w/ ↑ ICP & adequate ventilation, narcoanalysis* **Action:** Ultra–short-acting barbiturate, (hypnotic & anesthetic) **Dose:** *Adults. Anesthesia, slow induction:* 50–75 mg IV q 20–40 s, then 25–50 mg IV PRN pt moves *Anesthesia, rapid induction:* 3–4 mg/kg IV ÷ in 2–4 doses *Anesthesia, maint:* 0.2–0.4% IV, adjust to effect *Szs post-anesthesia:* 75–125 mg IV, may ↑ to 250 mg over 10 min *Neurosurg w/ ↑ ICP:* 1.5–3.5 mg/kg IV PRN *Narcoanalysis:* 100 mg/min IV, D/C when pt confused counting backwards from 100; 0.2% in D₅W at 50 mL/min max. 25–75 mg IV over 60 s to assess tolerance **Caution:** [C; +/−] Levels as low as 1 mg/dL, may be lethal **CI:** Hypersensitivity, porphyria, poor IV access **Disp:** Inj **SE:** ↓ Resp, myocardial depression, ↓ BP, hangover, laryngospasm **Interactions:** ↑ Effects *W/* probenecid; ↑ risk of hypotension *W/* diazoxide; ↓ effects *W/* zimelidine, aminophylline **NIPE:** Slow Inj ↓ risk of OD & resp depression; do not use conc < 2% in SWFI

Thioridazine (Mellaril) [Antipsychotic/Phenothiazine] WARNING:
Dose-related QT prolongation **Uses:** *Schizophrenia*, psychosis **Action:** Phenothiazine antipsychotic **Dose:** *Adults.* **Initial:** 50–100 mg PO tid; maint 200–800 mg/24 h PO in 2–4 ÷ doses *Peds > 2 y.* 0.5–3 mg/kg/24 h PO in 2–3 ÷ doses **Caution:** [C, ?] Phenothiazines, QTc-prolonging agents, Al **CI:** Phenothiazine sensitivity **Disp:** Tabs 10, 15, 25, 50, 100, 150, 200 mg; PO conc 30, 100 mg/mL **SE:** Low incidence of EPS; ventricular arrhythmias; ↓ BP, dizziness, drowsiness, neuroleptic malignant synd, Szs, skin discoloration, photosensitivity, constipation, sexual dysfunction, blood dyscrasias, pigmentary retinopathy, hepatic impair **Interactions:** ↑ Effects *W/* BBs; ↑ effects *OF* anticholinergics, antihypertensives, antihistamines, CNS depressants, nitrates, EtOH; ↓ effects *W/* barbiturates, Li, tobacco; ↓ effects *OF* levodopa **Labs:** ↑ Serum LFTs; ↓ HMG, Hct, plts, WBC **NIPE:** ↑ Risk of photosensitivity—use sunblock, take w/ food; ⊘ D/C abruptly; ↓ temperature regulation; urine color change to reddish brown; avoid EtOH, dilute PO conc in 2–4 oz Liq; monitor ECG for ↑ QT interval

Thiothixene (Navane) [Antipsychotic/Thioxanthene] WARNING: Not for dementia-related psychosis; ↑ mortality risk in elderly on antipsychotics **Uses:** *Psychosis* **Action:** ?; Antagonizes DA receptors **Dose:** *Adults & Peds > 12 y.* **Mild–mod psychosis:** 2 mg PO tid, up to 20–30 mg/d *Severe psychosis:* 5 mg PO bid; to max of 60 mg/24 h PRN *IM use:* 16–20 mg/24 h ÷ bid–qid; max 30 mg/d *Peds < 12 y.* 0.25 mg/kg/24 h PO ÷ q6–12h **Caution:** [C, ?] Avoid w/ ↑ QT interval or meds that can ↑ QT **CI:** Phenothiazine sensitivity **Disp:** Caps 1, 2, 5, 10, 20 mg; PO conc 5 mg/mL; Inj 10 mg/mL **SE:** Drowsiness, EPS most common; ↓ BP, dizziness, drowsiness, neuroleptic malignant synd, Szs, skin discoloration, photosensitivity, constipation, sexual dysfunction, blood dyscrasias, pigmentary retinopathy, hepatic impair **Interactions:** ↑ Effects *W/* BBs; ↑ effects *OF* anticholinergics, antihistamines, antihypertensives, CNS depressants, nitrates, EtOH; ↓ effects *W/* barbiturates, Li, tobacco, caffeine; ↓ effects *OF* levodopa **Labs:** ↑ LFTs **NIPE:** ↑ Risk of photosensitivity—use sunblock; take w/ food; ⊘ D/C abruptly; ↓ temperature regulation; darkens urine color to reddish brown; dilute PO conc stat before use

Thiotriethylenephosphoramide (Thiotepa, Thioplex, Tespa, TSPA) [Alkylating Agent] Uses: *Hodgkin Dz & NHLs; leukemia; breast, ovarian CAs, preparative regimens for allogeneic & ABMT w/ high doses, intravesical for bladder CA* **Action:** Polyfunctional alkylating agent **Dose:** 0.5 mg/kg q1–4wk, 6 mg/m² IM or IV × 4 d q2–4wk, 15–35 mg/m² by IV Inf over 48 h; 60 mg in bladder & retained 2 h q1–4wk; 900–125 mg/m² in ABMT regimens (max dose w/o ABMT 180 mg/m²); 1–10 mg/m² (typical 15 mg) IT 1–2×/wk; 0.8 mg/kg in 1–2 L of soln intraperitoneally; ↓ w/ renal failure **Caution:** [D, –] **CI:** Component allergy **Disp:** Inj 15, 30 mg **SE:** ↓ BM, N/V, dizziness, HA, allergy, paresthesias, alopecia; fatigue **Interactions:** ↑ Risk of tox w/ or stat following other alkylating agents (nitrogen mustards, cyclophosphamide), radiation, myelosuppressants; risk of apnea w/ succinylcholine **Labs:** Monitor CBC & plts weekly & for 3 wk post therapy; D/C if WBC < 3000 cells/mm³ or plt < 150,000 cells/mm³ **NIPE:** Intravesical use in bladder CA infrequent today; Inj site Rxns

Tiagabine (Gabitril) [Anticonvulsant] Uses: *Adjunct in partial Szs*, bipolar disorder **Action:** Antiepileptic, enhances activity of GABA **Dose:** *Adults & Peds ≥ 12 y.* Initial 4 mg/d PO, by 4 mg during 2nd wk; PRN by 4–8 mg/d based on response, 56 mg/d max; take w/ food **Caution:** [C, M] May ↑ suicidal risk **CI:** Component allergy **Disp:** Tabs 2, 4, 12, 16, 20 mg **SE:** Dizziness, HA, somnolence, memory impair, tremors **Interactions:** ↑ Effects W/ valproate; ↑ effects *OF* CNS depressants, EtOH; ↓ effects W/ barbiturates, carbamazepine, phenobarbital, phenytoin, primidone, rifampin, ginkgo **NIPE:** Take w/ food; ⊘ D/C abruptly—use gradual withdrawal; used in combo w/ other anticonvulsants

Ticarcillin/Potassium Clavulanate (Timentin) [Antibiotic/Penicillin, Beta-Lactamase Inhibitor] Uses: *Infxns of the skin, bone, resp & urinary tract, abdomen, sepsis* **Action:** Carboxy-PCN; bactericidal; ↓ cell wall synth; clavulanic acid blocks β-lactamase *Spectrum:* Good gram(+), not MRSA; good gram(−) & anaerobes **Dose:** *Adults.* 3.1 g IV q4–6h max 24 g ticarcillin component/d *Peds.* 200–300 mg/kg/d IV ÷ q4E26h; ↓ in renal failure **Caution:** [B, ±] PCN sensitivity **Disp:** Inj ticarcillin/clavulanic acid 3.1-g/0.1-g vial **SE:** Hemolytic anemia, false(+) proteinuria **Interactions:** ↑ Effects *OF* anticoagulants, MTX; ↓ effects W/ tetracyclines, ↓ effects *OF* aminoglycosides, OCPs **Labs:** False ↑ urine glucose, false(+) urine proteins **NIPE:** Monitor for S/Sxs super Infxn; frequent loose stools may be d/t pseudomembranous colitis; use barrier contraception; often used in combo w/ aminoglycosides; penetrates CNS w/ meningeal irritation

Ticlopidine (Ticlid) [Antiplatelet/Platelet Aggregation Inhibitor]
WARNING: Neutropenia/agranulocytosis, TTP, aplastic anemia reported **Uses:** *↓ Risk of thrombotic stroke*, protect grafts status postcoronary artery bypass graft, diabetic microangiopathy, ischemic heart Dz, DVT prophylaxis, graft prophylaxis after renal transplant **Action:** Plt aggregation Inhib **Dose:** 250 mg PO bid w/ food **Caution:** [B, ?/–], ↑ Tox of ASA, anticoagulation, NSAIDs, theophylline **CI:** Bleeding, hepatic impair, neutropenia, thrombocytopenia **Disp:** Tabs 250 mg **SE:** Bleeding, GI upset, rash **Interactions:** ↑ Effects W/ anticoagulants, cimetidine, dong quai, evening primrose oil, feverfew, garlic, ginkgo, ginseng, red clover; ↑ effects *OF* ASA, phenytoin, theophylline; ↓ effects W/ antacids; ↓ effects *OF* cyclosporine, digoxin **Labs:** ↑ LFTs; ↓ plts, RBCs, WBCs; monitor CBC for 1st 3 mo **NIPE:** Take w/ food; minimize or avoid invasive procedures (IV insertion, IM Inj etc), compress venipuncture sites up to 30 min

Tigecycline (Tygacil) [Antibiotic/Related to Tetracycline]
Uses: *Rx comp skin & soft-tissue Infxns & comp intra-Abd Infxns* **Action:** New class, related to tetracycline *Spectrum:* Broad gram(+), (−), anaerobic, some mycobacterial; *E coli, E faecalis* (vancomycin-susceptible isolates), *S aureus*

(methicillin-susceptible/resistant), *Streptococcus* (*agalactiae, anginosus* group, *pyogenes*), *C freundii, E cloacae, B fragilis* group, *C perfringens, Peptostreptococcus* **Dose:** *Adults.* 100 mg, then 50 mg q12h IV over 30–60 min q12h **Caution:** [D, ?] Hepatic impair, monotherapy w/ intestinal perforation, not OK in peds, w/ tetracycline allergy **CI:** Component sensitivity **Disp:** Inj 50-mg vial **SE:** N/V, Inj site Rxn **Interactions:** ↑ Risk of bleeding **W/** warfarin; ↓ effectiveness **OF** hormonal contraceptives **Labs:** ↑ LFTs, BUN, Cr, PT, PTT, INR; ↓ K⁺, HMG, Hct, WBCs **NIPE:** ⊘ w/ Children; ↑ risk of photosensitivity; monitor ECG for hypokalemia (flattened T waves)

Timolol (Blocadren) [Antihypertensive/Beta-Blocker] WARNING: Exacerbation of ischemic heart Dz w/ abrupt D/C **Uses:** *HTN & MI* **Action:** Adrenergic receptor blocker, 1, 2 **Dose:** *HTN:* 10–20 mg bid, up to 60 mg *MI:* 10 mg bid **Caution:** [C (1st tri; D if 2nd or 3rd tri), +] **CI:** CHF, cardiogenic shock, bradycardia, heart block, COPD, asthma **Disp:** Tabs 5, 10, 20 mg **SE:** Sexual dysfunction, arrhythmia, dizziness, fatigue, CHF **Interactions:** ↑ Effects **W/** antihypertensives, ciprofloxacin, fentanyl, nitrates, quinidine, reserpine; ↑ bradycardia & myocardial depression **W/** cardiac glycosides, diltiazem, reserpine, tacrine, verapamil; ↑ effects **OF** epinephrine, ergots, flecainide, lidocaine, nifedipine, phenothiazine, prazosin, verapamil; ↓ effects **W/** barbiturates, cholestyramine, colestipol, NSAIDs, penicillin, rifampin, salicylates, sulfinpyrazone, theophylline; ↓ effects **OF** hypoglycemics, sulfonylureas, theophylline **Labs:** ↑ BUN, K⁺, LFTs, uric acid **NIPE:** ⊘ D/C abruptly; ↑ cold sensitivity; monitor ECG for hyperkalemia (peaked T waves)

Timolol, Ophthalmic (Timoptic) [Antiglaucoma Agent/Beta-Blocker] **Uses:** *Glaucoma* **Action:** BB **Dose:** 0.25% 1 gt bid; ↓ to daily when controlled; use 0.5% if needed; 1 gtt/d gel **Caution:** [C (1st tri; D 2nd or 3rd), ?/+] **Disp:** Soln 0.25%/0.5%; Timoptic XE (0.25%, 0.5%) gel-forming soln **SE:** Local irritation **NIPE:** Depress lacrimal sac 1 min after administration to lessen systemic absorption; administer other drops 10 min before gel

Tinidazole (Tindamax) [Antiprotozoal/Anti-Infective] WARNING: Off-label use discouraged (animal carcinogenicity w/ other drugs in class) **Uses:** *Adults/children > 3 y: *Trichomoniasis & giardiasis; intestinal amebiasis or amebic liver abscess* **Action:** Antiprotozoal imidazole **Spectrum:** *Trichomonas vaginalis, Giardia duodenalis, Entamoeba histolytica* **Dose:** *Adults. Trichomoniasis:* 2 g PO; Rx partner *Giardiasis:* 2 g PO *Amebiasis:* 2 g PO daily × 3 d *Amebic liver abscess:* 2 g PO daily × 3–5 d *Peds. Trichomoniasis:* 50 mg/kg PO, 2 g/d max *Giardiasis:* 50 mg/kg PO, 2 g/d max *Amebiasis:* 50 mg/kg PO daily × 3 d, 2 g/d max *Amebic liver abscess:* 50 mg/kg PO daily × 3–5 d, 2 g/d max; take w/ food **Caution:** [C, D in 1st tri; –] May be cross-resistant w/ metronidazole; Sz/peripheral neuropathy may require D/C; w/ CNS/hepatic impair **CI:** Metronidazole allergy, 1st tri PRG, w/ EtOH use **Disp:** Tabs 250, 500 mg **SE:** CNS disturbances; blood dyscrasias, taste disturbances, N/V, darkens urine **Interactions:** ↑ Effects **OF** anticoagulants, cyclosporine, 5-FU, Li, phenytoin, tacrolimus; ↑ effects W/ cimetidine, ketoconazole; ↑ effects of Abd cramping, N/V, HA; ⊘ EtOH during & for 3 d after use; ⊘ w/in 2 wk of disulfiram; ↓ effects W/ cholestyramine, oxytetracycline, phenobarbital, rifampin **Labs:** ↑ LFTs **NIPE:** Crush & disperse in cherry syrup for peds; removed by HD

Tinzaparin (Innohep) [Anticoagulant/LMW Heparin] WARNING: Risk of spinal/epidural hematomas development w/ spinal anesthesia or LP **Uses:** *Rx of DVT w/ or w/o PE* **Action:** LMW heparin **Dose:** 175 units/kg SQ daily at least 6 d until warfarin dose stabilized **Caution:** [B, ?] Pork allergy, active bleeding, mild–mod renal impair, morbid obesity **CI:** Allergy to sulfites, heparin, benzyl alcohol; HIT **Disp:** Inj 20,000 units/mL **SE:** Bleeding, bruising, ↓ plts, Inj site pain **Interactions:** ↑ Bleeding W/ anticoagulants, NSAIDs, salicylates, thrombolytics **Labs:** ↑ LFTs; monitor via anti-Xa levels; no effect on bleeding time, plt Fxn, PT, aPTT **NIPE:** ⊘ Rub Inj site, administer deep SQ Inj, rotate Abd Inj sites; causes Inj site pain

Tioconazole (Vagistat) [Antifungal] Uses: *Vag fungal Infxns* **Action:** Topical antifungal **Dose:** 1 applicator-full intravag hs (single dose) **Caution:** [C, ?] **CI:** Component allergy **Disp:** Vag oint 6.5% **SE:** Local burning, itching, soreness, polyuria **Interactions:** Risk OF inactivation of nonoxynol-9 spermacidal **NIPE:** Insert high into Vag canal; may cause staining of clothing; refrain from intercourse during drug therapy; risk of latex breakdown of condoms & diaphragm

Tiotropium (Spiriva) [Bronchodilator/Anticholinergic] Uses: Bronchospasm w/ COPD, bronchitis, emphysema **Action:** Synthetic anticholinergic like atropine **Dose:** 1 caps/d inhaled using HandiHaler, *do not* use w/ spacer **Caution:** [C, ?/–] BPH, NAG, MyG, renal impair **CI:** Acute bronchospasm **Disp:** Inh caps 18 mcg **SE:** URI, xerostomia **Interactions:** ↑ Effects W/ other anticholinergic drugs **Labs:** Monitor FEV_1 or peak flow **NIPE:** ⊘ For acute resp episode; take daily at same time

Tipranavir (Aptivus) [Antiretroviral/Protease Inhibitor] WARNING: Coadministration w/ ritonavir in association w/ hep & hepatic decompensation w/ fatalities. D/C w/ S/Sxs of hep **Uses:** HIV-1 Infxn w/ highly Tx-experienced pts or HIV-1 strains resistant to multiple protease Inhibs. Must be used w/ ritonavir 200 mg **Action:** Antiretroviral HIV-1 protease Inhib **Dose:** 500 mg PO bid w/ food, administration w/ ritonavir 200 mg PO bid **Caution:** [C, –] Sulfa allergy, liver Dz **CI:** Mod–severe hepatic Insuff; concomitant use w/ amiodarone, astemizole, bepridil, cisapride, ergots, flecainide, lovastatin, midazolam, pimozide, propafenone, quinidine, rifampin, simvastatin, terfenadine, triazolam, St. John's wort **Disp:** Soft gel cap 250 mg **SE:** HA, GI distress, rash, fatigue, fat redistribution, hyperglycemia, hep, liver Dz, lipid elevations **Interactions:** ↑ Effects OF anticoagulants, antiplts, azole antifungals, CCB, clarithromycin, NNRTIs, rifabutin, sildenafil, statins, tadalafil, vardenafil; ↓ effects W/ antacids, didanosine; ↓ effects OF estrogens, methadone **Labs:** ↑ BS, LFTs, lipids, monitor baseline & periodically **NIPE:** ↑ Bioavailability w/ high-fat meals; monitor for bleeding in pts w/ hemophilia

Tirofiban (Aggrastat) [Antiplatelet Agent] Uses: *Acute coronary synd* **Action:** Glycoprotein IIB/IIIA Inhib **Dose:** Initial 0.4 mcg/kg/min for 30 min, followed by 0.1 mcg/kg/min 12–24 h; use in combo w/ heparin *ECC 2010:* ACS or PCI: 0.4 mcg/kg/min IV for 30 min, then 0.1 mcg/kg/min for 18–24 h post PCI ↓ in renal Insuff **Caution:** [B, ?/–] **CI:** Bleeding, intracranial neoplasm, vascular malformation, stroke/surgery/trauma w/in last 30 d, severe HTN **Disp:** Inj 50, 250 mcg/mL **SE:** Bleeding, bradycardia, coronary dissection, pelvic pain, rash **Interactions:** ↑ Bleeding risks W/ anticoagulants, antiplts, NSAIDs, salicylates, dong quai, feverfew, garlic, ginger, ginkgo, horse chestnut; ↓ effects W/ levothyroxine, omeprazole **Labs:** ↓ HMG, Hct, plts **NIPE:** ⊘ Breast-feeding

Tizanidine Hydrochloride (Zanaflex) [Alpha-2-Adrenergic Agonist] Uses: Muscle spasticity **Action:** Agonist at central α-adrenergic receptor sites **Dose:** *Adults.* 4 mg q6–8h PRN to a max of 3 doses/24 h; ↑ by 2–4 mg reaching optimum dose by 2–4 wk; max is 36 mg/d; ↓ w/ CrCl < 25 mL/min *Peds:* Not recommended **Caution:** [C, ?/–] **CI:** Concomitant fluvoxamine, ciprofloxacin **Disp:** Caps 2,4,6 mg; tabs 2,4 mg **SE:** Dry mouth, somnolence, dizziness, constipation, blurred vision, hypotension, bradycardia, hallucinations/psychosis, UTI **Interactions:** ↑ Hypotension W/ other antihypertensives; ↑ CNS depression W/ baclofen, benzodiazepines, other CNS depressants; EtOH; ↑ effects W/ CYP1A2 Inhibs (amiodarone, mexiletine, propafenone, verapamil, cimetidine, famotidine, other fluoroquinolones, acyclovir, ticlopidine, zileuton, OCP) **Labs:** ↑ AST, ALT, ✓ LFT **NIPE:** Monitor BP; do not D/C abruptly; taper dose; tabs ≠ caps

Tobramycin (Nebcin) [Antibiotic/Aminoglycoside] Uses: *Serious gram(–) Infxns* **Action:** Aminoglycoside; ↓ protein synth *Spectrum:* Gram(–) bacteria (including *Pseudomonas*) **Dose:** *Adults.* Conventional dosing: 1–2.5 mg/kg/dose IV q8–12h *Once-daily dosing:* 5–7 mg/kg/dose q24h *Peds.* 2.5 mg/kg/dose IV q8h; ↓ w/ renal Insuff **Caution:** [C, M] **CI:** Aminoglycoside sensitivity **Disp:** Inj 10, 40 mg/mL **SE:** Nephro- & ototox Notes: Levels: *Peak:* 30 min after Inf *Trough:* < 0.5 h before next dose *Therapeutic conventional: Peak:* 5–10 mcg/mL *Trough:* < 2 mcg/mL **Interactions:** ↑ Effects W/ indomethacin; ↑ nephro-, neuro-, and/or ototox effects W/ aminoglycosides, amphotericin B, cephalosporins, cisplatin, IV loop diuretics, methoxyflurane, vancomycin **Labs:** ↑BUN, Cr; ↓ serum K^+, Na^+, Ca^{2+}, Mg^{2+}, plt, WBC; follow CrCl & levels **NIPE:** ↑ Fluids to 2–3 L/d; monitor for super Infxn; monitor ECG for hypokalemia (flattened T waves)

Tobramycin Ophthalmic (AKTob, Tobrex) [Antibiotic/Aminoglycoside] Uses: *Ocular bacterial Infxns* **Action:** Aminoglycoside **Dose:** 1–2 gtt q4h; oint bid–tid; if severe, use oint q3–4h, or 2 gtt q30–60 min, then less frequently **Caution:** [C, M] **CI:** Aminoglycoside sensitivity **Disp:** Oint & soln tobramycin 0.3% **SE:** Ocular irritation **NIPE:** Depress lacrimal sac for 1 min to prevent systemic absorption; ↑ risk of blurred vision & burning

Tobramycin & Dexamethasone Ophthalmic (TobraDex) [Antibiotic/Anti-Inflammatory] Uses: *Ocular bacterial Infxns associated w/ sig inflammation* **Action:** Antibiotic w/ anti-inflammatory **Dose:** 0.3% Oint apply q3–8h or soln 0.3% apply 1–2 gtt q1–4h **Caution:** [C, M] **CI:** Aminoglycoside sensitivity **Disp:** Oint & susp 2.5, 5, 10 mL tobramycin 0.3% & dexamethasone 0.1% **SE:** Local irritation/edema **NIPE:** Eval IOP & lens if prolonged use; use under ophthalmologist's direction

Tocilizumab (Actemra)[Interleukin-6 Receptor Inhibitor] **WARNING:** May cause serious Infxn (TB, bacterial, invasive fungal, viral, opportunistic); w/ serious Infxn D/C tocilizumab until Infxn controlled **Uses:** *Mod/severe RA, SJIA* **Action:** IL-6 receptor Inhib **Dose:** RA 4–8 mg/kg; SJIA if < 30 kg 12 mg/ kg; if > 30 kg 8 mg/kg **Caution:** [C; ?/–] **CI:** ANC < 2000/mm³, plt count < 100,000, AST/ALT > 1.5 ULN; serious Infxn; high-risk bowel perforation **Disp:** Inj **SE:** URI, nasopharyngitis, HA, HTN **Interactions:** ↑ Risk of Infxn W/ concomitant immunosuppressants (eg, TNF antagonists IL-1R antagonists, anti-CD20 MoAb, selective costimulation modulators) **Labs:** ↑ALT, ↑AST, ↑LDL ↓ANC; ✓ CBC/plt counts, LFTs, lipids; monitor lipids 4–8 wk after initiation, then every 6 mo **NIPE:** Do not give live vaccines; PPD, if + treat before starting, w/ prior Hx retreat unless adequate Tx confirmed, monitor for TB, even if –PPD; ↓ mRNA expression of several CYP450 isoenzymes (CYP3A4)

Tolazamide (Tolinase) [Hypoglycemic/Sulfonylurea] Uses: *Type 2 DM* **Action:** Sulfonylurea; ↑ pancreatic insulin release; ↑ peripheral insulin sensitivity; ↓ hepatic glucose output **Dose:** 100–500 mg/d (no benefit > 1 g/d) **Caution:** [C, +/–] Elderly, hepatic or renal impair **Disp:** Tabs 100, 250, 500 mg **SE:** HA, dizziness, GI upset, rash, hyperglycemia, photosensitivity, blood dyscrasias **Interactions:** BB may mask hypoglycemia; ↑ effects W/ chloramphenicol, cimetidine, clofibrate, insulin, MAOIs, phenylbutazone, probenecid, salicylates, sulfonamides, garlic, ginseng; ↓ effects W/ diuretics **NIPE:** Risk of disulfiram-type Rxn w/ EtOH; take w/ food; use sunblock

Tolazoline (Priscoline) [Alpha-Adrenergic Antagonist] Uses: *Peripheral vasospastic disorders, persistent pulm hypertension of newborn* **Action:** Competitively blocks α-adrenergic receptors **Dose:** *Adults.* 10–50 mg IM/ IV/SQ qid *Neonates.* 1–2 mg/kg IV over 10–15 min, then 1–2 mg/kg/h (adjust w/ ↓ renal Fxn) **Caution:** [C, ?] Avoid alcohol, w/ CAD, renal impair, CVA, PUD, ↓ BP **CI:** CAD **Disp:** Inj 25 mg/mL **SE:** ↓ BP, peripheral vasodilation, tachycardia, arrhythmias, GI upset & bleeding, blood dyscrasias, renal failure **Interactions:** ↓ BP W/ epinephrine, norepinephrine, phenylephrine **NIPE:** Risk of disulfiram-type Rxn w/ EtOH

Tolbutamide (Orinase) [Hypoglycemic/Sulfonylurea] Uses: *Type 2 DM* **Action:** Sulfonylurea; ↑ pancreatic insulin release; ↑ peripheral insulin sensitivity; ↓ hepatic glucose output **Dose:** 500–1000 mg bid; 3 g/d max; ↓ in hepatic failure **Caution:** [C, +] **CI:** Sulfonylurea sensitivity **Disp:** Tabs 250, 500 mg **SE:** HA, dizziness, GI upset, rash, photosensitivity, blood dyscrasias, hypoglycemia, heartburn **Interactions:** ↑ Effects W/ anticoagulants, azole antifungals, chloramphenicol, insulin, H₂-antagonists, MAOIs, metformin, phenylbutazone, probenecid, salicylates, sulfonamides, TCAs; ↓ effects W/ BBs (can mask hypoglycemia), CCBs, cholestyramine, corticosteroids, hydantoins, INH, OCPs, phenothiazine, phenytoin, rifampin, sympathomimetics, thiazides, thyroid drugs NIPE: Risk of disulfiram-type Rxn w/ EtOH; take w/ food; use barrier contraception; ↑ risk of photosensitivity—use sunblock

Tolcapone (Tasmar) [Anti-Parkinson Agent/COMT Inhibitor]
WARNING: Cases of fulminant liver failure resulting in death have occurred Uses: *Adjunct to carbidopa/levodopa in Parkinson Dz* Action: COMT Inhib slows levodopa metabolism Dose: 100 mg PO tid w/ 1st daily levodopa/carbidopa dose, then dose 6 & 12 h later; ↓ w/ renal Insuff Caution: [C, ?] CI: Hepatic impair; w/ nonselective MAOI Disp: Tabs 100, 200 mg SE: Constipation, xerostomia, vivid dreams, hallucinations, anorexia, N/D, orthostasis, liver failure, rhabdomyolysis Interactions: ↑ Effects OF CNS depressants, SSRIs, TCAs, warfarin, EtOH; ↑ risk of hypertensive crisis W/ nonselective MAOIs (phenelzine, tranylcypromine) Labs: Monitor LFTs NIPE: May give w/o regard to food but food ↓ bioavailability of drug; may experience hallucinations; do not abruptly D/C or ↓ dose

Tolmetin (Tolectin) [Analgesic, Anti-Inflammatory, Antipyretic/NSAID] WARNING: May ↑ risk of CV events & GI bleeding Uses: *Arthritis & pain* Action: NSAID; ↓ prostaglandins Dose: 200–600 mg PO tid; 2000 mg/d max Caution: [C (D in 3rd tri or near term), +] CI: NSAID or ASA sensitivity; use for pain postcoronary artery bypass graft Disp: Tabs 200, 600 mg; caps 400 mg SE: Dizziness, rash, GI upset, edema, GI bleeding, renal failure Interactions: ↑ Effect OF aminoglycosides, anticoagulants, cyclosporine, digoxin, insulin, Li, MRX, K⁺-sparing diuretics, sulfonylureas; ↓ effect W/ ASA, food; ↓ effect OF furosemide, thiazides Labs: ↑ ALT, AST, serum K⁺, BUN, ↓ HMG, Hct NIPE: Take w/ food if GI upset; ↑ risk of photosensitivity—use sunblock; monitor ECG for hyperkalemia (peaked T waves)

Tolnaftate (Tinactin) [OTC] [Antifungal] Uses: *Tinea pedis, cruris, corporis, manus, versicolor* Action: Topical antifungal Dose: Apply to area bid for 2–4 wk Caution: [C, ?] CI: Nail & scalp Infxns Disp: OTC 1% Liq; gel; powder; topical cream; oint, powder, spray soln SE: Local irritation NIPE: Avoid ocular contact; Infxn should improve in 7–10 d; ⊘ w/ children < 2 y

Tolterodine (Detrol, Detrol LA) [Anticholinergic/Muscarinic Antagonist] Uses: *OAB (frequency, urgency, incontinence)* Action: Anticholinergic Dose: Detrol: 1–2 mg PO bid Detrol LA: 2–4 mg PO daily Caution: [C, ?/–] w/ CYP2D6 & 3A3/4 Inhib (Table 10) CI: Urinary retention, gastric retention, or uncontrolled NAG Disp: Tabs 1, 2 mg; Detrol LA tabs 2, 4 mg SE: Xerostomia, blurred vision, HA, constipation Interactions: ↑ Effects W/ azole antifungals, macrolides, grapefruit juice, food; ↑ anticholinergic effects W/ amantadine, amoxapine, bupropion, clozapine, cyclobenzaprine, disopyramide, olanzapine, phenothiazine, TCAs NIPE: May cause blurred vision; LA form may see "intact" pill in stool

Tolvaptan (Samsca) [Vasopressin V₂-Receptor Antagonist]
WARNING: Hospital use only w/ close monitoring of Na⁺ **Uses:** *Hypervolemic or euvolemic ↓ Na⁺** **Action:** Vasopressin V₂-receptor antagonist **Dose:** *Adults.* 15 mg PO daily; after ≥ 24 h, may ↑ to 30 mg × 1 daily; max 60 mg ×1 daily; titrate at 24-h intervals to Na⁺ goal **Caution:** [C, −] Monitor Na⁺, vol, neurologic status; GI bleed risk w/ cirrhosis, avoid w/ CYP3A inducers & mod Inhib, ↓ dose w/ P-gp Inhib, ↑ K⁺ (monitor K⁺) **CI:** Hypovolemic hyponatremia; urgent need to raise Na⁺; in pts incapable of sensing/reacting to thirst; anuria; w/ strong CYP3A Inhib **Disp:** Tabs 15, 30 mg **SE:** N, xerostomia, pollakiuria, polyuria, thirst, weakness, constipation, hyperglycemia **Interactions:** Do not use **W/** strong Inhibs of CYP3A (amiodarone, amprenavir, atazanavir, ciprofloxacin, cisapride, clarithromycin, dilttiazem, erythromycin, fluconazole, fluvoxamine, indinavir, itraconazole, ketoconazole, nefazodone, verapamil, grapefruit juice); avoid concomitant use **W/** CYP3A inducers (carbamazepine, efavirenz, glucocorticoids, macrolides, nevirapine, phenytoin, phenobarbital, rifabutin, rifampicine, rifampin, St. John's wort) (see Table 10) **NIPE:** Pts can & should drink in response to thirst; too rapid correction of serum Na (> 12 mEq/L/24 h) can cause serious neurologic sequelae (osmotic demyelination resulting in dysarthria, mutism, dysphagia, lethargy, effective changes, spastic quadriparesis, Szs, coma & death)

Topiramate (Topamax) [Anticonvulsant] **Uses:** *Adjunctive Rx for complex partial Szs & tonic–clonic Szs*, bipolar disorder, neuropathic pain, migraine prophylaxis **Action:** Anticonvulsant **Dose:** *Adults.* Neuropathic pain, *Szs:* Total dose 400 mg/d; see package insert for 8-wk titration schedule *Migraine prophylaxis:* Titrate 100 mg/d total *Peds 2–16 y.* Initial: 1–3 mg/kg/d PO qhs; titrate per insert to 5–9 mg/kg/d; ↓ w/ renal impair **Caution:** [C, ?/−] **CI:** Component allergy **Disp:** Tabs 25, 50, 100, 200 mg; caps sprinkles 15, 25, 50 mg **SE:** Wgt loss, memory impair, metabolic acidosis, kidney stones, fatigue, dizziness, psychomotor slowing, paresthesias, GI upset, tremor, nystagmus, acute glaucoma requiring D/C **Interactions:** ↑ CNS effects **W/** CNS depressants, EtOH; ↑ effects **OF** phenytoin; ↓ effects **W/** carbamazepine, phenytoin, valproate, ginkgo; ↓ effects **OF** digoxin, OCPs **Labs:** ↑ LFTs **NIPE:** Take w/o regard to food; ⊘ D/C abruptly; use barrier contraception; ↑ fluids to 2–3 L/d; metabolic acidosis responsive to ↓ dose or D/C; D/C w/ taper

Topotecan (Hycamtin) [Antineoplastic] **WARNING:** Chemotherapy precautions, for use by physicians familiar w/ chemotherapeutic agents, BM suppression possible **Uses:** *Ovarian CA (cisplatin-refractory), cervical CA, NSCLC*, sarcoma, ped NSCLC **Action:** Topoisomerase I Inhib **Dose:** 1.5 mg/m²/d as a 1-h IV Inf × 5 d, repeat q3wk; ↓ w/ renal impair **Caution:** [D, −] **CI:** PRG, breast-feeding **Disp:** Inj 4-mg vials **SE:** ↓ BM, N/V/D, drug fever, skin rash **Interactions:** ↑ Myelosuppression **W/** cisplatin, other neoplastic drugs, radiation therapy; ↑ in duration of neutropenia **W/** filgrastim **Labs:** ↑ AST, ALT, bilirubin; ↓ HMG, Hct, plt, WBCs **NIPE:** Monitor CBC; ⊘ PRG, breast-feeding, immunizations; ⊘ exposure to Infxn; use barrier contraception

Torsemide (Demadex) [Antihypertensive/Loop Diuretic] Uses: *Edema, HTN, CHF, & hepatic cirrhosis* Action: Loop diuretic; ↓ reabsorption of Na^+ & Cl^- in ascending loop of Henle & distal tubule Dose: 5–20 mg/d PO or IV; 200 mg/d max Caution: [B, ?] CI: Sulfonylurea sensitivity Disp: Tabs 5, 10, 20, 100 mg; Inj 10 mg/mL SE: Orthostatic ↓ BP, HA, dizziness, photosensitivity, lytes imbalance, blurred vision, renal impair Interactions: ↑ Risk of ototox W/ aminoglycosides, cisplatin; ↑ effects W/ thiazides; ↑ effects OF anticoagulants, antihypertensives, Li, salicylates; ↓ effects W/ barbiturates, carbamazepine, cholestyramine, NSAIDs, phenytoin, phenobarbital, probenecid, dandelion Labs: Monitor lytes, BUN, Cr, glucose, uric acid NIPE: Take w/o regard to food; monitor for S/Sxs tinnitus; 10–20 mg torsemide = 40 mg furosemide = 1 mg bumetanide; monitor ECG for hypokalemia (flattened T waves)

Tramadol (Rybix ODT, Ryzolt ER, Ultram, Ultram ER) [Centrally Acting Analgesic/Nonnarcotic] Uses: *Mod–severe pain* Action: Centrally acting analgesic Dose: Adults. 50–100 mg PO q4–6h PRN, start 25 mg PO qAM, ↑ q3d to 25 mg PO qid; ↑ 50 mg q3d, 400 mg/d max (300 mg if > 75 y); ER 100–300 mg PO daily; Rybix ODT individualize ↑ 50 mg/d q3d to 200 mg/d or 50 mg qid; after titration 50–100 mg q4–6h PRN, 400 mg/d max Peds. (ER form not recorded) 0.5–1 mg/kg PO q4–6h PRN; ↓ w/ renal Insuff Caution: [C, ?/–] CI: Opioid dependency; w/ MAOIs; sensitivity to codeine Disp: Tabs 50 mg; ER 100, 200, 300 mg;Rybix ODT 50 mg SE: Dizziness, HA, somnolence, GI upset, resp depression, anaphylaxis Interactions: ↑ Effects W/ antihistamines, CNS depressants, phenothiazine, quinidine, TCAs, EtOH; ↑ risk of serotonin synd W/ MAOIs, St. John's wort; ↑ effects OF digoxin, warfarin; ↓ effects W/ carbamazepine Labs: ↑ Cr, LFTs; ↑ HMG NIPE: Take w/o regard to food; do not cut, chew ODT tabs; ↓ Sz threshold; tolerance/dependence may develop; has mu-opioid agonist activity; monitor for abuse

Tramadol/Acetaminophen (Ultracet) [Centrally Acting Analgesic/Nonnarcotic] Uses: *Short-term Rx acute pain (< 5 d)* Action: Centrally acting analgesic; nonnarcotic analgesic Dose: 2 tabs PO q4–6h PRN; 8 tabs/d max Elderly/renal impair: Lowest possible dose; 2 tabs q12h max if CrCl < 30 mL/min Caution: [C, –] Szs, hepatic/renal impair, or h/o addictive tendencies CI: Acute intoxication Disp: Tab 37.5 mg tramadol/325 mg APAP SE: SSRIs, TCAs, opioids, MAOIs ↑ risk of Szs; dizziness, somnolence, tremor, HA, N/V/D, constipation, xerostomia, liver tox, rash, pruritus, ↑ sweating, physical dependence Interactions: ↑ Effects W/ CNS depressants, MAOIs, phenothiazines, quinidine, TCAs, EtOH; ↑ risk of serotonin synd W/ MAOIs, St. John's wort; ↑ effects OF digoxin, warfarin; ↓ effects W/ carbamazepine Labs: ↑ Cr, LFTs, ↓ HMG NIPE: Take w/o regard to food; ⊘ take other APAP-containing drugs; avoid EtOH; has mu-opioid agonist activity; monitor for abuse

Trandolapril (Mavik) [Antihypertensive/ACEI] WARNING: Use in PRG in 2nd/3rd tri can result in fetal death Uses: *HTN*, HF, LVD, post-AMI

Action: ACE Inhib **Dose:** *HTN:* 1–4 mg/d *HF/LVD:* Start 1 mg/d, titrate to 4 mg/d; ↓ w/ severe renal/hepatic impair **Caution:** [D, +] ACE Inhib sensitivity, angioedema w/ ACE Inhibs **Disp:** Tabs 1, 2, 4 mg **SE:** ↓ BP, bradycardia, dizziness, GI upset, renal impair, cough, angioedema **Interactions:** ↑ Effects *W/* diuretics; ↑ effects *OF* insulin, Li; ↓ effects *W/* ASA, NSAIDs **Labs:** ↑ K⁺ **NIPE:** ◎ Take if PRG or breast-feeding; ⊘ K⁺-containing salt substitutes; African Americans minimum dose is 2 mg vs 1 mg in whites; monitor ECG for hyperkalemia (peaked T waves)

Tranexamic Acid (Lysteda) [Antifibrinolytic] **Uses:** *↓ Cyclic heavy menstrual bleeding* **Action:** ↓ Dissolution of hemostatic fibrin by plasmin **Dose:** 2 Tabs tid (3900 mg/d) 5 d max during monthly menstruation; ↓ w/ renal impair (see label) **Caution:** [B, +/–] ↑ Thrombosis risk; w/ subarachnoid hemorrhage **CI:** Component sensitivity; active or ↑ thrombosis risk **Disp:** Tabs 650 mg **SE:** HA, sinus & nasal Sxs, Abd pain, back/musculoskeletal/Jt pains, cramps, migraine, anemia, fatigue, retinal/ocular occlusion; allergic RXns **Interactions:** ↑ Risk of MI/ CVA *W/* hormonal contraceptives, Factor IX products, anti-Inhib coagulant concentrates, oral tretinoin

Tranylcypromine (Parnate) [MAOI] **WARNING:** Antidepressants ↑ risk of suicidal thinking & behavior in children & adolescents w/ major depressive & other psychiatric disorders **Uses:** *Depression* **Action:** MAOI **Dose:** 30 mg/d PO ÷ doses, may ↑ 10 mg/d over 1–3 wk to max 60 mg/d **Caution:** [C; +/–] Buspirone, bupropion **CI:** CV Dz, cerebrovascular defects, Pheo **Disp:** Tabs 10 mg **SE:** Orthostatic hypotension, ↑ HR, sexual dysfunction, xerostomia **Interactions:** ↑ Risk of hypertensive crisis *W/* sympathomimetics (eg, amphetamines, pseudoephedrine), levodopa, high-tyramine foods (eg, cheese, salami, chocolate, wine, beer, yogurt, broad beans, yeast); ↑ CNS depression *W/* other CNS depressants (eg, MAOIs, TCAs, SSRI, SNRIs, EtOH, opiates, buspirone); ↑ risk of psychosis *W/* dextromethorphan; ↑ risk of circulatory collapse, coma/ death *W/* meperidine **Labs:** False(+) amphetamine drug test **NIPE:** Minimize foods *W/* tyramine; do not abruptly D/C; may mask angina pain; may potentiate anxiety or agitation

Trastuzumab (Herceptin) [Antineoplastic/Monoclonal Antibody] **WARNING:** Can cause cardiomyopathy & ventricular dysfunction; Inf Rxns & pulm tox reported **Uses:** *Mets breast CA that overexpress the HER2/neu protein*, breast CA adjuvant, w/ doxorubicin, cyclophosphamide, & paclitaxel if pt HER2/ neu(+) **Action:** MoAb; binds human EGFR 2 protein (HER2); mediates cellular cytotox **Dose:** Per protocol, typical 2 mg/kg/IV/wk **Caution:** [B, ?] CV dysfunction, allergy/Inf Rxns **CI:** Live vaccines **Disp:** Inj form 21 mg/mL **SE:** Anemia, cardiomyopathy, nephrotic synd, pneumonitis **Interactions:** ↑ Risk of cardiac dysfunction *W/* anthracyclines, cyclophosphamide, doxorubicin, epirubicin **Labs:** Monitor cardiac Fxn cardiomyopathy, ventricular dysfunction, & pulm tox have been reported; ↓ HMG, Hct, WBCs **NIPE:** ⊘ Use dextrose Inf soln; ⊘ breast-feed for 6 mo following drug therapy; Inf-related Rxns minimized w/ APAP, diphenhydramine, & meperidine

Trazodone (Desyrel, Oleptro) [Antidepressant] WARNING: Closely monitor for worsening depression or emergence of suicidality, particularly in pts < 24 y; Oleptro not approved in peds Uses: *Depression*, hypnotic, augment other antidepressants Action: Antidepressant; ↓ reuptake of serotonin & norepinephrine Dose: *Adults & Adolescents. Desyrel:* 50–150 mg PO daily–qid; max 600 mg/d *Sleep:* 50 mg PO, qhs, PRN *Adults. Oleptro:* Start 150 mg PO qd, may ↑ by 75 mg q3d; take qhs on empty stomach Caution: [C, ?/–] Serotonin/neuroleptic malignant synds reported; ↑ QTc; may activate manic states; syncope reported; may ↑ bleeding risk; avoid w/in 14 d of MAOI CI: Component allergy Disp: *Desyrel* tabs 50, 100, 150, 300 mg; *Oleptro* scored tabs 150, 300 mg SE: Dizziness, HA, sedation, N, xerostomia, syncope, confusion, tremor, hep, EPS Interactions: ↑ Effects *W/* fluoxetine, phenothiazines; ↑ risk of serotonin synd *W/* MAOIs, SSRIs, venlafaxine, St. John's wort; ↑ CNS depression *W/* barbiturates, CNS depressants, opioids, sedatives, EtOH; ↑ hypotension *W/* antihypertensive, neuroleptics; nitrates, EtOH; ↑ effects *OF* clonidine, digoxin, phenytoin; ↓ effects *W/* potent CYP3A4 inducers (carbamazepine) (Table 10); CYP3A4 Inhibs to ↑ trazodone conc (nefazodone, ritonavir, indinavir, ketoconazole, itraconazole) (see Table 10) NIPE: ↑ Fluids to 2–3 L/d; ⊘ D/C abruptly; takes 1–2 wk for Sx improvement

Treprostinil Sodium (Remodulin, Tyvaso) [Antihypertensive/Vasodilator] Uses: *NYHA Class II–IV pulm arterial HTN* Action: Vasodilation, inhibits plt aggregation Dose: *Remodulin* 0.625–1.25 ng/kg/min cont Inf/SQ (preferred), titrate to effect *Tyvaso:* Initial: 18 mcg (3 Inhs) q4h 4 times/d; if not tolerated, ↓ to 1–2 Inhs, then ↑ to 3 Inhs *Maint:* ↑ additional–3 Inhs 1–2 wk intervals; 54 mcg (or 9 Inhs) 4 × /d max Caution: [B, ?/–] CI: Component allergy Disp: *Remodulin:* Inj 1, 2.5, 5, 10 mg/mL *Tyvaso:* 0.6 mg/mL (2.9 mL) ~ 6 mcg/Inh SE: Inf site Rxns; D (25%), N (22%), HA (27%), ↓ BP Interactions: ↑ Effects *W/* CYP2C8 Inhibs (eg, gemfibrozil); ↑ risk of hypotension *W/* antihypertensives, diuretics, other vasodilators; ↑ risk of bleeding *W/* anticoagulants; ↓ effects *W/* CYP2C8 inducers (eg, rifampin) NIPE: Teach care of Inf site & pump; use barrier contraception; once med vial used discard after 14 d; initiate in monitored setting; do not D/C or ↓ dose abruptly (risk of rebound HTN)

Tretinoin, Topical [Retinoic Acid] (Avita, Retin-A, Renova, Retin-A Micro) [Retinoid/Antineoplastic] Uses: *Acne vulgaris, sun-damaged skin, wrinkles* (photo aging), some skin CAs Action: Exfoliant retinoic acid derivative Dose: *Adults & Peds > 12 y.* Apply daily hs (w/ irritation, ↓ frequency) *Photoaging:* Start w/ 0.025%, ↑ to 0.1% over several mo (apply only q3d if on neck area; dark skin may require bid use) Caution: [C, ?] CI: Retinoid sensitivity Disp: Cream 0.02%, 0.025%, 0.05%, 0.1%; gel 0.01%, 0.025%; microformulation gel 0.1%, 0.04%; Liq 0.05% SE: Avoid sunlight; edema; skin dryness, erythema, scaling, changes in pigmentation, stinging, photosensitivity Interactions:

↑ Photosensitivity W/ quinolones, phenothiazines, sulfonamides, tetracyclines, thiazides, dong quai, St. John's wort; ↑ skin irritation W/ topical sulfur, resorcinol, benzoyl peroxide, salicylic acid; ↑ effects W/ vit A supl & foods W/ excess vit A such as fish oils NIPE: ⊘ Apply to mucous membranes, wash skin & apply med after 30 min, wash hands after application; ⊘ breast-feeding, PRG use contraception; use sunblock

Triamcinolone (Azmacort) [Anti-Inflammatory/Corticosteroid]
Uses: *Chronic asthma* Actions: Topical steroid Dose: 2 Inh tid–qid or 4 Inh bid Caution: [C, ?] CI: Component allergy Disp: Aerosol, metered inhaler 100-mcg spray SE: Cough, oral candidiasis Interactions: ↑ Risk of GI bleed W/ ASA, NSAIDs; ↑ effects W/ salmeterol, troleandomycin; ↓ effects W/ barbiturates, hydantoins, phenytoin, rifampin; ↓ effects OF diuretics, insulin, oral hypoglycemics, K+ supl, salicylates, somatrem, live virus vaccines Labs: ↑ Glucose, cholesterol; ↓ serum Ca, K+ NIPE: Use bronchodilator several min before triamcinolone; allow 1 min between repeat Inhs; instruct pts to rinse mouth after use; not for acute asthma; monitor ECG for hypokalemia (flattened T waves)

Triamcinolone & Nystatin (Mycolog-II) [Anti-Inflammatory, Antifungal/Corticosteroid]
Uses: *Cutaneous candidiasis* Action: Antifungal & anti-inflammatory Dose: Apply lightly to area bid; max 25 mg/d Caution: [C, ?] CI: Varicella; systemic fungal Infxns Disp: Cream & oint 15, 30, 60, 120 mg SE: Local irritation, hypertrichosis, pigmentation changes Interactions: ↓ Effects W/ barbiturates, phenytoin, rifampin; ↓ effects OF salicylates, vaccines NIPE: ⊘ Eyes; ⊘ apply to open wounds/mucous membranes; for short-term use (< 7 d)

Triamterene (Dyrenium) [Diuretic/Potassium-Sparing Agent]
Uses: *Edema associated w/ CHF, cirrhosis* Action: K+-sparing diuretic Dose: Adults. 100–300 mg/24 h PO ÷ daily–bid Peds. HTN: 2–4 mg/kg/d in 1–2 ÷ doses; ↓ w/ renal/hepatic impair Caution: [B (manufacturer; D ed. opinion), ?/–] CI: ↑ K+, renal impair; caution w/ other K+-sparing diuretics Disp: Caps 50, 100 mg SE: ↑ K+, blood dyscrasias, liver damage, other Rxns Interactions: ↑ Risk of hyperkalemia W/ ACEIs, K+ supls, K+-sparing drugs, K+-containing drugs, K+ salt substitutes; ↑ effects W/ cimetidine, indomethacin; ↑ effects OF amantadine, antihypertensives, Li; ↓ effects OF digitalis Labs: ↑ LFTs, BUN, Cr, glucose, uric acid; ↓ HMG, Hct, plt, K+ NIPE: Take w/ food, blue discoloration of urine, ↑ risk of photosensitivity—use sunblock

Triazolam (Halcion) [C-IV] [Sedative/Hypnotic/Benzodiazepine]
Uses: *Short-term management of insomnia* Action: Benzodiazepine Dose: 0.125–0.25 mg/d PO hs PRN; ↓ in elderly Caution: [X, ?/–] CI: NAG; cirrhosis; concurrent fosamprenavir, ritonavir, nelfinavir, itraconazole, ketoconazole, nefazodone Disp: Tabs 0.125, 0.25 mg SE: Tachycardia, CP, drowsiness, fatigue, memory impair, GI upset Interactions: ↑ Effects W/ azole antifungals, cimetidine, clarithromycin, ciprofloxin, CNS depressants, disulfiram, digoxin, erythromycin, fluvoxamine, INH, protease Inhibs, troleandomycin, verapamil, EtOH, grapefruit

juice, kava kava, valerian; additive CNS depression W/ EtOH & other CNS depressants; ↓ effects OF levodopa; ↓ effects W/ carbamazepine, phenytoin, rifampin, theophylline NIPE: ⊘ PRG or breast-feeding; ⊘ D/C abruptly after long-term use; do not prescribe > 1 mo supply

Triethanolamine (Cerumenex) [OTC] [Ceruminolytic Agent] Uses: *Cerumen (ear wax) removal* Action: Ceruminolytic agent Dose: Fill ear canal & insert cotton plug; irrigate w/ H_2O after 15 min; repeat PRN Caution: [C, ?] CI: Perforated tympanic membrane, otitis media Disp: Soln 10, 16, 12 mL SE: Local dermatitis, pain, erythema, pruritus NIPE: Warm soln to body temperature before use for better effect

Triethylenethiophosphoramide (Thiotepa, Thioplex, Tespa, TSPA) [Alkylating Agent] Uses: *Hodgkin Dz & NHLs; leukemia; breast, ovarian CAs, preparative regimens for allogeneic & ABMT w/ high doses, intravesical for bladder CA* Action: Polyfunctional alkylating agent Dose: 0.5 mg/kg q1 alkylating agent breast, ova q25 mg/kg q1 alkylating agent breast, ova 8 h; 60 mg into the bladder & retained 2 h q1/kg q1 alkylating agent breast, ova 8 h; 60 mg into the bladder 180 mg/m². 1 alkylating agent breast, ova 8 h; 60 mg into the bladder & retain soln may be instilled intraperitoneally; ↓ in renal failure Caution: [D, –] CI: Component allergy Disp: Inj 15, 30 mg SE: ↓ alopecia Interactions: ↑ Tox W/ concomitant or sequential alkylating agents (nitrogen mustards, cyclophosphamide), radiation, myelosuppressants Labs: Monitor LFT, BUN, Scr; Monitor HMG & plts weekly during Tx & 3wks> therapy; D/C if WBC ≤ 3000/mm³ or plt ≤ 150,000/mm³ NIPE: Intravesical use in bladder CA infrequent today; avoid fluids 8–12 h prior to Tx; use contraception

Trifluoperazine (Stelazine) [Antipsychotic/Phenothiazine] Uses: *Psychotic disorders* Action: Phenothiazine; blocks postsynaptic CNS dopaminergic receptors Dose: Adults. 2–10 mg PO bid Peds 6–12 y. 1 mg PO daily–bid initial, gradually ↑ to 15 mg/d; ↓ in elderly/debilitated pts Caution: [C, ?/–] CI: h/o Blood dyscrasias; phenothiazine sensitivity Disp: Tabs 1, 2, 5, 10 mg; PO conc 10 mg/mL; Inj 2 mg/mL SE: Orthostatic ↓ BP, EPS, dizziness, neuroleptic malignant synd, skin discoloration, lowered Sz threshold, photosensitivity, blood dyscrasias Interactions: ↑ CNS depression W/ barbiturates, benzodiazepines, TCAs, EtOH; ↑ effects OF antihypertensives, propranolol, ↓ effects OF anticoagulants ↓ effects W/ antacids Labs: ↑ LFTs; ↓ WBCs NIPE: ↑ Risk of photosensitivity—use sunblock; urine color may change to pink to reddish-brown; PO conc must be diluted to 60 mL or more prior to administration; requires several wk for onset of effects

Trifluridine Ophthalmic (Viroptic) [Antiviral] Uses: *Herpes simplex keratitis & conjunctivitis* Action: Antiviral Dose: 1 gtt q2h, max 9 gtt/d; ↓ to 1 gtt q4h after healing begins; Rx up to 21 d Caution: [C, M] CI: Component allergy Disp: Soln 1% SE: Local burning, stinging NIPE: ⊘ < 6 y of age; reeval if no improvement in 7 d

Trihexyphenidyl (Artane) [Anti-Parkinson Agent/Anticholinergic]
Uses: *Parkinson Dz* **Action:** Blocks excess ACH at cerebral synapses **Dose:** 2–5 mg PO daily–qid **Caution:** [C, +] **CI:** NAG, GI obst, MyG, bladder obsts **Disp:** Tabs 2, 5 mg; elixir 2 mg/5 mL **SE:** Dry skin, constipation, xerostomia, photosensitivity, tachycardia, arrhythmias **Interactions:** ↑ Effects W/ MAOIs, phenothiazine, antihistamine, TCAs; ↑ effects *OF* amantadine, anticholinergics, digoxin; ↓ effects W/ antacids, tacrine; ↓ effects *OF* chlorpromazine, haloperidol, tacrine **NIPE:** Take w/ food; monitor for urinary hesitancy or retention; ⊘ D/C abruptly; ↑ risk of heat stroke; ↑ risk of CNS depression w/ concurrent EtOH use

Trimethobenzamide (Tigan) [Antiemetic/Anticholinergic] Uses: *N/V* **Action:** ↓ Medullary chemoreceptor trigger zone **Dose:** *Adults.* 300 mg PO or 200 mg IM tid–qid PRN *Peds.* 20 mg/kg/24 h PO in 3–4 ÷ doses **Caution:** [C, ?] **CI:** Benzocaine sensitivity **Disp:** Caps 300 mg; Inj 100 mg/mL **SE:** Drowsiness, ↓ BP, dizziness; hepatic impair, blood dyscrasias, Szs, parkinsonian-like synd **Interactions:** ↑ CNS depression W/ antidepressants, antihistamines, opioids, sedatives, EtOH; ↑ risk *OF* extrapyramidal effects **NIPE:** In the presence of viral Infxns, may mask emesis or mimic CNS effects of Reye synd

Trimethoprim (Primsol, Proloprim, Trimpex) [Antibiotic/Folate Antagonist] Uses: *UTI d/t susceptible gram(+) & (−) organisms; Rx PCP w/ dapsone* **Action:** ↓ Dihydrofolate reductase *Spectrum:* Many gram(+) & (−) except *Bacteroides, Branhamella, Brucella, Chlamydia, Clostridium, Mycobacterium, Mycoplasma, Nocardia, Neisseria, Pseudomonas,* & *Treponema* **Dose:** *Adults.* 100 mg PO bid or 200 mg PO qd; PCP 5 mg/kg tid × 21 d w/ dapsone *Peds.* 4 mg/kg/d in 2 ÷ doses; ↓ w/ renal failure **Caution:** [C, +] **CI:** Megaloblastic anemia d/t folate deficiency **Disp:** Tabs 100 mg; PO soln 50 mg/5 mL **SE:** Rash, pruritus, megaloblastic anemia, hepatic impair, blood dyscrasias **Interactions:** ↑ Effects W/ dapsone; ↑ effects *OF* dapsone, phenytoin, procainamide; ↓ efficacy W/ rifampin **Labs:** ↑ BUN, Cr, bilirubin **NIPE:** ↑ Fluids to 2–3 L/d; ↑ risk of folic acid deficiency (fatigue, pale skin, paranoia, wgt loss)

Trimethoprim (TMP)–Sulfamethoxazole (SMX) [Co-Trimoxazole] (Bactrim, Septra) [Antibiotic/Folate Antagonist] Uses: *UTI Rx & prophylaxis, otitis media, sinusitis, bronchitis, prevent PCP pneumonia (w/ CD4 count < 200 cells/mm³)* **Action:** SMX ↓ synth of dihydrofolic acid; TMP ↓ dihydrofolate reductase to impair protein synth *Spectrum:* Includes *Shigella,* PCP, & *Nocardia* Infxns, *Mycoplasma, Enterobacter* sp, *Staphylococcus, Streptococcus,* & more **Dose:** *Adults.* 1 DS tab PO bid or 5–20 mg/kg/d (based on TMP) in 3–4 ÷ doses *PCP:* 15–20 mg/kg/d IV or PO (TMP) in 4 ÷ doses *Nocardia:* 10–15 mg/kg/d IV or PO (TMP) in 4 ÷ doses *UTI prophylaxis:* 1 PO daily *Peds.* 8–10 mg/kg/24 h (TMP) PO ÷ into 2 doses or 3–4 doses IV; do not use in newborns; ↓ in renal failure; maint hydration **Caution:** [B (D if near term), +] **CI:** Sulfonamide sensitivity, porphyria, megaloblastic anemia w/ folate deficiency, sig hepatic impair **Disp:** Regular tabs 80 mg TMP/400 mg SMX; DS tabs 160 mg TMP/800 mg SMX;

PO susp 40 mg TMP/200 mg SMX/5 mL; Inj 80 mg TMP/400 mg SMX/5 mL **SE:** Allergic skin Rxns, photosensitivity, GI upset, Stevens–Johnson synd, blood dyscrasias, hep **Interactions:** ↑ Effect *OF* dapsone, MTX, phenytoin, sulfonylureas, warfarin, zidovudine; ↓ effects *W*/ rifampin; ↓ effect *OF* cyclosporine **Labs:** ↑ Serum bilirubin, alk phos, BUN, Cr **NIPE:** ↑ Risk of photosensitivity—use sunscreen; ↑ fluids to 2–3 L/d; synergistic combo

Trimetrexate (NeuTrexin) [Anti-Infective, Antiprotozoal/Folic Acid Antimetabolite] WARNING: Must be used w/ leucovorin to avoid tox
Uses: *Mod–severe PCP* **Action:** ↓ Dihydrofolate reductase **Dose:** 45 mg/m² IV q24h for 21 d; administer w/ leucovorin 20 mg/m² IV q6h for 24 d; ↓ in hepatic impair **Caution:** [D, ?/–] **CI:** MTX sensitivity **Disp:** Inj 25, 200 mg/vial **SE:** Sz, fever, rash, GI upset, anemias, peripheral neuropathy, renal impair **Interactions:** ↑ Effects *W*/ azole antifungals, cimetidine, erythromycin; ↓ effects *W*/ rifabutin, rifampin; ↓ effects *OF* pneumococcal immunization **Labs:** ↑ LFTs, SCr **NIPE:** ⊘ PRG, breast-feeding use contraception; ⊘ exposure to Infxn; use cytotoxic cautions; Infuse over 60 min

Triptorelin (Trelstar 3.75, Trelstar 11.25, Trelstar 22.5) [Antineoplastic/Gonadotropin-Releasing Hormone]
Uses: *Palliation of advanced PCa* **Action:** LHRH analogue; ↓ GnRH w/ cont dosing; transient ↑ in LH, FSH, testosterone, & estradiol 7–10 d after 1st dose; w/ chronic/cont use (usually 2–4 wk), sustained ↓ LH & FSH w/ ↓ testicular & ovarian steroidogenesis similar to surgical castration **Dose:** 3.75 mg IM q4wk or 11.25 mg IM q12wk or 22.5 mg q24wk **Caution:** [X, N/A] **CI:** Not indicated in females **Disp:** Inj Depot 3.75 mg; 11.25 mg; 22.5 mg **SE:** Dizziness, emotional lability, fatigue, HA, insomnia, HTN, D, V, ED, retention, UTI, pruritus, anemia, Inj site pain, musculoskeletal pain, osteoporosis, allergic Rxns **Interactions:** ↑ Risk of severe hyperprolactinemia *W*/ antipsychotics, metoclopramide **Labs:** ✓ Periodic testosterone levels; suppression of pituitary-gonadal Fxn; monitor for ↑ glucose **NIPE:** May cause hot flashes; initial ↑ bone pain & may cause spinal cord compression leading to paralysis & death; only 6 mo formulation

Trospium (Sanctura, Sanctura XR) [Antispasmodic/Anticholinergic]
Uses: *OAB w/ Sx of urge incontinence, urgency, frequency* **Action:** Muscarinic antagonist, ↓ bladder smooth muscle tone **Dose:** 20 mg tabs PO bid; 60 mg ER caps PO qd ᴀᴍ, 1 h ac or on empty stomach. ↓ w/ CrCl < 30 mL/min & elderly **Caution:** [C, +/–] w/ EtOH use, in hot environments, UC, MyG, renal/hepatic impair **CI:** Urinary/gastric retention, NAG **Disp:** Tab 20 mg; caps ER 60 mg **SE:** Dry mouth, constipation, HA, rash **Interactions:** ↑ Effects *W*/ amiloride, digoxin, morphine, metformin, procainamide, tenofovir, vancomycin; ↑ effects *OF* anticholinergics, amiloride, digoxin, morphine, metformin, procainamide, tenofovir, vancomycin **NIPE:** Take w/o food 1 h ac; ↑ risk of heat exhaustion/stroke; ↑ drowsiness w/ EtOH

Ulipristal Acetate (Ella) [Progesterone Agonist/Antagonist]
Uses: *Emergency contraceptive for PRG prevention (unprotected sex/contraceptive

failure)* **Action:** Progesterone agonist/antagonist, delays ovulation **Dose:** 1 Tab PO ASAP w/in 5 d of unprotected sex or contraceptive failure **Caution:** [X; −] **CI:** PRG **Disp:** Tab 30 mg **SE:** HA, N, Abd, dysmenorrhea **Interactions:** ↑ Effects w/ CYP3A4 Inhibs (eg, ketoconazole, itraconazole); ↓ effectiveness **W/** CYP3A4 inducers (barbiturates, bosentan, carbamazepine, felbamate, griseofulvin, oxcarbazepine, phenytoin, rifampin, topiramate, St. John's wort) **NIPE:** Not for routine contraception; fertility after use unchanged, maintain routine contraception; use any d of menstrual cycle

Urokinase (Abbokinase) [Thrombolytic Enzyme] Uses: *PE, DVT, restore patency to IV catheters* **Action:** Converts plasminogen to plasmin; causes clot lysis **Dose:** *Adults & Peds. Systemic effect:* 4400 units/kg IV over 10 min, then 4400–6000 units/kg/h for 12 h *Restore catheter patency:* Inject 5000 units into catheter & aspirate up to 2 doses **Caution:** [B, +] **CI:** Do not use w/in 10 d of surgery, delivery, or organ biopsy; bleeding, CVA, vascular malformation **Disp:** Powder for Inj, 250,000-unit vial **SE:** Bleeding, ↓ BP, dyspnea, bronchospasm, anaphylaxis, cholesterol embolism **Interactions:** ↑ Risk of bleeding **W/** anticoagulants, ASA, heparin, indomethacin, NSAIDs, phenylbutazone, feverfew, garlic, ginger, ginkgo; ↓ effects **W/** aminocaproic acid **Labs:** ↑ PT, PTT, INR; ↓ Hct **NIPE:** Monitor for bleeding q15min for 1st h & q30min for next 7 h; aPTT should be < 2 × nl before use & before starting anticoagulants after

Ustekinumab (Stelara) [Interleukin-12 & Interleukin-23 Antagonist] Uses: *Mod–severe plaque psoriasis * **Action:** Human IL-12 & IL-23 antagonist **Dose:** Wgt < 100 kg, 45 mg SQ initially & 4 wk later, then 45 mg q12wk. Wgt > 100 kg, 90 mg SQ initially & 4 wk later, then 90 mg q12 wk **Caution:** [B/?] **Disp:** Prefilled syringe & SDV 45 mg/0.5 mL, 90 mg/1 mL **SE:** Nasopharyngitis, URI, HA, fatigue **Interactions:** **W/** Concomitant live vaccines, other immunosuppressants, phototherapy **NIPE:** Do not use w/ live vaccines; do not give BCG vaccines during or w/in 1 y of starting or stopping ustekinumab

Valacyclovir (Valtrex) [Antiviral/Synthetic Purine Nucleoside] Uses: *Herpes zoster; genital herpes; herpes labialis* **Action:** Prodrug of acyclovir; ↓ viral DNA replication *Spectrum:* Herpes simplex I & II **Dose:** *Zoster:* 1 g PO tid × 7 d *Genital herpes (initial episode):* 1 g bid × 7–10 d, *(recurrent)* 500 mg PO bid × 3 d or 1 g PO qd × 5 d *Herpes prophylaxis:* 500 mg PO bid *Herpes labialis:* 2 g PO q12h × 1 d ↓ w/ renal failure **Caution:** [B, +] **Disp:** Caplets 500, 1000 mg **SE:** HA, GI upset, dizziness, pruritus, photophobia **Interactions:** ↑ Effects **W/** cimetidine, probenecid **Labs:** ↑ LFTs, Cr ↓ HMG, Hct, plt, WBCs **NIPE:** Take w/o regard to food; ↑ fluids to 2–3 L/d; begin drug at 1st sign of S/Sxs

Valganciclovir (Valcyte) [Antiviral/Synthetic Nucleoside] **WARNING:** Granulocytopenia, anemia, & thrombocytopenia reported. Carcinogenic, teratogenic, & may cause aspermatogenesis Uses: *CMV retinitis & CMV prophylaxis in solid-organ transplantation* **Action:** Ganciclovir prodrug; ↓ viral DNA synth **Dose:** *CMV retinitis induction:* 900 mg PO bid w/ food × 21 d, then 900 mg

PO daily *CMV prevention:* 900 mg PO qd × 100 d posttransplant, ↓ w/ renal dysfunction **Caution:** [C, ?/–] Use w/ imipenem/cilastatin, nephrotoxic drugs **CI:** Allergy to acyclovir, ganciclovir, valganciclovir; ANC < 500 cells/mm³; plt < 25,000 cells/mm³; Hgb < 8 g/dL **Disp:** Tabs 450 mg **SE:** BM suppression, HA, GI upset **Interactions:** ↑ Effects *W/* cytotoxic drugs, immunosuppressive drugs, probenecid; ↑ risks of nephrotox *W/* amphotericin B, cyclosporine; ↑ effects *W/* didanosine **Labs:** ↑ Cr; monitor CBC & Cr, monitor glucose for hypoglycemia **NIPE:** Take w/ food; ⊘ PRG, breast-feeding, EtOH, NSAIDs; use contraception for at least 3 mo after drug Rx

Valproic Acid (Depakene, Depakote, Stavzor) [Anticonvulsant/ Carboxylic Acid Derivative]

WARNING: Fatal hepatic failure (usually during 1st 6 mo of Tx, peds < 2 y high risk, monitor LFTs at baseline & frequent intervals), teratogenic effects, & life-threatening pancreatitis reported **Uses:** *Rx epilepsy, mania; prophylaxis of migraines*, Alzheimer disorder **Action:** Anticonvulsant; ↑ availability of GABA **Dose:** *Adults & Peds. Szs:* 30–60 mg/kg/ 24 h PO ÷ tid (after initiation of 10–15 mg/kg/24 h) *Mania:* 750 mg in 3 ÷ doses, ↑ 60 mg/kg/d max *Migraines:* 250 mg bid, ↑ 1000 mg/d max; ↓ w/ hepatic impair **Caution:** [D, +] Multiple drug interactions **CI:** Severe hepatic impair, urea cycle disorder **Disp:** Caps 250 mg; caps w/ coated particles 125 mg; tabs DR 125, 250, 500 mg; tabs ER 250, 500 mg; caps DR (Stavzor) 125, 250, 500 mg; syrup 250 mg/5 mL; Inj 100 mg/mL **SE:** Somnolence, dizziness, GI upset, diplopia, ataxia, rash, thrombocytopenia, hep, pancreatitis, ↑ bleeding times, alopecia, wgt ↑, hyperammonemic encephalopathy in pts w/ urea cycle disorders *Notes: Trough:* Just before next dose *Therapeutic: Peak:* 50–100 mcg/mL *Toxic trough:* > 100 mcg/mL; *1/2-life:* 5–20 h; phenobarbital & phenytoin may alter levels **Interactions:** ↑ Effects *W/* clarithromycin, erythromycin, felbamate, INH, phenytoin, salicylates, troleandomycin; ↑ effects *OF* anticoagulants, lamotrigine, nimodipine, phenobarbital, phenytoin, primidone, zidovudine; ↑ CNS depression *W/* CNS depressants, haloperidol, loxapine, maprotiline, MAOIs, phenothiazine, thioxanthenes, TCAs, EtOH; ↓ effects *W/* cholestyramine, colestipol; ↓ effects *OF* clozapine, rifampin **Labs:** ↑ LFTs; altered TFTs; monitor LFTs & serum levels **NIPE:** Take w/ food for GI upset; ⊘ PRG, breast-feeding; ⊘ D/C abruptly—↑ risk of Szs

Valsartan (Diovan) [Antihypertensive/ARB]

WARNING: Using during 2nd/3rd tri of PRG can cause fetal harm **Uses:** HTN, CHF, DN **Action:** Angiotensin II receptor antagonist **Dose:** 80–160 mg/d, max 320 mg/d **Caution:** [D, ?/–] w/ K⁺-sparing diuretics or K⁺ supls **CI:** Severe hepatic impair, biliary cirrhosis/ obst, primary hyperaldosteronism, bilateral RAS **Disp:** Tabs 40, 80, 160, 320 mg **SE:** ↓ BP, dizziness, HA, viral Infxn, fatigue, Abd pain, D, arthralgia, fatigue, back pain, hyperkalemia, cough **Interactions:** ↑ Effects *W/* diuretics, Li; ↑ risk of hyperkalemia *W/* K⁺-sparing diuretics, K⁺ supls, TMP **Labs:** ↑ K⁺, ↑ Cr **NIPE:** Take w/o regard to food; ⊘ PRG, breast-feeding; use contraception; monitor ECG for hyperkalemia (peaked T waves)

Vancomycin (Vancocin, Vancoled) [Antibiotic/Glycopeptide]
Uses: *Serious MRSA Infxns; enterococcal Infxns; PO Rx of *S aureus* & *C difficile* pseudomembranous colitis* Action: ↓ Cell wall synth *Spectrum:* Gram(+) bacteria & some anaerobes (includes MRSA, *Staphylococcus* sp, *Enterococcus* sp, *Streptococcus* sp, *C difficile*) Dose: *Adults.* 1 g IV q12h or 15–20 mg/kg/dose *C difficile:* 125–500 mg PO q6h × 7–10 d *Peds.* 40–60 mg/kg/d IV in ÷ doses q6–12 h *C difficile:* 40–60 mg/kg/d PO × 7–10 d *Neonates.* 10–15 mg/kg/dose q12h; ↓ w/ renal Insuff Caution: [C, M] CI: Component allergy; avoid in h/o hearing loss Disp: Caps 125, 250 mg; powder 250 mg/5 mL, 500 mg/6 mL for PO soln; powder for Inj 500, 1000 mg, 10 g/vial SE: Oto-/nephrotox, GI upset (PO) Notes: Levels: *Peak:* 1 h after Inf; *Trough:* < 0.5 h before next dose *Therapeutic: Peak:* 20–40 mcg/mL *Trough:* 10–20 mcg/mL *Toxic peak:* > 50 mcg/mL *Trough:* > 20 mcg/mL *1/2-life:* 6–8 h Interactions: ↑ Ototox & nephrotox W/ ASA, aminoglycosides, cyclosporine, cisplatin, loop diuretics; ↓ effects *OF* MRX Labs: ↑ BUN, Cr; ↓ WBC NIPE: Take w/ food, ↑ fluid to 2–3 L/d; not absorbed PO, local effect in gut only; give IV dose slowly (over 1–3 h) to prevent "red-man synd" (flushing of head/neck/upper torso); IV product used for colitis

Vardenafil (Levitra, Staxyn) [Anti-Impotence Agent/PDE5] Uses: *ED* Action: PDE5 Inhib, ↑ cyclic guanosine monophosphate (cGMP) & NO levels; relaxes smooth muscles, dilates cavernosal arteries Dose: *Levitra* 10 mg PO 60 min before sexual activity; titrate; max × 1 = 20 mg; 2.5 mg w/ CYP3A4 Inhibs (Table 10); *Staxyn* 1 (10 mg ODT) 60 min before sex Caution: [B, –] w/ CV, hepatic, or renal Dz or if sex activity not advisable CI: w/ Nitrates Disp: *Levitra* tabs 2.5, 5, 10, 20 mg; *Staxyn* 10 mg ODT (contains phenylalanine) SE: ↑ QT interval ↓ BP, HA, dyspepsia, priapism, flushing, rhinitis, sinusitis, flu synd, sudden ↓/loss of hearing, tinnitus, NIAON Interactions: ↑ Effects W/ erythromycin, ketoconazole indinavir, ritonavir; ↑ risk of hypotension W/ α-blockers, nitrates NIPE: Take w/o regard to food; ↑ risk of priapism; transient global amnesia reports; place Staxyn on tongue to disintegrate w/o Liqs; ODT not equal to oral pill; gets higher levels)

Varenicline (Chantix) [Nicotinic Acetylcholine Receptor Partial Agonist] WARNING: Serious neuropsychiatric events (depression, suicidal ideation/attempt) reported Uses: *Smoking cessation* Action: Nicotine receptor partial agonist Dose: *Adults.* 0.5 mg PO daily × 3 d, 0.5 mg bid × 4 d, then 1 mg PO bid for 12 wk total; after meal w/ glass of H₂O Caution: [C, ?/–] ↓ Dose w/ renal impair Disp: Tabs 0.5, 1 mg SE: Serious psychological disturbances, N, V, insomnia, flatulence, unusual dreams Interactions: May affect metabolism of warfarin, theophylline, insulin; ↑ effects W/ nicotine-replacement drugs NIPE: Slowly ↑ dose to ↓ N; initiate 1 wk before desired smoking cessation date; monitor for changes in behavior; use of additional smoking cessation OTC nicotine-replacement drugs may ↑ adverse effects

Varicella Immune Globulin (VarZIG) [investigational, call (800) 843-7477] Uses: Postexposure prophylaxis for persons w/o immunity, exposure likely to result in Infxn (household contact, > 5 min) & ↑ risk for severe Dz (immunosuppression, PRG) **Action:** Passive immunization **Dose:** 125 units/10 kg up to 625 units IV (over 3–5 min) or IM (deltoid or proximal thigh); give w/in 4–5 d (best < 72 h) of exposure **Caution:** [?, –] Indicated for PRG women exposed to varicella **CI:** IgA deficiency **Disp:** Inj 125-mg vials **SE:** Inj site Rxn, dizziness, fever, HA, N; ARF, thrombosis rare **NIPE:** Wait 5 mo before varicella vaccination after varicella immune globulin; may ↓ vaccine effectiveness; observe for varicella for 28 d; if VariZIG administration not possible w/in 96 h of exposure, consider administration of IGIV (400 mg/kg)

Varicella Virus Vaccine (Varivax) [Vaccine] Uses: *Prevent varicella (chickenpox)* **Action:** Active immunization w/ live attenuated virus **Dose:** *Adults & Peds > 12 mo.* 0.5 mL SQ, repeat 4–8 wk **Caution:** [C, M] **CI:** Immunocompromise; PRG, fever, untreated TB, neomycin-anaphylactoid Rxn **Disp:** Powder for Inj **SE:** Varicella rash, generalized or at Inj site, arthralgia/myalgias, fatigue, fever, HA, irritability, GI upset **Interactions:** ↓ Effects W/ acyclovir, immunosuppressant drugs **NIPE:** OK for all children & adults who have not had chickenpox; ⊘ salicylates for 6 wk after immunization; ⊘ PRG for 3 mo after immunization; OK for all children & adults who have not had chickenpox; do not give w/in 3 mo of immunoglobulin (IgG) & no IgG w/in 2 mo of vaccination; avoid high-risk people for 6 wk after vaccination

Vasopressin [Antidiuretic Hormone, ADH] (Pitressin) [Antidiuretic Hormone/Posterior Pituitary Hormone] Uses: *DI; Rx post-op Abd distention*; adjunct Rx of GI bleeding & esophageal varices; asystole & PEA, pulseless VT & VF, adjunct vasopressor (IV drip) **Action:** Posterior pituitary hormone, potent GI & peripheral vasoconstrictor **Dose:** *Adults & Peds. DI:* 2.5–10 units SQ or IM tid–qid *GI hemorrhage:* 0.2–0.4 units/min; ↓ in cirrhosis; caution in vascular Dz *VT/VF:* 40 units IV push × 1 **Peds:** *ECC 2010:* Cardiac arrest: 0.4–1 unit/kg IV/IO bolus; max dose 40 units Hypotension: 0.2–2 MU/kg/min cont Inf **Caution:** [B, +] w/ Vascular Dz **CI:** Allergy **Disp:** Inj 20 units/mL **SE:** HTN, arrhythmias, fever, vertigo, GI upset, tremor **Interactions:** ↑ Vasopressor effects W/ guanethidine, neostigmine; ↑ antidiuretic effects W/ carbamazepine, chlorpropamide, clofibrate, phenformin urea, TCAs; ↓ antidiuretic effects W/ demeclocycline, epi, heparin, Li, phenytoin, EtOH **Labs:** ↑ Cortisol level **NIPE:** Take 1–2 glasses H₂O w/ drug; addition of vasopressor to concurrent norepinephrine or epi Infs

Vecuronium (Norcuron) [Skeletal Muscle Relaxant/Nondepolarizing Neuromuscular Blocker] WARNING: To be administered only by appropriately trained individuals Uses: *Skeletal muscle relaxation* **Action:** Nondepolarizing neuromuscular blocker; onset 2–3 min **Dose:** *Adults & Peds.* 0.1–0.2 mg/kg IV bolus (also rapid intubation *ECC 2005*); maint 0.010–0.015 mg/kg after 25–40 min; additional doses q12–15min PRN; ↓ w/ severe renal/hepatic impair **Caution:** [C, ?] Drug interactions cause ↑ effect (eg, aminoglycosides, tetracycline, succinylcholine)

Disp: Powder for Inj 10, 20 mg **SE:** Bradycardia, ↓ BP, itching, rash, tachycardia, CV collapse **Interactions:** ↑ Neuromuscular blockade *W/* amikacin, clindamycin, gentamicin, neomycin, streptomycin, tobramycin, general anesthetics, quinidine, tetracyclines; ↑ resp depression *W/* opioids; ↓ effects *W/* phenytoin **NIPE:** Will not provide pain relief or sedation; fewer cardiac effects than succinylcholine

Venlafaxine (Effexor, Effexor XR) [Antidepressant/Serotonin, Norepinephrine, & Dopamine Reuptake Inhibitor] WARNING: Monitor for worsening depression or emergence of suicidality, particularly in ped pts **Uses:** *Depression, generalized anxiety*, social anxiety disorder; panic disorder*, obsessive-compulsive disorder, chronic fatigue synd, ADHD, autism **Action:** Potentiation of CNS neurotransmitter activity **Dose:** 75–225 mg/d ÷ into 2–3 equal doses (IR) or qd (ER); 375 mg IR or 225 mg ER max/d ↓ w/ renal/hepatic impair **Caution:** [C, ?/–] **CI:** MAOIs **Disp:** Tabs IR 25, 37.5, 50, 75, 100 mg; ER caps 37.5, 75, 150 mg **SE:** HTN, ↑ HR, HA, somnolence, GI upset, sexual dysfunction; actuates mania or Szs **Interactions:** ↑ Effects *W/* cimetidine, desipramine, haloperidol, MAOIs; ↑ risk of serotonin synd *W/* sumatriptan, trazodone, St. John's wort **NIPE:** XR caps swallow whole—⊘ chew; take w/ food; ⊘ use EtOH; ⊘ D/C abruptly; D/C MAOI 14 d before start of this drug; ↑ fluids to 2–3 L/d; may take 2–3 wk for full effects; frequent edema & wgt gain; may ↑ risk of mania & hypomania

Verapamil (Calan, Covera HS, Isoptin, Verelan) [Antihypertensive, Antianginal, Antiarrhythmic/CCB] Uses: *Angina, HTN, PSVT, AF, atrial flutter*, migraine prophylaxis, hypertrophic cardiomyopathy, bipolar Dz **Action:** CCB **Dose:** *Adults. Arrhythmias:* 2nd line for PSVT w/ narrow QRS complex & adequate BP 2.5–5 mg IV over 1–2 min; repeat 5–10 mg in 15–30 min PRN (30 mg max) *Angina:* 80–120 mg PO tid, ↑ 480 mg/24 h max *HTN:* 80–180 mg PO tid or SR tabs 120–240 mg PO daily to 240 mg bid *ECC 2010:* Reentry SVT w/ narrow QRS: 2.5–5 mg IV over 2 min (slower in older pts); repeat 5–10 mg, in 15–30 min PRN max of 20 mg; or 5 mg bolus q15min (max 30 mg) *Peds < 1 y.* 0.1–0.2 mg/kg IV over 2 min (may repeat in 30 min) *1–16 y.* 0.1–0.3 mg/kg IV over 2 min (may repeat in 30 min); 5 mg max *PO: 1–5 y.* 4–8 mg/kg/d in 3 ÷ doses *> 5 y.* 80 mg q6–8h; ↓ in renal/hepatic impair **Caution:** [C, +] Amiodarone/BB/ flecainide can cause bradycardia; statins, midazolam, tacrolimus, theophylline levels may be ↑; w/ elderly pts **CI:** Conduction disorders, cardiogenic shock; BB/thiazide combo, dofetilide, pimozide, ranolazine **Disp:** Tabs 40, 80, 120 mg; tabs ER 120, 180, 240 mg; tabs ER 24-h 180, 240 mg; caps SR 120, 180, 240, 360 mg; caps ER 100, 200, 300 mg; Inj 5 mg/2 mL **SE:** Gingival hyperplasia, constipation, ↓ BP, bronchospasm, HR or conduction disturbances **Interactions:** ↑ Effects *W/* antihypertensives, nitrates, quinidine, EtOH, grapefruit juice; ↑ effects *OF* buspirone, carbamazepine, cyclosporine, digoxin, prazosin, quinidine, theophylline; ↓ effects *W/* antineoplastics, barbiturates, NSAIDs; ↓ effects *OF* Li, rifampin; ↓ BP & bradyarrhythmias taken *W/* telithromycin **Labs:** ↑ ALT, AST, alk phos **NIPE:** Take w/ food; ↑ fluids & bulk foods to prevent constipation

Vigabatrin (Sabril) [Antiepileptic] WARNING: Vision loss reported **Uses:** * Refractory complex partial Sz disorder, infantile spasms* **Action:** ↓ GABA-transaminase (GABA-T) to ↑ levels of brain GABA **Dose:** *Adults.* Initially 500 mg 2 × /d, then ↑ daily dose by 500 mg at weekly intervals based on response & tolerability *Peds. Szs:* 10–15 kg: 0.5–1 g/d ÷ 2 × /d; 31–50 kg: 1.5–3 g/d ÷ 2 × /d; > 50 kg: 2–3 g/d ÷ 2 × /d *Infantile spasms:* Initially 50 mg/kg/d bid, ↑ 150 mg/kg/d max **Caution:** [C, +/–] ↓ Dose by 25% w/ CrCl > 50–80 mL/min, ↓ dose 50% w/ CrCl > 30–50 mL/min, ↓ dose 75% w/ CrCl > 10–30 mL/min, MRI signal changes reported in some infants **Disp:** Tabs 500 mg, powder/oral soln 500 mg/packet **SE:** Vision loss/blurring, anemia, peripheral neuropathy, fatigue, somnolence, nystagmus, tremor, memory impair, ↑ wgt, arthralgia, abnormal coordination, confusion **Interactions:** May ↓ phenytoin levels **Labs:** Monitor LFTs **NIPE:** Taper slowly to avoid withdrawal Szs; restricted distribution, to register call (888) 233-2334

Vilazodone HCL (Viibryd) [Selective Serotonin Reuptake Inhibitor + 5-HT$_{1A}$ Receptor Partial Agonist] WARNING: ↑ Suicide risk in children/adolescents/young adults on antidepressants for MDD & other psychological disorders **Uses:** *MDD* **Action:** SSRI & 5HT$_{1A}$ receptor partial agonist **Dose:** 40 mg/d; start 10 mg PO/d × 7 d, then 20 mg/d × 7 d, then 40 mg/d; ↓ to 20 mg w/ CYP3A4 Inhib **Caution:** [C; ?/–] **CI:** MAOI, < 14 d between D/C MAOI & start **Disp:** Tabs 10, 20, 40 mg **SE:** Serotonin synd, neuroleptic malignant synd, N/V/D, dry mouth, dizziness, insomnia, restlessness, abnormal dreams, sexual dysfunction **Interactions:** ↑ Risk of serotonin synd W/ concomitant triptans, MAOIs, SSRIs, SNRIs, buspirone, tramadol, antidopaminergic drugs; ↑ risk of bleeding W/ ASA, NSAIDs, warfarin, other anticoagulants, ↑ effects W/ CYP3A4 Inhibs; ↓ effects W/ CYP3A4 inducers **NIPE:** NOT approved for peds; w/ D/C, ↓ dose gradually, do not take w/in 14 d of MAOI

Vinblastine (Velban, Velbe) [Antineoplastic/Vinca Alkaloid] WARNING: Chemotherapeutic agent; handle w/ caution **Uses:** *Hodgkin Dz & NHLs, mycosis fungoides, CAs (testis, renal cell, breast, NSCLC), AIDS-related Kaposi sarcoma*, choriocarcinoma, histiocytosis **Action:** ↓ Microtubule assembly **Dose:** 0.1–0.5 mg/kg/wk (4–20 mg/m²); ↓ in hepatic failure **Caution:** [D, ?] **CI:** IT use **Disp:** Inj 1 mg/mL in 10-mg vial **SE:** ↓ BM (esp leukopenia), N/V, constipation, neurotox, alopecia, rash, myalgia, tumor pain **Interactions:** ↑ Effects W/ erythromycin, itraconazole; ↓ effects W/ glutamic acid, tryptophan; ↓ effects OF phenytoin **Labs:** ↑ Uric acid **NIPE:** ↑ Fluids to 2–3 L/d; ⊘ PRG or breast-feeding; use contraception for at least 2 mo after drug; photosensitivity— use sunblock; ⊘ administer immunizations; takes several wk for therapeutic effect; ↑ risk of Infxns

Vincristine (Oncovin, Vincasar PFS) [Antineoplastic/Vinca Alkaloid] WARNING: Chemotherapeutic agent; handle w/ caution; fatal if administered intrathecally **Uses:** *ALL, breast & SCLC, sarcoma (eg, Ewing tumor, rhabdomyosarcoma), Wilms tumor, Hodgkin Dz & NHLs, neuroblastoma, multiple myeloma* **Action:** Promotes disassembly of mitotic spindle, causing metaphase arrest **Dose:** 0.4–1.4 mg/m² (single doses 2 mg/max); ↓ in hepatic failure **Caution:** [D, ?] **CI:** IT use **Disp:** Inj 1 mg/mL, 5-mg vial **SE:** Neurotox commonly dose-limiting, jaw pain (trigeminal neuralgia), fever, fatigue, anorexia, constipation & paralytic ileus, bladder atony; no sig ↓ BM w/ standard doses; tissue necrosis w/ extrav **Interactions:** ↑ Effects W/ CCBs, azole antifungals; ↑ risk of bronchospasm W/ mitomycin; ↓ effects OF digoxin, phenytoin, quinolone antibiotics **Labs:** ↑ Uric acid; ↓ HMG, Hct, plt, WBC **NIPE:** ↑ Fluids to 2–3 L/d; reversible hair loss; ⊘ exposure to Infxn; ⊘ administer immunizations; ↑ risk of Infxns

Vinorelbine (Navelbine) [Antineoplastic/Vinca Alkaloid] WARNING: Chemotherapeutic agent; handle w/ caution **Uses:** *Breast CA & NSCLC* (alone or w/ cisplatin) **Action:** ↓ polymerization of microtubules, impairing mitotic spindle formation; semisynthetic vinca alkaloid **Dose:** 30 mg/m²/wk; ↓ in hepatic failure **Caution:** [D, ?] **CI:** IT use, granulocytopenia (< 1000 cells/mm³) **Disp:** Inj 10 mg **SE:** ↓ BM (leukopenia), mild GI, neurotox (6–29%); constipation/paresthesias (rare); tissue damage from extrav **Interactions:** ↑ Risk of granulocytopenia W/ cisplatin, ↑ pulm effects W/ mitomycin, paclitaxel **Labs:** ↑ LFTs **NIPE:** ⊘ PRG or breast-feeding; use contraception; avoid infectious environment; ↑ fluids to 2–3 L/d

Vitamin B₁ [See Thiamine]
Vitamin B₆ [See Pyridoxine]
Vitamin B₁₂ [See Cyanocobalamin]
Vitamin K [See Phytonadione]
Vitamin, Multi See Multivitamins (Table 12)

Voriconazole (VFEND) [Antifungal/Triazole] Uses: *Invasive aspergillosis, candidemia, serious fungal Infxns* **Action:** ↓ Ergosterol synth *Spectrum: Candida, Aspergillus, Scedosporium* sp, *Fusarium* sp **Dose:** *Adults & Peds > 12 y. IV:* 6 mg/kg q12h × 2, then 4 mg/kg bid; may ↓ to 3 mg/kg/dose *PO: < 40 kg:* 100 mg q12h, up to 150 mg > *40 kg:* 200 mg q12h, up to 300 mg; ↓ w/ mild–mod hepatic impair; IV w/ renal impair × 1 dose; PO w/o food **Caution:** [D, ?/–] **CI:** Severe hepatic impair, w/ CYP3A4 substrates (see Table 10) **Disp:** Tabs 50, 200 mg; susp 200 mg/5 mL; 200-mg Inj **SE:** Visual changes, fever, rash, GI upset **Interactions:** ↑ Effects W/ delavirdine, efavirenz; ↑ effects OF benzodiazepines, buspirone, CCBs, cisapride, cyclosporine, ergots, pimozide, quinidine, sirolimus, sulfonylureas, tacrolimus; ↓ effects W/ carbamazepine, mephobarbital, phenobarbital, rifampin, rifabutin **Labs:** ↑ LFTs **NIPE:** Take w/o food; ↑ risk of photosensitivity—use sunblock; ⊘ PRG or breast-feeding

Vorinostat (Zolinza) [Histone Deacetylase Inhibitor] Uses: *Rx cutaneous manifestations in cutaneous T-cell lymphoma* **Action:** Histone deacetylase Inhib **Dose:** 400 mg PO daily w/ food; if intolerant ↓ 300 mg PO d × 5 consecutive d each wk **Caution:** [D, ?/–] w/ warfarin (↑ INR) **Disp:** Caps 100 mg **SE:** N/V/D, dehydration, fatigue, anorexia, dysgeusia, DVT, PE, ↓ plt, anemia, hyperglycemia, QTc prolongation **Interactions:** ↑ Risk of thrombocytopenia & GI bleed *W/* HDAC Inhibs (valproic acid) **Labs:** Monitor CBC, lytes (K⁺, Mg, Ca), glucose, & SCr q2wk × 2 mo, then monthly; baseline, periodic ECGs **NIPE:** Drink 2 L fluid/d; ⊘ breast-feeding & < 18 y of age; may ↑ QT interval—monitor ECG; ↑ risk of DVT reported

Warfarin (Coumadin) [Anticoagulant/Coumarin Derivative]
WARNING: Can cause major or fatal bleeding **Uses:** *Prophylaxis & Rx of PE & DVT, AF w/ embolization*, other post-op indications **Action:** ↓ Vit K–dependent clotting factors in order: VII-IX-X-II **Dose:** *Adults.* Titrate, INR 2.0–3.0 for most; mechanical valves INR is 2.5–3.5 *American College of Chest Physicians guidelines:* 5 mg initial, may use 7.5–10 mg; ↓ if pt elderly or w/ other bleeding risk factors; maint 2–10 mg/d PO, follow daily INR initial to adjust dosage (Table 8) *Peds.* 0.05–0.34 mg/kg/24 h PO or IV; follow PT/INR to adjust dosage; monitor vit K intake; ↓ w/ hepatic impair/elderly **Caution:** [X, +] **CI:** Severe hepatic/renal Dz, bleeding, peptic ulcer, PRG **Disp:** Tabs 1, 2, 2.5, 3, 4, 5, 6, 7.5, 10 mg; Inj **SE:** Bleeding d/t overanticoagulation or injury & therapeutic INR; bleeding, alopecia, skin necrosis, purple toe synd **Interactions:** Caution pt on taking *W/* other meds, esp ASA *Common warfarin* **Interactions:** ↑ Action *W/* APAP, EtOH (w/ liver Dz), amiodarone, cimetidine, ciprofloxacin, cotrimoxazole, erythromycin, fluconazole, flu vaccine, INH, itraconazole, metronidazole, omeprazole, phenytoin, propranolol, quinidine, tetracycline. ↓ action *W/* barbiturates, carbamazepine, chlordiazepoxide, cholestyramine, dicloxacillin, nafcillin, rifampin, sucralfate, high-vit K foods **Labs:** ↑ PTT; false ↓ serum theophylline levels **NIPE:** Monitor vit K intake (↓ effect); INR preferred test; to rapidly correct overanticoagulation: vit K, fresh-frozen plasma, or both; highly teratogenic. Consider genotyping for VKORC1 & CYP2C9

Witch Hazel (Tucks Pads, Others [OTC]) **Uses:** After BM cleansing to ↓ local irritation or relieve hemorrhoids; after anorectal surgery, episiotomy, Vag hygiene **Dose:** Apply PRN **Caution:** [?, ?] External use only **CI:** None **Disp:** Pre-soaked pads **SE:** Mild itching or burning

Zafirlukast (Accolate) [Bronchodilator/Leukotriene Receptor Antagonist] **Uses:** *Adjunctive Rx of asthma* **Action:** Selective & competitive Inhib of leukotrienes **Dose:** *Adults & Peds > 12 y.* 20 mg bid *Peds 5–11 y.* 10 mg PO bid (empty stomach) **Caution:** [B, –] Interacts w/ warfarin, ↑ INR **CI:** Component allergy **Disp:** Tabs 10, 20 mg **SE:** Hepatic dysfunction, usually reversible on D/C; HA, dizziness, GI upset; Churg–Strauss synd, neuropsychological events (agitation, restlessness, suicidal ideation) **Interactions:** ↑ Effects *W/* ASA; ↑ effects *OF* CCBs, cyclosporine; ↑ risk of bleeding *W/* warfarin; ↓ effects *W/* erythromycin, theophylline, food **Labs:** ↑ ALT **NIPE:** Take w/o food; ⊘ use for acute asthma attack

Zaleplon (Sonata) [C-IV] [Sedative/Hypnotic] **Uses:** *Insomnia* **Action:** A nonbenzodiazepine sedative/hypnotic, a pyrazolopyrimidine **Dose:** 5–20 mg hs PRN; not w/ high-fat meal; ↓ w/ renal/hepatic Insuff, elderly **Caution:** [C, ?/–] w/ mental/psychological conditions **CI:** Component allergy **Disp:** Caps 5,

10 mg **SE:** HA, edema, amnesia, somnolence, photosensitivity **Interactions:** ↑ CNS depression W/ CNS depressants, imipramine, thoridazine, EtOH; ↓ effects W/ carbamazepine, phenobarbital, phenytoin, rifampin **NIPE:** Rapid effects of drug, take stat before onset; take w/o food; ⊘ D/C abruptly

Zanamivir (Relenza) [Antiviral/Neuramidase Inhibitor] Uses: *Influenza A & B w/ Sxs < 2 d; prophylaxis for influenza* **Action:** ↓ Viral neuraminidase **Dose:** *Adults & Peds > 7 y.* 2 Inh (10 mg) bid × 10 d, initiate w/in 48 h of Sxs *Prophylaxis household:* 10 mg qd × 10 d *Adults & Peds > 12 y. Prophylaxis community:* 10 mg qd × 28 d **Caution:** [C, M] Not recommended for pt w/ airway Dz **CI:** Pulm Dz **Disp:** Powder for Inh 5 mg **SE:** Bronchospasm, HA, GI upset, allergic Rxn, abnormal behavior, ear, nose, throat Sx **Labs:** ↑ ALT, AST, CPK **NIPE:** Does not reduce risk of transmitting virus; uses a Diskhaler for administering dose same time each d; 2009 H1N1 strains susceptible

Ziconotide (Prialt) [Pain Control Agent/Nonnarcotic] **WARNING:** Psychological, cognitive, neurologic impair may develop over several wk; monitor frequently; may necessitate D/C **Uses:** *IT Rx of severe, refractory, chronic pain* **Action:** N-type CCB in spinal cord **Dose:** 2.4 mcg/d IT at 0.1 mcg/h; may ↑ 2.4 mcg/d 3 × /wk to max 19.2 mcg/d (0.8 mcg/h) by d 21 **Caution:** [C, ?/–] w/ neuro-/psychological impair **CI:** Psychosis **Disp:** Inj 25, 100 mcg/mL **SE:** Dizziness, N/V, confusion, psychological disturbances, abnormal vision, meningitis; may require dosage adjustment **NIPE:** May D/C abruptly; uses specific pumps; do not ↑ more frequently than 2–3 × /wk

Zidovudine (Retrovir) [Antiretroviral/NRTI] **WARNING:** Neutropenia, anemia, lactic acidosis, myopathy, & hepatomegaly w/ steatosis Uses: *HIV Infxn, prevent maternal HIV transmission* **Action:** ↓ RT **Dose:** *Adults.* 200 mg PO tid or 300 mg PO bid or 1 mg/kg/dose IV q4h *PRG:* 100 mg PO 5×/d until labor; during labor 2 mg/kg IV over 1 h, then 1 mg/kg/h until cord clamped *Peds.* 160 mg/m^2/dose q8h; ↓ in renal failure **Caution:** [C, ?/–] **CI:** Allergy **Disp:** Caps 100 mg; tabs 300 mg; syrup 50 mg/5 mL; Inj 10 mg/mL **SE:** Hematologic tox, HA, fever, rash, GI upset, malaise, myopathy, fat redistribution **Interactions:** ↑ Effects W/ fluconazole, phenytoin, probenecid, valproic acid; ↑ hematologic tox W/ adriamycin, dapsone, ganciclovir, interferon-α; ↓ effects W/ rifampin, ribavirin, stavudine **NIPE:** Take w/o food; monitor for S/Sxs opportunistic infxn; monitor for anemia & liver tox/hep; w/ severe anemia/neutropenia dosage interruption may be needed

Recommended Pediatric Dosage of Retrovir

Dosage Regimen & Dose Body Weight (kg)	Total Daily Dose	bid–tid
4–< 9	24 mg/kg/d,	12 mg/kg, 8 mg/kg
≥ 9–< 30,	18 mg/kg/d,	9 mg/kg, 6 mg/kg
≥ 30,	600 mg/d,	300 mg, 200 mg

Zidovudine & Lamivudine (Combivir) [Antiretroviral/NRTI]
WARNING: Neutropenia, anemia, lactic acidosis, myopathy & hepatomegaly w/ steatosis **Uses:** *HIV Infxn* **Action:** Combo of RT Inhibs **Dose:** *Adults & Peds > 12 y.* 1 tab PO bid; ↓ in renal failure **Caution:** [C, ?/–] **CI:** Component allergy **Disp:** Tab zidovudine 300 mg/lamivudine 150 mg **SE:** Hematologic tox, HA, fever, rash, GI upset, malaise, pancreatitis **Interactions:** ↑ Effects W/ fluconazole, phenytoin, probenecid, valproic acid; ↑ hematologic tox W/ adriamycin, dapsone, ganciclovir, interferon-α; ↓ W/ rifampin, ribavirin, stavudine **NIPE:** Take w/o food; monitor for S/Sxs opportunistic Infxn; monitor for anemia; combo product ↓ daily pill burden

Zileuton (Zyflo, Zyflo CR) [Leukotriene Receptor Antagonist]
Uses: *Chronic Rx asthma* **Action:** Leukotriene Inhib (↓ 5-lipoxygenase) **Dose:** *Adults & Peds > 12 y.* 600 mg PO qid; CR 1200 mg bid w/in 1 h of AM/PM meal **Caution:** [C, ?/–] **CI:** Hepatic impair **Disp:** Tabs 600 mg; CR tabs 600 mg **SE:** Hepatic damage, HA, GI upset, leucopenia, neuropsychological events (agitation, restlessness, suicidal ideation) **Interactions:** ↑ Effects OF propranolol, terfenadine, theophylline, warfarin **Labs:** ↓ WBCs; ↑ LFTs; monitor LFTs qmo × 3, then q2–3mo **NIPE:** Take w/o regard to food; take on a regular basis; not for acute asthma; do not chew/crush CR

Ziprasidone (Geodon) [Antipsychotic/Piperazine Derivative]
WARNING: ↑ Mortality in elderly w/ dementia-related psychosis **Uses:** *Schizophrenia, acute agitation* **Action:** Atypical antipsychotic **Dose:** 20 mg PO bid, may ↑ in 2-d intervals up to 80 mg bid; agitation 10–20 mg IM PRN up to 40 mg/d; separate 10-mg doses by 2 h & 20-mg doses by 4 h (w/ food) **Caution:** [C, –] w/ ↑ Mg²⁺, ↓ K⁺ **CI:** QT prolongation, recent MI, uncompensated HF, meds that ↑ QT interval **Disp:** Caps 20, 40, 60, 80 mg; susp 10 mg/mL; Inj 20 mg/mL **SE:** Bradycardia; rash, somnolence, resp disorder, EPS, wgt gain, orthostatic ↓ BP **Interactions:** ↑ Effects W/ ketoconazole; ↑ effects OF antihypertensives; ↑ CNS depression W/ anxiolytics, sedatives, opioids, EtOH; TCAs, thioridazine; risk of prolonged QT W/ cisapride, chlorpromazine, clarithromycin, diltiazem, erythromycin, levofloxacin, mefloquine, pentamidine, TCAs, thioridazine; ↓ effects W/ amphetamines, carbamazepine; ↓ effects OF levodopa **Labs:** ↑ Glucose; monitor lytes **NIPE:** May take wk before full effects, take w/ food; ↑ risk of tardive dyskinesia; monitor ECG—may ↑ QT interval; ↑ risk of tardive dyskinesia

Zoledronic Acid (Zometa, Reclast) [Antihypercalcemic/Biphosphonate] **Uses:** *↑ Ca²⁺ of malignancy (HCM), ↑ skeletal-related events in CAP, multiple myeloma, & met bone lesions (Zometa)*; *prevent/Rx of postmenopausal osteoporosis, Paget Dz, ↑ bone mass in men w/ osteoporosis, steroid-induced osteoporosis (Reclast)* **Action:** Bisphosphonate; ↓ osteoclastic bone resorption **Dose:** *Zometa HCM:* 4 mg IV over ≥ 15 min; may retreat in 7 d w/ adequate renal Fxn *Zometa bone lesions/myeloma:* 4 mg IV over > 15 min, repeat q3–4wk PRN; extend w/ ↑ Cr *Reclast Rx osteoporosis:* 5 mg IV annually; *Reclast* prevent postmenopausal osteoporosis 5 mg IV q2y; Paget 5 mg IV × 1 **Caution:** [C, ?/−] Diuretics, aminoglycosides; ASA-sensitive asthmatics; avoid invasive dental procedures **CI:** Bisphosphonate allergy; urticaria, angioedema, w/ dental procedures **Disp:** Vial 4, 5 mg **SE:** All ↑ w/ renal dysfunction; fever, flu-like synd, GI upset, insomnia, anemia; lytes abnormalities, bone, Jt, muscle pain, AF, osteonecrosis of jaw **Interactions:** ↑ Risk of hypocalcemia W/ diuretics; ↑ risk of nephrotox W/ aminoglycosides, thalidomide **Labs:** Follow Cr; effect prolonged w/ Cr ↑ **NIPE:** ↑ Fluids to 2–3 L/d; requires vigorous prehydration; do not exceed recommended doses/Inf duration to ↓ renal dysfunction; avoid oral surgery; dental exam recommended prior to therapy; ↓ dose w/ renal dysfunction; give Ca^{2+} & vit D supls; may ↑ atypical subtrochanteric femur fxs

Zolmitriptan (Zomig, Zomig XMT, Zomig Nasal) [Analgesic Migraine Agent/5-HT₁ Receptor Agonist]

Uses: *Acute Rx migraine* **Action:** Selective serotonin agonist; causes vasoconstriction **Dose:** Initial 2.5 mg PO, may repeat after 2 h, 10 mg max in 24 h; nasal 5 mg; if HA returns, repeat after 2 h, 10 mg max 24 h **Caution:** [C, ?/−] **CI:** Ischemic heart Dz, Prinzmetal angina, uncontrolled HTN, accessory conduction pathway disorders, ergots, MAOIs **Disp:** Tabs 2.5, 5 mg; rapid tabs (*XMT*) 2.5, 5 mg; nasal 5 mg, **SE:** Dizziness, hot flashes, paresthesias, chest tightness, myalgia, diaphoresis **Interactions:** ↑ Effects W/ cimetidine, MAOIs, OPCs, propranolol; ↑ risk of prolonged vasospasms W/ ergots; ↑ risk of serotonin synd W/ sibutramine, SSRIs **NIPE:** Administer to relieve migraines; not for prophylaxis

Zolpidem Tartrate (Ambien IR, Ambien CR, Edluar, Zolpimist) [C-IV] [Sedative/Hypnotic]

Uses: *Short-term Rx of insomnia; Ambien & Edluar w/ difficulty of sleep onset; Ambien CR w/ difficulty of sleep onset and/or sleep maint* **Action:** Hypnotic agent **Dose:** Ambien: 5–10 mg or 12.5 mg CR PO hs PRN Edluar: 10-mg SL qhs Zolpimist: 10-mg spray qhs; ↓ in elderly, debilitated, & hepatic impair (5- or 6.25-mg CR) **Caution:** [C, −] May cause anaphylaxis, angioedema, abnormal thinking, CNS depression, withdrawal; eval for other comorbid conditions **CI:** None **Disp:** Ambien IR: Tabs 5, 10 mg; CR 6.25, 12.5 mg Edluar: SL tabs 5, 10 mg Zolpimist: Oral soln 5 mg/spray (60 actuations/unit) **SE:** HA, dizziness, drowsiness, drugged feeling, dry mouth, depression **Interactions:** ↑ CNS depression W/ CNS depressants, sertraline, EtOH; ↑ effects OF ketoconazole; ↓ effects OF rifampin **NIPE:** Take w/o food; be able to sleep 7–8 h Zolpimist: Prime w/ 5 sprays initially, & w/ 1 spray if not used in 14 d; store upright ⊘ D/C abruptly if long-term use; may develop tolerance to drug; may be habit-forming

Zonisamide (Zonegran) [Anticonvulsant/Sulfonamide]

WARNING: ↑ Risk of suicidal thoughts or behavior **Uses:** *Adjunct Rx complex partial Szs* **Action:** Anticonvulsant **Dose:** Initial 100 mg/D PO; may ↑ to 400 mg/d **Caution:** [C, −] ↑ tox w/ CYP3A4 Inhib; ↓ levels w/ carbamazepine, phenytoin, phenobarbital, valproic acid **CI:** Allergy to sulfonamides; oligohydrosis & hypothermia in peds **Disp:** Caps 25, 50, 100 mg **SE:** Dizziness, drowsiness, confusion, ataxia, memory impair, paresthesias, psychosis, nystagmus, diplopia, tremor, anemia, leukopenia; GI upset, nephrolithiasis, SJS **Interactions:** ↑ Tox **W/** CYP3A4 Inhib; ↓ effects **W/** carbamazepine, phenobarbital, phenytoin, valproic acid **Labs:** ↑ Serum alk phos, ALT, AST, Cr, BUN, ↓ glucose, Na **NIPE:** ⊘ D/C abruptly; swallow caps whole; monitor for ↓ sweating & ↑ body temperature

Zoster Vaccine, Live (Zostavax) [Vaccine] **Uses:** *Prevent varicella zoster in adults > 60 y* **Action:** Active immunization (live attenuated varicella virus) **Dose:** *Adults.* 0.65 mL SQ × 1 **CI:** Gelatin, neomycin anaphylaxis; fever, untreated TB, immunocompromise **Caution:** [C, ?/–] Not for peds **Disp:** SD vial **SE:** Inj site Rxn, HA **Interactions:** Risk of extensive rash **W/** corticosteroids **NIPE:** ⊘ PRG for at least 3 mo > vaccination; once reconstituted use stat; may be used if previous h/o zoster; do not use in place of varicella virus vaccine in children; contact precautions not necessary

COMMONLY USED NATURAL AND HERBAL AGENTS

The following is a guide to some common herbal products. These may be sold separately or in combination with other products. According to the FDA, "Manufacturers of dietary supplements can make claims about how their products affect the structure or function of the body, but they may not claim to prevent, treat, cure, mitigate, or diagnose a disease without prior FDA approval." These agents can have significant side effects that RNs & APNs should be aware of. The table below provides a listing of unsafe herbs with known toxicities

Unsafe Herbs with Known Toxicity

Agent	Toxicities
Aconite	Salivation, N/V, blurred vision, cardiac arrhythmias
Aristolochic acid	Nephrotox
Calamus	Possible carcinogenicity
Chaparral	Hepatotox, possible carcinogenicity, nephrotox
"Chinese herbal mixtures"	May contain ma huang or other dangerous herbs
Coltsfoot	Hepatotox, possibly carcinogenic
Comfrey	Hepatotox, carcinogenic
Ephedra/ma huang	Adverse cardiac events, stroke, Sz
Juniper	High-allergy potential, D, Sz, nephrotox
Kava kava	Hepatotox
Licorice	Chronic daily amounts (> 30 g/mo) can result in ↓ K+, Na/fluid retention w/ HTN, myoglobinuria, hyporeflexia
Life root	Hepatotox, liver CA
Ma huang/ephedra	Adverse cardiac events, stroke, Sz
Pokeweed	GI cramping, N/D/V, labored breathing, ↓ BP, Sz
Sassafras	V, stupor, hallucinations, dermatitis, abortion, hypothermia, liver CA
Usnic acid	Hepatotox
Yohimbine	Hypotension, Abd distress, CNS stimulation (mania/& psychosis in predisposed individuals)

Aloe Vera (*Aloe barbadensis*) **Uses:** Topically for burns, skin irritation, sunburn, wounds; internally used for constipation, amenorrhea, asthma, colds **Actions:** Multiple chemical components; aloinosides inhibit H_2O & lytes reabsorption & irritates colon which ↑ peristalsis & propulsion; wound healing d/t ↓ production of thromboxane A2, inhibiting bradykinin & histamine **Available forms:** Apply gel topically 3–5/d PRN; caps 100–200 mg PO hs **CI:** ⊘ Internally if PRG, lactating, or in children < 12 y **Notes/SE:** Abd cramping, D, edema, hematuria, hypokalemia, muscle weakness, dermatitis **Interactions w/ internal use:** ↑ K^+ loss W/ BB, corticosteroids, diuretics, licorice; ↑ effects OF antiarrhythmics, corticosteroids, digoxin, diuretics, hyperglycemias, jimsonweed **Labs:** ↓ K^+, BS **NIPE:** Assess for dehydration, lytes imbalance, Abd distress w/ internal use; stimulates uterine contractions & may cause spontaneous abortion

Arnica (*Arnica montana*) **Uses:** ↓ Swelling & inflammation from acne, blunt injury, bruises, rashes, sprains **Action:** Sesquiterpenoids have shown antibacterial, anti-inflammatory, & analgesic properties **Available forms:** Topical cream, spray, oint, tinc; for poultice dilute tinc 3–10 × w/ H_2O & apply PRN **CI:** Poisonous, ⊘ take internally; avoid if pt allergic to arnica, chrysanthemums, marigold, sunflowers **Notes/SE:** Arrhythmias, Abd pain, cardiac arrest, contact dermatitis, coma, death, hepatic failure, HTN, nervousness, restlessness **Interactions:** ↑ Risk of bleeding W/ ASA, heparin, warfarin, angelica, anise, asafetida, bogbean, boldo, capsicum, celery, chamomile, clove, danshen, fenugreek, feverfew, garlic, ginger, ginkgo, ginseng, horse chestnut, horseradish, licorice, meadowsweet, onion, papain, passion flower, poplar bark, prickly ash, quassia wood, red clover, turmeric, wild carrot, wild lettuce, willow; ↓ effects OF antihypertensives **Labs:** None **NIPE:** ⊘ Apply to broken skin, ⊘ use in PRG & lactation, serious liver & kidney damage w/ internal use, ingestion of flowers & root can cause death, prolonged topical use ↑ risk of allergic Rxn

Astragalus (*Astragalus membranaceus*) **Uses:** Rx of resp Infxns, enhancement of immune system, & HF **Action:** Root saponins ↑ diuresis, ↓ BP; anti-inflammatory action related to the stimulation of macrophages, ↑ Ab formation & ↑ T-lymphocyte proliferation **Available forms:** Caps/tabs 1–4 g tid, PO; Liq extract 4–8 mL/d (1:2 ratio) % doses; dry extract 250 mg (1:8 ratio) tid, PO **Notes/SE:** Immunosuppression w/ doses > 28 g **Interactions:** ↑ Effect OF acyclovir, anticoagulants, antihypertensives, antithrombotics, antiplts, IL-2, interferon; ↓ effect OF cyclophosphamide **Labs:** ↑ PT, INR **NIPE:** Use cautiously in immunosuppressed pts or those w/ autoimmune Dz

Bilberry (*Vaccinium myrtillus*) **Uses:** Prevent/Tx visual problems such as cataract, retinopathy, myopia, glaucoma, macular degeneration; treat vascular problems such as hemorrhoids, & varicose veins **Actions:** Contain anthocyanidins that ↓ vascular permeability, inhibit plt aggregation & thrombus formation, ↑ antioxidant effects on LDLs & liver, ↑ regeneration of rhodopsin in retina **Available forms:** Products should have 25% anthocyanoside content; caps, extracts, dried, or fresh fruit, leaves; eye/vascular problems 240–480 mg PO bid/tid; night vision

60–120 mg of extract PO OD **CI:** ⊘ PRG or lactation; caution in pts w/ DM & bleeding disorders **Notes/SE:** Constipation **Interactions:** ↑ Effects *OF* anticoagulants, antiplts, insulin, NSAIDs, oral hypoglycemics, ↓ effects *OF* Fe **Labs:** ↑ PT; ↓ glucose, plt aggregation **NIPE:** Large dose of leaves for long periods of time may be poisonous/fatal; take w/o regard to food

Black Cohosh (*Cimicifuga racemosa*) **Uses:** Antitussive; smooth-muscle relaxant; management of menopausal Sxs esp hot flashes, sleep disturbance, & anxiety, PMS, & dysmenorrhea. Anti-inflammatory, peripheral vasodilation, & sedative effects **Action:** Estrogenic activity w/ some studies showing ↓ in LH; vasodilation activity causing ↑ blood flow & hypotensive effects; antimicrobial activity **Available forms:** Dried root/rhizome caps 40–200 mg once/d; fluid extract (1:1) 2–4 mL or 1 tsp once/d; tinc (1:5) 3–6 mL or 1–2 tsp once/d; powdered extract (4:1) 250–500 mg once/d; Remifemin menopause (standardized extract brand name) 20 mg bid **Notes/SE:** ↓ Hypotension, bradycardia, N/V, anorexia, HA, miscarriage, nervous system & visual disturbances; liver damage/failure **Interactions:** ↑ Effects *OF* antihypertensives, estrogen HRT, OCPs, hypnotics, sedatives; tinc may cause a Rxn *W/* disulfiram & metronidazole; ↑ antiproliferative effect *W/* tamoxifen; ↓ effects *OF* ferrous fumarate, ferrous gluconate, ferrous sulfate **Labs:** May ↓ LH levels & plt counts **NIPE:** Tinc contains large % of EtOH, ⊘ use in PRG or lactation or give to children

Bogbean (*Menyanthes trifoliate*) **Uses:** ↑ Appetite; treat GI distress; anti-inflammatory for arthritis **Action:** Several chemical constituents include alkaloids (choline, gentianin, gentianidine), flavonoids (hyperin, kaempferol, quercetin, rutin, trifolioside) that act as an anti-inflammatory, & acids (caffeic, chlorogenic, ferulic, folic, palmitic, salicylic, vanillic); 2 compounds produce considerable inhibition of prostaglandin synth **Available forms:** Extract (1:1 dilution) 1–2 mL PO tid w/ fluid; dried leaf as tea 1–3 g PO tid **CI:** ⊘ PRG or lactating **Notes/SE:** N/V, bleeding **Interactions:** ↑ Risk of bleeding *W/* anticoagulants, antiplts, ANA, NSAIDs; ↑ effects *OF* stimulant laxatives; ↓ effects *OF* antacids, H₂-antagonists, PPIs, sucralfate **Labs:** None **NIPE:** May ↑ uterine contractions; extracts contain EtOH; monitor for S/Sxs bleeding or ↑ bruising; ⊘ if h/o colitis, anemia

Borage (*Borago officinalis*) **Uses:** Oil used for eczema & dermatitis & as a GLA supl; treat colds, coughs, & bronchitis; anti-inflammatory action used to treat arthritis **Action:** Oil contains GLA & its metabolites produce anti-inflammatory action; topical oil absorbed in skin ↑ fluid retention in stratum corneum; mucilage & malic acid components have expectorant & diuretic actions; contains alkaloids that are hepatotox **Available forms:** Caps w/ 10–25% GLA; 1.1–1.4 g GLA PO OD for Jt inflammation; oil topical application bid for dermatitis & eczema **CI:** ⊘ PRG, lactation, & pts w/ h/o liver Dz or Sz disorder **Notes/SE:** ↑ Constipation, flatulence, liver dysfunction, Sz **Interactions:** ↑ Risk of bleeding *W/* anticoagulants, antiplts; ↑ effects *OF* antihypertensives; ↓ effects *OF* anticonvulsants, phenothiazine, TCAs; ↓ effects *OF* herb *W/* NSAIDs **Labs:** Monitor LFTs; may ↑ LFTs, PT, & INR **NIPE:** Only use herb w/o UPA alkaloids

Bugleweed (*Lycopus virginicus*) **Uses:** ↓ Hyperthyroid Sxs, analgesic, astringent **Action:** Inhibits gonadotropin, prolactin, TSH & IgG Ab activity **Available forms:** Teas, extracts, dried herb **CI:** ⊘ PRG or lactation, pts w/ hypothyroidism, pituitary or thyroid tumors, hypogonadism, & CHF **Notes/SE:** Thyroid gland enlargement **Interactions:** ↑ Effects *OF* insulin, oral hypoglycemics, ↑ thyroid suppressing effects *W/* balm leaf & wild thyme plant; ↓ effects *OF* thyroid hormone **Labs:** ↓ FSH, LH, HCG, TSH; monitor BS **NIPE:** ⊘ Substitute for antithyroid drugs; avoid if undergoing Tx or diagnostic procedures w/ radioisotopes; ⊘ D/C abruptly

Butcher's Broom (*Ruscus aculeatus*) **Uses:** Rx of circulatory disorders such as PVD, varicose veins, & leg edema; hemorrhoids; diuretic; laxative; inflammation; arthritis **Action:** Vasoconstriction d/t direct activation of the α-receptors of the smooth-muscle cells in vascular walls **Available forms:** Raw extract 7–11 mg once/d, PO; tea 1 tsp in 1 cup H$_2$O; topical oint apply PRN **Notes/SE:** GI upset, N/V **Interactions:** ↑ Effects *OF* anticoagulants, MAOIs; ↓ effects *OF* antihypertensives **Labs:** None **NIPE:** Hypertensive crisis may occur if administer w/ MAOIs; ⊘ use in PRG & lactation

Capsicum (*Capsicum frutescens*) **Uses:** Topical use includes pain relief from arthritis, diabetic neuropathy, postherpetic neuralgia, postsurgical pain; internal uses include circulatory disorders, GI distress, HTN **Actions:** Stimulates skin pain receptors causing burning sensations; desensitization of pain receptors results in pain relief; ↓ lymphocyte production, Ab production, & plt aggregation **Available forms:** Topical creams 0.025–0.25% up to qid; caps 400–500 mg PO tid **CI:** ⊘ On open sores, in PRG, children < 2 y **Notes/SE:** GI irritation, sweating, bronchospasm, resp irritation, topical burning, stinging, erythema **Interactions:** ↑ Effects *OF* anticoagulants, antiplts, theophylline; ↑ risk of cough *W/* ACEIs; ↑ risk of anticoagulant effects *W/* feverfew, garlic, ginger, ginkgo, ginseng; ↑ risk of hypertensive crisis *W/* MAOIs; ↓ effects *OF* clonidine, methyldopa **Labs:** None **NIPE:** Pain relief may take several wk; ⊘ apply heat on areas w/ topical capsicum cream; avoid contact w/ eyes or mucous membranes

Cascara (*Rhamnus purshiana*) **Uses:** Laxative **Action:** Stimulates large intestine, ↑ bowel motility & propulsion **Available forms:** Liq extract 1–5 mL PO OD **CI:** ⊘ PRG, lactation, & IBD **Notes/SE:** N/V, Abd cramps, urine discoloration, osteomalacia **Interactions:** ↑ Effects *OF* antiarrhythmics, cardiac glycosides; ↑ K$^+$ loss *W/* diuretics, corticosteroids, cardiac glycosides; ↓ effects *W/* antacids, milk **Labs:** ↓ Serum K$^+$ **NIPE:** Short-term use; monitor lytes; caution w/ diuretics

Chamomile (*Matricaria recutita*) **Uses:** Anti-inflammatory, antipyretic, antimicrobial, antispasmodic, astringent, sedative **Action:** Ingredients include α-bisabolol oil, which ↓ inflammation, antispasmodic activity, ↑ healing times for burns & ulcers, & inhibits ulcer formation; apigenin contributes to the anti-inflammatory effect, antispasmodic & sedative effect; azulene inhibits histamine release; chamazulene reduces inflammation & has antioxidant & antimicrobial effects **Available forms:** Teas 3–5 g (1 tbsp) flower heads steeped in 250 mL hot H_2O tid–qid between meals, also use as a gargle or compress; fluid extract 1:1—45% EtOH 1–3 mL tid **Notes/SE:** Allergic Rxns w/ pt allergic to Compositae family (chrysanthemums, ragweed, sunflowers, asters) eg, angioedema, eczema, contact dermatitis, & anaphylaxis **Interactions:** ↑ Effects *OF* CNS depressants, EtOH, anticoagulants, antiplts; ↑ risk of miscarriage; ↓ effects *OF* drugs metabolized by CY4503A4, eg, alprazolam, atorvastatin, diazepam, ketoconazole, verapamil **Labs:** Monitor anticoagulant levels **NIPE:** ⊘ PRG, lactation, children < 2 y, pt w/ asthma or hay fever; delayed ↓ gastric absorption of meds if taken together (↓ GI motility)

Chondroitin Sulfate **Uses:** Combine w/ glucosamine to Rx arthritis; use as an anticoagulant; draws fluids/nutrients into Jt, "shock absorption" **Action:** Biological polymer, flexible matrix between protein filaments in cartilage; attracts fluid & nutrients into the Jts; inhibits thrombin **Available forms:** 1200 mg once/d, PO, & usually given w/ glucosamine 1500 mg once/d, PO for nl wgt adults **Notes/SE:** D, dyspepsia, HA, N/V, restlessness **Interactions:** ↑ Effects *OF* anticoagulants, ASA, NSAIDs **Labs:** None **NIPE:** ⊘ PRG & lactation

Comfrey (*Symphytum officinale*) **Uses:** Topical Tx of wounds, bruises, sprains, inflammation **Action:** Multiple chemical components, allantoin promotes cell division, rosmarinic acid has anti-inflammatory effects, tannin possesses astringent effects, mucilage is a demulcent w/ anti-inflammatory properties, UPA cause hepatotox **Available forms:** Topical application w/ 5–20% of herb applied on intact skin for up to 10 d **CI:** ⊘ Internally d/t hepatotox, ⊘ PRG or lactation **Notes/SE:** N/V, exfoliative dermatitis w/ topical use **Interactions:** ↑ Risk of hepatotox *W/* ingestion of borage, golden ragwort, hemp, petasites **Labs:** ↑ LFTs, total bilirubin, urine bilirubin **NIPE:** ⊘ Use for more than 6 wk in 1 y; ⊘ use on broken skin

Coriander (*Coriandrum sativum*) **Uses:** ↑ Appetite, treat D, dyspepsia, flatulence **Action:** Stimulates gastric secretions, spasmolytic effects **Available forms:** Tinc 10–30 gtts PO OD **CI:** ⊘ PRG or lactation **Notes/SE:** N/V, fatty liver tumors, allergic skin Rxns **Interactions:** ↑ Effects *OF* oral hypoglycemics **Labs:** Monitor BS **NIPE:** ↑ Risk of photosensitivity—use sunscreen

Cranberry (*Vaccinium macrocarpon*) **Uses:** Prevention UTI; urinary deodorizer in urinary incontinence **Actions:** Interferes w/ bacterial adherence to epithelial cells of the bladder **Available forms:** Caps 300–500 mg PO bid–qid; unsweetened juice 8–16 oz daily; tinc 3–5 mL or *tinc* 1/2–1 tsp up to 3 × /d, *tea* 2–3 tsps of dried flowers/cup; *creams* apply topically 2–3 × /d PO **SE:** D, irritation, nephrolithiasis if ↑ urinary Ca oxalate **Interactions:** ↑ Effects *OF* warfarin; ↑ excretion *OF* alkaline drugs such as antidepressants & methotrexate will cause ↓ effectiveness *OF* drug; ↓ effectiveness *OF* Uva-ursi **Labs:** ↑ Urine pH **NIPE:** Possibly effective in treating UTI; tinc contains up to 45% EtOH; only unsweetened form effective; regular use may ↓ frequency of bacteriuria w/ pyria

Dong Quai (Angelica polymorpha, sinensis) Uses: Uterine stimulant; dysmenorrhea, PMS, menorrhagia, chronic pelvic Infxn, irregular menstruation. Other reported uses include anemia, HTN, HA, rhinitis, neuralgia, hep, anti-inflammatory, vasodilator, CNS stimulant, immunosuppressant, analgesic, antipyretic, antiasthmatic **Action:** Root extracts contain at least 6 coumarin derivatives that have anticoagulant, vasodilating, antispasmodic, & CNS-stimulating activity. Studies demonstrate weak estrogen-agonist actions of the extract **Efficacy:** Possibly effective for menopausal Sx **Available forms:** Caps 500 mg, 1–2 caps PO, tid; Liq extract 1–2 gtt, tid; tea 1–2 g, tid **Notes/SE:** D, bleeding, photosensitivity, skin CA **Interactions:** ↑ Effects *OF* anticoagulants, antiplts, estrogens, warfarin; ↑ anticoagulant activity *W/* chamomile, dandelion, horse chestnut, red clover; ↑ risk of disulfiram-like Rxn *W/* disulfiram, metronidazole **Labs:** ↑ INR w/ warfarin **NIPE:** Photosensitivity—use sunscreen, ⊘ if breast-feeding or PRG; tincs & extracts contain EtOH up to 60%; D/C herb 14 d prior to dental or surgical procedures

Echinacea (Echinacea purpurea) Uses: Immune system stimulant; prevention/Rx of colds, flu; as supportive therapy for colds & chronic Infxns in the resp tract & lower urinary tract **Action:** Stimulates phagocytosis & cytokine production & ↑ resp cellular activity; topically exerts anesthetic, antimicrobial, & anti-inflammatory effects **Efficacy:** Not established; may ↓ severity & duration of URI **Available forms:** Caps w/ powdered herb equivalent to 300–500 mg, PO, tid; pressed juice 6–9 mL, PO, once/d; tinc 2–4 mL, PO, tid (1:5 dilution); tea 2 tsp (4 g) of powdered herb in 1 cup of boiling H_2O **Notes/SE:** Fever, taste perversion, urticaria, angioedema **CI:** ⊘ In pts w/ autoimmune Dz, collagen Dz, progressive systemic Dz (TB, MS, collagen-vascular disorders), HIV, leukemia, may interfere w/ immunosuppressive therapy **Interactions:** ↑ Risk of disulfiram-like Rxn *W/* disulfiram, metronidazole; ↑ risk of exacerbation of HIV or AIDS *W/* echinacea & amprenavir, other protease Inhibs; ↓ effects *OF* azathioprine, basiliximab, corticosteroids, cyclosporine, daclizumab, econazole Vag cream, muromonab-CD3, mycophenolate, prednisone, tacrolimus **Labs:** ↑ ALT, AST, lymphocytes, ESR **NIPE:** Large doses of herb interferes w/ sperm activity; ⊘ w/ breast-feeding or PRG; ⊘ continuously for longer than 8 wk w/o a 3-wk break in Rx-possible immunosuppression; 3 different commercial forms

Ephedra/Ma Huang Uses: Stimulant, aid in wgt loss, bronchial dilation **Dose:** Not OK d/t reported deaths (> 100 mg/d can be life-threatening). US sales banned by FDA in 2004; bitter orange w/ similar properties has replaced this compound in most wgt loss supls **Caution:** Adverse cardiac events, strokes, death **SE:** Nervousness, HA, insomnia, palpitations, V, hyperglycemia **Interactions:** Digoxin, antihypertensives, antidepressants, diabetic medications **Labs:** ↑ ALT, AST, total bilirubin, urine bilirubin, serum glucose **NIPE:** Tincs & extracts contain EtOH; linked to several deaths; monitor for behavioral mood changes

Evening Primrose Oil (Oenothera biennis) Uses: PMS, diabetic neuropathy, ADHD, IBS, RA, mastalgia **Action:** Anti-inflammatory, antispasmodic, diuretic, sedative effects related to a high conc of essential fatty acids esp GLA & CLA & their conversion into prostaglandins **Efficacy:** Possibly for PMS, not for menopausal Sx **Available forms:** Caps, gel-caps, Liq dose depends on GLA content *DM neuropathy:* 4000–6000 mg PO OD *Eczema:* 4000 mg PO OD *Mastalgia:* 3000–4000 mg PO OD *PMS:* 2000–4000 mg PO OD *RA:* Upto 5000 mg PO OD **Notes/SE:** Indigestion, N, soft stools, flatulence, HA, anorexia, rash **CI:** ⊘ PRG or lactation; ⊘ persons w/ Sz disorders **Interactions:** ↑ Phenobarbital metabolism, ↓ Sz threshold, ↑ effects *OF* diuretics, sedatives **Labs:** None **NIPE:** May take up to 4 mo for max effectiveness, take w/ food

Feverfew (*Tanacetum parthenium*)
Uses: Prevent/Rx migraine; fever; menstrual disorders; anti-inflammatory for arthritis, asthma, digestion problems, threatened abortion; toothache; insect bites **Action:** Active ingredient, parthenolide, inhibits serotonin release, prostaglandin synth, plt aggregation, & histamine release from mast cells; several ingredients inhibit activation of polymorphonuclear leukocytes & leukotriene synth **Efficacy:** Weak for migraine prevention **Available forms:** Freeze-dried leaf extract 25 mg once/d; caps 300–400 mg tid PO; tinc 15–30 gtt once/d to 0.2–0.7 mg of parthenolide **Notes/SE:** Mouth ulcers, muscle stiffness, Jt pain, GI upset, rash **CI:** ⊘ PRG & lactation or w/ ragweed allergy **Interactions:** ↑ Effects *OF* anticoagulants, antiplts, ↓ absorption *OF* Fe **Labs:** ↑ PT, INR, PTT **NIPE:** ⊘ D/C herb abruptly or may experience Jt stiffness & pain, HAs, insomnia

Fish Oil Supplements (*Omega-3 Polyunsaturated Fatty Acid*)
Uses: CAD, hypercholesterolemia, hypertriglyceridemia, type 2 DM, arthritis **Efficacy:** No definitive data on ↓ cardiac risk in general population; may ↓ lipids & help w/ secondary MI prevention **Dose:** 1 FDA approved (Lovaza); OTC 1500–3000 mg/d; AHA rec 1 g/d **Caution:** Mercury contamination possible, some studies suggest ↑ cardiac events **SE:** ↑ Bleed risk, dyspepsia, belching, aftertaste **Interactions:** Anticoagulants

Garlic (*Allium sativum*)
Uses: Antioxidant, Antithrombotic, antilipidemic, antitumor, antimicrobial, antiasthmatic, anti-inflammatory, HTN; anti-infective (antibacterial, antifungal); tick repellant (oral) **Action:** Inhibits gram(+) & (−) organisms, exerts cholesterol-lowering by preventing gastric lipase fat digestion & fecal excretion of sterols & bile acids & it inhibits free radicals **Efficacy:** ↓ Cholesterol by 4–6%; soln ↓ BP; possible ↓ GI/CAP risk **Available forms:** Teas, tabs, caps, extract, oil, dried powder, syrup, fresh bulb **Dose:** 2–5 g, fresh garlic; 0.4–1.2 g of dried powder; 2–5 mg oil; 300–1000 mg extract or other formulations = to 2–5 mg of allicin daily, 400–1200 mg powder (2–5 mg allicin) PO **Notes/SE:** ↑ Insulin/lipid/cholesterol levels, anemia, oral burning sensation, dizziness, diaphoresis, HA, N/V, hypothyroidism, contact dermatitis, allergic Rxns, systemic garlic odor, ↓ Hgb production, lysis of RBCs **Interactions:** ↑ Effects *OF* anticoagulants, antiplts, insulin, oral hypoglycemics; CYP450 3A4 inducer (may ↓ cyclosporine, HIV antivirals, OCPs; ↓ effects *W/* acidophilus **Labs:** ↓ Total cholesterol, LDL, triglycerides, plt aggregation, iodine uptake; ↑ PT, serum IgE; monitor CBC, PT

NIPE: ⊘ PRG—abortifacient, lactation, prior to surgery—D/C 7 d pre-op (bleeding risk), GI disorders; report bleeding, bruising, petechiae, tarry stools

Gentian (*Gentiana lutea*) **Uses:** ↑ Appetite, treat digestive disorders such as colitis, IBS, flatulence **Actions:** Chemical components stimulate digestive juices **Available forms:** Liq extract 2–4g PO OD, tinc 1–3 g PO OD, dried root 2–4 g PO OD **CI:** ⊘ PRG, lactation, & HTN **Notes/SE:** N/V, HA **Interactions:** ↑ CNS sedation *W/* barbiturates, benzodiazepines, EtOH if extract/tinc contains alcohol; ↓ absorption *OF* Fe salts **Labs:** None **NIPE:** Caution—many herb preps contain up to 60% EtOH

Ginger (*Zingiber officinale*) **Uses:** Prevent motion sickness; N/V d/t anesthesia; antiemetic ↓ N/V; anti-inflammatory relieves pain & swelling of muscle injury, OA & RA; antispasmodic action relieves colic, flatulence & indigestion; antiplt; antipyretic; antioxidant; anti-infective against gram(+) & (−) bacteria **Action:** Anti-inflammatory effect inhibits prostaglandin, thromboxane, & leukotriene biosynthesis; antiemetic effects d/t action on the GI tract; antiplt effect d/t the inhibition of thromboxane formation; + inotropic effect on CV system **Efficacy:** Benefit in ↓ N/V w/ motion or PRG; weak for post-op or chemotherapy **Available forms:** Dosage form & strength depends on Dz process, fluid extract 0.7–2 mL once/d, PO, (2:1 ratio); tabs 500 mg bid–qid, PO; tinc 1.7–5 mL once/d, PO, (1:5 ratio) **Caution:** Pt w/ gallstones; excessive dose (↑ depression, & may interfere w/ cardiac Fxn or anticoagulants) **SE:** Heartburn **Interactions:** ↑ Risk of bleeding *W/* anticoagulants, antiplts; ↑ risk of disulfiram-like Rxn *W/* disulfiram, metronidazole **Labs:** ↑ PT **NIPE:** Store herb in cool, dry area; ⊘ PRG, lactation; lack of standardization for herb dosing

Ginkgo (*Ginko biloba*) **Uses:** Effective w/ circulatory disorders, cerebrovascular Dz, & dementia; used to improve alertness & attention span; memory deficits, dementia, anxiety, improvement, Sx peripheral vascular Dz, vertigo, tinnitus, asthma/bronchospasm, antioxidant, premenstrual Sx (esp breast tenderness), impotence, SSRI-induced sexual dysfunction **Action:** Extract flavonoids, release neurotransmitters, & inhibit MAO, which enhances cognitive Fxn; vascular protective action results from relaxation of blood vessels, ↑ tissue perfusion, inhibition of plt aggregation; eradicates free radicals & ↓ polymorphonuclear neutrophils **Efficacy:** Small cognition benefit w/ dementia; no other demonstrated benefit in healthy adults **Available forms:** Dosage depends on diagnosis *General use:* Tabs & caps 40–80 mg tid, PO; tinc 0.5 mL tid, PO; extract 40–80 mg tid, PO **Caution:** ↑ Bleeding risk (antagonism of plt-activating factor), concerning w/ antiplt agents (D/C 3 d pre-op); reports of ↑ Sz risk **Notes/SE:** GI upset, dizziness, HA, heart palpitations, rash **Interactions:** ↑ Effect *OF* MAOIs; ↑ risk of bleeding *W/* anisindine, dalteparin, dicumarol garlic, heparin, salicylates, warfarin; ↑ risk of coma *W/* trazodone; ↑ effect *OF* carbamazepine, gabapentin, insulin, oral hypoglycemics, phenobarbital, phenytoin; ↓ Sz threshold *W/* bupropion, TCAs **Labs:** ↑ PT **NIPE:** ⊘ PRG & lactation; tincs contain up to 60% EtOH; ⊘ 2 wk prior to surgery

Ginseng (*Panax quinquefolius*) Uses: "Energy booster" general; ↑ physical endurance, conc, appetite, sleep, & stress resistance; ↓ fatigue; antioxidant; aids in glucose control—type 2 DM; also for pt undergoing chemotherapy, stress reduction, enhance brain activity, & physical endurance (adaptogenic), panax ginseng being studied for ED **Action:** Dried root contains ginsenosides, which ↑ natural killer cell activity, & nuclear RNA synth, & motor activity **Efficacy:** Not established **Available forms:** No standard dosage *General u*SE: Caps 200–500 mg once/d, PO; tea 3 g steeped in boiling H_2O tid PO, tinc 1–2 mg once/d, PO (1:1 dilution); 1–2 g of root or 100–300 mg of extract (7% ginsenosides) PO tid **Caution:** w/ Cardiac Dz, DM, ↓BP, HTN, mania, schizophrenia, w/ corticosteroids; avoid in PRG; D/C 7 d pre-op (bleeding risk) **Notes/SE:** Anxiety, anorexia, CP, D, HTN, N/V, palpitations **Interactions:** ↑ Effects *OF* estrogen, hypoglycemics, CNS stimulants, caffeine, ephedra; ↑ risk of bleeding *W/* ibuprofen; ↑ risk of HA, irritability & visual hallucinations *W/* MAOIs; ↓ effects *OF* anisindione, dicumarol, furosemide, heparin, warfarin **Labs:** ↑ Digoxin level falsely; ↓ glucose, PT, INR **NIPE:** ⊘ Use continuously for > 3 mo; ⊘ during PRG or lactation; eval for ginseng abuse synd w/ Sxs of D, depression, edema, HTN, insomnia, rash, & restlessness

Glucosamine Sulfate (*Chitosamine*) Uses: Used w/ chondroitin for the Rx of OA (glucosamine: rate-limiting step in glycosaminoglycan synth), ↑ cartilage rebuilding; **Action:** Stimulate the production of cartilage components **Available forms:** Caps/tabs 1500 mg once/d, PO & chondroitin sulfate 1200 mg once/d, PO for adults of wt lgwt **Caution:** Many forms come from shellfish, so avoid if have shellfish allergy **Notes/SE:** Abd pain, anorexia, constipation or D, drowsiness, HA, heartburn, N/V, rash **Interactions:** ↑ Effects *OF* hypoglycemics **Labs:** Monitor serum glucose levels in DM **NIPE:** Take w/ food to reduce GI effects; no uniform standardization of herb

Green Tea (*Camellia sinensis*) Uses: Antioxidant, antibacterial, diuretic; prevention of CA, hyperlipidemia, atherosclerosis, dental caries Actions: Chemical components include anti-inflammatory, anti-CA, polyphenol, epigallocatechin, & epigallocatechin-3-gallate which inhibit tumor growth; fluoride & tannins demonstrate antimicrobial action against oral bacteria; antioxidant activity delays lipid peroxidation; antimicrobial action d/t inhibition of growth of various bacteria including *S aureus* **Available forms:** Recommend 300–400 mg polyphenol PO OD (3 cups tea = 240–320 mg polyphenol) **CI:** Caution ↑ intake may cause tannin-induced asthma **Notes/SE:** Tachycardia, insomnia, anxiety, N/V, ↑ BP **Interactions:** ↑ Effects *OF* doxorubicin, ephedrine, stimulant drugs, theophylline; ↑ risk of hypertensive crisis *W/* MAOIs; ↑ bleeding risk *W/* anticoagulants, antiplts; ↓ effects *W/* antacids, dairy products **Labs:** ↑ PT, PTT **NIPE:** Contains caffeine—caution in PRG, infants, & small children & pts w/ CAD, hyperthyroidism & anxiety disorders; GI distress d/t tannins ↓ w/ the addition of milk; ↑ tannin content w/ ↑ brewing times

Guarana (*Paullinia cupana*)   Uses: Appetite suppressant, CNS stimulant, ↑ sexual performance, ↓ fatigue Actions: ↑ Caffeine content stimulates cardiac, CNS, & smooth muscle; ↑ diuresis; ↓ plt aggregation Available forms: Daily ÷ doses w/ max 3 g PO daily CI: Avoid in PRG & lactation, CAD, hyperthyroidism, anxiety disorders d/t high caffeine content Notes/SE: Insomnia, tachycardia, anxiety, N/V, HA, HTN, Sz Interactions: ↑ Effects OF anticoagulants, antiplts, BBs, bronchodilators; ↑ risk of hypertensive crisis W/ MAOIs; ↑ effects W/ cimetidine, ciprofloxacin, ephedrine, hormonal contraceptives, theophylline, cola, coffee; ↓ effects OF adenosine, antihypertensives, benzodiazepines, Fe, ↓ effects W/ smoking Labs: ↑ PT, PTT NIPE: Tincs contain EtOH; may exacerbate GI disorders & HTN

Hawthorn (*Crataegus laevigata*)   Uses: Rx of HTN, arrhythmias, HF, stable angina pectoris, insomnia Action: ↑ Myocardial contraction by ↓ oxygen consumption, ↓ peripheral resistance, dilating coronary blood vessels, ACE inhibition Available forms: Tinc 1–2 mL (1:5 ratio) tid, PO; Liq extract 0.5–1 mL, (1:1 ration) tid, PO Notes/SE: Arrhythmias, fatigue, hypotension, N/V, sedation Interactions: ↑ Effects OF antihypertensives, cardiac glycosides, CNS depressants, & herbs such as adonis, lily of the valley, squill; ↓ effects OF Fe Labs: False ↑ of digoxin NIPE: ⊘ PRG & lactation; many tincs contain EtOH

Horsetail (*Equisetum arvense*)   Uses: ↑ Strength of bones, hair, nails, & teeth; diuretic; treat dyspepsia, gout; topically used to treat wounds Actions: Multiple chemical components; flavonoids ↑ diuretic activity; contains silica which strengthens bones, hair, & nails Available forms: Extract 20–40 gtts in H₂O PO tid–qid; topically 10 g herb/L H₂O as compress PRN CI: ⊘ PRG, lactation, w/ children, CAD; contains nicotine & large amounts may cause nicotine tox Notes/SE: Nicotine tox (N/V, weakness, fever, dizziness, abnormal HR, wgt loss) Interactions: ↑ Effects OF digoxin, diuretics, Li, adonis, lily of the valley; ↑ CNS stimulation W/ CNS stimulants, theophylline, coffee, tea, cola, nicotine; ↑ K⁺ depletion W/ corticosteroids, diuretics, stimulant laxatives, licorice; ↑ risk of thiamine deficiency W/ EtOH use Labs: Monitor digoxin, lytes, thiamine levels NIPE: Tinc contains EtOH which may cause disulfiram-like Rxn if taken w/ benzodiazepines or metronidazole; short-term use only; active components of herb absorbed through skin

Kava Kava (*Piper methysticum*)   Uses: ↓ Anxiety, stress, restlessness & insomnia; sedative effect Action: Appears to act directly on the limbic system Available forms: Standardized extract (70% kavalactones) 100 mg bid–tid, PO Efficacy: Possible mild anxiolytic Caution: Hepatotox risk, banned in Europe/ Canada. Not OK in PRG, lactation. D/C 24 h pre-op (may ↑ sedative effect of anesthetics) Notes/SE: ↑ Reflexes, HA, dizziness, visual changes, red eyes, puggy face, muscle weakness, hematuria, SOB, mild GI disturbances; rare allergic skin/ rash Rxns Interactions: ↑ Effects OF antiplts, benzodiazepines, CNS depressants, MAOIs, phenobarbital; ↑ absorption when taken W/ food; ↑ in parkinsonian Sxs W/ kava kava & antiparkinsonian drugs Labs: ↑ ALT, AST, urinary RBCs; ↓ albumin, total protein, bilirubin, urea, plts, lymphocytes **NIPE:** ⊘ Take for > 3 mo; ⊘ during PRG & lactation

Licorice (*Glycyrrhiza glabra*) **Uses:** Expectorant, shampoo, GI complaints **Action:** ↑ Mucus secretions, ↓ peptic activity, ↓ scalp sebum secretion **Available forms:** Liq extract, bulk dried root, tea; 15 g once/d PO of licorice root; intake > 50 g once/d may cause tox **Notes/SE:** HTN, arrhythmias, edema, hypokalemia, HA, lethargy, rhabdomyolysis **Interactions:** ↑ Drug effects *OF* diuretics, corticosteroids, may prolong QT interval *W/* loratadine, procainamide, quinidine, terfenadine **Labs:** None **NIPE:** Monitor for lytes & ECG changes, HTN, mineralocorticoid-like effects; tox more likely w/ prolonged intake of small doses than 1 large dose

Melatonin (*MEL*) **Uses:** Insomnia, jet lag, antioxidant, immunostimulant **Action:** Hormone produce by the pineal gland in response to darkness; declines w/ age **Available forms:** XR caps 1–3 mg once/d 2 h before hs PO **Efficacy:** Sedation most pronounced w/ elderly pts w/ ↑ endogenous melatonin levels; some evidence for jet lag **Caution:** Use synthetic rather than animal pineal gland, "heavy head," HA, depression, daytime sedation, dizziness **Notes/SE:** HA, confusion, sedation, HTN, tachycardia, hyperglycemia **Interactions:** ↑ Anxiolytic effects *OF* benzodiazepines; ↑ risk of insomnia *W/* cerebral stimulants, methamphetamine, succinylcholine **Labs:** None **NIPE:** ⊘ during PRG & lactation

Milk Thistle (*Silybum marianum*) **Uses:** Prevent/Rx liver damage (eg, from alcohol, toxins, cirrhosis, chronic hep); preventive w/ chronic toxin exposure (painters, chemical workers, etc), dyspepsia; **Action:** Stimulates protein synth, which leads to liver cell regeneration **Available forms:** 80–200 mg PO tid; tinc 70–120 mg (70% silymarin) tid, PO **Efficacy:** Use before exposure more effective than use after damage has occurred **Notes/SE:** D, menstrual stimulation, N/V, GI intolerance **Interactions:** ↑ Effects *OF* drugs metabolized by the cytochrome P-450, CYP3A4, CYP2C9 enzymes **Labs:** ↑ PT; ↓ LFTs, serum glucose **NIPE:** ⊘ PRG & lactation; ⊘ pts allergic to ragweed, chrysanthemums, marigolds, daisies

Nettle (*Urtica dioica*) **Uses:** Allergic rhinitis, asthma, cough, TB, BPH, bladder inflammation, diuretic, antispasmodic, expectorant, astringent, & topically for oily skin, dandruff, & hair stimulant **Actions:** Multiple chemical components have different actions; scopoletin has anti-inflammatory action, root extract ↓ BPH, lectins display immunostimulant activity **Available forms:** Caps 150–300 mg PO OD; Liq extract 2–8 mL PO tid **CI:** ⊘ PRG or lactating or in children < 2 y **Notes/SE:** N/V, edema, Abd distress, D, oliguria, edema, local skin irritation **Interactions:** ↑ Effects *OF* diclofenac, diuretics, barbiturates, antipsychotics, opiates, EtOH; ↓ effects *OF* anticoagulants **Labs:** Monitor lytes **NIPE:** Skin contact w/ plant will result in stinging & burning; ↑ intake of foods high in K⁺

Red Yeast Rice (*Monascus purpureus*) **Uses:** Hyperlipidemia **Efficacy:** HMG-CoA reductase activity, naturally occurring lovastatin; ↓ LDL, ↓ triglycerides, ↑ HDL; ↓ secondary CAD events **Dose:** 1200–1800 mg bid **Caution:** CI w/ PRG, lactation; do not use w/ liver Dz, recent surgery, serious Infxn; may contain a mycotoxin, citrinin, can cause renal failure **Disp:** Caps 600–1200 mg **SE:** N, V, Abd pain, hep, myopathy, rhabdomyolysis **Interactions:** Possible interactions w/ many drugs, avoid w/ CYP3A4 Inhibs or EtOH NIPE : Use only in adults; generic lovastatin cheaper

Resveratrol **Uses:** Cardioprotective, prevent aging ? antioxidant **Efficacy:** Limited human research **Caution:** Avoid w/ Hx of estrogen responsive Ca or w/ CYP3A4 metabolized drugs **Disp:** Caps, tabs 20–500 mg, skins of red grapes, plums, blueberries, cranberries, red wine **SE:** D/N, anorexia, insomnia, anxiety, Jt pain, antiplt aggregation **Interactions:** Avoid w/ other antiplt drugs or anticoagulants; CYP3A4 Inhib

Rue (*Ruta graveolens*) **Uses:** Sedative, spasmolytic for muscle cramps, GI & menstrual disorders, promote lactation, promote abortion via uterine stimulation, anti-inflammatory effect for sports injuries, bruising, arthritis, Jt pain **Action:** Contains essential oils, flavonoids, & alkaloids; shown mutagenic & cytotoxic action on cells; produced CV effects d/t + chronotropic & inotropic effects on atria; vasodilatory effects reduce BP; shown strengthening effect on capillaries; alkaloids produce antispasmodic & abortifacient activity **Available forms:** Caps, extracts, teas, topical creams, topical oils; topical oil for earache; topical creams to affected areas PRN; teas use 1 tsp/1/4 L H$_2$O; extract 1/4–1 tsp PO tid w/ food; caps 1 PO tid w/ food **Notes/SE:** Dizziness, tremors, hypotension, bradycardia, allergic skin Rxns, spontaneous abortion **CI:** ⊘ During PRG or lactation or give to children; caution in pts w/ CHF, arrhythmias, or receiving antihypertensive medication **Interactions:** ↑ Inotropic effects *OF* cardiac glycosides; ↑ effects *OF* antihypertensives & warfarin; ↓ effects *OF* fertility drugs **Labs:** ↑ BUN, Cr, LFT **NIPE:** Large doses can be toxic or fatal; research does not establish a safe dose; tincs & extracts contain EtOH; no data w/ use in children; avoid if h/o EtOH abuse or liver Dz

Saw Palmetto (*Serenoa repens*) **Uses:** Rx of benign prostatic hypertrophy (BPH) stages 1 & 2 (inhibits testosterone-5-α-reductase), ↑ sperm production, ↑ breast size (estrogenic), ↑ sexual vigor, mild diuretic, treat chronic cystitis, hair tonic **Action:** Theorized that sitosterols inhibit conversion of testosterone to dihydrotestosterone (DHT), which reduces the prostate gland, also competes w/ DHT on receptor sites resulting in antiestrogenic effects **Available forms:** Caps/tabs 160 mg bid, PO; tinc 20–30 gtt qid (1:2 ration); fluid extract, standardized 160 mg bid PO or 320 mg once/d PO **Efficacy:** Small, no sig benefit for prostatic Sx **Caution:** Possible hormonal effects, avoid in PRG, w/ women of childbearing years **Notes/SE:** Abd pain, back pain, D, dysuria, HA, HTN, N/V, impotence **CI:** ⊘ PRG, lactation **Interactions:** ↑ Effects *OF* adrenergics, anticoagulants, antiplts, hormones, Fe **Labs:** May affect semen analysis, may cause false(−) PSA **NIPE:** Take w/ meals to ↓ GI upset, do baseline PSA prior to taking herb, no standardization of herb content

Spirulina (*Spirulina sp*) **Uses:** Rx of obesity & as a nutritional supl **Action:** Contains 65% protein, all amino acids, carotenoids, B-complex vits, essential fatty acids & Fe; has been shown to inhibit replicating viral cells **Available forms:**

Caps/tabs or powder administer 3–5 g ac, PO **Notes/SE:** Anorexia, N/V **Interactions:** ↑ Effects *OF* anticoagulants; ↓ effects *OF* thyroid hormones d/t high iodine content; ↓ absorption *OF* vit B₁₂ **Labs:** ↑ Serum Ca, alk phos; monitor PT, INR **NIPE:** May contain ↑ levels of Hg & radioactive ion content

St. John's Wort (*Hypericum perforatum*) **Uses:** Mild–mod depression, anxiety, anti-inflammatory, immune stimulant/anti-HIV/antiviral, gastritis, insomnia, vitiligo **Action:** MAOI in vitro, not in vivo; bacteriostatic & bactericidal, ↑ capillary blood flow, uterotonic activity in animals **Efficacy:** Variable; benefit w/ mild–mod depression in several trials, but not always seen in clinical practice **Available forms:** Teas, tabs, caps, tinc, oil extract for topical use **Dose:** 2–4 g of herb or 0.2–1 mg of total hypericin (standardized extract) daily *Common preps:* 300 mg PO tid (0.3% hypericin) **Notes/SE:** Photosensitivity (use sunscreen) rash, dizziness, dry mouth, GI distress **Interactions:** Enhance MAOI activity, EtOH, narcotics, sympathomimetics **Labs:** ↑ GH; ↓ digoxin, serum Fe, serum prolactin, theophylline **NIPE:** ⊘ PRG, breast-feeding, or in children; ⊘ w/ SSRIs, MAOIs, EtOH, ⊘ sun exposure

Stevia (*Stevia rebaudiana*) **Uses:** Natural sweetener, hypoglycemic & hypotensive properties **Actions:** Multiple chemical components; sweetness d/t glycoside stevioside; hypotensive effect may be d/t diuretic action or vasodilation action **Available forms:** Liq extract, powder, caps **Notes/SE:** HA, dizziness, bloating **Interactions:** ↑ Hypotensive effects *W/* antihypertensives esp CCB, diuretics **Labs:** Monitor BS **NIPE:** Monitor BP; does not encourage dental caries

Tea Tree (*Melaleuca alternifolia*) **Uses:** Rx of superficial wounds (bacterial, viral, & fungal), insect bites, minor burns, cold sores, acne **Action:** Broad-spectrum antibiotic activity against *E coli*, *S aureus*, *C albicans* **Available forms:** Topical creams, lotions, oint, oil apply topically PRN **Notes/SE:** Ataxia, contact dermatitis, D, drowsiness, GI mucosal irritation **Interactions:** ↓ Effects *OF* drugs that affect histamine release **Labs:** ↑ Neutrophil count **NIPE:** Caution pt to use externally only; ⊘ apply to broken skin

Valerian (*Valeriana officinalis*) **Uses:** Anxiolytic, antispasmodic, dysmenorrheal, restlessness, sedative **Action:** Inhibits uptake & stimulates release of GABA, which ↑ GABA conc extracellularly & causes sedation **Available forms:** Extract 400–900 mg PO 30 min < hs, tea 2–3 g (1 tsp of crude herb) qid, PRN, tinc 3–5 mL (1/2–1 tsp) (1:5 ratio) PO qid, PRN **Efficacy:** Probably effective sedative (reduces sleep latency) **Notes/SE:** GI upset, HA, insomnia, N/V, palpitations, restlessness, vision changes **Interactions:** ↑ Effects *OF* barbiturates, benzodiazepines, opiates, EtOH, catnip, hops, kava kava, passion flower, skullcap; ↓ effects *OF* MAOIs, phenytoin, warfarin **Labs:** ↑ ALT, AST, total bilirubin, urine bilirubin **NIPE:** Periodic intake of LFTs, unknown effects in PRG & lactation, full effect may take 2–4 wk, taper herb to avoid withdrawal Sxs after long-term use

Yohimbine (*Pausinystalia yohimbe*) **Uses:** Rx for impotence, aphrodisiac, Rx ED **Action:** Peripherally affects autonomic nervous system by ↓ adrenergic activity & ↑ cholinergic activity; ↑ blood flow **Efficacy:** Variable **Available forms:** Tabs 5.4 mg tid, PO; doses at 20–30 mg/d may ↑ BP & HR **Caution:** Do not use w/ renal/hepatic Dz; may exacerbate schizophrenia/mania (if pt predisposed). α₂-Adrenergic antagonist (↓ BP, Abd distress, weakness w/ high doses), OD can be fatal; salivation, dilated pupils, arrhythmias **SE:** Anxiety, tremors, dizziness, high BP, ↑ HR **Notes/SE:** Anxiety, dizziness, dysuria, genital pain, HTN, tachycardia, tremors **Interactions:** ↑ Effects *OF* CNS stimulants, MAOIs, SSRIs, caffeine, EtOH; ↑ risk of tox *W/* α-adrenergic blockers, phenothiazines; ↑ yohimbe tox *W/* sympathomimetics; ↑ BP *W/* foods containing tyramine **Labs:** ↑ BUN, Cr **NIPE:** ⊘ w/ caffeine-containing foods w/ herb, may exacerbate mania in pts w/ psychiatric disorders

Tables

TABLE 1
Local Anesthetic Comparison Chart for Commonly Used Injectable Agents

Agent	Proprietary Names	Onset	Duration	Maximum Dose mg/kg	Volume in 70-kg Adult[a]
Bupivacaine	Marcaine	7–30 min	5–7 h	3	70 mL of 0.25% solution
Lidocaine	Xylocaine, Anestacon	5–30 min	2 h	4	28 mL of 1% solution
Lidocaine with epinephrine (1:200,000)		5–30 min	2–3 h	7	50 mL of 1% solution
Mepivacaine	Carbocaine	5–30 min	2–3 h	7	50 mL of 1% solution
Procaine	Novocaine	Rapid	30 min–1 h	10–15	70–105 mL of 1% solution

[a] To calculate the maximum dose if not a 70-kg adult, use the fact that a 1% solution has 10 mg/mL drug.

TABLE 2
Comparison of Systemic Steroids

Drug	Relative Equivalent Dose (mg)	Relative Mineralo-corticoid Activity	Duration (h)	Route
Betamethasone	0.75	0	36–72	PO, IM
Cortisone (Cortone)	25	2	8–12	PO, IM
Dexamethasone (Decadron)	0.75	0	36–72	PO, IV
Hydrocortisone (Solu-Cortef, Hydrocortone)	20	2	8–12	PO, IM, IV
Methylprednisolone acetate (Depo-Medrol)	4	0	36–72	PO, IM, IV
Methylprednisolone succinate (Solu-Medrol)	4	0	8–12	PO, IM, IV
Prednisolone (Delta-Cortef)	5	1	12–36	PO, IM, IV
Prednisone (Deltasone)	5	1	12–36	PO

TABLE 3
Topical Steroid Preparations

Agent	Common Trade Names	Potency	Apply
Alclometasone dipropionate	Aclovate, cream, oint 0.05%	Low	bid/tid
Amcinonide	Cyclocort, cream, lotion, oint 0.1%	High	bid/bid
Betamethasone			
Betamethasone dipropionate	Diprosone cream 0.05%	High	qd/bid
	Diprosone aerosol 0.1%		
Betamethasone dipropionate, augmented	Diprolene oint, gel 0.05%	Ultrahigh	qd/bid
Betamethasone valerate	Valisone cream, lotion 0.01%	Low	qd/bid
Betamethasone valerate	Valisone cream 0.01, 0.1%, oint, lotion 0.1%	Intermediate	qd/bid
Clobetasol propionate	Temovate cream, gel, oint, scalp, soln 0.05%	Ultrahigh	bid (2 wk max)
Clocortolone pivalate	Cloderm cream 0.1%	Intermediate	qd–qid
Desonide	DesOwen, cream, oint, lotion 0.05%	Low	bid–qid
Desoximetasone			
Desoximetasone 0.05%	Topicort LP cream, gel 0.05%	Intermediate	qd–qid
Desoximetasone 0.25%	Topicort cream, oint	High	qd–bid
Dexamethasone base	Aeroseb-Dex aerosol 0.01%	Low	bid–qid
	Decadron cream 0.1%		
Diflorasone diacetate	Psorcon cream, oint 0.05%	Ultrahigh	bid/qid
Fluocinolone			
Fluocinolone acetonide 0.01%	Synalar cream, soln 0.01%	Low	bid/tid
Fluocinolone acetonide 0.025%	Synalar oint, cream 0.025%	Intermediate	bid/tid

388

Fluocinolone acetonide 0.2%	Synalar-HP cream 0.2%	High	bid/tid
Fluocinonide 0.05%	Lidex, anhydrous cream, gel, oint, soln 0.05%	High	bid/tid
	Lidex-E aqueous cream 0.05%		
Flurandrenolide	Cordran cream, oint 0.025%	Intermediate	bid/tid
	cream, lotion, oint 0.05%	Intermediate	bid/tid
	tape, 4 mcg/cm²	Intermediate	qd
Fluticasone propionate	Cutivate cream 0.05%, oint 0.005%	Intermediate	bid
Halcinonide	Halog cream 0.025%, emollient base 0.1% cream, oint, soln 0.1%	High	qd/tid
Halobetasol	Ultravate cream, oint 0.05%	Very high	bid
Hydrocortisone			
Hydrocortisone	Cortizone, Caldecort, Hycort, Hytone, etc—aerosol 1%, cream 0.5, 1, 2.5%, gel 0.5%, oint 0.5, 1, 2.5%, lotion 0.5, 1, 2.5%, paste 0.5%, soln 1%	Low	tid/qid
Hydrocortisone acetate	Corticaine cream, oint 0.5, 1%	Low	tid/qid
Hydrocortisone butyrate	Locoid oint, soln 0.1%	Intermediate	bid/tid
Hydrocortisone valerate	Westcort cream, oint 0.2%	Intermediate	bid/tid

(Continued)

TABLE 3 (Continued)
Topical Steroid Preparations

Agent	Common Trade Names	Potency	Apply
Mometasone furoate	Elocon 0.1% cream, oint, lotion	Intermediate	qd
Prednicarbate	Dermatop 0.1% cream	Intermediate	bid
Triamcinolone			
Triamcinolone acetonide 0.025%	Aristocort, Kenalog cream, oint, lotion 0.025%	Low	tid/qid
Triamcinolone acetonide 0.1%	Aristocort, Kenalog cream, oint, lotion 0.1%	Intermediate	tid/qid
	Aerosol 0.2-mg/2-spray		
Triamcinolone acetonide 0.5%	Aristocort, Kenalog cream, oint 0.5%	High	tid/qid

TABLE 4
Comparison of Insulins

Type of Insulin	Onset (h)	Peak (h)	Duration (h)
Ultra Rapid			
Apidra (glulisine)	< 0.25	0.5–1.5	3–4
Humalog (lispro)	< 0.25	0.5–1.5	3–4
NovoLog (aspart)	< 0.25	0.5–1.5	3–4
Rapid (regular insulin)			
Humulin R, Novolin R	0.5–1	2–3	4–6
Intermediate			
Humulin N, Novolin L	1–4	6–10	10–16
Prolonged			
Lantus (insulin glargine)	1–4	No peak	24
Levemir (insulin detemir)	1–4	No peak	24
Combination Insulins			
Humalog Mix 75/25 (lispro protamine/ lispro)	< 0.25	Dual	Up to 10–6
Humalog Mix 50/50 (lispro protamine/ lispro)	< 0.25	Dual	Up to 10–16
NovoLog Mix 70/30 (aspart protamine/ aspart)	< 0.25	Dual	Up to 10–16
Humulin 70/30, Novolin 70/30 (NPH/regular)	0.5–1	Dual	Up to 10–16

Note: Do not confuse Humalog, NovoLog, Humalog Mix, and NovoLog Mix with each other or with other agents as serious medication errors can result.

TABLE 5

Oral Contraceptives

(Note: 21 = 21 active pills; 24 = 24 active pills; standard for most products is 28 [unless specified] = 21 active pills + 7 Placebo[a])

Drug (Manufacturer)	Estrogen (mcg)	Progestin (mg)	Content of Additional Pills (d = days)
Monophasics			
Alesse 21, 28 (Wyeth)	Ethinyl estradiol [20]	Levonorgestrel [0.1]	
Apri (Barr)	Ethinyl estradiol [30]	Desogestrel [0.15]	
Aviane (Barr)	Ethinyl estradiol [20]	Levonorgestrel [0.1]	
Balziva (Barr)	Ethinyl estradiol [35]	Norethindrone [0.4]	
Beyaz (Bayer)[f]	Ethinyl estradiol [20]	Drospirenone [3.0]	0.451 mg levomefolate in all including 7 placebo
Brevicon (Watson)	Ethinyl estradiol [35]	Norethindrone [0.5]	
Cryselle (Barr)	Ethinyl estradiol [30]	Norgestrel [0.3]	
Demulen 1/35 21, 28 (Pfizer)	Ethinyl estradiol [35]	Ethynodiol diacetate [1]	
Demulen 1/50 21, 28 (Pfizer)	Ethinyl estradiol [50]	Ethynodiol diacetate [1]	
Desogen (Organon)	Ethinyl estradiol [30]	Desogestrel [0.15]	
Emoquette (Qualitest/Endo)	Ethinyl estradiol [30]	Desogestrel [0.15]	
Femcon Fe (Warner-Chilcott)	Ethinyl estradiol [35]	Norethindrone [0.4]	75 mg Fe × 7 d
Junel Fe 1/20, 21, 28 (Barr)	Ethinyl estradiol [20]	Norethindrone acetate [1]	75 mg Fe × 7 d
Junel Fe 1.5/30, 28 (Barr)	Ethinyl estradiol [30]	Norethindrone acetate [1.5]	75 mg Fe × 7 d
Kariva (Barr)	Ethinyl estradiol [20, 0, 10]	Desogestrel [0.15]	2 inert; 2 ethinyl estradiol [10]
Kelnor 1/35 (Barr)	Ethinyl estradiol [35]	Ethynodiol Diacetate [1]	

392

Brand (Manufacturer)	Estrogen	Progestin	Notes
Lessina (Barr)	Ethinyl estradiol (20)	Levonorgestrel (0.1)	
Levlen 21, 28 (Bayer)	Ethinyl estradiol (30)	Levonorgestrel (0.15)	
Levlite (Bayer)	Ethinyl estradiol (20)	Levonorgestrel (0.1)	
Levora (Watson)	Ethinyl estradiol (30)	Levonorgestrel (0.15)	
Loestrin 24 Fe (Warner-Chilcott)	Ethinyl estradiol (20)	Norethindrone (1)	75 mg Fe × 4 d
Loestrin 1/20 21 (Warner-Chilcott)	Ethinyl estradiol (20)	Norethindrone acetate (1)	
Loestrin 1.5/20 21 (Warner-Chilcott)	Ethinyl estradiol (20)	Norethindrone acetate (1.5)	
Loestrin Fe 1.5/30 21, 28 (Warner-Chilcott)	Ethinyl estradiol (30)	Norethindrone acetate (1.5)	75 mg Fe × 7 d in 28 d
Loestrin Fe 1/20 21, 28 (Warner-Chilcott)	Ethinyl estradiol (20)	Norethindrone acetate (1)	75 mg Fe × 7 d in 28 d
Lo/Ovral 21, 28 (Wyeth)	Ethinyl estradiol (30)	Norgestrel (0.3)	
Low-Ogestrel (Watson)	Ethinyl estradiol (30)	Norgestrel (0.3)	
Lutera (Watson)	Ethinyl estradiol (20)	Levonorgestrel (0.1)	
Microgestin 1/20 21, 28 (Watson)	Ethinyl estradiol (20)	Norethindrone acetate (1)	
Microgestin 1.5/30 21, 28 (Watson)	Ethinyl estradiol (30)	Norethindrone acetate (1.5)	
Microgestin Fe 1/20 21, 28 (Watson)	Ethinyl estradiol (20)	Norethindrone acetate (1)	75 mg Fe × 7 d in 28 d
Microgestin Fe 1.5/30 21, 28 (Watson)	Ethinyl estradiol (30)	Norethindrone acetate (1.5)	75 mg Fe × 7 d in 28 d
Mircette (Organon)	Ethinyl estradiol (20, 0, 10)	Desogestrel (0.15)	2 inert; 2 ethinyl estradiol (10)
Modicon (Ortho-McNeil)	Ethinyl estradiol (35)	Norethindrone (0.5)	
MonoNessa (Watson)	Ethinyl estradiol (35)	Norgestimate (0.25)	

(Continued)

TABLE 5 (Continued)
Oral Contraceptives

(Note: 21 = 21 active pills; 24 = 24 active pills; standard for most products is 28 [unless specified] = 21 active pills + 7 Placebo[a])

Drug (Manufacturer)	Estrogen (mcg)	Progestin (mg)	Content of Additional Pills (d = days)
Monophasics			
Necon 0.5/35 (Watson)	Mestranol (35)	Norethindrone (0.5)	
Necon 1/50 (Watson)	Mestranol (50)	Norethindrone (1)	
Necon 1/35 (Watson)	Ethinyl estradiol (35)	Norethindrone (0.5)	
Necon 1/35 (Watson)	Ethinyl estradiol (35)	Norethindrone (1)	
Nordette 21, 28 (King)	Ethinyl estradiol (30)	Levonorgestrel (0.15)	
Norinyl 1/35 (Watson)	Ethinyl estradiol (35)	Norethindrone (1)	
Norinyl 1/50 (Watson)	Mestranol (50)	Norethindrone (1)	
Nortrel 0.5/35 (Barr)	Ethinyl estradiol (35)	Norethindrone (0.5)	
Nortrel 1/35 21, 28 (Barr)	Ethinyl estradiol (35)	Norethindrone (1)	
Ocella (Barr)	Ethinyl estradiol (30)	Drosperinone (3)	
Ogestrel 0.5/50 (Watson)	Ethinyl estradiol (50)	Norgestrel (0.5)	
Ortho-Cept (Ortho-McNeil)	Ethinyl estradiol (30)	Desogestrel (0.15)	
Ortho-Cyclen (Ortho-McNeil)	Ethinyl estradiol (35)	Norgestimate (0.25)	
Ortho-Novum 1/35 (Ortho-McNeil)	Ethinyl estradiol (35)	Norethindrone (1)	
Ortho-Novum 1/50 2 (Ortho-McNeil)	Mestranol (50)	Norethindrone (1)	
Ovcon 35 21, 28 (Warner-Chilcott)	Ethinyl estradiol (35)	Norethindrone (0.4)	

394

Drug	Estrogen (mg)	Progestin (mcg)	Content of Additional Pills
Ovcon 35 FE (Warner-Chilcott)	Ethinyl estradiol (35)	Norethindrone (0.4)	75 mg Fe × 7 in 28 d
Ovcon 50 (Warner-Chilcott)	Ethinyl estradiol (50)	Norethindrone (1)	
Orval 21, 28 (Wyeth-Ayerst)	Ethinyl estradiol (50)	Norgestrel (0.5)	
Portia (Barr)	Ethinyl estradiol (30)	Levonorgestrel (0.15)	
Reclipsen (Watson)	Ethinyl estradiol (30)	Desogestrel (0.15)	
Safyral (Bayer)[f]	Ethinyl estradiol (30)	Drospirenone (3.0)	0.451 mg levomefolate in all including 7 placebo
Solia (Prasco)	Ethinyl estradiol (30)	Desogestrel (0.15)	
Sprintec (Barr)	Ethinyl estradiol (35)	Norgestimate (0.25)	
Sronyx (Watson)	Ethinyl estradiol (20)	Levonorgestrel (0.1)	
Yasmin (Bayer)[e] (generics: Ocella, Syeda, Zarah)	Ethinyl estradiol (30)	Drospirenone (3.0)	
Yaz (Bayer) 28 day[b,d,e] (generics: Gianvi,Loryna)	Ethinyl estradiol (20)	Drospirenone (3.0)	4 inert in 28 d
Zenchent (Watson)	Ethinyl estradiol (35)	Ethynodiol diacetate (0.4)	
Zovia 1/35 (Watson)	Ethinyl estradiol (35)	Ethynodiol diacetate (1)	
Drug	Estrogen (mg)	Progestin (mcg)	Content of Additional Pills

Multiphasics

Drug	Estrogen (mg)	Progestin (mcg)	
Aranelle (Barr)	Ethinyl estradiol (35)	Norethindrone (0.5, 1, 0.5)	
Cesia (Prasco)	Ethinyl estradiol (25)	Desogestrel (0.1, 0.125, 0.15)	
Cyclessa (Organon)	Ethinyl estradiol (25)	Desogestrel (0.1, 0.125, 0.15)	
Enpresse (Barr)	Ethinyl estradiol (30, 40, 30)	Levonorgestrel (0.05, 0.075, 0.125)	

(Continued)

TABLE 5 (Continued)
Oral Contraceptives

[Note: 21 = 21 active pills, 24 = 24 active pills; standard for most products is 28 [unless specified] = 21 active pills + 7 Placebo[a]]

Drug	Estrogen (mg)	Progestin (mcg)	Content of Additional Pills
Multiphasics			
Estrostep (Warner-Chilcott)[b]	Ethinyl estradiol [20, 30, 35]	Norethindrone acetate (1)	
Estrostep Fe (Warner-Chilcott)[b]	Ethinyl estradiol [20, 30, 35]	Norethindrone acetate (1)	75 mg Fe × 7 in 28 d
Generess Fe (Watson) (Note: Chewable tablets)	Ethinyl estradiol (25)	Norethindrone acetate (0.8)	75 mg Fe × 4 d
Leena (Watson)	Ethinyl estradiol (35)	Norethindrone [0.5, 1, 0.5]	
Lessina (Watson)	Ethinyl estradiol (20)	Levonorgestrel [0.1]	
Lutera (Watson)	Ethinyl estradiol (20)	Levonorgestrel [0.1]	
Natazia (Bayer) (see footnote g)			
Necon 10/11 21, 28 (Watson)	Ethinyl estradiol [35]	Norethindrone [0.5, 1]	
Necon 7/7/7 (Watson)	Ethinyl estradiol [35]	Norethindrone [0.5, 0.75, 1]	
Nortrel 7/7/7 (Barr)	Ethinyl estradiol [35]	Norethindrone [0.5, 0.75, 1]	
Orsythia (Qualitest)	Ethinyl estradiol [20]	Levonorgestrel [0.1]	
Ortho-Novum 10/11 (Ortho-McNeil)	Ethinyl estradiol [35]	Norethindrone [0.5, 1]	
Ortho-Novum 7/7/7 21 (Ortho-McNeil)	Ethinyl estradiol [35, 35, 35]	Norethindrone (0.5, 0.75, 1)	

396

Ortho Tri-Cyclen 21, 28 (Ortho-McNeil)[b]	Ethinyl estradiol (25)	Norgestimate (0.18, 0.215, 0.25)	
Ortho Tri-Cyclen Lo 21, 28 (Ortho-McNeil)	Ethinyl estradiol (35, 35, 35)	Norgestimate (0.18, 0.215, 0.25)	
Previfem (Teva)	Ethinyl estradiol (35)	Norgestimate (0.25)	
Tilia Fe (Watson)	Ethinyl estradiol (20, 30, 35)	Norethindrone (1)	75 mg Fe × 7 d in 28 d
Tri-Legest (Barr)	Ethinyl estradiol (20, 30, 35)	Norethindrone (1)	
Tri-Legest Fe (Barr)	Ethinyl estradiol (20, 30, 35)	Norethindrone (1)	75 mg Fe × 7 d in 28 d
Tri-Levlen (Bayer)	Ethinyl estradiol (30, 40, 30)	Levonorgestrel (0.05, 0.075, 0.125)	
Tri-Nessa (Watson)	Ethinyl estradiol (35)	Norgestimate (0.18, 0.215, 0.25)	
Tri-Norinyl 21, 28 (Watson)	Ethinyl estradiol (35, 35, 35)	Norethindrone (0.5, 1, 0.5)	
Triphasil 21, 28 (Wyeth)	Ethinyl estradiol (30, 40, 30)	Levonorgestrel (0.05, 0.075, 0.125)	
Tri-Previfem (Teva)	Ethinyl estradiol (35)	Norgestimate (0.18, 0.215, 0.25)	
Tri-Sprintec (Barr)	Ethinyl estradiol (35)	Norgestimate (0.18, 0.215, 0.25)	
Trivora 28 (Watson)	Ethinyl estradiol (30, 40, 30)	Levonorgestrel (0.05, 0.075, 0.125)	
Velivet (Barr)	Ethinyl estradiol (25)	Desogestrel (0.1, 0.125, 0.15)	

(Continued)

TABLE 5 (Continued)
Oral Contraceptives

(Note: 21 = 21 active pills; 24 = 24 active pills; standard for most products is 28 [unless specified] = 21 active pills + 7 Placebo[a])

Drug	Estrogen (mg)	Progestin (mcg)	Content of Additional Pills
Progestin Only (aka "mini-pills")			
Camila (Barr)	None	Norethindrone (0.35)	
Errin (Barr)	None	Norethindrone (0.35)	
Jolivette 28 (Watson)	None	Norethindrone (0.35)	
Micronor (Ortho-McNeil)	None	Norethindrone (0.35)	
Nora-BE (Ortho-McNeil)	None	Norethindrone (0.35)	
Nor-QD (Watson)	None	Norethindrone (0.35)	

Drug	Estrogen (mg)	Progestin (mcg)	Content of Additional Pills
Extended-Cycle Combination (aka COCP [combined oral contraceptive pills])			
Jolessa (Barr) 91-d pack	Ethinyl estradiol (30)	Levonorgestrel (0.15)	7 inert
Lybrel (Wyeth) 28-d pack[c]	Ethinyl estradiol (20)	Levonorgestrel (0.09)	None
Quasense (Watson)	Ethinyl estradiol (30)	Levonorgestrel (0.15)	7 inert
Seasonale (Duramed) 91-d pack	Ethinyl estradiol (30)	Levonorgestrel (0.15)	7 inert
Seasonique (Duramed) 91-d pack	Ethinyl estradiol (30)	Levonorgestrel (0.15)	7 (10 mcg ethinyl estradiol)

Based in part on data published in the *Medical Letter*, Volume 49 (Issue 1266) 2007, manufacturers insert and web sites as of August 29, 2009.

[a] The designations 21 and 28 refer to number of days in regimen available.

[b] Also approved for acne.

[c] First FDA-approved pill for 365 d dosing.

[d] Approved for premenstrual dysphoric disorder (PMDD) in women who use contraception for birth control.

[e] Avoid in patients with hyperkalemia risk.

[f] Raises folate levels to help decrease neural tube defect risk with eventual pregnancy.

[g] First "four phasic" OCP. Varies doses of estrogen (estradiol valerate) with progestin (dienogest) throughout cycle with 2 inert pills at end of cycle.

TABLE 6
Oral Potassium Supplements

Brand Name	Salt	Form	mEq Potassium/ Dosing Unit
Glu-K	Gluconate	Tablet	2 mEq/tab
Kaon Elixir	Gluconate	Liquid	20 mEq/15 mL
Kaon-Cl 10%	KCl	Tablet, SR	10 mEq/tab
Kaon-Cl 20%	KCl	Liquid	40 mEq/15 mL
K-Dur 20	KCl	Tablet, SR	20 mEq/tab
KayCiel	KCl	Liquid	20 mEq/15 mL
K-Lor	KCl	Powder	20 mEq/packet
K-Lyte/Cl	KCl/bicarbonate	Effervescent tablet	25 mEq/tab
Klorvess	KCl/bicarbonate	Effervescent tablet	20 mEq/tab
Klotrix	KCl	Tablet, SR	10 mEq/tab
K-Lyte	Bicarbonate/ citrate	Effervescent tablet	25 mEq/tab
Klor-Con/EF	Bicarbonate/ citrate	Effervescent tablet	25 mEq/tab
K-Tab	KCl	Tablet, SR	10 mEq/tab
Micro-K	KCl	Capsule, SR	8 mEq/capsule
Potassium Chloride 10%	KCl	Liquid	20 mEq/15 mL
Potassium Chloride 20%	KCl	Liquid	40 mEq/15 mL
Slow-K	KCl	Tablet, SR	8 mEq/tab
Tri-K	Acetate/ bicarbonate and citrate	Liquid	45 mEq/15 mL
Twin-K	Citrate/gluconate	Liquid	20 mEq/5 mL

SR = sustained release.

Note: Alcohol and sugar content vary between preparations.

TABLE 7
Tetanus Prophylaxis

History of Absorbed Tetanus Toxoid Immunization	Clean, Minor Wounds		All Other Wounds[a]	
	Td[b]	TIG[c]	Td[d]	TIG[c]
Unknown or < 3 doses	Yes	No	Yes	Yes
= 3 doses	No[e]	No	No[f]	No

[a]Such as, but not limited to, wounds contaminated with dirt, feces, soil, saliva, etc; puncture wounds; avulsions; and wounds resulting from missiles, crushing, burns, and frostbite.

[b]Td = tetanus-diphtheria toxoid (adult type), 0.5 mL IM.
• For children < 7 y, DPT (DT, if pertussis vaccine is contraindicated) is preferred to tetanus toxoid alone.
• For persons > 7 y, Td is preferred to tetanus toxoid alone.
• DT = diphtheria-tetanus toxoid (pediatric), used for those who cannot receive pertussis.

[c]TIG = tetanus immune globulin, 250 units IM.

[d]If only 3 doses of fluid toxoid have been received, then a fourth dose of toxoid, preferably an adsorbed toxoid, should be given.

[e]Yes, if >10 y since last dose.

[f]Yes, if > 5 y since last dose.

Based on guidelines from the Centers for Disease Control and Prevention and reported in *MMWR* (MMWR, December 1, 2006; 55[RR-15]:1-48).

TABLE 8
Oral Anticoagulant Standards of Practice

Thromboembolic Disorder	INR	Duration

Deep Venous Thrombosis and Pulmonary Embolism

Treatment single episode		
Transient risk factor	2–3	3 mo
Idiopathic[a]	2–3	long-term
Recurrent systemic embolism	2–3	long-term

Prevention of Systemic Embolism

AF cardioversion	2–3	3 wks prior; 4 wks post sinus rhythm
Atrial fibrillation (AF)[b]	2–3	long-term
Cardiomyopathy (usually ASA)[c]	2–3	long-term
Mitral valvular heart dx[d]	2–3	long-term

Acute Myocardial Infarction

High-risk[e]	2–3 + low-dose aspirin	long-term
All other infarcts[f] (usually ASA)		

TABLE 8 (Continued)
Oral Anticoagulant Standards of Practice

Thromboembolic Disorder	INR	Duration
Prosthetic Valves		
Bileaflet mechanical valves in aortic position[g]	2–3	long-term
Bioprosthetic heart valves		
Mitral position	2–3	3 mo
Aortic position[h]	2–3	3 mo
Other mechanical prosthetic valves[i]	2.5–3.5	long-term

[a]3 mo if mod or high risk of bleeding or distal DVT; if low-risk bleeding then long-term for proximal DVT/PE.

[b]Paroxysmal AF or ≥ 2 risk factors (age >75, Hx, BP, DM, mod-severe LV dysfunction or CHF) then warfarin; 1 risk factor warfarin or 75–325 mg ASA; 0 risk factors ASA.

[c]In adults only ASA; only indication for anticoagulation cardiomyopathy in children, to begin no later than their activation on transplant list.

[d]Mitral valve Dz: rheumatic if Hx systemic embolism, or AF or LA thrombus or LA > 55 mm; MVP: only if AF, systemic embolism or TIAs on ASA; Mitral valve calcification: warfarin if AF or recurrent embolism on ASA; aortic valve w/ calcification: warfarin not recommended.

[e]High risk = large anterior MI, significant CHF, intracardiac thrombus visible on TE, AF, and Hx of a thromboembolic event.

[f]If meticulous INR monitoring and highly skilled dose titration are expected and widely accessible then INR 3.5 (3.0-4.0) w/o ASA or 2.5 (2.0-3.0) w ASA long-term (4 y).

[g]Ttarget INR 2.5–3.5 if AF, large anterior MI, LA enlargement, hypercoagulable state, or low EF.

[h]Usually ASA 50–100 mg; warfarin if Hx embolism, LA thrombus, AF, low EF, hypercoagulable state, 3 mo or until thrombus resolves.

[i]Add ASA 50–100 mg if high risk (AF, hypercoagulable state, low EF, or Hx of ASCVD).

Based on data in *Chest; Antithrombotic and Thrombolytic Therapy*, 8th ed.

TABLE 9
Antiarrhythmics: Vaughn Williams Classification

Class I: *Sodium Channel Blockade*

A. **Class Ia:** Lengthens duration of action potential ($\uparrow$ the refractory period in atrial and ventricular muscle, in SA and AV conduction systems, and Purkinje fibers)
1. Amiodarone (also classes II, III, IV)
2. Disopyramide (Norpace)
3. Imipramine (MAO inhibitor)
4. Procainamide (Pronestyl)
5. Quinidine

B. **Class Ib:** No effect on action potential
1. Lidocaine (Xylocaine)
2. Mexiletine (Mexitil)
3. Phenytoin (Dilantin)
4. Tocainide (Tonocard)

C. **Class Ic:** Greater sodium current depression (blocks the fast inward Na^+ current in heart muscle and Purkinje fibers, and slows the rate of $\uparrow$ of phase 0 of the action potential)
1. Flecainide (Tambocor)
2. Propafenone

Class II: *Beta-Blocker*

D. Amiodarone (also classes Ia, III, IV)
E. Esmolol (Brevibloc)
F. Sotalol (also class III)

Class III: *Prolong Refractory Period via Action Potential*

G. Amiodarone (also classes Ia, II, IV)
H. Sotalol

Class IV: *Calcium Channel Blocker*

I. Amiodarone (also classes Ia, II, III)
J. Diltiazem (Cardizem)
K. Verapamil (Calan)

TABLE 10
Cytochrome P-450 Isoenzymes and Common Drugs They Metabolize, Inhibit, and Induce[a]

CYP1A2

Substrates:	Acetaminophen, caffeine, cyclobenzaprine, clozapine, imipramine, mexiletine, naproxen, theophylline, propranolol
Inhibitors:	Cimetidine, most fluoroquinolone antibiotics, fluvoxamine, verapamil
Inducers:	Tobacco smoking, charcoal-broiled foods, cruciferous vegetables, omeprazole

CYP2C9

Substrates:	Most NSAIDs (including COX-2), glipizide, irbesartan, losartan, phenytoin, warfarin
Inhibitors:	Amiodarone, fluconazole, ketoconazole, metronidazole
Inducers:	Barbiturates, rifampin

CYP2C19

Substrates:	Diazepam, amitriptyline, lansoprazole, omeprazole, phenytoin, pantoprazole, rabeprazole, clopidogrel
Inhibitors:	Omeprazole, lansoprazole, isoniazid, ketoconazole, fluoxetine, fluvoxamine
Inducers:	Barbiturates, rifampin

CYP2D6

Substrates:	**Antidepressants:** Most tricyclic antidepressants, clomipramine, fluoxetine, paroxetine, venlafaxine **Antipsychotics:** Aripiprazole, clozapine, haloperidol, risperidone, thioridazine **Beta blockers:** Carvedilol, metoprolol, propranolol, timolol **Opioids:** Codeine, hydrocodone, oxycodone, propoxyphene, tramadol **Others:** Amphetamine, dextromethorphan, duloxetine, encainide, flecainide, mexiletine, ondansetron, propafenone, selegiline tamoxifen
Inhibitors:	Amiodarone, bupropion, cimetidine, clomipramine, doxepin, duloxetine, fluoxetine, haloperidol, methadone, paroxetine, quinidine, ritonavir
Inducers:	Unknown

(Continued)

TABLE 10 (Continud)
Cytochrome P-450 Isoenzymes and Common Drugs
They Metabolize, Inhibit, and Induce[a]

CYP3A

Substrates: **Anticholinergics:** Darifenacin, oxybutynin, solifenacin, tolterodine
Benzodiazepines: Alprazolam, diazepam, midazolam, triazolam
Ca channel blockers: Amlodipine, diltiazem, felodipine, nimodipine, nifedipine, nisoldipine, verapamil
Chemotherapy: Cyclophosphamide, erlotinib, ifosfamide, paclitaxel, tamoxifen, vinblastine, vincristine
HIV protease inhibitors: Amprenavir, atazanavir, indinavir, nelfinavir, ritonavir, saquinavir
HMG-CoA reductase inhibitors: Atorvastatin, lovastatin, simvastatin
Immunosuppressive agents: Cyclosporine, tacrolimus
Macrolide-type antibiotics: Clarithromycin, erythromycin, telithromycin, troleandomycin
Opioids: Alfentanil, cocaine, fentanyl, methadone, sufentanil
Steroids: Budesonide, cortisol, 17-β-estradiol, progesterone
Others: Acetaminophen, amiodarone, carbamazepine, delavirdine, efavirenz, nevirapine, quinidine, repaglinide, sildenafil, tadalafil, trazodone, vardenafil

Inhibitors: Amiodarone, amprenavir, aprepitant, atazanavir, ciprofloxacin, cisapride, clarithromycin, diltiazem, erythromycin, fluconazole, fluvoxamine, grapefruit juice (in high ingestion), indinavir, itraconazole, ketoconazole, nefazodone, nelfinavir, norfloxacin, ritonavir, saquinavir, telithromycin, troleandomycin, verapamil, voriconazole

Inducers: Carbamazepine, efavirenz, glucocorticoids, modafinil, nevirapine, phenytoin, phenobarbital, rifabutin, rifapentine, rifampin, St. John's wort

[a]Increased or decreased (primarily hepatic cytochrome P-450) metabolism of medications may influence the effectiveness of drugs or result in significant drug-drug interactions. Understanding the common cytochrome P-450 isoforms (eg, CYP2C9, CYP2D9, CYP2C19, CYP3A4) and common drugs that are metabolized by (aka "substrates"), inhibit, or induce activity of the isoform helps minimize significant drug interactions. CYP3A is involved in the metabolism of > 50% of drugs metabolized by the liver.

Based on data from Katzung B (ed). *Basic and Clinical Pharmacology*, 11th ed. McGraw-Hill, New York, 2009; The Medical Letter, Volume 47, July 4, 2004; *N Engl J Med*. 2005:352:2211–2221.

TABLE 11
SSRIs/SNRI/Triptan and Serotonin Syndrome

A life-threatening condition, when selective serotonin reuptake inhibitors (SSRIs) and 5-hydroxytryptamine receptor agonists (triptans) are used together. However, many other drugs have been implicated (see below). Signs and symptoms of serotonin syndrome include the following:

Restlessness, coma, N/V/D, hallucinations, loss of coordination, overactive reflexes, ↑ HR/temperature, rapid changes in BP, increased body temperature

Class	Drugs
Antidepressants	MAOIs, TCAs, SSRIs, SNRIs, mirtazapine, venlafaxine
CNS stimulants	Amphetamines, phentermine, methylphenidate, sibutramine
5-HT$_1$ agonists	Triptans
Illicit drugs	Cocaine, methylenedioxymethamphetamine (ecstasy), lysergic acid diethylamide (LSD)
Opioids	Tramadol, pethidine, oxycodone, morphine, meperidine
Others	Buspirone, chlorpheniramine, dextromethorphan, linezolid, lithium, selegiline, tryptophan, St. John's wort

Management includes removal of the precipitating drugs and supportive care. To control agitation serotonin antagonists (cyproheptadine or methysergide) can be used. When symptoms are mild, discontinuation of the medication or medications and the control of agitation with benzodiazepines may be needed. Critically ill patients may require sedation and mechanical ventilation as well as control of hyperthermia. (Boyer EW, Shanon M. The serotonin syndrome. *N Engl J Med*. 2005;352(11):1112–1120.)
MOAI = monoamine oxidase inhibitor
TCA = tricyclic antidepressant
SNRI = serotonin-norepinephrine reuptake inhibitors

TABLE 12

Multivitamins, Oral OTC

Composition of Selected Multivitamins and Multivitamins with Mineral and Trace Element Supplements. Listings Show Vitamin Content (Part 1) and then Mineral Trace Element and other Components (Part 2) of Popular US Brands. Values Listed are a Percentage of Daily Value.

Part 1. Vitamins

	Fat Soluble				Water Soluble								
	A	D	E	K	C	B_1	B_2	B_3	B_6	Folate	B_{12}	Biotin	B_5
Centrum[a]	70	100	100	31	150	100	100	100	100	125	100	10	100
Centrum Performance[a]	70	100	200	31	200	300	300	200	300	100	300	17	100
Centrum Silver[a]	50	125	167	38	150	100	100	100	150	125	417	10	100
Nature Made Multi Complete	50	250	167	100	300	100	100	100	100	100	100	10	100
Nature Made Multi Daily	60	100	100	0	100	100	100	100	100	100	100	0	100
Nature Made Multi Max	60	100	500	50	500	3333	2941	250	2500	100	833	17	500
Nature Made Multi 50+	60	100	200	13	200	200	200	100	200	100	417	10	100
One-A-Day 50 Plus	50	100	110	25	200	300	200	100	300	100	417	10	150
One-A-Day Essential	60	100	100	0	100	100	100	100	100	100	100	0	100

One-A-Day Maximum[b]	50	100	100	31	100	100	100	100	100	100	100	100	10	100
Therapeutic Vitamin	100	100	100	0	150	200	200	100	100	100	150	150	10	100
Theragran-M Advanced High Protein	100	100	200	35	150	200	200	300	100	300	200	100	10	100
Theragran-M Premier High Potency	70	100	200	31	200	267	235	200	125	200	150	150	10	100
Theragran-M Premier 50 Plus High Potency	70	100	200	13	125	176	176	100	125	300	500	500	12	150
Therapeutic Vitamin + Minerals[b]	100	100	200	0	200	100	100	100	100	100	100	100	10	100
Unicap M	100	100	100	0	100	100	100	100	100	100	100	100	0	100
Unicap Sr.	100	50	100	NA	100	80	82	80	110	100	50	50	0	100
Unicap T	100	100	100	0	833	667	588	500	300	300	300	300	0	250

(Continued)

TABLE 12 (Continud)
Multivitamins, Oral OTC

Composition of Selected Multivitamins and Multivitamins with Mineral and Trace Element Supplements. Listings Show Vitamin Content (Part 1) and then Mineral Trace Element and other Components (Part 2) of Popular US Brands. Values Listed are a Percentage of Daily Value.

Part 2. Minerals, Trace elements, and Other Components

	Minerals						Trace Elements						Other
	Ca	P	Mg	Fe	Zn	I	Se	K	Mn	Cu	Cr	Mo	
Centrum[a]	20	11	25	100	73	100	79	2	115	45	29	60	Lutein, lycopene
Centrum Performance[a]	10	5	10	100	73	100	100	2	200	45	100	100	Gingko, ginseng
Centrum Silver[a]	22	11	13	0	73	100	79	2	115	45	38	60	Lutein, lycopene
Nature Made Multi Complete	16	NA	25	100	100	100	35	NA	200	100	100	100	
Nature Made Multi Daily	45	0	0	100	100	0	0	0	0	0	0	0	
Nature Made Multi Max	10	4	6	50	100	100	100	1	100	100	100	0	Lutein
Nature Made Multi 50+	20	5	25		100	100	71	2	100	100	100	33	Lutein
One-A-Day 50 Plus	12	0	25	0	150	100	150	1	200	100	150	120	Lutein
One-A-Day Essential	5	0	0	0	0	0	0	0	0	0	0	0	
One-A-Day Maximum	16	11	25	100	100	100	29	2	175	100	54	213	

Supplement													Other active ingredients
Therapeutic Vitamin[b]	0	0	0	0	0	0	0	0	0	0	0	0	
Theragran-M Advanced High Potency	4	3	25	50	100	100	100	1	100	100	42	100	Lutein, lycopene, coenzyme Q10
Theragran-M Premier High Protein	17	11	25		100	100	286	2	175	100		107	Lutein, coenzyme Q10
Theragran-M Premier 50 Plus High Potency	20	5	25	0	113		286	2	100	100	21	100	Lutein, coenzyme Q10
Therapeutic Vitamin + Minerals[b]	4	3	10	50	100	50	36	100	100	100	42	100	
Unicap M	6	5		100	100			<1	50	100	0	0	0
Unicap Sr.	10	8		56	100			<1	50	100	0	0	0
Unicap T	0	0		100	100		14	<1	50	100	0	0	0

Common multivitamins available without a prescription are listed. Most chain drug stores have generic versions of many of the multivitamin supplements listed above; thus, specific generic brands are not listed.[c] Many specialty vitamin combinations are available, but not included in this list (examples are B vitamins plus C, supplements for a specific condition or organ, pediatric and infant formulations, and prenatal vitamins). Values are listed as percentages of the Daily Value (also known as %DV) based on recommended Dietary Allowances of vitamins and minerals based on Dietary Reference Intakes (Food and Nutrition Board, Institute of Medicine, National Academy of Science). Additional information may be available for many other supplements from the NIH Dietary Supplements labels Database http://dietarysupplements.nih.gov/dietary

[a]New formulation October 2007.
[b]Formulations may vary. Consult with pharmacy for current product.
[c]Common generic brands (when other than the store name itself) are: Osco Drug Central-Vite (Albertson's); Spectravite (CVS); Kirkland Signature Daily Multivitamin (Costco); Whole Source, PharmAssure (Rite Aid); Central-Vite (Safeway); Member's Mark (Sam's Club); Vitasmart (Kmart); Century (Target); A thru Z Select, Super Ayrinol, Ultra Choice (Walgreens), Equate Complete or Spring Valley Sentury-Vite (Wal-Mart).

Vitamins: B_1 = thiamine; B_2 = riboflavin; B_3 = niacin; B_5 = pantothenic acid; B_6 = pyridoxine; B_{12} = cyanocobalamin. Elements: Ca = calcium; Cr = chromium; Cu = copper; Fe = iron; I = iodine; K = potassium; Mg = magnesium; Mn = manganese; Mo = molybdenum; P = phosphorus; Se = selenium; Zn = zinc; 0 = not applicable or not available.

Index

Index

413